COMPOUNDING STERILE PREPARATIONS

COMPOUNDING STERILE PREPARATIONS

5th Edition

RYAN A. FORREY, PharmD, MS, BCSCP, FFIP, FASHP

Global Clinical Solutions Director
Surgical Complication Solutions
Becton, Dickinson and Company
Clinical Assistant Professor
The Ohio State University, College of Pharmacy
Atlanta, Georgia

LINDSEY B. AMERINE, PharmD, MS, BCPS, CPEL, FASHP

System Executive Director of Pharmacy
UNC Health
Associate Professor of Clinical Education
UNC Eshelman School of Pharmacy
Morrisville, North Carolina

ANGELA W. YANIV, PharmD, BCSCP

Director of Pharmacy—Sterile Products
Cleveland Clinic
Cleveland, Ohio

ashp®

Any correspondence regarding this publication should be sent to the publisher, American Society of Health-System Pharmacists, 4500 East-West Highway, Suite 900, Bethesda, MD 20814, attention: Special Publishing.

The authors would like to acknowledge the contributions of The U.S. Pharmacopeial Convention (USP), including allowing the generous references throughout this book to the *United States Pharmacopeia* (USP) and the *National Formulary (USP–NF),* in particular use of one of the official USP General Chapters, <797> Pharmaceutical Compounding—Sterile Preparations, as well as Chapters <71>, <659>, <800>, <825>, and <1066>. The presentation and interpretation of USP Chapters provided by the authors do not necessarily reflect the views of USP or the requirements of USP <797>, and readers should be aware that USP <797>, like all USP standards, is subject to revision.

For ASHP guidelines on compounding sterile preparations and handling hazardous drugs, please visit the ASHP website to access the current version.

Senior Vice President, Professional Development and Publishing Office: Daniel J. Cobaugh, PharmD, DABAT, FAACT

Editorial Director, Special Publishing: Ryan E. Owens, PharmD, BCPS

Editorial Coordinator, Special Publishing: Güneş Turhanlı, MA

Director, Production and Platform Services, Publishing Operations: Johnna M. Hershey, BA

Production Services/Printing: KGL/Sheridan

Cover Design: DeVall Advertising

Cover Art: Shutterstock; photo contributor, Motorolka

Page Design: David Wade

Library of Congress Cataloging-in-Publication Data

Names: Forrey, Ryan A., editor. | Amerine, Lindsey B., editor. | Yaniv, Angela W., editor. | American Society of Health-System Pharmacists, issuing body.

Title: Compounding sterile preparations / [edited by] Ryan A. Forrey, Lindsey B. Amerine, Angela W. Yaniv.

Other titles: Principles of sterile product preparation

Description: Fifth edition. | Bethesda, MD : American Society of Health-System Pharmacists, [2023] | Includes bibliographical references and index. | Summary: "Now through four editions, this reference has served as both a professional reference guide for pharmacists and pharmacy technicians and a student textbook covering the regulation, technique, and quality assurance of compounding sterile preparations. All chapters in the fifth edition have been significantly revised due to new literature since the previous edition and the publication of the revised USP 797 standards. Additionally, this edition includes the new USP Chapter 825 which covers radiopharmaceutical compounding. This new edition will contain the most updated guidance for compounding sterile preparations. This resource would be considered an essential resource to help individuals learn more about and comply with the standards related to sterile compounding"—Provided by publisher.

Identifiers: LCCN 2023035185 | ISBN 9781585286485 (paperback) | ISBN 9781585286492 (Adobe PDF) | ISBN 9781585286508 (epub)

Subjects: MESH: Drug Compounding—standards | Sterilization—standards | Technology, Pharmaceutical—standards | Drug Contamination—prevention & control

Classification: LCC RS199.S73 | NLM QV 779 | DDC 615/.19—dc23/eng/20230828

LC record available at https://lccn.loc.gov/2023035185

Print ISBN: 978-1-58528-648-5
PDF ISBN: 978-1-58528-649-2
ePub ISBN: 978-1-58528-650-8
DOI: 10.37573/9781585286492

10 9 8 7 6 5 4 3 2 1

DEDICATION

*This edition is dedicated to all health-system staff
who met the challenging demands of the
COVID-19 global pandemic while ensuring the safety
and accuracy of compounded sterile preparations for their patients.*

Ryan A. Forrey
Lindsey B. Amerine
Angela W. Yaniv

TABLE OF CONTENTS

DOI 10.37573/9781585286492.FM

ACKNOWLEDGMENTS

Every day many pharmacists and pharmacy technicians participate in compounding sterile preparations. In the vast majority of cases, their preparations are accurate, stable, pure, and free of contamination. We salute these health professionals who maintain essential high standards. Such work requires great attention to detail and genuine care for patients. Safe compounding of sterile preparations also requires strong leadership and recognition of the importance of compounding to patient safety and outcomes.

We are grateful to Angela Cassano, Ryan Owens, Daniel Cobaugh, and the many other ASHP staff members who reviewed and edited each chapter of this text. We would also like to thank past ASHP staff members Elaine Jimenez and Ruth Bloom for their assistance early in the process of starting this edition. The journey to update and publish this 5th edition was long and winding, with delays from the revisions to USP Chapter <797>, the appeal and remand of the chapter, the final release of the chapter in November 2022, and the impact of the COVID-19 pandemic from 2020 to 2023. The idea and work to bring this latest edition began in November 2018, nearly 5 years to the month of first publication. Without the encouragement of ASHP, the authors, and each other, our work would not have been possible.

Finally, to our family members and friends who gave us the space and emotional support to start, stop, restart, and finally finish, we express our heartfelt appreciation.

Ryan A. Forrey
Lindsey B. Amerine
Angela W. Yaniv

DOI 10.37573/9781585286492.FM

PREFACE

This professional reference for pharmacists and pharmacy technicians who compound sterile preparations serves well as a textbook for student pharmacists and pharmacy technicians. There is a robust list of references at the end of each chapter for those scholars who wish to dig deeper into this rich material.

Much has changed with the standards and guidelines for sterile compounding since *Compounding Sterile Preparations, 4th Edition.* In 2019, the United States Pharmacopeial Convention (USP) released a revised version of USP Chapter <797> as well as the new chapter, USP Chapter <825> Radiopharmaceuticals—Preparation, Compounding, Dispensing, and Repackaging. The 2019 revision to USP Chapter <797> as well as USP Chapter <825> were appealed. At the end of the appeals process, USP Chapter <797> was remanded back to the USP Compounding Expert Committee, but USP Chapter <825> was allowed to become official. During this time, there were slight changes to USP Chapter <800> Hazardous Drugs—Handling in Healthcare Settings to align with proposed revisions to the National Institute for Occupational Safety and Health (NIOSH) hazardous drug list. Those changes were proposed in 2018, 2020, and 2022, yet, at the time of this writing, the 2016 list is still official. Around the time of the challenges to USP Chapter <797>, USP also changed the way that USP Chapters were considered enforceable, using a term called "compendial applicability." A general chapter numbered below 1000 becomes compendially applicable and thus is considered a required standard only when one of the following requirements are met:

1. The chapter is referenced in a monograph;
2. The chapter is referenced in another General Chapter below 1000; or
3. The chapter is referenced in General Notices.

The consequence of all of these changes is that USP Chapter <800> and USP Chapter <825> do not become enforceable until the official date of the revision to USP Chapter <797> in which they are referenced. These nuances and the question of official versus compendially applicable should be resolved and the appropriate standards are incorporated into this text as they relate to sterile compounding. Of course, these USP standards are the *minimum* that must be in place for safe sterile compounding. However, the authors of the chapters in this text often provide information based on additional best practices and practical experience in compounding.

All chapters have been updated, and several new chapters and chapter authors have been added. New chapters include the following:

- Allergenic Extracts
- Corrective and Preventative Action (CAPA) Plans

Chapters that have an updated scope and title include:

- Establishing Beyond-Use Dates (formerly Storage and Beyond-Use Dating)
- Receipt, Storage, Movement, and Disposal of Compounded Sterile Preparation Components and Finished Preparations in the Pharmacy (formerly Handling Sterile Commercial Products and Compounded Sterile Preparations Within the Pharmacy)
- Secondary Engineering Controls and Cleanroom Design (formerly Secondary Engineering Controls)
- Point of Care Compounding and Preparation for Administration (formerly Immediate-Use Compounding)
- Biologicals, Biosimilars, and Vaccines (formerly Special Considerations in Compounding Biologicals)
- Handling and Compounding of Hazardous Drugs (formerly Hazardous Drugs as Compounded Sterile Preparations)

Over two-thirds of the authors for this edition are new from the previous one. New authors include Lindsey B. Amerine, Paul M. Baker, Hallie Barr, Erich Brechtelsbauer, Matthew M. Brown, Angela T. Cassano, Ashley M. Duty, Varsha Gaitonde, Chuck Gaziano, Kevin N. Hansen, Joshua S. Ilenin, Joyce S. Jih, Lynda Kiliany, F. Kurt Last, Nicholas A. Link, Ben R. Lopez, Matthew Madurski, Mary C. McManamon, Christina Michalek, Patricia A. Roberts, Abby Roth, David Short, Robert Shrewsbury, David A. South, and Elaine Strauss. Sadly, one of the authors, Chuck Gaziano, passed away during the development and writing of this chapter. All chapter authors are listed with their credentials in the Contributors section and anyone who compounds sterile preparations will recognize the experts assembled for this work.

DOI 10.37573/9781585286492.FM

In addition to the author refresh, two-thirds of the editors for this edition are new. Both E. Clyde Buchanan and Philip J. Schneider have retired from practice and are enjoying their well-deserved rest after a lifetime of contributions to the profession. To fill the gap, we welcome Lindsey B. Amerine, System Executive Director of Pharmacy for UNC Health, and Angela W. Yaniv, Director of Pharmacy—Sterile Products for Cleveland Clinic, as co-editors in addition to their roles as authors of chapters for this text.

Many challenges face all who compound sterile preparations, and in particular the pharmacy staff who perform the vast majority of compounding in health systems. Let us meet those challenges by providing our patients with the safest compounded sterile preparations possible and by protecting the healthcare employees who handle hazardous drugs. Our professional reputation depends on it.

Ryan A. Forrey
Lindsey B. Amerine
Angela W. Yaniv
October 2023

CONTRIBUTORS

Lindsey B. Amerine, PharmD, MS, BCPS, CPEL, FASHP
System Executive Director of Pharmacy
UNC Health
Associate Professor of Clinical Education
UNC Eshelman School of Pharmacy
Morrisville, North Carolina

Paul M. Baker, PharmD, BCSCP
Compounding Quality and Compliance Coordinator
Massachusetts General Hospital
Boston, Massachusetts

Hallie Barr, PharmD, MBA, BCOP
Pharmacy Manager, Investigational Drug Service
The Ohio State University Wexner Medical Center and James Cancer Hospital
Columbus, Ohio

Craig A. Boyce, BSPharm
Principal
Acumity Consulting
Asheville, North Carolina

Erich Brechtelsbauer, PharmD, MS, BCPS
Associate Director, Value, Evidence, and Outcomes
Eli Lilly and Co
Atlanta, Georgia

Matthew M. Brown, PharmD, DPLA, MLS (ASCP)
Manager
Duke Compounding Facility
Durham, North Carolina

Todd W. Canada, PharmD, BCNSP, BCCCP, FASHP, FTSHP, FASPEN
Clinical Pharmacy Services Manager and Nutrition Support Team Coordinator
The University of Texas MD Anderson Cancer Center
Houston, Texas

Richard C. Capps, PharmD, DPLA
Pharmacy Manager and Pharmacist in Charge
Prisma Health Oconee Memorial Hospital
Seneca, South Carolina

Angela T. Cassano, PharmD, MS, BCSCP, FASHP
President
Pharmfusion Consulting, LLC
Midlothian, Virginia

Ashley M. Duty, PharmD, MS, BCSCP, FASHP
Director of Inpatient Pharmacy Operations
Nationwide Children's Hospital
Columbus, Ohio

Bruce A. Erickson, RPh, MS
Pharmacy Automation Consultant (Ret.)
Director of Pharmacy (Ret.)
VA Medical Center, Minneapolis
Placida, Florida

Ryan A. Forrey, PharmD, MS, BCSCP, FFIP, FASHP
Global Clinical Solutions Director, Surgical Complication Solutions
Becton, Dickinson and Company
Clinical Assistant Professor
The Ohio State University, College of Pharmacy
Atlanta, Georgia

Varsha Gaitonde, PharmD, PhD, BCPS, BCSCP, FACHE
Vice President, Pharmacy Services
QuVa Pharma, Inc.
Sugarland, Texas

Chuck Gaziano, PE, MBA (in memoriam)
Managing Director and Principal
WorkingBuildings, LLC—Trinity Consultants
Atlanta, Georgia

Kathleen M. Gura, PharmD, BCNSP, FASHP, FPPAG, FPPA, FASPEN, FMSHP
Pharmacy Clinical Research Program Manager
Boston Children's Hospital
Boston, Massachusetts

Kevin N. Hansen, PharmD, MS, BCSCP
Pharmacy Director, 503B Program
Premier Inc.
Charlotte, North Carolina

George H. Hinkle, RPh, MS, BCNP
Medical Health Physicist
The Ohio State University
Columbus, Ohio

Joshua Ilenin, PharmD, MS
Pharmacy Manager, Operations
OhioHealth Riverside Methodist Hospital
Columbus, Ohio

DOI 10.37573/9781585286492.FM

Joyce S. Jih, PharmD, BCPS
Clinical Pharmacist
Stanford Health Care
Stanford, California

Patricia C. Kienle, RPh, MPA, BCSCP, FASHP
Director, Accreditation and Medication Safety
Cardinal Health
Wilkes-Barre, Pennsylvania

Lynda Kiliany, PharmD, BCSCP
IV Therapy Coordinator
Cleveland Clinic Akron General
Akron, Ohio

F. Kurt Last
Executive VP and Practice Leader
WorkingBuildings, LLC—Trinity Consultants
Atlanta, Georgia

Nicholas A. Link, PharmD, MBA, BCOP
Pharmacy Manager, Oncology Clinical Services
University Hospitals
Cleveland, Ohio

Ben R. Lopez, PharmD, MS, MHA, BCPS
Director of Pharmacy Operations
The Ohio State University Wexner Medical Center
Columbus, Ohio

Matthew Madurski, PharmD, MS, BCPS
Pharmacy Operations Manager
Saint Vincent Hospital
Erie, Pennsylvania

Linda F. McElhiney, PharmD, RPh, MS
Senior Compounding Pharmacist
Indiana University Health
Plainfield, Indiana

Mary C. McManamon, PharmD
Clinical Pharmacist
Cleveland Clinic
Cleveland, Ohio

Christina Michalek, BS, FASHP
Director of Membership and Patient Safety Organization (PSO)
ISMP
Plymouth Meeting, Pennsylvania

Patricia A. Roberts, PharmD, MS, BCPS, BCSCP
Director of Pharmacy, Oncology
University Hospitals
Cleveland, Ohio

Abby Roth, CMQ/OE
Owner/Microbiologist
Pure Microbiology
Allentown, Pennsylvania

David Short, BA
Chief Quality Officer
QuVa Pharma, Inc.
Sugar Land, Texas

Robert Shrewsbury, PhD
Associate Professor
UNC Eshelman School of Pharmacy
Chapel Hill, North Carolina

David A. South, PharmD, BCSCP
Pharmacy Director
Encompass Health Rehabilitation Hospital of North Alabama
Huntsville, Alabama

Elaine Strauss, PharmD, MS, BCSCP
Senior Consultant, Cleanrooms and Sterile Compounding
WorkingBuildings, LLC—Trinity Consultants
Atlanta, Georgia

Mary Ann Stuhan, PharmD, RPh
Pharmacy Program Director (Ret.)
Cuyahoga Community College
Cleveland, Ohio

Angela W. Yaniv, PharmD, BCSCP
Director of Pharmacy—Sterile Products
Cleveland Clinic
Cleveland, Ohio

REVIEWERS

Michael J. Freudiger, PharmD, APh, BCPS, BCSCP
Compounding and Regulatory Compliance Supervisor
Valley Children's Healthcare
Madera, California

Raynold Yin, PharmD, BCACP, APh, CDCES
Clinical Pharmacy Supervisor
Sharp Grossmont Hospital
San Diego, California

DOI 10.37573/9781585286492.FM

SECTION 1: Introduction to Sterile Compounding

DOI 10.37573/9781585286492

1

IMPERATIVE FOR CHANGE: ADVERSE STERILE COMPOUNDING EVENTS

Christina Michalek

INTRODUCTION

Today, sterile compounding is an essential component of pharmacy practice for pharmacists and pharmacy technicians. Efforts to identify and reduce adverse events during the preparation of sterile products are imperative in order to provide safe, optimal patient care. Unfortunately, adverse events related to sterile compounding practices have been occurring for more than thirty years. Identifying the causative factors that trigger these events is crucial to eliminating repeat occurrences, preventing harm, and improving patient care.[1;2;3]

RATIONALE FOR THE PHARMACY'S ROLE IN STERILE COMPOUNDING

Historically, sterile compounding was not a pharmacy established role. Until the late 1960s, a nurse was the primary practitioner who prepared sterile doses of medications for patients. These drugs, meant to be administered via intravenous (IV), subcutaneous, or intramuscular routes, were prepared in a nonsterile environment by a nurse, likely in a medication room or at a patient's bedside. These medication doses were usually administered in an unlabeled volume control chamber between a large volume parenteral solution and the patient or by IV push, subcutaneous, or intramuscular injection using an unlabeled syringe.[4]

One of the foundational works that charted the growth of pharmacy practice in the hospital setting was *Mirror to Hospital Pharmacy*, which was published in 1964 by the American Society of Hospital Pharmacists. This groundbreaking publication called for the expanded role of hospital pharmacists based on a national audit of pharmaceutical services in hospitals. One recommendation stated "hospitals to be encouraged to assign to pharmacists the responsibility and to provide the necessary facilities for the preparation and quality control of sterile medicinal products produced in hospitals even when these products are produced in another department."[5]

Following the publication of *Mirror to Hospital Pharmacy,* problems with the safety of IV drug therapies were reported as justification for pharmacy-based programs. Patterson et al. expressed concerns about drug incompatibilities and the length of time between preparation and administration of medications prepared in patient care areas. They found that 60% of IV fluids used at their hospital contained more than one drug, and many were administered more than one hour after preparation.[6] These authors, similar those who wrote the recommendations set forth in *Mirror to Hospital Pharmacy,* called for pharmacy to assume responsibility for compounding IV doses to resolve these problems.

Flack et al. reported requests for "technical help from the pharmacy service" by surgeons investigating the effectiveness and safety of parenteral nutrition. They sought to resolve problems with contamination and incompatibilities with formulas that were being manually prepared in open lab surroundings.[7] Thur et al. reported a 21% error rate when observing nurses preparing parenteral products in patient care areas. Errors included wrong dose (9%), incompatible drugs mixed together (6%), wrong drug or solution (3%), and preparation of drugs not ordered (3%). Additionally, the researchers observed numerous deviations from accepted sterile practices, including counters not being cleaned (99%), hands not washed (97%), touching critical site areas (47%), and not cleaning vial or bottle stoppers (31%).[8]

O'Hare et al. used a disguised observer methodology to evaluate physician and nurse preparations and administration of IV medications. They found that physicians made at least one error in 98% of the doses prepared and 83% of these doses were administered by nurses.[9] Taxis and Barber observed nurses who prepared and administered IV medications in 10 wards in a hospital in the United Kingdom. The researchers observed 430 doses of drugs and found a total of 249 errors. Most errors occurred when bolus doses were prepared and administered or when a dose required multiple preparation steps. One of the error prevention recommendations set forth by this research team was to reduce the amount of sterile preparation in the ward.[10]

DOI 10.37573/9781585286492.001

Thompson et al. evaluated the concentration of infusions prepared at the bedside and found evidence of incomplete mixing of drugs in IV solutions. They also found that there was more uniformity of concentration of potassium chloride when these doses were prepared by the pharmacy.[11] Calculation errors were also found to be a root cause of error in doses prepared by nurses. Pearlstein et al. found that one in twelve doses calculated by nurses had an error that resulted in a 10-fold dose compared with what was ordered. Pediatricians made errors in 1 in 26 computations, and pharmacists made fewer errors than nurses or physicians.[12]

In addition to the issues mentioned in the studies, the risk of microbial contamination of parenteral doses prepared under aseptic techniques in clinical and pharmacy environments cannot be overlooked. In a meta-analysis of 16,552 doses that came from a compilation of 34 studies, it was found that a significantly higher frequency of contaminated doses were prepared in clinical settings than in pharmaceutical environments. The authors concluded that the amount of contaminated orders grossly exceeded acceptable reference standards, and that it may cause increased infection risks. They further noted that the data supported dose preparation in pharmaceutical rather than clinical environments.[13]

As a result of these reports, pharmacy-based sterile compounding emerged as a potentially safer method than compounding in a clinical setting.

SAFETY IS NOT STATIC

Safety is everyone's job. Regardless of one's profession or the industry in which one works, we all need to be on guard for threats to the safety of ourselves and others. Safety work is never finished. It is not something for which we can check a box and then move on to the next item. No matter what we do or what well-designed safety process, policy, or plan is developed and put in place, it will always need to be monitored, revisited, and updated periodically. Based on safety science and quality improvement, it is known that conditions will change, and everyone needs to be prepared. Drifting from identified best practice workflows, standard processes, policies, or procedural steps is human nature.[14] Safety efforts to prevent, reduce, and eliminate medication errors should be vigilantly observed and updated, including efforts associated with compounding sterile preparations.

STERILITY ISSUES AND COMPOUNDING ERRORS

Prescribing sterile preparations is rather ubiquitous in acute care and ambulatory procedural settings. In fact, in these settings it might be a bit of a challenge to find a patient who has not received a medication. And it may be even more challenging to find someone who has not received an injectable medication during their stay. There is good reason for the use of injectable medications. IV, epidural, intrathecal, intramuscular, intradermal, and subcutaneous routes of administration have apparent advantages over medications that are administered orally, topically, rectally, or via inhalation. In fact, some medications are only available in a parenteral form. Since many injectable sterile medications are not in a dose or dosage form that is commercially available and ready to administer, and there is variability in patient specific doses of most injectable sterile medications, it is understandable that many of these drugs would need to be compounded.

Adverse events related to preparation of parenteral products have frequently been reported to the Institute for Safe Medication Practices (ISMP) National Medication Errors Reporting Program (MERP) and National Vaccine Errors Reporting Program (VERP). These cases have often been a topic of discussion in various *ISMP Medication Safety Alert!* newletters.[15-23] *Pharmacy Purchasing & Products* magazine annually polls a sample of health-system pharmacy directors across the United States on the state of pharmacy compounding in the U.S. In 2022, 29% of these pharmacy leaders indicated that in the past 5 years their facility experienced a patient incident involving a compounding error.[24] The data also indicated a positive relationship between compounding volumes and compounding errors, as pharmacies that reported higher daily compounding volumes were more likely to be aware of patient incidents. Forty-four percent of pharmacies preparing more than 500 compounded sterile preparations (CSPs) a day reported experiencing a patient incident, whereas only 21% of organizations preparing 51 to 100 CSPs per day reported incidents.[24] It is, however, important to note that risk identification, reporting systems, safety culture, and other factors play a role in error identification. When the same group of pharmacy directors was asked about changes to the volume of preparations expected to be compounded in the next year, nearly 60% of the directors from organizations over 100 beds in size projected an increase in compounding volume, which could lead to an increase in adverse events.[24]

Harmful or fatal infections linked to sterile compounding practices in the U.S. began to be reported in the 1990s. Over the past three decades, there have been variety of contaminated products that reached patients after breaches in sterile compounding practices. In 1998, 11 children became septic, with 10 testing positive for *Enterobacter cloacae* blood-stream infections associated with contaminated prefilled saline syringes.[25] In 2001, 4 children contracted *Enterobacter cloacae* infections from IV ranitidine compounded in a hospital pharmacy.[26] In 2005, 10 patients died after exposure to cardioplegia solutions contaminated with gram negative rods. In 2011, 19 patients received parenteral nutrition solutions contaminated with *Serratia marcescens* when nonsterile components were used to prepare amino acids, 9 of which died from their infection.[1] In March 2012, 9 cases of clinically diagnosed fungal endophthalmitis were linked to the mold *Fusarium incarnatum-equiseti* species complex, which was in contaminated compounded Brilliant Blue-G dye. This investigation expanded to include compounded intravitreal injections of triamcinolone-containing products prepared by the same compounding lab. Overall, a total of 33 confirmed and probable cases in 7 different states were identified.[27] The largest scale outbreak due to breaches in sterile compounding occurred during the nationwide fungal meningitis outbreak of 2012 that affected more than 750 patients, causing the death of 64 people due to *Exserohilum* and *Aspergillus* species contaminated methylprednisolone acetate injections.[28] According to the U.S. Food and Drug Administration (FDA), the outbreak represents "the largest public health crisis caused by a pharmaceutical product" to date.[1;29]

The United States Pharmacopeia (USP) Chapter <797> Pharmaceutical Compounding—Sterile Preparations was introduced in 2004 as the first enforceable sterile preparation compounding requirements, and it has since gone through several revisions. USP seeks to provide guidance in the form of minimum standards to follow when preparing CSPs in order to minimize harm (including death) to human and animal patients that can result from microbial contamination (nonsterility), excessive bacterial endotoxins, variability from the intended strength of correct ingredients, physical and chemical incompatibilities, chemical and physical contaminants, and/or use of ingredients of inappropriate quality.[30] It is promising that 87% of the U.S. pharmacy directors surveyed in 2022 reported mostly meeting, meeting, or exceeding USP Chapter <797> standards for compounding, further assuring that these identified minimum standards are being followed and, in some cases, being exceeded.[24] These practice standards are further supported and enforced through inspections by state boards of pharmacy and accreditation agencies (see Chapter 2).

Events linked to sterility and infection from contamination are only one type of medication safety risk related to sterile compounding. In addition to harmful and fatal infections associated with lapses in sterile compounding, there are also several compounding-related medication errors that have caused harm to patients or have resulted in death in the past couple of decades. In 1997, Flynn and colleagues, in their observational study of accuracy in compounding at 5 hospitals, identified a mean daily sterile compounding error rate of 9%, which meant almost 1 in 10 products dispensed at the time of their observations were prepared incorrectly. The most common error type at that time was wrong dose. Parenteral nutrition had the highest error rate when prepared manually or with a partially automated process.[31]

Calculation errors are also a commonly reported cause of harmful events. In 2006, an infant died of a 1,000-fold overdose of zinc that they received from a hospital-prepared parenteral nutrition infusion. In this event, an order was written to add 330 mcg of zinc/100 mL of parenteral nutrition solution. However, the sterile products automated compounder was programmed to accept zinc additives in mcg/kg. Although the pharmacist correctly converted the ordered dose to mcg/kg, it was incorrectly entered into the compounder as milligrams and not micrograms by selecting milligram from a drop-down list. The pharmacy technician who prepared the solution did not appreciate the large volume of zinc required to prepare the parenteral nutrition, and although they thought it was unusual, they did not mention it to another pharmacy technician or pharmacist at the time of compounding.[7]

In that same year, a child died after a chemotherapy infusion was prepared with 23.4% sodium chloride instead of 0.9% sodium chloride. When this event occurred, routine information system maintenance during the prior shift had caused several hours of delay in printing infusion labels. This caused production to be backed up, so staff were pressed to prepare and verify the chemotherapy product quickly in a small, crowded area of the pharmacy. The error was missed during the verification process.[22] In 2007, 3 patients received compounded IV colchicine in a 4 mg/mL concentration instead of 0.5 mg/mL concentration. Two of these patients died from an overdose.[16] One child died in 2010 after receiving an overdose of sodium chloride when a compounding error lead to them receiving 60 times the intended amount.[1]

In 2010, an infusion of valproate was mistakenly prepared with vecuronium. In this event, shortly after initiation of the infusion, the patient had trouble breathing and was able to alert their nurse who stopped the infusion very soon after it began.[32] Four years later, in 2014, a patient received IV rocuronium instead of IV fosphenytoin due to a compounding error. Unfortunately, this patient experienced cardiopulmonary arrest and died as a result of the mistake.[23] In 2019, another 1,000-fold zinc overdose very similar to the event from 2006 was reported. However, when the compounding staff recognized the significant volume of zinc solution needed to prepare the parenteral nutrition product, the error was identified and caught before reaching the patient.[33] These and other similar events have repeatedly shown that manual processes for the inspection and verification of CSPs is not a sufficient strategy for preventing preparation and dispensing errors.[3]

SYMPTOMS OF A BROKEN SYSTEM: COMPOUNDING OUTSIDE A PHARMACY

In 2020, an ISMP survey provided insights into compounding practices occurring outside a pharmacy environment.[34] Over 400 practitioners participated in the survey, which provided an in-depth look at sterile, injectable medication preparation practices occurring outside the pharmacy setting. Nurses, anesthesia providers, and decentralized technicians and pharmacists working primarily in the acute care or specialty hospital setting reported that the most frequently prepared sterile injectables were IV push medications, IV intermittent infusions, and intramuscular injections. More than 25% of respondents also reported often or always preparing IV continuous infusions, including titratable infusions, with an additional 20% of respondents reporting sometimes preparing these medications. Most respondents reported rarely or never preparing epidural and neuraxial injections or infusions. However, 7% of respondents (mostly anesthesia providers) reported always preparing these medications. When asked about five best practices associated with preparing sterile products (eg, preparing one product at a time, following a standard process for preparation and labeling, a requirement for training and competency assessment for those preparing sterile products), the majority of respondents agreed or strongly agreed with the practices. However, few strongly agreed that these procedures were actually being followed. Identified locations where compounding was occurring included medication rooms, at a patient's bedside, on a counter or desk in a nursing station, on an anesthesia workstation, on a computer workstation, in a patient's home, in an ambulance, and in an operating or procedure room. Thirty-one percent of respondents were aware of or personally experienced errors when compounding during the prior twelve months. Sixty-nine percent were uncertain or unaware of errors. Given that in these settings the practitioner preparing sterile medications is often the one administering them, the detection of an error is less likely. The types of errors most cited included use of an expired drug, use of the wrong drug, wrong dose, wrong concentration, wrong diluent or diluent volume, failure to label the preparation or other labeling error, and following the wrong preparation process (eg, improper use of multidose vials, failure to use a filter when necessary).[34]

Prior ISMP surveys related to IV push medication practices revealed similar concerning results. In 2018, findings from a survey of over 900 practitioners (mostly nurses) noted that five unsafe practices associated with IV push medications had persisted or worsened since prior surveys in 2010 and 2014. Using prefilled syringes or cartridges as vials, unnecessarily diluting medications, using prefilled flush syringes to dilute or reconstitute medications and then administer them to patients, failing to properly label syringes, and performing these compounding activities outside a pharmacy environment were common practices that put patients at risk for harm.[35]

ANATOMY OF AN ERROR

The first item that should be tackled when working on error prevention is addressing false beliefs, such as a tendency to attribute good outcomes to skill and bad outcomes to bad luck. If you read the previous adverse event stories with an uneasy feeling, that is to be expected. Although the events are compelling, perhaps you reasoned why the same can't happen to you or why they won't happen at your practice site. That too is common, it's a protection mechanism, we are attempting to protect our own self-image. In order to learn from the events of others and prevent the same events from reoccurring, we have to remove the bias that "it can't happen to me" and recognize that we may be overly optimistic in thinking that we would be less vulnerable to the exact same conditions should they be present in our practice site. We must admit our vulnerability to sterile compounding adverse events that have happened to others and move our thinking from "Could this happen here?" to encouraging everyone to instead challenge themselves to ask and answer, "*How* could this happen here?"[36]

There are many factors that contribute to an error reaching a patient. It is important to understand these causal factors to design safer systems that make it more difficult to err. Root causes are factors that contribute to an event. They are the most fundamental reason why an event has occurred. These causes are primarily system and process issues and not human performance concerns.[37] There are also active and latent failures. *Active failures* are usually human errors. *Latent failures* are conditions that exist in the design, environment, or equipment that are not apparent until they contribute to errors or allow errors to go undetected until they harm a patient. These are considered accidents waiting to happen. In the event where the chemotherapy infusion was prepared with 23.4% sodium chloride instead of 0.9% sodium chloride, the active failure is the failure of the pharmacist to detect the wrong concentration and the latent failure is the extended information system downtime that caused staff to get behind on their work. When several latent conditions align and are combined with active failures by individuals, it usually results in an adverse event.[38]

When reviewing an adverse event, it is relatively easy to identify human errors (active failures), but it is more challenging to find latent system failures. Systematic changes carry more leverage in the prevention of sterile compounding errors than approaches that rely on improving human performance. It is better to understand and implement strategies that prevent pharmacists and pharmacy technicians from being involved in an adverse event than trying to make them perform flawlessly. For example, introducing a policy that states pharmacists and pharmacy technicians should read the label of a vial of medication three times before withdrawing the dose needed to compound a sterile product carries less safety weight than instituting a workflow process that prompts for the scan of the vial's barcode or RFID code, which then matches that scan to the product being prepared. Robust error prevention models should favor identification of system interventions to help facilitate changes that can prevent medication errors.

SAFE STERILE PREPARATION CONSIDERATIONS

Based on detailed analysis of reported sterile compounding errors, *ISMP Guidelines for Safe Preparation of Compounded Sterile Preparations* was published in 2013 (revised and updated in 2016) as a result of a national invitational sterile preparation compounding summit.[3] The guidelines attempted to fill the gap between USP Chapter <797> standards, which are primarily designed to ensure compounded products are sterile at the time of dispensing, and what were identified as safe practices to avoid medication errors during sterile compounding.

In the safety hierarchy for sterile preparations (see **Figure 1-1**), providing manufacturer-prepared, patient specific doses of parenteral products in a ready-to-administer form is a high-leverage approach. However, due to the

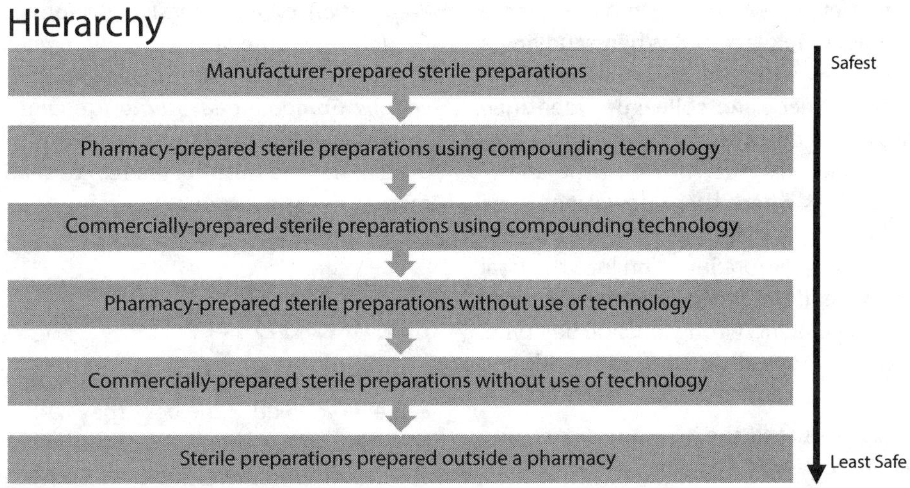

FIGURE 1-1. Safety hierarchy for sterile preparations

variety of drugs, doses, and dosage forms, availability of products filling all these criteria are limited. Therefore, it is necessary to rely on compounded products. Since published data have repeatedly shown that manual processes for verification of sterile compounding process steps is insufficient for detecting and preventing medication errors, the ISMP guidelines recommended that "technology solutions are utilized to augment manual processes for preparing and verifying compounded sterile preparations."[3] Similarly, in 2019, the American Society of Health-System Pharmacists (ASHP) advocated for the adoption of "automation and information technology to facilitate in-process and final verification of compounded sterile preparations to ensure quality."[39] ISMP's 2022–2023 *Targeted Medication Safety Best Practices for Hospitals* Best Practice number 11 calls for organizations compounding sterile preparations to "perform an independent verification to ensure that the proper ingredients are added, including confirmation of the proper amount of each ingredient prior to its addition to the final container."[40] It specifically calls for organizations to "eliminate the use of proxy methods of verification for compounded sterile preparations of medications" (eg, the syringe pull-back method or checking only a compounding record and not the ingredients and amounts used in the compounding process) and to "use technology to assist in the verification process to augment manual processes."[40] In 2019, the ASHP House of Delegates decided that ASHP should "advocate that until such time as automation or technology can be implemented, independent in-process and final verification of compounded sterile preparations be performed."[39] They also decided to "advocate to oppose the use of the syringe pull-back method or other proxy methods of compounded sterile preparation verification."[39] The use of automated workflow and other technology for sterile compounding is discussed in greater detail in Chapter 9.

While introducing technology is a strong strategy to prevent errors and improve and standardize processes, there are other strategies that support prevention of adverse events during sterile compounding. Initial and ongoing training with competency assessment is equally important to the safe preparation of sterile products (see Chapters 3, 4, and 5). For those who routinely perform sterile compounding, certificate programs and certification (specifically for sterile compounding leads) are also a recommended strategy. Foundational elements, such as policies, standard operating procedures, and master formulation records, that help guide practices are of equal significance (see Chapters 33 and 30). Based on ISMP MERP data, one of the most commonly identified contributing factors to medication mix-ups is look-alike packaging. Therefore, consideration should also be given to how sterile drug inventory is stored and managed (see Chapter 19). Intermingling of products, insufficient space to provide segregation of drugs and different drug concentrations, lack of space for the volume of work being done in the compounding area, incorrect or incomplete labeling of storage locations, poor lighting, and distractions have all been implicated in adverse sterile compounding medication events. Observation should be made of the workspace in order to identify and mitigate these risks where they exist. The use of bins for assembling products to be prepared; segregating, sequestering, and differentiating high-alert medications such as neuromuscular blocking agents; segregating concentrated electrolytes; and using barcode verification during stock replenishment are all recommended strategies to reduce risks related to wrong medication selection.[3]

TECHNOLOGY HOLDS PROMISE

With strong advocacy for the adoption and use of sterile compounding technology, several groups have studied the impact of introducing automated workflows that incorporate barcode verification of drugs and diluents as well as volumetric and gravimetric analysis of medication amounts to the manual sterile compounding process. In these studies, the addition of automation identified and prevented error types that had previously gone undetected in publicized medication compounding errors when only manual sterile compounding processes were in place.[41-43] When studying a newly implemented workflow software system in an oncology ambulatory pharmacy, Reece and colleagues identified a 7.1% error rate (1,126 errors detected in 15,843 doses prepared) during sterile compounding activities. In the analysis of the steps in the process where these deviations were identified, they found that 71% of the total errors were recognized in the drug weighing step before injection into the final bag; 26% of the errors were identified in the barcode scanning step as errors of wrong diluent, wrong infusion bag type, wrong infusion bag size, or wrong drug were captured; and 3% of the errors were identified during vial reconstitution.[41]

Eckel and colleagues evaluated the efficiency, cost, and safety benefits of technology-assisted sterile compounding workflow compared to manual workflow processes in a total of 341,138 compounded sterile preparations across 8 U.S. hospitals. Technology-assisted sterile compounding workflow provided a safety benefit, detecting 14 times more errors than the manual systems, and it was also associated with lower costs per compounded sterile preparation and faster turnaround times.[42] Similarly, use of a workflow software system in a large U.S. pediatric hospital intercepted 72% of identified errors during sterile compounding of 421,730 prepared doses over the course of 12 months.[43] Researchers Yihong and colleagues found that the most common error types identified by the workflow software system were incorrect diluent and incorrect drug. This research team also found that certain staff shifts and certain days of the week correlated to higher error rates. In their data analysis, the first (morning) shift had the highest error rate compared with second or third shift, and errors were more likely to occur on Sunday or Monday.[43] Although USP Chapter <797> provides enforceable standards to avoid sterility related events during sterile compounding, there is currently no enforceable standard or state or regulatory requirement for practitioners to follow identified best practices related to medication error prevention during sterile compounding.

As more organizations began to adopt use of sterile compounding technologies, it became imperative to identify and support safe practices related to the use of these technologies. In 2021, ISMP convened an invitational sterile compounding safety summit to address safe practices related to the use of sterile compounding workflow management systems, automated compounding devices, and robotic compounding automation. The resulting document, *Guidelines for Sterile Compounding and the Safe Use of Compounding Technology*, which replaced the 2016 *Guidelines for Safe Preparation of Compounded Sterile Preparations*, identifies best practices for the safe use of various forms of technology and automation in sterile compounding processes and recommends best practices associated with sterile compounding when technology cannot be used.[44] ASHP also addressed selection, safe implementation, and utilization of compounding technology in *ASHP Guidelines on the Safe Use of Automated Compounding Devices for the Preparation of Parenteral Nutrition Admixtures* and *ASHP Guidelines on the Selection, Implementation, and Utilization of Workflow and Robotic Technologies for Preparing Intravenous Compounded Sterile Preparations.*[45;46] Others have sought to address recommendations for vendors, drug manufacturers, and hospital leaders to support successful implementation of compounding robotic technology in order to maximize patient safety.[47]

WE'VE GOT THIS

When it comes to safety, it is a constantly evolving endeavor and everyone does the best they can do with the knowledge that they have today. To avoid adverse events related to sterile compounding, the best way to apply current knowledge includes compliance with USP Chapter <797> standards, ASHP and ISMP guidelines, and other regulatory standards as applicable. Pharmacy staff need time for adequate training, and their competency must be assessed prior to independently working and re-evaluated annually. Robust standard operating procedures and work standards must be in place to support safety. This includes proper engineering controls, equipment, and the adoption of sterile compounding technology to improve accuracy and reliability, something organizations such as ISMP and ASHP have long advocated for. Sterile compounding operations should be supported by an overarching infrastructure that holds staff and the organization accountable for meeting current standards of practice and quality outcomes.

While compounding procedures have come a long way, and people have learned a lot about avoiding adverse events and errors through the analysis of sterile compounding incidents and identification of best practices, there is still more work to do. People and organizations must make every effort toward adopting safer systems for pharmacists and pharmacy technicians in order to protect patients from harm. As stewards of medication use, pharmacists and pharmacy technicians are in the best position, as they provide the most knowledgeable about reliable and safe sterile compounding to meet the needs of the patients they serve.

REFERENCES

1. Institute for Safe Medication Practices (ISMP). Sterile compounding tragedy is a symptom of a broken system on many levels. *ISMP Medication Safety Alert!* 2012;17(21):1–4.

2. Hughes CF, Grant AF, Leckie BD, Baird DK. Cardioplegic solution: a contamination crisis. *J Thorac Cardiovasc Surg* 1986;91(2):296–302.

3. Institute for Safe Medication Practices (ISMP). *ISMP Guidelines for Safe Preparation of Compounded Sterile Preparations.* **https://www.ismp.org/sites/default/files/attachments/2017-11/Guidelines%20for%20Safe%20Preparation%20of%20Compounded%20**

Sterile%20Preperations_%20revised%202016.pdf. Published 2013. Revised 2016. Accessed March 11, 2023.

4. Buchanan EC, McKinnon BT, Scheckelhoff DJ, et al. *Principles of sterile product preparation*. Bethesda, MD: American Society of Health-System Pharmacists; 1995.
5. Francke DE, Latiolais CJ, Francke GN, et al. *Mirror to hospital pharmacy*. Washington DC: American Society of Hospital Pharmacists; 1964:4.
6. Patterson TR, Nordstrom KA. An analysis of IV additive procedures on nursing units. *Am J Hosp Pharm.* 1968;25:134–137.
7. Flack HL, Gans JA, Serlick SE, et al. The current status of parenteral hyperalimentation. *Am J Hosp Pharm.* 1971;28:326–335.
8. Thur MP, Miller WA, Latiolais CJ. Medication errors in a nurse-controlled parenteral admixture program. *Am J Hosp Pharm.* 1972;29:298–304.
9. O'Hare MCB, Bradley AM, Gallagher T, et al. Errors in the administration of intravenous drugs. *Br Med J.* 1995;310:1536–1537.
10. Taxis, K, Barber N. Ethnographic study of incidence and severity of intravenous drug errors. *Br Med J.* 2003;326:684–687.
11. Thompson WL, Feer TD. Incomplete mixing of drugs in intravenous solutions. *Crit Care Med.* 1980;8:603–607.
12. Perlstein PH, Callison C, White M, et al. Errors in drug computations during newborn intensive care. *Am J Dis Child.* 1979;133:376–379.
13. Austin PK, KS Hand, E Marinos. Systematic review and meta-analysis of the risk of microbial contamination of parenteral doses prepared under aseptic techniques in clinical and pharmaceutical environments. *J Hosp Infec.* 2015;91:306–318.
14. Institute for Safe Medication Practices (ISMP). Just culture and its critical link to patient safety (Part I). *ISMP Medication Safety Alert!* 2012;17(10):1–4.
15. Institute for Safe Medication Practices (ISMP). Unfortunately, this time it wasn't the equipment. *ISMP Medication Safety Alert!* 2005;10(20):1–2.
16. Institute for Safe Medication Practices (ISMP). Colchicine deaths. *ISMP Medication Safety Alert!* 2007;12(21):1–3.
17. Institute for Safe Medication Practices (ISMP). Fatal 1,000-fold overdoses can occur, particularly to neonates, by transposing mcg and mg. *ISMP Medication Safety Alert!* 2007;12(18):1–4.
18. Institute for Safe Medication Practices (ISMP). Post-production IV admixture checks less than ideal. *ISMP Medication Safety Alert!* 2010;15(13):3.
19. Institute for Safe Medication Practices (ISMP). TPN-related deaths call for FDA guidance and pharmacy board oversight of USP Chapter <797>. *ISMP Medication Safety Alert!* 2011;16(7):1–3.
20. Institute for Safe Medication Practices (ISMP). Another tragic parenteral nutrition compounding error. *ISMP Medication Safety Alert!* 2011;16(8):1–3.
21. Institute for Safe Medication Practices (ISMP). Safe practices in pharmacy sterile compounding areas. *ISMP Medication Safety Alert!* 2011;16(11):1–4.
22. Institute for Safe Medication Practices (ISMP). Failed check system for chemotherapy leads to pharmacist's no contest plea for involuntary manslaughter. *ISMP Medication Safety Alert!* 2009;14(8):1–2.
23. Institute for Safe Medication Practices (ISMP). Tragic error with neuromuscular blocker should prompt risk assessment by all hospitals. *ISMP Medication Safety Alert!* 2014;19(25):1,4.
24. *Pharmacy Purchasing & Products'* State of Pharmacy Compounding 15th Annual National Survey. *Pharmacy Purchasing & Products.* April 2022;19(4):s1–60.
25. Centers for Disease Control and Prevention (CDC). Notice to readers Enterobacter cloacae bloodstream infections associated with contaminated prefilled saline syringes–California, November 1998. *MMWR Weekly.* November 13, 1998;47(44):959–960.
26. Selenic D, Dodson DR, Jensen B, et al. Enterobacter cloacae bloodstream infections in pediatric patients traced to a hospital pharmacy. *Am J Health Syst Pharm* 2003;60(14):1440–1446.
27. Centers for Disease Control and Prevention (CDC). Notes from the field: multistate outbreak of postprocedural fungal endophthalmitis associated with a single compounding pharmacy—United States, March–April 2012. *MMWR Weekly.* May 4, 2012;61(17):310–311.
28. Centers for Disease Control and Prevention (CDC). Multistate fungal meningitis outbreak investigation. **https://www.cdc.gov/hai/outbreaks/meningitis.html**. Updated October 30, 2015. Accessed March 12, 2023.
29. Owner of New England compounding center convicted of racketeering leading to nationwide fungal meningitis outbreak [press release]. Washington, DC: Food and Drug Administration Office of Criminal Investigations, U.S. Department of Justice; March 22, 2017. **https://www.justice.gov/opa/pr/owner-new-england-compounding-center-convicted-racketeering-leading-nationwide-fungal#:~:text=Barry%20Cadden%2C%20the%20owner%20and,outbreak%2C%20the%20Justice%20Department%20announced**. Accessed August 18, 2023.

30. USP <797> Pharmaceutical compounding—sterile preparations. In: 2023: *USP Compounding Compendium*. Rockville, MD: The United States Pharmacopeial Convention. doi:10.31003/USPNF_M99925_07_01.

31. Flynn BA, Pearson RE, Barker KN. Observational study of accuracy in compounding i.v. admixtures at five hospitals. *Am J Health Syst Pharm* 1997;54(8):904–912.

32. Institute for Safe Medication Practices (ISMP). Neuromuscular blocker mix-up in the pharmacy. *ISMP Medication Safety Alert!* 2010;15(1):3.

33. Institute for Safe Medication Practices (ISMP). Too close for comfort: fatal zinc overdose narrowly avoided. *ISMP Medication Safety Alert!* 2019;24(13):1–4.

34. Institute for Safe Medication Practices (ISMP). ISMP survey provides insights into preparation and admixture practices outside the pharmacy. *ISMP Medication Safety Alert!* 2020;25(22):1–5.

35. Institute for Safe Medication Practices (ISMP). Part II: survey results suggest action is needed to improve safety with adult IV push medications. *Nurse AdviseERR*. 2018;16(12):1–4.

36. Institute for Safe Medication Practices (ISMP). Using external errors to signal a clear and present danger. *ISMP Medication Safety Alert!* 2008;13(22):1–2.

37. Institute for Safe Medication Practices (ISMP). Root cause analysis workbook for community/ambulatory care pharmacy. **https://www.ismp.org/sites/default/files/attachments/2018-01/FINAL%20ISMP52-RCA-011414.pdf**. Published 2013. Accessed August 18, 2023.

38. Institute for Safe Medication Practices (ISMP). Multiple latent failures align to allow a serious drug interaction to harm a patient. *ISMP Medication Safety Alert!* 2011;16(9):1–3.

39. American Society of Health-System Pharmacists. House of Delegates Session—2019. Proceedings of the 71st annual session of the ASHP House of Delegates, June 9 and 11, 2019; June 9–11, 2019; Boston, MA. **https://www.ashp.org/-/media/4D2DBE635E5947478111A5E1504B9107.ashx**. Accessed August 18, 2023.

40. Institute for Safe Medication Practices (ISMP). Targeted medication safety best practices for hospitals. **https://www.ismp.org/guidelines/best-practices-hospitals**. Published 2022. Accessed March 12, 2023.

41. Reece KM, Lozano MA, Roux R, et al. Implementation and evaluation of a gravimetric i.v., workflow system in an oncology ambulatory care pharmacy. *Am J Health-Syst Pharm*. 2016;73(3):165–173.

42. Eckel SF, Higgins JP, Hess E. Multicenter study to evaluate the benefits of technology-assisted workflow on i.v. room efficiency, costs, and safety. *Am J Health-Syst Pharm*. 2019;76(12):895–901.

43. Yihong D, Lin AC, Hingl J, et al. Risk factors for i.v. compounding errors when using an automated workflow management system. *Am J Health-Syst Pharm*. 2016;73(12):887–893.

44. Institute for Safe Medication Practices (ISMP). Guidelines for sterile compounding and the safe use of sterile compounding technology. Published May 4, 2022. **https://www.ismp.org/resources/guidelines-sterile-compounding-and-safe-use-sterile-compounding-technology**.

45. Iredell B, Mourad H, Nickman N, et al. ASHP guidelines on the safe use of automated compounding devices for the preparation of parenteral nutrition admixtures. *Am J Health-Syst Pharm*. 2022;79(10):730–735.

46. American Society of Health-System Pharmacists (ASHP). ASHP guidelines on the selection, implementation, and utilization of workflow and robotic technologies for preparing intravenous compounded sterile preparations. **https://www.ashp.org/-/media/assets/policy-guidelines/docs/guidelines/compounding-sterile-preparations.ashx**.

47. Long J, Calabrese S, Al-jedai A, et al. Cleveland Clinic International IV Robotics Summit. *Am J Health-Syst Pharm*. 2021;78(9):800–805.

STANDARDS FOR COMPOUNDED STERILE PREPARATIONS

Ryan A. Forrey

INTRODUCTION

Poor sterile compounding practices have caused much patient harm and many deaths, but it was the New England Compounding Center tragedy, which caused 64 deaths and 753 illnesses across 20 states in 2012, that changed the world of sterile compounding laws, regulations, and standards (Chapter 1).[1] Such changes included the federal Drug Quality and Security Act (DQSA) of 2013 and renewed emphasis on the compounding and outsourcing of sterile preparations by accrediting agencies.

This chapter will teach compounding personnel the standards and regulations involved in their work. It will also instruct them about the enforcement bodies that will impact their training, practices, and facilities. Relevant standards and regulations are summarized, followed by a listing of relevant enforcement agencies. Agencies are arranged in descending order based on the likelihood that they will enforce standards for pharmacists and pharmacies that compound sterile preparations. Make no mistake, citations by agencies such as these can lead to revoked licenses, ruined reputations and careers, bankrupted businesses, and even imprisonment for perpetrators.[2-7] In the case of the New England Compounding Center, the compounding supervisor and president were given extended 10.5- and 14.5-year sentences after their less harsh sentences were appealed by prosecutors and overturned by an appellate court.[8;9]

According to a 2022 survey of pharmacy compounding at 315 hospitals, regulators visited hospitals asking about nonhazardous sterile compounding at rates similar to prepandemic, with the exception of Centers for Medicare & Medicaid Services (CMS). The rates were 75% of hospitals by state board of pharmacy inspectors, 74% by accrediting surveyors, and 18% by CMS surveyors.[10] For hazardous sterile compounding, inspections for compliance with hazardous drug standards were much lower at 47% by state board of pharmacy inspectors, 46% by accrediting surveyors, and 14% by CMS sureyors.[10] However, at the time of this survey, U.S. Pharmacopeial Convention (USP) Chapter <800> Hazardous Drugs—Handling in Healthcare Settings was only informational, therefore not a regulatory requirement.

STANDARDS AND REGULATIONS

United States Pharmacopeia–National Formulary

The U.S. Pharmacopeial Convention (USP) is a scientific nonprofit organization that sets standards for the identity, strength, quality, and purity of medicines, food ingredients, and dietary supplements manufactured, distributed, and consumed worldwide.[11] USP is a standard setting organization and has no enforcement role for the standards it sets, but its standards are legally recognized in more than 140 countries.[12] Standards in the United States Pharmacopeia-National Formulary *USP–NF* for compounded preparations may be enforced by state boards of pharmacy, health-system accrediting agencies, and the FDA. In the late 1980s, USP decided that compounding sterile IV preparations for home use involved special concerns (eg, extended parenteral nutrition storage and patient manipulations prior to use). Therefore, they established a Home Healthcare Advisory Panel in 1989 to draft a chapter on compounding sterile preparations for home use. USP Chapter <1206> Sterile Drug Products for Home Use appeared in the 1995 *USP–NF* and was revised in the 2000 *USP–NF*.[13;14]

USP Chapter <797> Pharmaceutical Compounding—Sterile Preparations

In March 2002, USP changed Chapter <1206> to USP Chapter <797>, and the first official version was published in USP's *Pharmacopeial Forum*.[15] USP Chapter <797> became official on January 1, 2004. Unlike USP Chapter <1206>, which was limited to home care, USP Chapter <797> describes requirements for all sterile compounding

Note: The author acknowledges E. Clyde Buchanan who authored this chapter in the previous edition.

DOI 10.37573/9781585286492.002

conducted by workers (eg, pharmacists, technicians, nurses, physicians, veterinarians, dentists, naturopaths, and chiropractors) in all places (eg, hospitals and other healthcare institutions, medical and surgical patient treatment sites, infusion facilities, pharmacies, and physician or veterinarian practice sites).[16] This chapter does not pertain to actual clinical administration of compounded sterile preparations (CSPs) to patients, however other standards, such as the Centers for Disease Control and Prevention (CDC) Safe Injection Practices, may apply. The intent of USP Chapter <797> is to minimize harm, including death, to human and animal patients that could result from the following[16]:

- Microbial contamination [nonsterility]
- Excessive bacterial endotoxins
- Variability from the intended strength of correct ingredients
- Physical and chemical incompatibilities
- Chemical and physical contaminants
- Use of ingredients of inappropriate quality

The Food, Drug, and Cosmetic (FD&C) Act of 1938 established the FDA as the enforcement authority for therapeutic drugs and recognized USP as the official compendia of standards. When the compounding chapter <1206> was revised and renumbered to <797>, it became a federally enforceable chapter. All *USP–NF* chapters numbered under 1,000 are considered "applicable general chapters" and are enforceable, whereas chapters between 1000 and 1999 are intended to provide information on, give definition to, or describe a particular subject and are considered "informational general chapters."[17] In other words, the FDA can use USP Chapter <797> to determine whether CSPs have been contaminated, misbranded, or adulterated.[18]

Because the first edition of USP Chapter <797> resulted in hundreds of comments from professional organizations, healthcare institutions, and individual pharmacists, USP appointed a new committee of experts to review and improve USP Chapter <797>. This committee, the Sterile Compounding Committee (SCC), served from 2005 to 2010 and was composed of 12 persons representing pharmacy academia, institutional pharmacy, home care, microbiology, and controlled environments. Based on the USP standard development process, the SCC took more than 500 comments into consideration and published the revised USP Chapter <797> on December 3, 2007 as a revision bulletin. The chapter became official and enforceable on June 1, 2008, replacing the original USP Chapter <797> that had become official on January 1, 2004.[15]

The 2008 revision to USP Chapter <797> provided more extensive information and focused on personnel training, garbing, and cleaning. Sections were added on HDs (see USP Chapter <800> below), radiopharmaceuticals (see USP Chapter <825> below), and allergen extracts as CSPs. There were new sections on definitions, immediate-use CSPs, single-dose and multiple-dose containers, personnel training, competency and evaluation of garbing, aseptic work practices and cleaning/disinfection, elements of quality control, and abbreviations and acronyms. All previous sections were revised (eg, environmental sampling included microbial air and surface testing), and there were four new appendixes.[19]

In June 2019, USP published a revision to USP Chapter <797> that was to become official on December 1, 2019. This revision represented a significant change to the standard, including the removal of some provisions for extending beyond-use dates (BUDs) of CSPs, which had become common practice for some compounders. An appeal was filed with USP according to their bylaws, and hearings were held to review the appellants concerns.[20] In March 2020, the USP appeals panel found in favor of the appellants and remanded USP Chapter <797> back to the Compounding Expert Committee with the recommendation of further engagement of stakeholders in the revision process.[21;22]

After stakeholder feedback sessions, review and revisions, the Compounding Expert Committee of USP published a revised Chapter <797> in November 2022, with an official date of November 1, 2023.[16] This revision took into account the concerns of compounders raised during the appeal process. The most notable change was the addition of provisions to extend the BUDs of CSPs beyond the defaults given in the chapter. Chapter 16 provides more detail on BUDs as specified by USP Chapter <797>.

Responsibility of Compounding Personnel

USP Chapter <797> outlines 21 sections relevant to the safe compounding of sterile preparations that qualified licensed healthcare professionals who compound or supervise compounding and dispensing of CSPs must ensure.[16] The chapter sections are listed below.

1. Introduction and Scope
2. Personnel Training and Evaluation
3. Personal Hygiene and Garbing
4. Facilities and Engineering Controls
5. Certification and Recertification
6. Microbiological Air and Surface Monitoring
7. Cleaning, Disinfecting, and Applying Sporicidal Disinfectants
8. Introducing Items into the SEC and PEC
9. Equipment, Supplies, and Components
10. Sterilization and Depyrogenation
11. Master Formation and Compounding Records
12. Release Inspections and Testing
13. Labeling
14. Establishing Beyond-Use Dates
15. Use of Conventionally Manufactured Products as Components
16. Use of CSPs as Components

17. SOPs
18. Quality Assurance and Quality Control
19. CSP Handling, Storage, Packaging, Shipping, and Transport
20. Documentation
21. Compounding Allergenic Extracts

Each compounding facility must have one or more persons assigned to oversee compliance with the requirements of USP Chapter <797>. This person is called the "designated person," and they are responsible for the facility operation and are accountable for the performance of all compounding personnel preparing CSPs and performing other functions required by the chapter.[16]

USP Chapter <800> Hazardous Drugs—Handling in Healthcare Settings

Published in final form on February 1, 2016, USP Chapter <800> consolidates the requirements for healthcare personnel who handle HDs.[23] The purpose of USP Chapter <800> is to minimize exposure to HDs for patients, healthcare personnel, and the environment. USP Chapter <800> builds on standards established by the existing USP Chapter <795> and USP Chapter <797>, setting standards for HD containment in both nonsterile and sterile handling processes so as to minimize personnel exposure to HDs to a limit as low as reasonably achievable (ALARA). USP Chapter <800> incorporates standards from the Occupational Safety and Health Administration (OSHA), the National Institute for Occupational Safety and Health (NIOSH), and the American Society of Health-System Pharmacists (ASHP). The chapter includes standards for the receipt, storage, mixing, preparing, compounding, dispensing, administering, disposing, and otherwise altering, counting, crushing, or pouring of HDs. These standards apply to all personnel who handle HDs and to all places where HDs are prepared, stored, transported, and administered. The official date of USP Chapter <800> was December 1, 2019, however, because of the appeal to USP Chapter <797>, it became informational only on that date.[20] For USP Chapter <800> to become compendially applicable (enforceable) another official compounding chapter, in the case of sterile preparations USP Chapter <797>, was required to reference it. When the appeal to USP Chapter <797> was settled and the chapter became official, USP Chapter <800> also become official.

Sections within USP Chapter <800> include the following[23]:

1. List of HDs (see NIOSH below)
2. Types of Exposure
3. Responsibilities of Personnel Handling HDs
4. Facilities and Engineering Controls (Chapters 6 and 7)
5. Environmental Quality and Control
6. Personal Protective Equipment (Chapter 13)
7. Hazard Communication Program
8. Personnel Training
9. Receiving
10. Labeling, Packaging, Transport, and Disposal
11. Dispensing Final Dosage Forms
12. Compounding
13. Administering
14. Deactivating, Decontaminating, Cleaning, and Disinfecting (Chapter 14)
15. Spill Control
16. Documentation and Standard Operating Procedures
17. Medical Surveillance
18. Appendix 1: Acronyms and Definitions
19. Appendix 2: Examples of Design for HD Compounding Areas
20. Appendix 3: Types of Biological Safety Cabinets
21. References

More details on USP Chapter <800> are supplied in Chapter 27 and many other chapters in this book.

To ensure compliance with USP Chapter <800>, each entity must have a designated person who is qualified and trained to be responsible for developing and implementing appropriate procedures; overseeing entity compliance with this chapter and other applicable laws, regulations, and standards; ensuring competency of personnel; and ensuring environmental control of the storage and compounding areas. The designated person must thoroughly understand the rationale for risk-prevention policies, risks to themselves and others, risks of noncompliance that may compromise safety, and the responsibility to report potentially hazardous situations to the management team. The designated person must also be responsible for the oversight of monitoring the facility, maintaining reports of testing/sampling performed in facilities, and acting on the results.[23]

USP Chapter <825> Radiopharmaceuticals—Preparation, Compounding, Dispensing, and Repackaging

As the 2008 version of USP Chapter <797> was being revised, the decision was made to remove radiopharmaceuticals from the chapter and create a separate compounding chapter specifically for radiopharmaceuticals. This new standard was designated USP Chapter <825>. Since it is numbered less than 1000, the chapter is therefore compendially applicable and enforceable since it is cross-referenced by USP Chapter <797>. The new USP Chapter <825> was published in June 2019, with an official date of December 2019. Like the 2019 revision to USP Chapter <797>, it was appealed. However, the appeal was denied by the USP appeals panel and it was assigned a new official date of December 2020.[24] USP Chapter <825> provides standards for radiopharmaceutical compounding that take into account the unique requirements for handling radioactive materials (RAMs) as defined by the Nuclear Regulatory Commission (NRC) as well as the requirements for sterile and nonsterile compounding. The chapter is divided into the following sections[25]:

1. Introduction
2. Radiation Safety Considerations
3. Immediate Use of Sterile Radiopharmaceuticals
4. Personnel Qualifications, Training, and Hygiene
5. Facilities and Engineering Controls
6. Microbiological Air and Surface Monitoring
7. Cleaning and Disinfecting
8. Assessing BUD
9. Documentation
10. Preparation
11. Compounding
12. Dispensing
13. Repackaging
14. Quality Assurance and Quality Control

More details on USP Chapter <825> are provided in Chapter 25 of this book.

Other USP Chapters

The following are some of the other USP general chapters that relate to pharmacy compounding practice:

- General Notices
- <795> Pharmaceutical Compounding—Nonsterile Preparations
- <823> Positron Emission Tomography Drugs for Compounding, Investigational, and Research Uses
- <1151> Pharmaceutical Dosage Forms
- <1160> Pharmaceutical Calculations in Pharmacy Practice
- <1163> Quality Assurance in Pharmaceutical Compounding
- <1168> Compounding for Phase I Investigational Studies
- <1176> Prescription Balances and Volumetric Apparatus
- <1231> Water for Pharmaceutical Purposes
- <1265> Written Prescription Drug Information—Guidelines
- <7> Labeling
- <11> USP Reference Standards
- <17> Prescription Container Labeling
- <41> Balances
- <51> Antimicrobial Effectiveness Testing
- <71> Sterility Tests
- <85> Bacterial Endotoxins Test
- <381> Elastomeric Components in Injectable Pharmaceutical Product Packaging/Delivery Systems
- <659> Packaging and Storage Requirements
- <660> Containers—Glass
- <661> Plastic Packaging Systems and their Materials of Construction
- <661.1> Plastic Materials of Construction
- <661.2> Plastic Packaging Systems for Pharmaceutical Use
- <671> Containers—Performance Testing
- <731> Loss on Drying
- <785> Osmolality and Osmolarity
- <788> Particulate Matter in Injections
- <791> pH
- <821> Radioactivity
- <831> Refractive Index
- <852> Atomic Absorption Spectroscopy
- <853> Fluorescence Spectroscopy
- <854> Mid-Infrared Spectroscopy
- <857> Ultraviolet-Visible Spectroscopy
- <1066> Physical Environments That Promote Safe Medication Use
- <1072> Disinfectants and Antiseptics
- <1079> Risks and Mitigation Strategies for the Storage and Transportation of Finished Drug Products
- <1085> Guidelines on Endotoxins Test
- <1112> Application of Water Activity Determination to Nonsterile Pharmaceutical Products
- <1113> Microbial Characterization, Identification, and Strain Typing
- <1116> Microbiological Control and Monitoring of Aseptic Processing Environments
- <1178> Good Repackaging Practices
- <1191> Stability Considerations in Dispensing Practice
- <1197> Good Distribution Practices for Bulk Pharmaceutical Excipients
- <1207> Package Integrity Evaluation—Sterile Products

- <1223> Validation of Alternative Microbiological Methods
- <1228> Depyrogenation
- <1228.1> Dry Heat Depyrogenation
- <1228.3> Depyrogenation by Filtration
- <1228.4> Depyrogenation by Rinsing
- <1228.5> Endotoxin Indicators for Depyrogenation
- <1229.5> Biological Indicators for Sterilization
- <1229.9> Physicochemical Integrators and Indicators for Sterilization
- <1229.12> New Sterilization Methods
- <1229.13> Sterilization-in-Place
- <1229.14> Sterilization Cycle Development
- <1229.15> Sterilizing Filtration of Gasses
- <1251> Weighing on an Analytical Balance
- <1821> Radioactivity—Theory and Practice

Federal Regulations

U. S. Food and Drug Administration

Since 1990, the FDA has sent warning letters to pharmacies that manufacture, distribute, and promote unapproved drugs for human use outside the bounds of licensed pharmacy practice.[26] The U.S. Congress passed the Food and Drug Administration Modernization Act in 1997 (FDAMA) to clarify the roles of compounding pharmacies versus pharmaceutical manufacturers by adding Section 503A to the FD&C Act. Lawsuits resulted in the invalidation of Section 503A of the act, leaving uncertainty on roles of compounding pharmacies and for enforcement. The fungal meningitis tragedy brought large compounding operations into national headlines and caused the U.S. Congress to enact the Drug Quality and Security Act on November 27, 2013.[27]

Drug Quality and Security Act

The DQSA contains two titles. Title I covers drug compounding, and Title II relates to drug supply chain security. Title I creates a "safe harbor" for traditional pharmacy compounding pursuant to a specific patient prescription under Section 503A. The act leaves jurisdiction of traditional compounding to the states, thereby exempting this type of compounding from FDA regulations, such as current good manufacturing practices (CGMP), drug product labeling, and FDA approval prior to selling. DQSA applies to all pharmacies, although some medications are not covered under the act (eg, radiopharmaceuticals that are regulated by the Nuclear Regulatory Commission, investigational drugs, and veterinary compounds).

Health-system pharmacies and community pharmacies generally operate within the safe harbor of Section 503A as long as such operations include drug compounding allowed under 503A. DQSA defines what drugs can be compounded under Section 503A and the FDA has a guidance document that presents the agency's current thinking on the topic of compounding under 503A[28]:

1. The drug product is compounded for an identified individual patient based on the receipt of a valid prescription order, or a notation, approved by the prescribing practitioner, on the prescription order that a compounded product is necessary for the identified patient...
2. The compounding of the drug product is performed:
   - By a licensed pharmacist in a state licensed pharmacy or a federal facility, or by a licensed physician on the prescription order for an individual patient made by a licensed physician or other licensed practitioner authorized by state law to prescribe drugs.
   - By a licensed pharmacist or licensed physician in limited quantities before the receipt of a valid prescription order for such individual patient and:
     - is based on a history of the licensed pharmacist or licensed physician receiving valid prescription orders for the compounding of the human drug product.
     - those orders that been generated solely within an established relationship between the licensed pharmacist or licensed physician and either such patient for whom the prescription order will be provided or the physician or other licensed practitioner who will write the prescription order.
3. The drug product is compounded in compliance with the United States Pharmacopoeia (USP) chapters on pharmacy compounding using bulk drug substances, as defined in 21 CFR 207.3(a)(4), that comply with the standards of an applicable USP or National Formulary (NF) monograph, if one exists.

   If such a monograph does not exist, the drug substance(s) must be a component of an FDA-approved human drug product. If a monograph does not exist and the drug substance is not a component of an FDA-approved human drug product, it must appear on a list of bulk drug substances for use in compounding developed by FDA through regulation (section 503A(b)(1)(A)(i) of the FD&C Act)...
4. The drug product is compounded using bulk drug substances that are manufactured by an establishment that is registered under section 510 of the FD&C Act (including a foreign establishment that is registered under section 510(i) of the FD&C Act) (section 503A(b)(1)(A)(ii) of the FD&C Act).
5. The drug product is compounded using bulk drug substances that are accompanied by valid certificates of analysis for each bulk drug substance (section 503A(b)(1)(A)(iii) of the FD&C Act).

6. The drug product is compounded using ingredients (other than bulk drug substances) that comply with the standards of an applicable USP or NF monograph, if one exists, and the USP chapters on pharmacy compounding (section 503A(b)(1)(B) of the FD&C Act).
7. The drug product does not appear on the list, published at 21 CFR 216.24, that includes drug products that have been withdrawn or removed from the market because such drug products or components of such drug products have been found to be unsafe or not effective (section 503A(b)(1)(C) of the FD&C Act)...
8. The licensed pharmacist or licensed physician does not compound regularly or in inordinate amounts any drug products that are essentially copies of commercially available drug products (section 503A(b)(1)(D) of the FD&C Act).
9. The drug product is not a drug product identified by FDA by regulation as a drug product that presents demonstrable difficulties for compounding that reasonably demonstrate an adverse effect on the safety or effectiveness of that drug product (section 503A(b)(3)(A) of the FD&C Act)...
10. The drug product is compounded in a state that has entered into a memorandum of understanding (MOU) with FDA that addresses the distribution of inordinate amounts of compounded drug products interstate and provides for appropriate investigation by a state agency of complaints relating to compounded drug products distributed outside such state; or, in states that have not entered into such an MOU with FDA, the licensed pharmacist, licensed pharmacy, or licensed physician does not distribute, or cause to be distributed, compounded drug products out of the state in which they are compounded, more than 5% of the total prescription orders dispensed or distributed by such pharmacy or physician (sections 503A(b)(3)(B)(i) & (ii) of the FD&C Act)...[28]

Under 503A, compounding does not include mixing, reconstituting, or other acts necessary in following the directions on a manufacturer's label.[29]

Title I also gives compounding pharmacies the option of registering with the FDA as outsourcing facilities governed under section 503B (see Chapter 34).[30] An FDA-registered outsourcing facility must adhere to CGMP, but they do not need to receive FDA approval for their compounded products prior to marketing and can qualify for exemptions regarding labeling products with adequate directions for use. In addition, outsourcing facilities must adhere to the following:

- They are not required to be state-licensed pharmacies.
- They must compound under the supervision of a licensed pharmacist or physician.
- They may or may not obtain patient-specific prescriptions.
- They may only use drugs from a bulk ingredients list.
- They are not allowed to compound products already commercially available unless the products are in short market supply.
- They must undergo regular FDA inspections on a risk-based schedule.
- They must submit information about products compounded within the facility to the FDA every 6 months.
- They must report product-related adverse events to the FDA.
- They must pay an annual fee of $15,000 (to increase annually with inflation; $17,823 in FY23)[31] to the FDA to cover inspection costs.[32]

Pharmacy compounders that choose not to register with the FDA as an outsourcing facility and who are not traditional compounders under 503A are subject to the same requirements as conventional manufacturers under the FD&C Act (eg, new drug approval, adequate directions for use, and CGMP requirements).[33] When a 503A compounding pharmacy cannot prepare a CSP, the FDA encourages healthcare systems and providers to buy compounded medications from registered outsourcing facilities.[33] The FDA provides a regularly updated list of registered outsourcing facilities.[34]

In consultation with the National Association of Boards of Pharmacy (NABP), the secretary of the U.S. Department of Health and Human Services (HHS) is required to receive information from state boards of pharmacy about compounding pharmacies and outsourcing facilities. This information can include descriptions of actions they have taken against these entities, such as imposing sanctions or penalties, suspending or revoking a pharmacy license or registration, or the recall of a compounded drug. A state board of pharmacy can also submit any concerns to HHS about a compounding pharmacy that might be acting contrary to Section 503A. The secretary of HHS is required to notify all state boards of pharmacy when information is received from a state board regarding actions taken against a compounding pharmacy or when the secretary determines a pharmacy is acting contrary to Section 503A.[30]

The secretary of HHS convened with the Advisory Committee on Compounding to issue regulations that identify the drugs that are demonstrably difficult to compound and are likely to lead to adverse effects.[35] Pharmacists can compound substances unlikely to be on the bulk drug substances list by submitting treatment investigational new drug (IND) applications. With a standing treatment IND, individual healthcare providers will not have to pursue the approval of an institutional review board before having a patient use the drug.[36]

To enforce its inspections and actions, the FDA may issue warning letters, seize products, obtain court injunctions against pharmacies, and support criminal prosecutions for compounding violations. Although compounding performed by health-system pharmacies is not changed under DQSA, regional compounding centers operated by a health system are in a gray area and could fall under 503A or 503B. Drug products compounded in accordance with 503A are exempt from certain requirements in the FD&C Act, as described above. However, the products remain subject to all other provisions of the FD&C Act that apply to conventional drug manufacturers, including but not limited to the prohibition of preparing, packing, or holding drugs under insanitary conditions.[37] In 2020, the FDA released a final guidance on insanitary conditions at compounding facilities that are subject to regulatory action for 503A facilities.[38] This guidance offers insight on the conditions that cause a compounded drug to be considered adulterated in violation of the FD&C Act and the corrective actions that should be taken if these conditions are found.

Since pharmacies located within a hospital or standalone pharmacies that are part of a health system frequently provide compounded drug products for administration within the hospital or health system, the FDA has also provided guidance (draft at the time of this writing) on hospital and health-system compounding under 503A.[39] This draft guidance addresses the prescription requirement within health systems as well as compounding drug products that are essentially copies of a commercial drug product.

ENFORCEMENT AGENCIES

State Boards of Pharmacy

As of February 2018, 32 states require direct compliance with USP Chapter <797> Pharmaceutical Compounding—Sterile Preparations, while another 11 states have compounding regulations although they do not directly refer to USP Chapter <797>.[40] These numbers are up from a 2015 study which only showed 26 states requiring compliance with USP Chapter <797>.[40] Compliance with this chapter was a strong focus in 75% of the most recent state board inspections.[10]

As accreditation and regulatory bodies have become more familiar with inspecting for sterile compounding, use of personal protective equipment (PPE), hand hygiene, and aseptic technique observations are virtually guaranteed in any visit. More focus is being placed on documentation within the sterile compounding areas and personnel. Examples of the types of documentation being inspected include engineering control certification reports, environmental monitoring logs, cleaning logs, and competency documentation.[10] Moreover, inspectors are reviewing the documentation in much more detail than done previously, sometimes with inspection checklists that are shared in advance.[10]

National Association of Boards of Pharmacy

Founded in 1904, NABP is an impartial professional organization that supports the state boards of pharmacy in protecting public health. NABP's member boards of pharmacy are grouped into eight districts that include all 50 United States, the District of Columbia, Guam, Puerto Rico, the Virgin Islands, ten Canadian provinces, and the Bahama Islands.[41] Because the 50 state boards of pharmacy and the District of Columbia are members of the NABP, the NABP has much influence on the rules and regulations that the respective state boards create. The NABP has long held that prescription compounding is a pharmacist's responsibility and should be regulated by state boards of pharmacy.[42] As mentioned previously in the chapter, NABP is recognized as having a consulting role in the DQSA. To distinguish between compounding and manufacturing, NABP defines these terms in its Model State Pharmacy Practice Act:

> "Compounding" means the preparation, mixing, assembling, altering, packaging, and Labeling of a Drug, Drug-Delivery Device, or Device in accordance with a Licensed Practitioner's Prescription Drug Order, Medical Order, or initiative based on the Practitioner/patient/Pharmacist/compounder relationship in the course of professional practice. Compounding includes the following:
>
> 1. preparation of Drug dosage forms for both human and animal patients;
> 2. preparation of Drugs or Devices in anticipation of Prescription Drug Orders based on routine, regularly observed prescribing patterns; and
> 3. manipulation of commercial Products for patient-specific needs beyond FDA-approved Labeling.
>
> "Manufacturing" means the production, preparation, propagation, conversion, or processing of a Drug or Device, either directly or indirectly, by extraction from substances of natural origin or independently by means of chemical or biological synthesis. Manufacturing includes the packaging or repackaging of a Drug or Device or the labeling or relabeling of the container of a Drug or Device for resale by pharmacies, Practitioners, or other Persons.[43]

Although NABP strives for uniformity in state board of pharmacy regulations, the boards themselves run the gamut of oversight of sterile compounding. In 2018, Pew Charitable Trusts repeated a survey first conducted in 2015 to assess the national landscape of state policies on compounding sterile drugs.[40] Authors of the study used public websites and developed a questionnaire sent to all 50 states and the District of Columbia. Forty-three of the state and the District of Columbia boards of pharmacy responded to the survey. Alarming inconsistencies surfaced among state policies.

- Only 62% of states required full compliance with USP Chapter <797>.

- Only 47% required pharmacies that ship or dispense compounded drugs into their state for patients or healthcare providers to comply with their own state's sterile compounding standards.
- Twenty-two percent allowed pharmacies to compound without patient-specific prescriptions for office stock (in conflict with the DQSA).
- Nearly 75% required licensing or registration for 503B outsourcing facilities.
- Only 43% conducted annual inspections of traditional pharmacies that perform sterile compounding, which is less frequent than in 2015.

In understating the matter, the authors of the study concluded, "The significant progress in adopting USP Chapter <797> quality standards and aligning with federal law on compounding without prescriptions suggests a key opportunity for jurisdictions that have not yet adopted these best practices. Improvements in rigor and frequency of inspection of facilities that perform sterile compounding will require resources, but interim measures such as harmonizing inspection forms and processes among states may allow for optimal use of existing capacity and enhance efficiencies."[40]

Accrediting Agencies for Healthcare Organizations

Via the Social Security Act, hospitals accredited by CMS-approved agencies must meet CMS Conditions of Participation (CoP) to serve Medicare and Medicaid patients and thereby receive reimbursement for those services.[44] Four accrediting bodies (ie, with deeming authority) accredit hospitals for participation in Medicare and Medicaid services: The Joint Commission (TJC), the Accreditation Commission for Health Care (ACHC), Det Norske Veritas Healthcare (DNV), and the Center for Improvement in Healthcare Quality (CIHQ).[45] TJC accredits the majority of accredited hospitals, critical access hospitals, and ambulatory surgery centers. Few U.S. hospitals can afford not to be accredited because of the large number of Medicare and Medicaid patients.

According to a 2022 survey of hospital pharmacists, 77% of the accreditation surveys resulted in no findings or actions taken against hospital pharmacy sterile compounders. However, surveyors did make recommendations for improvements in sterile compounding in 14% of surveys and issued citations in 9% of surveys.[10]

All four accreditation agencies survey for details contained in USP Chapter <797> and USP Chapter <800>. In January 2015, the Office of the Inspector General made two recommendations to CMS[46]:

- Ensure that hospital surveyors receive training on standards from nationally recognized organizations related to safe compounding practices.
- Amend its interpretive guidelines to address hospital contracts with standalone compounding pharmacies.

Centers for Medicare & Medicaid Services

Following the Office of Inspector General (OIG) recommendations in an October 15, 2015, memorandum to state survey agency directors, the CMS Director of Survey and Certification Group stated the following:

> ***Pharmaceutical Services***: Revisions were made to portions of the pharmaceutical services CoP to bring them into alignment with current accepted standards of practice. To improve clarity, the revised guidance addresses: accepted professional pharmacy principles, including United States Pharmacopeia (USP) standards; compounding of medications, particularly compounded sterile preparations (CSPs); determining beyond-use dates (BUDs); safe and appropriate storage and use of medications; and, policies and procedures related to high-alert medications and minimizing drug errors.[47]

The OIG further "clarified that a hospital must have pharmaceutical services administered in accordance with accepted professional principles, such as those found in the U.S. Pharmacopeia/National Formulary (USP/NF)... We have expanded our hospital guidance on the requirements for compounding of medications, particular for CSPs."[47] To confirm that deeming agencies are performing effectively, state agencies conduct surveys following the guidance outlined in the interpretive guidelines maintained by CMS.[48] Based on the 2022 State of Pharmacy Compounding survey, state boards of pharmacy and accreditation agencies are inspecting for sterile compounding compliance with USP Chapter <797> at a significantly higher rate (75%) than CMS inspectors are (18%).[10] This suggests that the changes recommended by OIG in 2015 have improved enforcement of sterile compounding standards in hospital inspections.

The Joint Commission

As an independent, not-for-profit organization, TJC accredits and certifies more than 23,000 U.S. healthcare organizations and programs. TJC accreditation and certification is recognized nationwide as an organization's commitment to meeting certain quality performance standards.[49] See **Table 2-1** for a description of sterile compounding locations that TJC often accredits.

TJC expects organizations to comply with USP Chapter <797> and will survey for compliance with provisions of USP Chapter <797> that overlap with their standards, including those in the 2016 Hospital Accreditation Manual (medication management, infection control, environment of care, human resources, provision of care, treatment and services leadership, and performance improvement).[50] See **Table 2-2** for a list of USP Chapter <797> requirements.

Accreditation Commission for Health Care

The ACHC is a nationally recognized accreditation organization with deeming authority from CMS. It was formed with the merger of the Healthcare Facilities Accreditation Program

TABLE 2-1. The Joint Commission: Accredited Healthcare Sites with Operations (eg, pharmacies) That Compound Sterile Preparations

Ambulatory Care	Critical Access Hospitals	Home Care	Hospitals
Ambulatory centers	Definition: Maintains no more than 25 total beds; keeps patients hospitalized no longer than 96 hours; receives critical access designation by a state agency	Home health	General hospitals
Outpatient surgery centers		Hospice	Children's hospitals
Physician office-based surgery		Personal care	Long-term acute care
Imaging centers		Infusion pharmacy	Oncology hospitals
Urgent care centers		Specialty compounding pharmacy	Psychiatric hospitals Rehabilitation hospitals Specialty hospitals (eg, cardiac, orthopedic, surgical)

(HFAP) and the Accreditation Association for Hospitals/Health Systems (AAHHS).[51] Their mission is to advance high quality patient care and safety through objective application of recognized standards. The ACHC follows CMS guidance. In April 2016, HFAP (now ACHC) approved several accreditation standards that directly affect the compounding of sterile preparations in hospitals.[52] The most recent version of the ACHC standards should be consulted to identify areas where sterile compounding will be surveyed.

Center for Improvement in Healthcare Quality

Serving healthcare organizations since 1999, the CIHQ is a member-based organization comprised of hospitals and other healthcare entities throughout the United States.[53] CIHQ is a CMS-approved deeming authority for acute care hospitals.[45] Their accreditation program is designed to ensure that hospitals comply with Medicare CoP and improve the quality of care, treatment, and service in their communities. CIHQ accreditation is awarded to an organization for a maximum of 36 months. CIHQ has medication management standards very similar to those of TJC. In the 2023 standards, sterile compounding is explicitly mentioned in standards CE-11: Ventilation, Lighting & Temperature Control, MM-1: Establishment of a Pharmacy Service, MM-24: Preparation of Medications, and MM-26: Labeling of Medications.[54]

Det Norkse Veritas Healthcare

A merger between DNV and Germanischer Lloyd (GL) was cleared by international competition authorities, and the new company DNV GL Healthcare became operational on September 12, 2013. In March 2021, DNV GL was renamed to DNV.[55] In 2008, DNV received CMS deeming authority, and since then it has accredited over 550 hospitals of all sizes in every region of the United States and is the second largest of the four accrediting bodies with deeming authority.[56] DNV melds the healthcare accreditation survey process with a gradual compliance with the International Organization for Standardization (ISO) 9001 standard, which is the international standard for quality management systems. DNV accreditation requires an annual survey and the organization's continual compliance with the DNV accreditation process.

DNV accreditation standards cover the following key aspects of organizational governance and clinical care.

- Quality management system and governance
- Proactive risk management
- Higher risk services, such as anesthesia, obstetrics, and ER
- Medication management
- Patient rights
- Physical environment
- Accreditation standards developed for the following types of healthcare organizations:
    - Hospitals
    - Primary care providers
    - Specialist outpatient clinics

DNV surveyors have a healthcare background, and they specialize in one of three areas: management systems, clinical care, or physical environment.[57]

TABLE 2-2. USP Chapter <797> Crosswalk with The Joint Commission 2023 Standards

USP Chapter <797> Requirements	TJC 2023 Hospital Standards and National Patient Safety Goals
Adequate training of personnel	HR.01.04.01 and HR. 01.05.03
ADR and error reporting	MM.07.01.03
Air quality and environmental monitoring of sterile compounding area	EC.02.04.01 and EC.02.04.03
Beyond-use dating	MM.05.01.09
Cleaning and disinfecting of sterile compounding area	IC.02.02.01
Competence assessment	HR.01.06.01 and HR.01.07.01
Construction and renovation	EC.02.06.05
Contaminants	EC.02.05.01 and MM.05.01.07
Emergency power/critical equipment	EC.02.05.01 and EC.02.05.03
Environmental design of the sterile compounding area	MM.05.01.07
Equipment testing and maintenance	EC.02.04.01 and EC.02.04.03
Facilities Space and equipment ISO 5 compliance	 LD.04.01.11 and EC.02.05.01 MM.05.01.07
Hand hygiene	IC.01.04.01 and NPSG.07.01.01
Hazardous drugs	EC. 02.02.01, EC.04.01.01 and MM.01.01.03
High-alert medications	MM.01.01.03
Infection prevention and control	IC.01.05.01
Look-alike and sound-alike medications	MM.01.02.01
Labels	MM.05.01.09 and NPSG.03.04.01
Patient education	PC.02.03.01
Patient monitoring	MM.05.01.01
Patient's own medications	MM.03.01.05
Quality assurance and performance improvement Responsibility for safe and quality care Evaluates effectiveness of system Monitors performance Compiles and analyzes data Improves performance	 LD.01.03.01 MM.08.01.01 PI.01.01.01 PI.02.01.01 PI.03.01.01
Radiopharmaceuticals	MM.05.01.07
Recalls	MM.05.01.17
Redispensing preparations	MM.05.01.19
Regulation and compliance with laws	LD.04.01.01 and MM.05.01.11
Supplies (garb, disposables, etc.)	IC.01.02.01
Temperature testing and documentation	EC.02.05.03 and MM.03.01.01

ISO = International Organization for Standardization.

Source: Adapted with permission of Uselton JP, Kienle PC, Murdaugh LB. United States Pharmacopeia (USP) Compounding Standards: Chapters <795>, <797>, <800>, and <825>. In: *Meeting Accreditation Standards: a pharmacy preparation guide.* Bethesda, MD: ASHP; 2019:313-25.

Accrediting Agencies for Standalone Compounding Pharmacies

Three agencies accredit and provide certifications to pharmacies that are not a part of a hospital or health system (ie, independent or standalone compounding pharmacies). Many pharmacies seek these accreditations and certifications on a voluntary basis. Some examples of these pharmacies are home infusion pharmacies, large or small outsourcing facilities, specialty compounding pharmacies, community compounding pharmacies, and other types of pharmacies that compound and dispense based on an individual patient prescription or on wholesale orders from other healthcare entities. Each standalone pharmacy accrediting agency has distinct standards and methods of survey. The most recently established and most powerful of these surveyors is the FDA.

Accreditation Commission for Health Care

Preceding its merger with HFAP when acute care standards were added, the ACHC was a national organization developed by home care and alternate-site healthcare providers to establish a standard of care for those types of facilities. It is uniquely concerned with healthcare providers from a wide array of practicing locations, and it focuses on helping them deliver optimum care for their patients. ACHC specializes in accrediting not just pharmacies but also home health (Medicare-certified), community retail pharmacies, hospice, durable medical equipment, prosthetics, orthotics and supplies, private duty nurses (non-Medicare certified), sleep labs, and behavioral health organizations. ACHC collaborates with industry experts to create standards to ensure that quality is maintained throughout all aspects of the organization.

Onsite surveys are conducted every 3 years by healthcare experts. A comprehensive review is conducted of organizational structure, policies and procedures, compliance with federal/state/local laws, leadership, patient rights and responsibilities, fiscal operations, human resource management, provision of care, patient records, quality outcomes, performance improvement, infection control, and patient and employee safety. At the time of survey, organizations demonstrate how they have maintained continuous compliance with ACHC's standards for accreditation.[58]

ACHC is a recognized leader in the area of pharmacy accreditation. ACHC pharmacy surveyors are licensed pharmacists who draw on relevant experience to provide a comprehensive assessment of an organization and offer helpful, consultative advice. ACHC accredits pharmacies that dispense medications pursuant to a prescription order for an individually identified patient for the following pharmacy services[58]:

- *Infusion pharmacy*: The infusion pharmacy continuum of care includes intravenous (IV) drug admixture preparation, IV administration, therapy monitoring, and client/patient counseling and education. It is the administration of medications using IV, subcutaneous, and epidural routes. Accreditation for sterile compounding includes compliance with USP Chapter <797>.
- *Ambulatory infusion center (AIC)*: An AIC is a centralized location where a patient can receive infusion therapy administered by appropriate clinical personnel.
- *Specialty pharmacy*: A specialty pharmacy dispenses medications (injectable, IV, or oral) in a client or patient's home, physician's office, or clinic specializing in certain disease states. These medications target a specific population with a chronic and sometimes life-threatening disease. Specialty pharmacy includes disease-specific clinical monitoring as well as patient compliance and adherence programs.
- *Long-term care pharmacy*: Long-term care pharmacy is the management of medications for residents of institutional facilities to ensure proper drug therapy as well as packaging and delivery of medications.

Pharmacy Compounding Accreditation Board

The Pharmacy Compounding Accreditation Board (PCAB) is a voluntary accrediting organization founded in 2004. PCAB was formed by eight national pharmacy organizations, including USP, to serve as a voluntary accrediting body for the practice of pharmacy compounding. This type of accreditation is suitable for a smaller compounding pharmacy that is not part of a large health system or outsourcing facility. Beginning July 1, 2014, PCAB became a service of ACHC.

ACHC administers PCAB accreditation for nonsterile and sterile pharmacy compounding. PCAB accreditation assesses the compounding process based on a specific set of standards that concentrate on the quality and consistency of medications produced. The ACHC and PCAB describe the presurvey process, the onsite process, the postsurvey process, standards, and informational resources.[59]

The Joint Commission Medication Compounding Certification Program

In early 2017, TJC announced the development of a new medication compounding certification program. The certification is open to all compounding pharmacies operating or shipping to states with regulations that require compliance with USP Chapters <795> and/or <797>. The certification program is awarded for a two-year period and is designed to help organizations[60]:

- Reduce risk and harm
- Ensure USP standard compliance related to the process, testing, and verification of compounded sterile and nonsterile preparations

- Find and fix gaps in policies and procedures, focusing on the following:
    - People: training, competency, proper use of PPE, and aseptic technique
    - Product: sterility of base products, expiration dates, and labeling
    - Environment: airflow, buffer areas, guidelines for cleaning and documentation, and storage
- Demonstrate excellence through complying with both TJC and USP standards

It is unclear whether many standalone sterile compounding pharmacies will seek TJC certification, however those pharmacies performing in Michigan must have some certification, such as that from TJC.[61]

Occupational Safety and Health Administration

The Occupational Safety and Health Act of 1970 created both NIOSH and OSHA. Under the U.S. Department of Labor, OSHA has authority to go into workplaces, inspect worksite conditions, cite employers found in violation of agency standards, and levy fines. Under the General Duty Clause, OSHA may cite employers for "recognized hazards that are causing or are likely to cause death or serious physical harm."[62] Specific OSHA standards of concern to healthcare organizations include PPE, blood-borne pathogens, hazard communication, ergonomics, and others. OSHA has identified worker exposure to HDs as a problem of increasing health concern.[63]

Highlights of OSHA standards and standard interpretations include the following:

- 29 CFR 1910.1020[64] is the standard that allows for access to employee exposure and medical records. OSHA requires the reporting of employee exposure to hazardous medications and allows employees access to these records.
- 29 CFR 1910.1200[65] is the standard for hazard communication, which requires any drugs posing a health hazard, with the exception of those in solid, final form for direct administration to the patient (eg, tablets or pills) to be included on lists of hazardous chemicals to which employees are exposed. In compliance with this standard, all personnel involved in any aspect of the handling of covered hazardous medications must receive information and training to apprise them for hazards in the work area.
- Safety Data Sheets (SDS), previously known as Material Safety Data Sheets (MSDS), must be provided to employees who package and process drugs for distribution into final form if they contain hazardous chemicals.[66]
- An OSHA standard interpretation for the hazard communication standard and pharmaceuticals explains that the pharmaceutical manufacturer and the importer have the primary duty for the evaluation of chemical hazards, and that the employer may rely on the hazard determination performed by the pharmaceutical manufacturer or importer.[67]
- OSHA standard interpretation letter for the hazard communication standard clarifies that an SDS is required and must be mainained by the employer for drugs which are determined to be hazardous by the manufacturer.[68]

OSHA standards for storing, handling, preparation, administration, and disposal of HDs are covered in Chapter 27.

Centers for Disease Control and Prevention's NIOSH Alert

NIOSH, a part of the CDC, is an agency that was established to help ensure safe and healthful working conditions for workers by providing research, information, education, and training in the field of occupational safety and health. In September 2004, NIOSH published an alert entitled "Preventing Occupational Exposures to Antineoplastic and Other Hazardous Drugs in Health Care Settings."[69]

The purpose of this alert is to increase awareness among healthcare workers and their employers about the health risks posed by working with HDs and to provide them with measures for protecting their health. Healthcare workers who prepare or administer HDs or who work in areas where these drugs are used may be exposed to these agents in the air, on work surfaces, contaminated clothing, medical equipment, patient excreta, and other surfaces. The health risk is influenced by the extent of the exposure and the potency and toxicity of the HD. This alert applies to all workers who handle HDs (eg, pharmacy and nursing personnel, physicians, operating room personnel, environmental services workers, workers in research laboratories, veterinary care workers, and shipping and receiving personnel). Under USP Chapter <800>, the NIOSH list of HDs becomes a minimum standard, so a healthcare organization must include all items on this list on its own list (provided that the use of the HD is allowed at the organization). NIOSH updates the list typically every 2 years based on new drugs that come to market and comments from stakeholders. As of this writing, the list from September 2016 is the most recent.[70]

This NIOSH list is sorted into three different HD groups, which includes antineoplastics, non-antineoplastic HDs, and reproductive hazardous medications. The list also provides links that detail why the drug is included on the list. A draft list was released in 2018 and again in 2020, but it was never finalized by NIOSH. The 2020 list proposed a different structure than the 2016 list, with only two tables.[71] Healthcare facilities should consider the officially approved

NIOSH HD list when creating their own facility-specific HD list. Each pharmacy needs to prepare itself by identifying which of the drugs on the list they handle. USP Chapter <800> makes the NIOSH Alert and HD list enforceable by incorporating parts of the alert into the chapter itself. The handling, preparation, administration, and disposal of HDs are covered in Chapter 27.

American Society of Health-System Pharmacists

ASHP is the national professional association that represents pharmacists and pharmacy technicians who practice in hospitals, health maintenance organizations, long-term care facilities, home care, and other components of healthcare systems. ASHP has continually promoted appropriate pharmacy compounding in the institutional setting since the 1940s. ASHP developed a practice standard for the quality assurance of pharmacy CSPs. First published in 1993 as a technical assistance bulletin, this standard was updated and republished in 2000.[72] This guideline has been superseded by USP Chapter <797>, which is an enforceable sterile compounding standard.

Guidelines

To harmonize with USP Chapter <797>, ASHP updated its guidelines on compounding sterile preparations in 2014.[73] ASHP also published a technical assistance bulletin on compounding ophthalmic preparations and guidelines on the safe use of automated compounding devices for compounding of parenteral nutrition admixtures.[74;75] In a follow-up to the NIOSH Alert, ASHP published guidelines on handling hazardous drugs.[76] In response to the DQSA and the FDA's desire for health systems to utilize 503B, which describes outsourcing facilities for sterile products that cannot be compounded by the health system, ASHP created guidelines on outsourcing sterile compounding services.[77] Additional detail on the outsourcing of CSPs can be found in Chapter 34.

ASHP Accreditation of Pharmacy Residency Programs

The ASHP accreditation standard for postgraduate year 1 and 2 (PGY1 and PGY2) pharmacy residency programs says that pharmacies where residents are trained must meet high standards. These standards include the following[78]:

> 5.2.b Medication-use policies reflect current best practices and guidelines and include but are not limited to
>
> > 5.2.b.1 Management of secure storage for all medications
> >
> > 5.2.b.2 Identification, storage and labeling of high risk/high alert medications
> >
> > 5.2.b.3 Management of medications that have specific regulatory, compliance, or reporting requirements
> >
> > 5.2.b.4 Management of medications in automated systems
> >
> > 5.2.b.5 Management of hazardous medications
> >
> > 5.2.b.6 Procedures to ensure that all medications are dispensed in a ready-to-administer dose
> >
> > 5.2.b.7 Management of pharmaceutical waste

ASHP residency accreditation surveyors inspect pharmacy and other practice setting facilities for compliance with national standards of practice, such as USP Chapter <797> and USP Chapter <800>.

ASHP Accreditation of Pharmacy Technician Training Programs

The ASHP Accreditation Standard for Pharmacy Technician Training programs includes standards that pertain to sterile compounding.[79]

> 5.1 Describes and applies state and federal laws pertaining to processing, handling, and dispensing of medications, including controlled substances.
>
> 5.5 Describes pharmacy compliance with professional standards and relevant legal, regulatory, formulary, contractual, and safety requirements.
>
> 5.6 Describes OSHA, NIOSH, and USP requirements for prevention and treatment of exposure to hazardous substances (eg, risk assessment, PPE, eyewash, spill kit).
>
> 10.4 Experiential training sites are recognized by an organization(s) appropriate to the practice setting (eg, licensed by the State Board of Pharmacy).

Where the state board of pharmacy requires full or partial compliance with USP Chapter <797> and USP Chapter <800>, these standards become a requirement for ASHP-accredited pharmacy technician training programs in those states.

ASHP Resources on Sterile Compounding

The ASHP website has a compilation of tools and resources to help pharmacists ensure the quality of CSPs.[80]

Miscellaneous Organizations and Agencies

American Society for Parenteral and Enteral Nutrition Guidelines for Parenteral Nutrition

Recognizing the importance of safe practices associated with these preparations, the American Society for Parenteral and Enteral Nutrition (ASPEN) publishes their guidelines. They are organized under 12 questions that include background evidence to support specific recommendations.[81]

A few of the questions touch on sterile compounding. For example, question 12 answers the question, "What beyond-use date should be used for (a) intravenous fat emulsion (IVFE) dispensed for separate infusion in the original container and (b) repackaged IVFE?"

American Society for Testing and Materials

American Society for Testing and Materials International (ASTM) is a globally recognized leader in developing voluntary consensus standards. ASTM standards are used to improve product quality, enhance health and safety, strengthen market access and trade, and build consumer confidence. Through more than 140 technical standard writing committees, ASTM serves a broad range of industries, inluding metals, construction, petroleum, consumer products, and many more.[82]

According to USP Chapter <800>, when chemotherapy gloves are required, they must meet ASTM Standard D6978 (or its successor).[23] Chemotherapy gloves should be worn for handling all HDs, including nonantineoplastics, and for reproductive risk only HDs. Chemotherapy gloves must be powder-free because powder can contaminate the work area and can adsorb and retain HDs. When used for sterile compounding, the outer chemotherapy gloves must be sterile (see Chapter 27).

In February 2023, ASTM released standard F3267 Standard Specification for Protective Clothing for Use Against Liquid Chemotherapy and Other Liquid Hazardous Drugs. This standard covers the design, performance, documentation, and labeling requirements and provides test methods for protective clothing used in preventing exposure to liquid chemotherapy and other liquid hazardous drugs.[83] While not required by USP Chapter <800>, it is important that chemotherapy gowns used in the handling of HDs conform to this new standard.

Controlled Environment Testing Association

The Controlled Environment Testing Association (CETA) is devoted to promoting and developing quality assurance within the controlled environment testing industry. The 2008 version of USP Chapter <797> made specified CETA guidelines enforceable by inclusion. While the most recent revision to USP Chapter <797> removed any reference to CETA explicitly, its guidelines are important for sterile compounding nonetheless.[16] CETA guidelines related to sterile compounding and HDs include the following:

- CAG-001-2008: Applications Guide for the Use of Compounding Aseptic Isolators in Compounding Sterile Preparations in Healthcare Facilities (revised December 2008)
- CAG-002-2008: Compounding Isolator Testing Guide (revised December 2008)
- CAG-003-2022: Certification of Sterile Compounding Facilities for USP Compliance (revised October 2022)
- CAG-004-2020: Biological Decontamination and Disinfection of Accessible Surfaces in Biosafety Cabinets (revised September 2020)
- CAG-005-2007: Servicing Hazardous Drug Compounding Primary Engineering Controls (revised 2007)
- CAG-006-2010: CETA High Efficiency Filter Application Guide (revised February 2010)
- CAG-007-2020: Exhaust System Requirements of Class II Biosafety Cabinets (revised September 2020)
- CAG-008-2022: Certification Matrix for Sterile & Nonsterile USP Compounding Facilities (revised March 2022)
- CAG-009-2020: Viable Environmental Monitoring for Sterile Compounding Facilities (revised September 2020)
- CAG-010-2011: CETA Application Guide for Informational Notes to Meet the NSF/ANSI 49:2010a Standard Requirements (revised July 2011)
- CAG-011-2021: Gloved Fingertip Testing for Sterile Compounding Personnel (revised February 2021)
- CAG-013-2021: Media Fill Testing for Sterile Compounding Personnel (revised August 2021)
- CAG-014-2022: Airflow Visualization Study (revised April 2022)

As of January 2012, CETA application guides are available to CETA members as a free download. Nonmembers may access the guides for a nominal fee. CETA has a national board of testing for cleanroom certification professionals.[84]

Environmental Protection Agency

The U.S. Environmental Protection Agency (EPA) regulates the disposal of hazardous wastes under the Resource Conservation and Recovery Act (RCRA) of 1977.[85] In 2019, a final rule titled Management Standards for Hazardous Waste Pharmaceuticals and Amendment to the P075 Listing for Nicotine was published by the EPA. This rule contains three sections, with Part 266 Subpart P including many of the key changes that affect sterile compounding. This section of the rule is considered more stringent than the previous RCRA regulations. As a result, states must adopt these new regulations. Hazardous waste pharmaceuticals must be managed in accordance with this section by all healthcare facilities except for very small quantity generators that may opt out using a conditional exemption.[86] See Chapters 19 and 27 for a full discussion of the strong implications of this act for virtually all health-system pharmacies.

Institute for Environmental Sciences and Technology

The Institute for Environmental Sciences and Technology (IEST), founded in 1953, is a multidisciplinary international society whose members are recognized for their contributions to the environmental sciences in the areas of contamination control in electronics manufacturing and pharmaceutical processes; design, test, and evaluation of commercial and military equipment; and product reliability issues associated with commercial and military systems.[87] IEST has recommended practices for cleanroom design and compliance with USP Chapter <797> (see Chapter 7).[88]

Institute for Safe Medication Practices

The Institute for Safe Medication Practices (ISMP) is a nonprofit organization that aims to educate the healthcare community and consumers about safe medication practices. In 2013, ISMP published guidelines for the safe preparation of CSPs. Experts developed these guidelines to provide procedures and safe practices for reducing errors in CSP preparation.[89] The guidelines address drug storage, compounding, product labeling, and staff management. CMS specifically cites the ISMP guidelines for review by accredited health systems and pharmacies.[46] These guidelines were revised in 2022 and retitled Guidelines for Sterile Compounding and the Safe Use of Sterile Compounding Technology to place emphasis on the role of technology in safe sterile compounding.[90] In the 2016-2017 release, ISMP published targeted medication safety best practices for hospitals that included sterile compounding. This best practice has remained on the ISMP targeted best practice list since that time, and it is most recently included on the 2022-2023 list.[91] **Table 2-3** illustrates a best practice to improve sterile compounding accuracy along with its rationale.

International Organization for Standardization

The (ISO) is a nongovernmental organization (ie, its members are not delegations of national governments). ISO occupies a position between the public and private sectors. Some member institutes are part of the governmental structure of their countries or are mandated by their government. Other members have their roots in the private sector, which were set up by national partnerships of industry associations. ISO has published a series of standards for cleanrooms and associated controlled environments. The U.S. federal government now uses the terminology set forth by the ISO in place of its former standard (Federal Standard 209e; Chapters 6 and 7). **Table 2-4** summarizes the ISO monographs on cleanrooms and associated controlled environments.

NSF International

Founded in 1944 as the National Sanitation Foundation, this organization's name changed to NSF International in 1990,

TABLE 2-3. ISMP: Best Practice for Sterile Compounding

Best Practice
When compounding sterile preparations, perform an independent verification to ensure that the proper ingredients (medications and diluents) are added, including confirmation of the proper amount (volume) of each ingredient prior to its addition to the final container. • Specifically, eliminate the use of proxy methods of verification for compounded sterile preparations of medications (eg, the "syringe pull-back method," checking a label rather than the actual ingredients). • Except in an emergency, perform this verification in all locations where compounded sterile preparations are made, including patient care units. • Use technology to assist in the verification process (eg, machine-readable coding [eg, barcode scanning, radio frequency identification] of ingredients, gravimetric verification, robotics, IV workflow software) to augment the manual processes. When technology is in use, it is important that processes are in place to ensure it is maintained, the software is updated, and that the technology is always used in a manner that maximizes the medication safety features of these systems.
Rationale
• The goal of this Best Practice is to prevent medication errors during sterile compounding of drugs that are not detected with proxy checks, such as the "syringe pull-back method" or other retrospective verification processes. • ISMP has reported multiple serious compounding errors that caused patient harm or death mostly due to preparation of the wrong concentration/strength or using the wrong product or diluent. Many of these would have been identified prior to dispensing if preproduction checks or sterile processing technology would have been utilized. • ISMP has received reports of errors that were specifically attributed to a failed check system when using the "syringe pull-back method." • This error-prone method has been used in pharmacies during the sterile compounding process for years. Using this method, an ingredient is injected from the syringe into the final container, and the plunger is then pulled back to the amount on the syringe that was injected. It is this "pulled-back" syringe that is checked to determine the accuracy of the amount injected. Errors may not be detected if the syringe does not reflect the actual amount added or when the pulled-back syringes are partnered with the wrong container of medication.

ISMP = Institute for Safe Medication Practices.

Source: Reprinted with permission of ISMP. 2022–2023 targeted medication safety best practices for hospitals. www.ismp.org/tools/bestpractices/TMSBP-for-Hospitals.pdf.

TABLE 2-4. ISO Standards for Cleanrooms and Associated Environments[a]

ISO Standards
• ISO 14644-1:2015 Cleanrooms and associated controlled environments—Part 1: Classification of air cleanliness by particle concentration
• ISO 14644-2:2015 Cleanrooms and associated controlled environments—Part 2: Monitoring to provide evidence of cleanroom performance related to air cleanliness by particle concentration
• ISO 14644-3:2005 Cleanrooms and associated controlled environments—Part 3: Test methods
• ISO 14644-4:2022 Cleanrooms and associated controlled environments—Part 4: Design, construction, and start-up
• ISO 14644-5:2004 Cleanrooms and associated controlled environments—Part 5: Operations
• ISO 14644-7:2004 Cleanrooms and associated controlled environments—Part 7: Separative devices (clean air hoods, gloveboxes, isolators, and mini-environments)
• ISO 14644-8:2022 Cleanrooms and associated controlled environments—Part 8: Assessment of air cleanliness by chemical concentration (ACC)
• ISO 14644-9:2022 Cleanrooms and associated controlled environments—Part 9: Assessment of surface cleanliness for particle concentration
• ISO 14644-10:2022 Cleanrooms and associated controlled environments—Part 10: Assessment of surface cleanliness for chemical contamination

ISO = International Organization for Standardization.

[a] See www.iso.org for more information.

as services expanded beyond sanitation. The letters no longer represent any specific words. NSF International develops public health standards and certification programs to protect food, water, consumer products, and environment. NSF International's mission is to protect and improve global human health. The international standard for Class II biological safety cabinets is NSF Standard 49 (Chapter 6).[92]

SUMMARY

Pharmacists who are responsible for compounding sterile preparations face many issues that were unknown 40 years ago. With current publicity, governmental scrutiny, and technological changes, pharmacists are greatly challenged to meet this responsibility. To compound sterile preparations appropriately, pharmacists must understand the guidelines and standards of state boards of pharmacy, accrediting agencies, FDA, USP, OSHA, CDC, NIOSH, ASHP, ASPEN and other agencies. USP Chapter <797>, USP Chapter <800>, and USP Chapter <825> have become the de facto national standards that licensing and accreditation bodies use to judge if pharmacies and other healthcare organizations are in compliance with set standards when compounding sterile preparations.

REFERENCES

1. Centers for Disease Control and Prevention. Multistate fungal meningitis outbreak investigation. **www.cdc.gov/hai/outbreaks/meningitis.html**. Accessed August 18, 2023.
2. Collins S. Two years after meningitis outbreak: Massachusetts passes compounding overhaul. *Pharm Today*. 2014;20:61.
3. Belz KH. Tennessee health officials warn about drugs from Cleveland pharmacy. *Times Free Press*. September 24, 2014.
4. Reuters staff. U.S. seizes $18 million from owners of pharmacy tied to meningitis outbreak. *Reuters*. January 6, 2015. **https://www.reuters.com/article/us-usa-health-meningitis/u-s-seizes-18-million-from-owners-of-pharmacy-tied-to-meningitis-outbreak-idUSKBN0KF25Z20150106**. Accessed August 18, 2023.

5. The United States Department of Justice. Two pharmacists sentenced to prison for adulteration of drugs in connection with Alabama-based compounding pharmacy. **www.justice.gov/opa/pr/two-pharmacists-sentenced-prison-adulteration-drugs-connection-alabama-based-compounding**. Published June 2016. Accessed August 18, 2023.
6. Associated Press. Judge approves $200M settlement in 2012 meningitis outbreak. *CBS News*. May 20, 2015. **https://www.cbsnews.com/news/judge-approves-200-million-settlement-over-meningitis-outbreak/**. Accessed August 18, 2023.
7. Maddox W. Dallas pharmacist pleads guilty to adulterating compounded medication. *D Magazine*. October 15, 2021. **https://www.dmagazine.com/healthcare-business/2021/10/dallas-pharmacist-pleads-guilty-to-adulterating-compounded-medication/**. Accessed August 18, 2023.
8. Raymond N. Pharmacist in deadly U.S. meningitis outbreak resentenced to 10-1/2 years in prison. *Reuters*. July 21, 2021. **https://www.reuters.com/legal/litigation/pharmacist-deadly-us-meningitis-outbreak-resentenced-10-12-years-prison-2021-07-21/**. Accessed August 18, 2023.
9. Raymond N. Pharmacy exec in deadly U.S. meningitis outbreak gets stiffer, 14-1/2 year prison term. *Reuters*. July 7, 2021. **https://www.reuters.com/world/us/pharmacy-exec-deadly-us-meningitis-outbreak-gets-stiffer-14-12-year-prison-term-2021-07-07/**. Accessed August 18, 2023.
10. Halvorsen D, Halvorsen RM. State of pharmacy compounding—2022. *Pharm Purch Prod*. 2022;19(4):S1–S56. **https://www.pppmag.com/article/2902**. Accessed January 8, 2023.
11. About the U.S. pharmacopeia (USP). USP website. **https://www.usp.org/about**. Accessed January 8, 2023.
12. Legal recognition of USP standards. **https://www.usp.org/about/legal-recognition**. Accessed January 8, 2023.
13. USP <1206> Sterile drug products for home use. In: *1994: USP Compounding Compendium*. Rockville, MD: The United States Pharmacopeial Convention; 1994:1963–1975.
14. USP <1206> Sterile drug products for home use. In: *2000: USP Compounding Compendium*. Rockville, MD: The United States Pharmacopeial Convention; 2000:2130–2143.
15. USP <797> Pharmaceutical compounding—sterile preparations. *Pharmacopia Forum*. 2003;29:940–965.
16. USP <797> Pharmaceutical compounding—sterile preparations. In: *2023: USP Compounding Compendium*. Rockville, MD: The United States Pharmacopeial Convention. doi:10.31003/USPNF_M99925_07_01.
17. USP General notices and requirements. In: *2023: USP Compounding Compendium*. Rockville, MD: The United States Pharmacopeial Convention. doi:10.31003/USPNF_M99989_09_01.
18. Thompson C. USP publishes enforceable chapter on sterile compounding. *Am J Health-Syst Pharm*. 2003; 60:1814, 1817-8, 1822.
19. USP <797> Pharmaceutical compounding—sterile preparations. In: *2020: USP Compounding Compendium*. Rockville, MD: The United States Pharmacopeial Convention. doi:10.31003/USPNF_M99925_06_01.
20. USP. FAQs on the compounding appeals. **https://www.usp.org/sites/default/files/usp/document/our-work/compounding/faqs-on-compounding-appeals.pdf**. Published March 2020. Accessed January 15, 2023.
21. USP. Appeals panel decisions on USP <795>, <797>, and <825>. **https://www.usp.org/sites/default/files/usp/document/our-work/compounding/decisions-appeals-fs.pdf**. Published March 2020. Accessed August 18, 2023.
22. USP Revision Bulletin. General chapters <797> Pharmaceutical compounding—sterile reparations. **https://www.uspnf.com/sites/default/files/usp_pdf/EN/USPNF/revisions/gc-797-rb-notice-20200424.pdf**. Published April 2020. Accessed January 8, 2023.
23. USP <800> Hazardous drugs—handling in healthcare settings. In: *2020: USP Compounding Compendium*. Rockville, MD: The United States Pharmacopeial Convention. doi:10.31003/USPNF_M7808_07_01.
24. USP Revision Bulletin. General chapter <825> radiopharmaceuticals—preparation, compounding, dispensing, and repackaging. **https://www.uspnf.com/sites/default/files/usp_pdf/EN/USPNF/revisions/gc-825-rb-notice-20200529.pdf**. Published May 2020. Accessed January 8, 2023.
25. USP. Radiopharmaceuticals—preparation, compounding, dispensing, and repackaging <825>. Rockville, MD: USP; Dec 1, 2020. **https://doi.org/10.31003/USPNF_M11915_04_01**.
26. Teshome BF, Reveles KR, Lee GC, et al. How gaps in regulation of compounding pharmacy set the stage for a multistate fungal meningitis outbreak. *J Am Pharm Assoc*. 2014;54(4):441–445. doi:10.1331/JAPhA.2014.14011.
27. Drug quality and security act of 2013. **https://www.govinfo.gov/content/pkg/BILLS-113hr3204eh/pdf/BILLS-113hr3204eh.pdf**. Accessed January 15, 2023.
28. Center for Drug Evaluation and Research. Pharmacy compounding of human drug products under section 503A of the Federal Food, Drug and Cosmetic Act.

https://www.fda.gov/regulatory-information/search-fda-guidance-documents/pharmacy-compounding-human-drug-products-under-section-503a-federal-food-drug-and-cosmetic-act. Published July 2014. Accessed January 15, 2023.

29. American Society of Health-System Pharmacists. The drug quality and security act (H.R. 3204) section 503A of the food, drug and cosmetic act. **https://www.ashp.org/-/media/assets/advocacy-issues/docs/drug-quality-and-security-act-section-503a-of-the-food-drug-cosmetic-act.ashx?la=en**. Published November 2013. Accessed January 15, 2023.

30. The Drug Quality and Security Act. (H.R. 3204) section 503B of the Food, Drug and Cosmetic Act (2013 November 13). **www.ashp.org/-/media/assets9/advocacy-issues/docs/drug-quality-and-security-act-section-503b-of-the-food-drug-cosmetic-act.ashx?la=en**. Accessed January 15, 2023.

31. U.S. Food and Drug Administration. Outsourcing facility fee rates for fiscal year 2023. *Federal Regiser*. 2023; 87(144); 45335–9. **https://www.federalregister.gov/documents/2022/07/28/2022-16170/outsourcing-facility-fee-rates-for-fiscal-year-2023**. Accessed January 15, 2023.

32. Gabay M. The drug quality and security act. *Hosp Pharm*. 2014; 49(7):615, 676. doi:10.1310/hpj4907-615.

33. U.S. Food and Drug Administration. Letter from Margaret A. Hamburg, MD, Commissioner of Food and Drugs, to hospital pharmacists. January 8, 2014. **https://web.archive.org/web/20140630095703/http:/www.fda.gov:80/downloads/Drugs/GuidanceComplianceRegulatoryInformation/PharmacyCompounding/UCM380599.pdf**. Accessed January 15, 2023.

34. U.S. Food and Drug Administration. Registered outsourcing facilities: facilities registered as human drug compounding outsourcing facilities under section 503B of the federal food, drug, and cosmetic act (FD&C Act). Updated January 3, 2023. **https://www.fda.gov/drugs/human-drug-compounding/registered-outsourcing-facilities**. Accessed January 15, 2023.

35. Traynor K. FDA revives compounding advisory committee. *Am J Health Syst Pharm*. 2015;72(8): 598–599. doi:10.2146/news150030.

36. Thompson CA. Substances doubtful for bulk drug substances list could be INDs. *Am J Health Syst Pharm*. 2016;73(8):512–514. doi:10.2146/news150030.

37. U.S. Department of Health and Human Services. Notice of FDA change to 503A of FD&C act. **https://www.fda.gov/downloads/drugs/guidancecomplianceregulatoryinformation/pharmacycompounding/ucm510684.pdf**. Accessed January 15, 2023.

38. U.S. Food and Drug Administration. Insanitary conditions at compounding facilities: guidance for industry. **https://www.fda.gov/regulatory-information/search-fda-guidance-documents/insanitary-conditions-compounding-facilities-guidance-industry**. Published November 2020. Accessed January 15, 2023.

39. U.S. Food and Drug Administration. Hospital and health system compounding under section 503A of the federal food, drug, and cosmetic act guidance for industry. **https://www.fda.gov/regulatory-information/search-fda-guidance-documents/hospital-and-health-system-compounding-under-section-503a-federal-food-drug-and-cosmetic-act**. Revised October 2021. Accessed January 15, 2023.

40. Urahn S, Coukell A, Jungman E et al. *State Oversight of Drug Compounding: Major Progress since 2015, but opportunities remain to better protect patients*. Philadelphia: The Pew Charitable Trusts; February 2018. **https://www.pewtrusts.org/-/media/assets/2018/02/drug_safety_assesment_web.pdf**. Accessed January 15, 2023.

41. National Association of Boards of Pharmacy. About. NABP. **https://nabp.pharmacy/about/**. Accessed August 18, 2023.

42. Delegates approve 20 resolutions at annual meeting, resolution No. 89-1-93. *NABP News*. 1993; 22:57.

43. National Association of Boards of Pharmacy. Model state pharmacy act and model rules of the national association of boards of pharmacy. Published August 2022. **https://nabp.pharmacy/members/board-resources/model-pharmacy-act-rules/**. Accessed August 18, 2023.

44. Social Security Act. 1865, 42 U.S.C. 1395bb; 42 CFR 488.12.

45. Centers for Medicare & Medicaid Services. CMS-approved accrediting organizations. **https://www.cms.gov/Medicare/Provider-Enrollment-and-Certification/SurveyCertificationGenInfo/Downloads/Accrediting-Organization-Contacts-for-Prospective-Clients-.pdf**. Published July 2022. Accessed January 15, 2023.

46. U.S. Department of Health and Human Services. Medicare's oversight of compounded pharmaceuticals used in hospitals. Office of Inspector General. **https://www.oig.hhs.gov/oei/reports/oei-01-13-00400.asp**. Published January 2015. Accessed January 15, 2023.

47. Centers for Medicare & Medicaid Services. Revised hospital guidance for pharmaceutical services and expanded guidance related to compounding of medications. **https://www.hhs.gov/guidance/document/sc1601hospital-pharmaceutical-services**. Published October 2015. Accessed January 15, 2023.

48. Centers for Medicare & Medicaid Services. State operations manual appendix a – survey protocol, regulations and interpretive guidelines for hospitals. **https://www.cms.gov/Medicare/Provider-Enrollment-and-Certification/GuidanceforLawsAndRegulations/Hospitals**. Revised February 2020. Accessed January 15, 2023.

49. Facts about the joint commission. The Joint Commission website. **https://www.jointcommission.org/who-we-are/facts-about-the-joint-commission/**. Accessed January 15, 2023.

50. Uselton JP, Kienle PC, Murdaugh LB. United States pharmacopeia (USP) compounding standards: chapters <795>, <797>, <800>, and <825>. In: *Meeting Accreditation Standards: A Pharmacy Preparation Guide*. 9th ed. Bethesda, MD: ASHP; 2019:313–325.

51. About us. Accreditation Commission for Health Care. **https://www.hfap.org/about/**. Accessed January 16, 2023.

52. Anonymous. HFAP Revises Pharmacy and Nursing Standards for Hospitals. HNX Healthcare Update. February 12, 2016. **https://hcupdate.wordpress.com/2016/02/12/hfap-revises-pharmacy-and-nursing-standards-for-accredited-hospitals/**. Accessed July 17, 2023.

53. About our organization. Center for Improvement in Healthcare Quality. **https://cihq.org/about_our_organization.asp**. Accessed January 16, 2023.

54. Center for Improvement in Healthcare Quality. Welcome: Hospitals. **https://www.cihq.org/acc-default-hospitals.asp**. Published January 2023. Accessed January 16, 2023.

55. Our history. Det Norske Veritas (DNV). **https://www.dnv.com/about/in-brief/our-history.html** Accessed January 16, 2023.

56. Accreditation organizations with hospitals with recent substantial deficiencies. Quality Certification & Oversight Reports. **https://qcor.cms.gov/hosp_cop/8.html**. Published January 2023. Accessed January 16, 2023.

57. Hospital accreditation. Det Norske Veritas (DNV). **https://www.dnv.com/services/hospital-accreditation-7516**. Accessed January 16, 2023.

58. Pharmacy accreditation. Accreditation Commission for Health Care. **https://www.achc.org/pharmacy/**. Accessed January 16, 2023.

59. Pharmacy Compounding Accreditation Board. Compounding pharmacy accreditation. Accreditation Commission for Health Care. **https://www.achc.org/compounding-pharmacy/**. Accessed January 16, 2023.

60. Medication compounding certification fact sheet. The Joint Commission. **https://www.jointcommission.org/resources/news-and-multimedia/fact-sheets/facts-about-medication-compounding-certification/**. Accessed January 16, 2023.

61. Medication compounding certification benefits state boards of pharmacy. The Joint Commission. **https://www.jointcommission.org/what-we-offer/certification/certifications-by-setting/hospital-certifications/medication-compounding-certification/medication-compounding-state-pharmacy-boards-stakeholders/**. Accessed January 16, 2023.

62. Occupational Safety and Health Administration, Department of Labor. *Title 29 USC Chapter 15 Section 654 Part (a)(1). Duties of Employers and Employees*. Washington, DC: U.S. Government Printing Office; 2020. **https://www.govinfo.gov/content/pkg/USCODE-2020-title29/pdf/USCODE-2020-title29-chap15-sec654.pdf**. Accessed January 16, 2023

63. Occupational Safety and Health Administration. Hazardous drugs. U.S. Department of Labor. **https://www.osha.gov/hazardous-drugs**. Accessed January 16, 2023.

64. Occupational Safety and Health Administration. Toxic and hazardous substances: access to employee exposure and medical records. U.S. Department of Labor. **https://www.osha.gov/laws-regs/regulations/standardnumber/1910/1910.1020**. Accessed January 16, 2023.

65. Occupational Safety and Health Administration. Toxic and hazardous substances: hazard communication. U.S. Department of Labor. **https://www.osha.gov/laws-regs/regulations/standardnumber/1910/1910.1200**. Accessed January 16, 2023.

66. Fairfax RE. Letter of standard interpretation. Dated May 8, 2005. U.S. Department of Labor. **https://www.osha.gov/laws-regs/standardinterpretations/2005-02-08-0**. Accessed January 16, 2023.

67. Coe CP. Letter of standard interpretation: hazard communication and pharmaceuticals. U.S. Department of Labor. Dated January 3, 1994. **https://www.osha.gov/laws-regs/standardinterpretations/1994-01-03**. Accessed January 16, 2023.

68. Clark RA, Ewing TW, Willey JD. Letters of standard interpretation: MSDS requirements for drugs. Dated August 13, 1993. U.S. Department of Labor. **https://www.osha.gov/laws-regs/standardinterpretations/1993-08-13**. Accessed January 16, 2023.

69. National Institute for Occupational Safety and Health. Preventing occupational exposures to antineoplastic and other hazardous drugs in healthcare settings. Centers for Disease Control and Prevention. **www.cdc.gov/niosh/docs/2004-165/**. Accessed January 16, 2023.

70. National Institute for Occupational Safety and Health. NIOSH list of antineoplastic and other hazardous drugs in healthcare settings, 2016. Centers for Disease Control and

Prevention. **https://www.cdc.gov/niosh/docs/2016-161/default.html**. Accessed January 16, 2023.

71. Centers for Disease Control and Prevention. Hazardous drugs: draft NIOSH list of hazardous drugs in healthcare dettings, 2020; procedures; and risk management information. *Federal Register*. 2020; 85(85); 25439-51. **https://www.govinfo.gov/content/pkg/FR-2020-05-01/pdf/2020-09332.pdf**.

72. American Society of Health System Pharmacists. ASHP guidelines on quality assurance for pharmacy-prepared sterile products. *Am J Health Syst Pharm*. 2000;57(12):1150–1169. doi:10.1093/ajhp/57.12.1150.

73. American Society of Health System Pharmacists. ASHP guidelines on compounding sterile preparations. *Am J Health Syst Pharm*. 2014;71(2):145–166. doi:10.2146/sp140001.

74. American Society of Hospital Pharmacists. ASHP technical assistance bulletin on pharmacy-prepared ophthalmic products. *Am J Hosp Pharm*. 1993;50(7):1462–1463. **https://pubmed.ncbi.nlm.nih.gov/8362884/**.

75. Iredell B, Mourad H, Nickman NA, et al. ASHP guidelines on the safe use of automated compounding devices for the preparation of parenteral nutrition admixtures. *Am J Health Syst Pharm*. 2022;79(10): 730–735. doi:10.1093/ajhp/zxac004.

76. Power LA, Coyne JW. ASHP guidelines on handling hazardous drugs. *Am J Health Syst Pharm*. 2018;75(24):1996–2031. doi:10.2146/ajhp180564.

77. American Society of Health-System Pharmacists. ASHP guidelines on out-sourcing sterile compounding services. *Am J Health Syst Pharm*. 2015;72(19): 1664–1675. doi:10.2146/sp150024.

78. American Society of Health-System Pharmacists. ASHP accreditation standard for postgraduate residency programs. **https://www.ashp.org/-/media/assets/professional-development/residencies/docs/examples/ASHP-Accreditation-Standard-for-Postgraduate-Residency-Programs-effective-July-2023.pdf**. Published July 2023. Accessed January 16, 2023.

79. American Society of Health-System Pharmacists, Accreditation Council for Pharmacy Education. ASHP / ACPE accreditation standard for pharmacy technician education and training programs. **https://www.ashp.org/-/media/assets/professional-development/technician-program-accreditation/docs/ashp-acpe-pharmacy-technician-accreditation-standard-2018.pdf**. Published July 2018. Accessed January 16, 2023.

80. Catalog American Society of Health-System Pharmacists. **https://elearning.ashp.org/catalog/default**. Accessed January 16, 2023.

81. Boullata JI, Gilbert K, Sacks G, et al. A.S.P.E.N. clinical guidelines: parenteral nutrition ordering, order review, compounding, labeling, and dispensing. *JPEN*. 2014;38(3):334–377. doi:0.1177/0148607114521833.

82. Detailed Overview. American Society for Testing of Materials. **https://www.astm.org/about/overview/detailed-overview.html**. Accessed January 16, 2023.

83. New Standard Will Help Improve Protective Clothing for Healthcare Professionals. News Release #11624. February 17, 2023. American Society for Testing of Materials. **https://newsroom.astm.org/newsroom-articles/new-standard-will-help-improve-protective-clothing-healthcare-professionals**. Accessed July 17, 2023.

84. CETA Application Guides. Controlled Environment Testing Association. **https://coeta.memberclicks.net/current-cags**. Accessed January 16, 2023.

85. Resource Conservation and Recovery Act of 1976. 42 U.S.C. 82 §6901-92.

86. Brechtelsbauer E, Shah S. Update on pharmaceutical waste disposal regulations: Strategies for success. *Am J Health Syst Pharm*. 2020;77(7):574–582. doi:10.1093/ajhp/zxz360.

87. About IEST. Institute of Environmental Sciences and Technology. **https://www.iest.org/About-IEST**. Accessed January 17, 2023.

88. USP <797> Compliance Handbook. Institute of Environmental Sciences and Technology. **https://www.iest.org/Standards-RPs/USP-797/USP-797-Handbook**. Accessed January 16, 2023.

89. Proceedings from the ISMP sterile preparation compounding safety summit: guidelines for SAFE preparation of sterile compounds 2013. Institute for Safe Medication Practices. **https://www.ismp.org/sites/default/files/attachments/2017-11/Guidelines%20for%20Safe%20Preparation%20of%20Compounded%20Sterile%20Preperations_%20revised%202016.pdf**. Accessed August 10, 2023.

90. Institute for Safe Medication Practices (ISMP). *ISMP Guidelines for Sterile Compounding and the Safe Use of Sterile Compounding Technology*. Plymouth Meeting, PA: ISMP; 2022. **https://www.ismp.org/resources/guidelines-sterile-compounding-and-safe-use-sterile-compounding-technology**. Accessed January 16, 2023.

91. Institute for Safe Medication Practices. ISMP 2022-2023 targeted medication safety best practices for hospitals. **https://www.ismp.org/system/files/resources/2022-02/2022-2023%20TMSBP%20final.pdf**. Accessed January 16, 2023.

92. NSF/ANSI Standard 49—2020: biosafety cabinetry: design, construction, performance, and field certification. Ann Arbor, MI: NSF International and American National Standards Institute; 2021.

SECTION 2: Sterile Compounding Training and Competency

DOI 10.37573/9781585286492

3

PHARMACIST EDUCATION

Joyce S. Jih and Robert P. Shrewsbury

INTRODUCTION

The adoption of the Doctor of Pharmacy degree as the entry-level degree for pharmacists shifted the emphasis of pharmacy education toward biological sciences and clinical practice rather than distributive processes, such as nonsterile and sterile compounding. Yet pharmacy compounding is defined as the art and science of preparing personalized medications for patients.[1] Compounding allows pharmacists to collaborate with patients and prescribers to individualize a medication that will meet a patient's specific need.

Pharmacy schools offer limited compounding instruction since the skill set is not required for all prescriptions filled in the United States.[2] However, the practice of compounding in pharmacy education continues to be mandated by three national organizations, which are the Accreditation Council for Pharmacy Education (ACPE), American Association of Colleges of Pharmacy (AACP), and National Association of Boards of Pharmacy (NABP).[3-5] Compounding practice standards have been established by the United States Pharmacopeia (USP), which are legally enforceable by the Food and Drug Administration (FDA) and state boards of pharmacy.[6]

The scope of compounding also continues to expand, driven by technological developments such as 3-D printing,[7-9] pharmacogenomics,[10-12] and pharmaceutical development. Additionally, most medical information is now processed through computer technology, making medication usage and monitoring accessible at any time from any place.

Compounding is the only avenue to obtain personalized medications for patients because there is not and will not be a "one size fits all" medication answer for patients. Compounding is one skill that pharmacists must possess because it integrates into all future practice developments to provide optimal medication management for patients. Therefore, it is reasonable that schools of pharmacy, as the purveyors of pharmacy education, re-evaluate the adequacy of their compounding training for their students, pharmacists, and technicians, as they are to competently assume roles as compounding practitioners in the future.

ACADEMIC EDUCATION

In the past years, some schools of pharmacy began expanding their curricular instruction models as they explored different pedagogical methods for sterile compounding education.[13-16] However, the scope, frequency, timing, and methods of this academic curricular transition were slow to occur and highly individualized in each institution. Results of a study published in 2007 found that only 13% of schools reported that their students had adequate training in compounding sterile preparations before graduation.[15] A survey of compounding education in AACP member institutions published in 2012 indicated that only 27% of respondents' institutions had compounding education facilities for sterile compounding.[17]

Improvement in the adoption of sterile compounding education within schools of pharmacy was evaluated again in 2017.[18] When compared with a study from 2007, significantly more pharmacy programs had purchased sterile solutions and supplies for student instruction ($P = .022$), made students garb before compounding sterile preparations ($P = .0009$), and assessed students' compounding skills by both observation and written examination ($P = .0129$). Analysis suggested that programs offering a standalone course in compounding sterile preparations and training conducted inside a cleanroom were significantly more likely to have students believe they received adequate training before graduation. The survey data also suggested that postgraduate on-the-job training was the most influential factor that students believed developed their competency in preparing sterile preparations. As of 2019, 70% of Doctor of Pharmacy programs in the United States required students to be able to independently

DOI 10.37573/9781585286492.003

compound sterile preparations prior to starting advanced pharmacy practice experience (APPEs); only 33% of pharmacy programs had a standalone course devoted to sterile compounding.

ASSESSMENT METHODS

In teaching compounding science, there are three factors to consider in a school of pharmacy course: engineering controls, personnel responsibility and controls, and process control. Schools of pharmacy primarily focus on teaching process control (ie, aseptic techniques). In teaching aseptic techniques, some schools of pharmacy have standalone sterile compounding courses while others have compounding topics spread throughout a group of skills-based courses. Some programs have advanced sterile compounding experiences beyond the usual laboratory teaching pedagogical styles, such as immersive and live virtual simulations[19] and remote and virtual learning experiences that became common due to the COVID-19 pandemic.[20] Schools have also adopted a variety of assessment schemes to evaluate student competency. **Table 3-1** provides examples of designs and assessment schemes used in schools of pharmacy for instruction and evaluation of aseptic techniques.

Some general comments about representative studies are the following:

- Begley et al. designed a repetitive measures lab where students used a checklist to examine an order and the compounded preparation for errors.[21] The scenario was repeated four or more times. From 2009 to 2012, scores on preparation sterile verification improved with repeated trials ($P = .002$) but plateaued after the third trial.
- A required hands-on laboratory exercise was incorporated into an introductory pharmacy practice experience (IPPE) for third-year pharmacy students.[22] Students first prepared a modified low risk compounded sterile preparation (CSP) media fill test. During the media fill test, students were observed by an instructor in 10 areas. The CSPs were incubated and inspected for microbial contamination. Contamination of the media fill test was less than 1%.
- A preceptor survey showed that 21% did not permit APPE students to prepare sterile preparations in their facilities.[23] The most common reasons for not allowing students to prepare sterile preparations were lack of training for the institution's requirements (63%), liability concerns (56%), and the cost and time associated with media-fill and glove fingertip testing (38% and 31% respectively). Of the facilities that allowed students to prepare sterile preparations, 89% provided training, 32% required students to pass a media-fill test, 26% required students to pass a glove fingertip test, and 37% required students to pass a written competency test. Some schools have attempted to address the lack of general training in sterile compounding by giving students additional instruction in their third professional IPPE experiences.[24]
- Patel et al. developed a voluntary virtual environment to teach USP Chapter <797> requirements.[25] Pharmacy students used 3D glasses and a wireless controller to identify violations in standards of practice for CSPs. Two virtual laboratory sessions were offered to the students. For the first offering, students were asked to identify items in the IV room, evaluate an IV preparation for accuracy, select an appropriate product for an IV preparation, and provide a recommendation for IV fluids. In the second offering, students simulated an IV preparation in a virtual clean room and needed to identify at least one inappropriate item in the virtual clean room. They also needed to select the appropriate medication vial and diluents to prepare their preparation.
- Dennis et al. studied second- and third-year students who reviewed sterile preparation course materials using online aseptic technique videos.[26] The second-year students completed compounding protocols with nine low-risk aseptic preparations, while the third-year students completed sixteen low-risk aseptic preparations. These aseptic preparations were considered low risk according

TABLE 3-1. Examples of Course Designs and Assessment Methods Used in Aseptic Technique Education of School of Pharmacy Students

Assessment Method	Example References
Grading rubrics	21, 24
Direct instructor observation	22
Improvement in media-fill, glove fingertip test pass rates	23
Online teaching media	25
Compounding practice protocols with instructor feedback	26
Flexible learning via online video review	27
Topic video, demonstration video	28
Analytical potency of preparation	32
Immersive simulation	19
Live virtual simulation	25
Remote virtual learning	20

to USP Chapter <797> standards at the time the study was conducted. For the final assessment, all students prepared a simulated small volume parenteral with a single additive while instructors noted major or minor errors via a checklist. Additional aseptic compounding materials were added, and the students had a lower probability of committing minor and major errors as compared with students before the curriculum change.

- At the University of Georgia, researchers decided to show five 5-minute videos on aseptic compounding to first year pharmacy students on selecting the diluent, gowning and garbing, sterilizing the hood, preparing the preparation, and checking the final preparation.[27] Students were evaluated compounding a gentamicin parenteral in 0.9% sodium chloride (NS). Sixty-nine percent (69%) of the students reviewed at least one video link before making the preparation. Students who clicked on at least one video link did not perform significantly different on the assessment than students who did not access the video.
- In another study, an open-source website available to pharmacy students was updated and fully integrated with additional videos, animations, and study questions.[28] Students were surveyed about the expanded video library regarding accessibility, functionality, and usefulness, and how using the library impacted their learning of compounding. Videos were used by 386/391 students. Thirty-four percent (34%) of students used the videos an average of 30 minutes or less per week; 56% used the videos 1–2 hours per week. Approximately 80% of the students were satisfied with the functionality and accessibility of the videos. All students, regardless of professional year or campus affiliation, surveyed their compounding confidence and competence levels at 70% at the end of the course.

Other teaching methods have been investigated in compounding as a discipline, though several strategies have not been directly applied to sterile compounding instruction. Podcasts,[29] lecture videos,[30;31] and observational assessments at the end of all compounding instruction[26] are three such examples. One methodology rarely found in the pharmacy education literature to assess student compounding competency is the use of quantitative analysis of the final preparation's potency.[32] The AACP member institution survey of compounding curricula in schools of pharmacy found that most respondents cited direct observation as their primary assessment approach, while only a small percentage (8%) of institutions used a quantitative method to evaluate student preparations.[17] Kosinski et al. used potency analysis to assess the retention of sterile compounding skills over a three-semester period.[24] There was no significant difference between the potency accuracy of the two student groups.

Course Designs

Numerous course designs and evaluation schemes have attempted to maximize compounding instruction outcomes.[19;27;33] Newer technologies have also made use of simulations to optimize instruction time. One innovation company has developed a virtual interactive cleanroom simulation as an instructional adjunct or alternative for students to become familiar with the complexities of a cleanroom environment. This virtual interaction also allows students to gain an overview of aseptic manipulation techniques.[25;34] A student satisfaction and perception survey suggested that virtual sterile compounding experiences might be marginally effective since only 57% of the students felt that the virtual compounding experience prepared them for clinical rotations.[35] Another simulated community pharmacy environment was developed to teach students about dispensing medication. The goal of the program is to help students develop skills in accuracy of prescription dispensing (drug strength, route, and dosing) and the five Rs (right drug, right route, right time, right dose, right patient).[36]

Sterile compounding training is often expensive to conduct, which leads to inadequate training in using aseptic techniques. Consequently, most sterile compounding instruction is limited to one semester and is typically taught in the P1 year. This creates a real possibility that upon entering the workforce, graduates are three years removed from their initial training and may no longer possess the basic knowledge or skills of sterile preparation. It has been reported that graduates entering the workforce possessed assorted levels of sterile compounding skills.[26]

The impact of prior experience in sterile compounding and the importance of repeated assessment within a short period of time have been reported to improve aseptic compounding skills.[21;24;33;37;38] As a corollary to experience and repeated testing within a small period of time, the issue of how frequently aseptic technique training should be included within an entire curriculum and the optimal points to include such training have also been discussed.[23;26]

NON-ACADEMIC EDUCATION

Pharmacists compounding CSPs must possess the adequate training and skill necessary to ensure the quality and safety of the preparations. Moreover, as different practice environments have different standards and policies, training should be customized to best suit the needs of each institution and location. As discussed earlier, schools of pharmacy have been slow to increase the number of compounding courses in pharmacy curriculums, and pharmacy residency programs have given little emphasis to compounding CSPs. Consequently, the area that has grown the most in the education and training of compounding pharmacists lies outside schools of pharmacy.

Sources

Nonacademic compounding education can be provided by government agencies, professional associations, educational companies, and institution-specific employee training programs. Federal regulatory agencies, accreditation agencies, and state boards of pharmacy may all impose external requirements on the practice of sterile compounding.[39] While these standards are intended to ensure the quality of CSPs, the directives can also serve as an educational resource for institutions and pharmacists.

Many professional organizations, such as the American Society of Health-System Pharmacists (ASHP) and the American College of Apothecaries (ACA), host online tools, courses, and resources to educate practitioners on sterile compounding.[40;41] Some organizations offer intensive boot camps that combine online coursework with in-person practical skills training and assessment. Sponsored lectures and seminars at professional meetings are other common methods of obtaining information about compounding.

Educational companies provide the most comprehensive training in many different formats, ranging from in-person intensive training camps to on-demand internet-based video instruction and written materials.[41] Many compounding education companies are associated with pharmaceutical manufacturers or chemical distributers.

Regardless of the educational experience, there is a common core of sterile compounding topics covered in non-academic source materials[42]:

- Aseptic technique: use of syringes, needles, vials, ampules, filters, working in primary engineering controls (PECs), secondary engineering controls (SECs)
- Component and testing of final preparations
- Critical area contamination factors
- Environmental monitoring: microbial surface and air particle sampling
- Equipment and supplies
- Facility design
- General personnel conduct in a controlled area
- Good manufacturing practices versus good compounding practices
- Proper gowning and gloving techniques
- Quality assurance procedures
- Sterile compounding documentation: formulation records, compounding records, labeling, beyond-use dating
- Sterile preparation calculations and terminology
- Sterilization techniques

Given that pharmacists must learn and keep current knowledge of the increasing complexities of the standards, technology, and regulatory requirements in the sterile compounding arena, it is inevitable that some form of credentialing will evolve. Such a certificate program or board certification may become the standard requirement for employment in jobs that emphasize sterile compounding. As a case in point, the Board of Pharmacy Specialties (BPS) has created a new specialty for Board Certified Sterile Compounding Pharmacists (BCSCP).[43]

Employee Education

It is standard practice for new pharmacist hires to undergo new employee orientation and training, including training in sterile compounding. In some cases, the pharmacist is not well educated in compounding CSPs due to a lack of academic training. In other cases, there are site-specific requirements that are unknown to the new employee that must be learned before assuming their responsibilities. In either case, the education generally consists of two components. The first component is providing information for the employee. The second component is measuring the employee baseline performance.

Employee education should ideally be provided by a pharmacist well-experienced in compounding CSPs, and employers should utilize training standards to ensure all staff is adequately and comprehensively prepared.[44] USP recommends training "by expert personnel and through audio-video instructional sources and professional publications in the theoretical principles and practical skills of aseptic manipulations and in achieving and maintaining ISO Class 5 environmental conditions before they begin to prepare CSPs."[45]

This education can be delivered by several means which include the following:

- Demonstration and observation by expert personnel
- Audio-video instructional sources
- Professional publications in theoretical principles and practical skills of compounding CSPs
- Didactic review and written test
- Media fill testing of aseptic manipulative skills

The core elements of employee education typically include the following:

- Dress code and garb requirements
- Handwashing techniques, personal hygiene
- Procedures for entering and leaving critical and controlled areas
- Locations of medications and supplies
- Procedures for recording orders and generating labels
- Documentation of work
- Types and locations of drug information resources
- Methods for transmitting medication orders

- Policies for storing CSPs
- Dispensing methods to patients
- Policies for reusing returned doses
- Special procedures for chemotherapy agents and total parenteral nutrition
- Quality management procedures including process validation and environmental monitoring
- Problem resolution, spill management

A checklist is recommended for documenting the satisfactory completion of the employee education. Checklists, templates are available from credentialing agencies and commercial vendors. A checklist ensures that the education is comprehensive and has been correctly completed. In this manner, the CSP compounding pharmacist can be both competent and confident of the abilities and skills.[46]

CONTINUING EDUCATION

To maintain proper quality assurance, pharmacy personnel should regularly receive didactic and experiential training and competency evaluation.[47] In addition, some state boards of pharmacy require several contact hours of sterile compounding continuing education for pharmacists who oversee or directly engage in compounding sterile preparations. Helpful continuing education topics about CSPs for pharmacists include the following:

- Aseptic technique
- Component and testing of final preparations
- Critical area contamination factors
- Environmental monitoring
- Environmental quality control
- Equipment and supplies
- Facilities
- General conduct in a controlled area
- Good manufacturing practices
- Proper gowning and gloving techniques
- Quality assurance procedures
- Sterile compounding documentation
- Sterile preparation calculations and terminology
- Sterilization techniques

SUMMARY

Pharmacists do not always receive adequate education to compound CSPs during their years in pharmacy school. Colleges of pharmacy should recognize the regulatory and public scrutiny being placed on them to appropriately educate students in this essential skill. Though curricular progress has begun in colleges of pharmacy, it is slow to gain momentum and lacks standardization. The commercial education sector has become a major player in this space, but it lacks the instructional innovation afforded by colleges of pharmacy. The result of these shortcomings in both education sectors is that new pharmacist hires typically lack a full understanding of sterile compounding science, technology, and skill. The resulting burden falls to the individual employer to remedy the education gap. But a pathway forward has begun to be defined, and it offers an exciting opportunity for pharmacists in their patient care provider role.

REFERENCES

1. Roark AM, Anksorus HN, Shrewsbury RP. Long-term results of an analytical assessment of student compounded preparations. *Am J Pharm Educ*. 2014;78(9):164. doi:10.5688/ajpe789164
2. Allen LV Jr. Editorial: should all pharmacists compound? *Int J Pharm Compd*. 2022;26(1):24–28. **https://pubmed.ncbi.nlm.nih.gov/35081041/**.
3. Accreditation Council for Pharmacy Education. Accreditation standards and guidelines for the professional program in pharmacy leading to the doctor of pharmacy, standards 2016. **https://www.acpe-accredit.org/pdf/Standards2016FINAL.pdf**. Released February 2015. Accessed August 18, 2023.
4. Medina MS, Plaza CM, Stowe CD, et al. Center for the advancement of pharmacy education 2013 educational outcomes. *Am J Pharm Educ*. 2013;77(8):162. doi:10.5688/ajpe778162.
5. NABP launches accreditation program for compounding pharmacies. National Association of Boards of Pharmacy. **https://nabp.pharmacy/news/news-releases/nabp-launches-accreditation-program-for-compounding-pharmacies/**. Published January 2020. Accessed August 18, 2023.
6. USP General notices and requirements. In: *2023: USP Compounding Compendium*. Rockville, MD: The United States Pharmacopeial Convention. doi:10.31003/USPNF_M99989_09_01.
7. Allen LV Jr. Basics of compounding: 3D printing—pharmacy applications, part 1. *Int J Pharm Compd*. 2017;21(2):127–130. **https://pubmed.ncbi.nlm.nih.gov/28346208/**.
8. Allen LV Jr. Basics of compounding: 3D printing—pharmacy applications, part 2. *Int J Pharm Compd*. 2017;21(3):215–220. **https://pubmed.ncbi.nlm.nih.gov/28557783/**.

9. Allen LV Jr. Basics of compounding: 3D printing—pharmacy applications, part 3: compounding, formulation considerations, and the future. *Int J Pharm Compd*. 2017;21(4):293–298. **https://pubmed.ncbi.nlm.nih.gov/28719372/**.

10. Allen LV Jr. Biotechnology, nanotechnology, and pharmacogenomics and pharmaceutical compounding, Part 1. *Int J Pharm Compd*. 2015;19(1):38–40. **https://pubmed.ncbi.nlm.nih.gov/25902626/**.

11. Allen LV Jr. Biotechnology, nanotechnology, and pharmacogenomics and pharmaceutical compounding, Part 2. *Int J Pharm Compd*. 2015;19(4):280–287. **https://pubmed.ncbi.nlm.nih.gov/26625563/**.

12. Drummond J, Bennet D, Allen LV Jr. Pharmacogenomics: precision pharmacy in 503A compounding. *Int J Pharm Compd*. 2018;22(2):95–107. **https://pubmed.ncbi.nlm.nih.gov/29877857/**.

13. Miller CM, Cordova MA, Hladik WB. The status of undergraduate instruction in parenteral products at U.S. colleges of pharmacy. *Am J Pharm Educ*. 1983;47:48–51. doi:10.5688/ajpe7338.

14. Monk MR, Brown TR, Garner DD, Smith MC. The status of home intravenous therapy instruction provided by U.S. schools and colleges of pharmacy. *Am J Pharm Educ*. 1991;55(2):120–124. doi:10.5688/ajpe80112.

15. Hellums M, Alverson SP, Monk-Tutor MR. Instruction on compounded sterile preparations at U.S. schools of pharmacy. *Am J Health Syst Pharm*. 2007;64(21): 2267–2274. doi:10.2146/ajhp060531.

16. Brown MC, Conway J, Sorensen TD. Development and implementation of a scoring rubric for aseptic technique. *Am J Pharm Educ*. 2006;70(6):133. doi:10.5688/aj7006133.

17. Shrewsbury R, Augustine S, Birnie C, et al. Assessment and recommendations of compounding education in AACP member institutions. *Am J Pharm Educ*. 2012;76(7):S9. doi:10.5688/ajpe767S9.

18. Dana KN, Hertig JB, Scott CR, Briscoe-Dwyer L. Instruction on compounded sterile preparations at schools of pharmacy. *Am J Health Syst Pharm*. 2018;75(12):847–849. doi:10.2146/ajhp170636.

19. Monestime S, Thomas D, Hooper CD, et al. Instructional and assessment redesign of a sterile compounding course using immersive simulation. *Am J Pharm Educ*. 2020;84(2):7473. doi:10.5688/ajpe7473.

20. Higbea A, Bald E, Isaacs AN, et al. Forging ahead from adaptions of teaching during the COVID-19 pandemic: perspectives from multiple pharmacy programs. *JACCP*. 2021;4(1):101–112. doi:10.1002/jac5.1349.

21. Begley K, Monaghan MS, Qi Y. Repeated testing to improve skills in a pharmacy practice laboratory course. *Am J Pharm Educ*. 2013;77(6):130. doi:10.5688/ajpe776130.

22. Cretton-Scott E, Cruthirds D, Coward L. Incorporation of hands-on sterile technique instruction in an introductory pharmacy practice experience. *Am J Pharm Educ*. 2015;79(2):28. doi:10.5688/ajpe79228.

23. Wuller WR, Kwasiborski CL. Developing entry-level competencies in sterile product preparation: an emerging challenge for pharmacy schools and experiential practice sites. *Am J Health Syst Pharm*. 2012;69(12):1072–1075. doi:10.2146/ajhp110366.

24. Kosinski TM, Brown MC, Valdovinos K, Zavala PJ. Acquisition and retention of sterile compounding accuracy skills. *Am J Pharm Educ*. 2017;81(6):115. doi:10.5688/ajpe816115.

25. Patel S, Vincent AH, Abel SR, et al. A virtual clean room to teach USP 797 regulations for intravenous medications. *Am J Pharm Educ*. 2011;75(1):7. doi:10.5688/ajpe7517.

26. Dennis VC, Owora AH, Kirkpatrick AE. Comparison of aseptic compounding errors before and after modified laboratory and introductory pharmacy practice experiences. *Am J Pharm Educ*. 2015;79(10):158. doi:10.5688/ajpe7910158.

27. Neville MW, Palmer R, Elder D, et al. Evaluating the effects of flexible learning about aseptic compounding on first-year students in a pharmacy skills laboratory. *Am J Pharm Educ*. 2015;79(6):91. doi:0.5688/ajpe79691.

28. Park HL, Shrewsbury RP. Student evaluation of online pharmaceutical compounding videos. *Am J Pharm Educ*. 2016;80(2):30. doi:10.5688/ajpe80230.

29. Abdous M, Facer BR, Yen CJ. Academic effectiveness of podcasting: a comparative study of integrated versus supplemental use of podcasting in second language classes. *Comput Educ*. 2012;58(1):43–52. doi:10.1016/j.compedu.2011.08.021.

30. Pierce R, Fox J. Vodcasts and active-learning exercises in a "flipped classroom" model of a renal pharmacotherapy module. *Am J Pharm Educ*. 2012;76(10):196. doi:10.5688/ajpe7610196.

31. Moore WA, Smith AR. Effects of video podcasting on psychomotor and cognitive performance, attitudes, and study behavior of student physical therapists. *Innov Educ Teach Int*. 2012;49(4):401–414. doi:10.1080/14703297.2012.728876.

32. Lee RK, Shrewsbury RP. Potency analysis provides insight to student aseptic compounding technique errors. *Am J Pharm Educ*. 2019;83(9):7338. doi:10.5688/ajpe7338.

33. Nemec EC, Petraglia C, Mattison MJ. Design considerations of a compounded sterile preparations course. *Am J Pharm Educ*. 2016;80(1):12. doi:10.5688/ajpe80112.

34. **https://penguin-innovations.com/**. Penguin Innovations website. Accessed August 18, 2023.

35. Mohammad I, Lobkovich A, Nardolillo J, Wilhelm S. Pharmacy student satisfaction and perceptions following a virtual sterile compounding exercise. *Int J Pharm Compd*. 2022;26(1):10–17. **https://pubmed.ncbi.nlm.nih.gov/35081039/**.

36. McDowell J, Styles K, Sewell K, et al. A simulated learning environment for teaching medicine dispensing skills. *Am J Pharm Educ*. 2016;80(1):11. doi:10.5688/ajpe80111.

37. Isanhart CM, McCall KL, Kretschmer D, Grimes BA. Parenterals laboratory course to reduce microbial contamination rates in media fill tests performed by pharmacy students. *Am J Pharm Educ*. 2008;72(2):27. doi:10.5688/aj720227.

38. Ratka A, Demps E, Mack A. The effect of prior experience with aseptic techniques on learning outcomes in a sterile compounding laboratory course. *Curr Pharm Teach Learn*. 2012;4(1):19–28. doi:10.1016/j.cptl.2011.10.008.

39. Douglass K. Training and competency considerations for pharmacies providing compounded sterile preparations. *Int J Pharm Compd*. 2006;10(4):253–261. **https://pubmed.ncbi.nlm.nih.gov/23974256/**.

40. McElhiney LF. Education, training, and evaluation of hospital compounding personnel. *Int J Pharm Compd*. 2006;10(5):361–368. **https://pubmed.ncbi.nlm.nih.gov/23974256/**.

41. Stevens JT. Summary of educational offerings provided by compounding support companies in 2019. *Int J Pharm Compd*. 2019;23(3):188–191. **https://pubmed.ncbi.nlm.nih.gov/31085786/**.

42. The ecourses in sterile compounding. CriticalPoint website. **https://www.criticalpoint.info/course/the-course-in-sterile-compounding/**. Accessed August 18, 2023.

43. Compounded sterile preparation pharmacy. Board of Pharmacy Specialties. **https://www.bpsweb.org/bps-specialties/compounded-sterile-preparations-pharmacy/**. Accessed August 18, 2023.

44. Penzien CE, Tharp JC, Mulzer K, et al. Development of a sterile compounding training and competency program at a large academic medical center. *Am J Health Syst Pharm*. 2020;77(24):2089–2100. doi:10.1093/ajhp/zxaa326.

45. Newton G. Should just any pharmacist compound? *Int J Pharm Compd*. 1997;1(5):362.

46. Jih JS, Shrewsbury RP. Student self-analysis of their nonsterile preparations and its effect on compounding confidence. *Am J Pharm Educ*. 2018;82(10):6473. doi:10.5688/ajpe6473.

47. American Society of Health-System Pharmacists. ASHP guideline on quality assurance for pharmacy-prepared sterile products. *Am J Health Syst Pharm*. 2000;57:1150–1169.

4 PHARMACY TECHNICIAN EDUCATION, CERTIFICATION, TRAINING, EVALUATION, AND REGULATION

Mary Ann Stuhan

INTRODUCTION

Pharmacy technicians have been assisting in compounding sterile preparations since the early years of formal sterile admixture programs, and their performance has been studied and documented for over 40 years.[1] In 1991, the American Society of Health-System Pharmacists (ASHP; then known as the American Society of Hospital Pharmacists) held a conference on quality assurance for pharmacy-prepared sterile preparations.[2] Conference proceedings listed several problems related to pharmacy technician training for compounding sterile preparations:

- Many pharmacy technicians lacked education and training on the preparation of sterile preparations.
- Many pharmacy technicians did not understand applicable quality assurance principles.
- Mere experience in the preparation of sterile preparations did not impart the knowledge and understanding necessary to ensure their accurate and safe preparation.

ADVANCES IN TECHNICIAN EDUCATION, CERTIFICATION, TRAINING, AND REGULATION

In the thirty-odd years that have followed, there have been many advances in training and evaluating pharmacy technicians, including improved education and training in compounded sterile preparations (CSPs):[3]

- 1991: The Pharmacy Technician Educators Council (PTEC) was formed.
- 1994: The Scope of Pharmacy Practice Project was completed, including a task analysis of what technicians do.[4]
- 1995: ASHP, the American Pharmaceutical Association (now the American Pharmacists Association [APhA]), the Illinois Council of Health-System Pharmacists, and the Michigan Pharmacists Association created the Pharmacy Technician Certification Board (PTCB) as an independent body to develop and administer national voluntary pharmacy technician certification examinations.[5]
- 1996: ASHP and APhA prepared a White Paper on pharmacy technicians, urging planning for uniform national standards for pharmacy technician training.[6]
- 1997: ASHP, APhA, the American Association of Colleges of Pharmacy (AACP), the American Association of Pharmacy Technicians (AAPT), and PTEC collaborated to create the Model Curriculum for Pharmacy Technician Training.
- 1999: The PTCB conducted an updated task analysis of what pharmacy technicians do.[7]
- 2001: The second edition of the *Model Curriculum for Pharmacy Technician Training* was published.[8]
- 2003: The *White paper on pharmacy technicians 2002: Needed changes can no longer wait* was published.[9]
- 2008: The ASHP Pharmacy Technician Training Program Directory listed 116 accredited programs.[10]
- 2008: In response to the tragic death of a two-year-old that involved a pharmacy technician sterile compounding error, U.S. Representative Steven LaTourette (*R*-Ohio) introduced legislation that would require standardized training and

Note: The author acknowledges E. Clyde Buchanan who authored this chapter in the previous edition.

DOI 10.37573/9781585286492.004

registration for pharmacy technicians. (This legislation was not enacted.)[11]

- 2009: The Council on Credentialing in Pharmacy (CCP) published a resource paper on contemporary pharmacy practice, which included an examination of the roles, responsibilities, and functions of pharmacy technicians.[12]
- 2009: CCP published a detailed plan for a uniform national system of regulating pharmacy technician registration, training, and competency assessments in the United States.[13]
- 2011: ASHP announces Pharmacy Practice Model Initiative with a statement on advancing the roles of pharmacy technicians and a call for the certifications for specialized technician practice areas, such as sterile compounding.[14]
- 2014: ASHP and the Accreditation Council for Pharmacy Education (ACPE) formed the Pharmacy Technician Accreditation Commission (PTAC) and adopted a new accreditation standard.[15]
- 2015: ASHP published the fourth edition of *Model Curriculum for Pharmacy Technician Education and Training Programs*.[16]
- 2016: ASHP/ACPE implemented an updated accreditation standard (previously interpreted as requiring simulated or experiential training in IV admixture), allowing accredited pharmacy technician education and training programs to choose whether they provide hands-on training in sterile compounding, nonsterile compounding, or both.[17]
- 2017: PTCB established a specialized certification for compounded sterile preparation technicians.[18]
- 2018: ASHP/ACPE issued a revised accreditation standard (effective 2019) to distinguish two levels of technician training programs. Only the advanced level standard requires competency and experience in sterile compounding and hazardous drugs.[19]
- 2018: ASHP published the fifth edition of *Model Curriculum for Pharmacy Technician Education and Training* Programs.[20]
- 2020: PTCB announced the launch of a hazardous drug management certificate program for certified pharmacy technicians.[21]
- 2022: ASHP lists 248 technician training programs with accredited or candidate status, including 62 offering advanced level education.[22]

TECHNICIAN INVOLVEMENT IN STERILE PREPARATIONS

Pharmacy technicians are actively involved in all aspects of pharmaceutical care. CCP, in its report on the scope of pharmacy practice, found that 66% of a certified technician's time was being spent in assisting the pharmacist and serving patients, with 22% maintaining medication and inventory control systems, and 12% participating in pharmacy practice management and administration.[12] Among health-system pharmacy technicians, preparing IV admixtures was among the primary responsibilities listed.

The fifth edition of the *Model Curriculum for Pharmacy Technician Education and Training Programs* lists 77 key elements for competencies corresponding to the five knowledge/skill areas of the 2018 Accreditation Standard.[20] Although many of these goals are applicable to a wide range of technician skills (eg, demonstrate ethical conduct and apply patient- and medication-safety practices), some of those associated with Standards 3 and 5 have specific relevance to training pharmacy technicians to compound sterile preparations (see **Table 4-1**).

TABLE 4-1. Pharmacy Technician Training Elements Related to Sterile Preparations

Standard 3: Processing and Handling of Medications and Medication Orders

• 3.8 (entry-level) Maintain pharmacy facilities and equipment, including
  • policies and procedures for sanitation management and hazardous waste handling
  • appropriate techniques for cleaning laminar flow biological safety cabinets
  • importance of maintaining a clean and neat work environment
  • how to accurately calibrate . . . fluid compounders, or syringe pumps
• 3.15 (entry-level) Describe basic concepts related to preparation for sterile and nonsterile compounding.
• 3.23 (advanced-level) Prepare compounded sterile preparations per applicable, current USP Chapters.
• 3.25 (advanced-level) Prepare or simulate chemotherapy/hazardous drug preparations per applicable, current USP Chapters.

Standard 5: Regulatory and Compliance Knowledge and Skills
• 5.6 (entry-level) Describe Occupational Safety and Health Administration (OSHA), National Institute of Occupational Safety and Health (NIOSH), and United States Pharmacopeia (USP) requirements for prevention and treatment of exposure to hazardous substances (eg, risk assessment, personal protective equipment, eyewash, spill kit).

Source: Adapted with permission of American Society of Health-System Pharmacists, Accreditation Council for Pharmacy Education. Model curriculum for pharmacy technician education and training programs. 5th ed. https://www.ashp.org/-/media/assets/professional-development/technician-program-accreditation/docs/modelcurriculum-for-pharmacy-technician-educationtraining-programs-final-2018.pdf. Published 2018. Accessed August 8, 2022.

Technician Education

Technician Educators

PTEC was organized in 1991 with a mission to assist the profession of pharmacy in preparing "high quality, well-trained technical personnel through education and practical training."[23] PTEC members instruct and administer a variety of technician training programs with a membership that includes pharmacists, pharmacy technicians, allied health educators, nurses, and consultants. PTEC representatives have been consulted on and actively involved with pharmacy technician program accreditation, the Scope of Pharmacy Practice Project, and the National Voluntary Pharmacy Technician Certification Exam.[23]

Although qualifications of instructors in technician training and education programs vary widely, faculty in programs accredited by the PTAC must "have demonstrated expertise with at least three years of experience, and current knowledge in the areas in which they are instructing," and "adhere to state regulations for licensure or registration to practice as a pharmacist or pharmacy technician."[19]

Educational Programs

Until the early 21st century, pharmacy technicians typically learned their duties through on-the-job training.[10] For a variety of reasons, many employers began to prefer technicians who had relevant training and experience prior to hire. The armed forces were the first to offer formalized pharmacy technician education, but postsecondary programs are currently available at many teaching hospitals, community colleges, and career and technical schools.

Most formal programs include didactic and practical training in areas, such as medical and pharmaceutical terminology, pharmacology, dosage forms, pharmacy laws and record-keeping, pharmaceutical calculations, nonsterile and sterile compounding, and dispensing of medications. Graduates of educational programs may receive a certificate, a diploma, or an associate degree depending on the length, nature, and site of the program.

Accreditation of Pharmacy Technician Educational Programs

Accreditation is a system of recognition for programs or institutions that meet established quality standards. Since 1983, ASHP has encouraged the formal education of pharmacy technicians in either hospitals or academic settings by means of accrediting these educational programs. ASHP is the only nationally recognized nongovernmental, nonprofit pharmacy association that grants programmatic accreditation to pharmacy technician training programs in the United States.[24] In 2014, ASHP and ACPE collaborated to create PTAC. This alliance was formed to involve the expertise of the organization charged with oversight of professional pharmacist (Doctor of Pharmacy) education programs in the accreditation process for technician education. The accreditation standard for pharmacy technician training programs was most recently updated on January 1, 2019.[19]

Pharmacy technician training programs must include a minimum of 400 hours of training (contact) time, extending over a period of 8 weeks or longer for entry level accreditation, and at least 600 hours over 15 or more weeks for advanced level status. The period of training must include time allocated for didactic, simulated/laboratory, and experiential training. Program directors, faculty, and experiential sites must meet the qualifications set out in the accreditation standard, and surveyors must conduct an onsite visit. The accreditation standard requires programs to base the training on meeting a list of key elements (Standards 1 through 5) that include understanding the preparation and process for sterile compounding, assisting pharmacists in preparing medications requiring special handling, and preparing patient-specific medication therapy. Additionally, accreditation at advanced level requires instruction and experience in preparing CSPs and HDs, while programs accredited at entry level have the option of selecting to give detailed laboratory instruction on CSPs and/or preparing chemotherapy and hazardous products. The *Model Curriculum*[20] referenced earlier, is recommended for guidance in fulfilling these goals. Currently, PTAC accreditation is the only established mechanism for ensuring a minimum quality for pharmacy technician education.

Technician Certification

PTCB offers voluntary, national pharmacy technician certification examinations. The certified pharmacy technician (CPhT) credential certifies the competence of persons who demonstrate the knowledge required to practice as pharmacy technicians. The goal of the CPhT is to maintain a national standard for pharmacy technician certification that is consistent with the approach used by other health professions, including the pharmacist licensure process. PTCB's mission is to advance "medication safety by certifying technicians who are qualified to support pharmacists and patient care teams in all practice settings."[25] Pharmacy technician certification is also available through at least one other organization, the National Healthcareer Association.[26] The CPhT is a general credential, however, and is based on passing a written multiple choice examination on a wide variety of pharmacy topics, including some sterile compounding knowledge. While completion of a technician training program and/or work experience is currently required of candidates for certification, knowledge of and training in sterile compounding are not specific prerequisites. Since its inception in 1995, PTCB has certified more than 760,000 technicians, and currently more than 280,000 maintain active certification.[27] Certification is recognized or required for pharmacy technicians in some capacity by more than 40 state boards of pharmacy.

PTCB awards a Certified Compounded Sterile Preparation Technician™ (CSPT) certification to PTCB-certified pharmacy technicians who have established their education and experience in sterile compounding and passed an examination with specialized content related to sterile preparations (see **Table 4-2** for a full list of requirements).[28]

TABLE 4-2. Compounded Sterile Preparation Technician Requirements

Eligibility Requirements
Active PTCB CPhT in good standing
Education and Experience Requirements • Pathway 1: Completion of or enrollment in, a PTCB-recognized education/training program for the CSPT Program, AND one year of full-time continuous compounded sterile preparation (CSP) work experience. • Pathway 2: Three years of full-time continuous compounded sterile preparation (CSP) work experience. • Work experiences must be within the last 8 years. Sterile compounding experience must have been completed in a U.S. facility and subject to USP Chapter <797> and USP Chapter <800> regulations.
Competency Attestation Form: Must be completed by a qualified supervisor who directly observed the skill and competency assessments of the CSPT candidate/certificant.
CSPT Exam Content Outline Domains
1.0 Medications and Components (17%)
2.0 Facilities and Equipment (22%)
3.0 Sterile Compounding Procedures (53%)
4.0 Handling, Packaging, Storage, and Disposal (8%)

Source: Adapted with permission of Credentialing guidelines and requirements: a candidate guidebook. Pharmacy Technician Certification Board. https://www.ptcb.org/guidebook. Updated May 2023. Accessed November 12, 2022.[41] Used with permission from PTCB.

The examination content includes medications and components of sterile preparations (17%), sterile compounding facilities and equipment (22%), sterile compounding procedures (53%), and handling/packaging/storage/disposal of sterile medications and associated waste. Annual renewal for the CSPT credential requires maintenance of the PTCB CPhT certification, a supervisor's competency attestation, and a minimum of 5 hours of sterile compounding-specific continuing education. According to PTCB, "CSPT-certified technicians are valuable for compliance with USP Chapter <797> sterile compounding standards."[18]

In 2020, PTCB launched a new certificate program in hazardous drug management, documenting competency in safe handling of hazardous drugs.[21] Candidates for this certification are required to document completion of a recognized hazardous drug training course. As of this writing, PTCB only recognizes the hazardous drug management programs offered by the American College of Apothecaries, ASHP, and Critical Point. The examination blueprint includes engineering controls, facility cleaning, personal protective equipment (PPE), transport and receiving, dispensing, and administrative procedures.[29]

Technician Employee Competency and Evaluation

Although it is easier to train new employees for their jobs if they already have formal education, certification, and experience, all employees must be oriented to any new workplace, and their training must continue as pharmacy policies and procedures change. Pharmacy employers are obligated to have competent employees, especially when their work involves patient care. *The U.S. Pharmacopeial Convention* (USP) Chapter <797> Pharmaceutical Compounding—Sterile Preparations sets specific standards for training and evaluating compounding personnel.[30]

According to USP Chapter <797>, all personnel who compound or have direct oversight of compounding must initially be trained and qualified by demonstrating knowledge and competency in compounding CSPs before being allowed to perform their job functions independently. Personnel who compound or have direct oversight of compounding personnel must complete an initial training and continue training at least every 12 months in appropriate sterile compounding principles and practices. Each compounding facility must develop a written training program that describes the required training, the frequency of training, and the process for evaluating the performance of individuals who compound, have direct oversight of compounding personnel, perform in-process checks, final verification, and dispensing of CSPs.[30]

Orientation

Because pharmacy technician knowledge of sterile compounding principles and practice may vary as widely as the types of training programs detailed earlier, each new employee should receive proper orientation that provides facility-specific information about the following:

- Dress code and garb requirements
- Hand-washing techniques, including where and when to wash hands, and personal hygiene
- Procedures for entering and leaving environmentally controlled areas

- Locations of medications and supplies
- How orders are recorded and labels are generated
- Documentation of work, including who made a dose and what was used
- Types and locations of drug information resources
- Policies for storing CSPs
- Methods for sending doses to patients
- Policies for reusing returned doses
- Special procedures for hazardous drugs and total parenteral nutrition (TPN)
- Quality management procedures, including media fill testing, fingertip glove testing, and environmental monitoring
- Problem resolution, including spill management
- Staffing and scheduling

Focus Areas and Resources

Following this orientation, detailed instruction (including appropriate study materials), appropriate competency demonstration, and documentation should include, at minimum, the core areas listed in USP Chapter <797>.[30]

- Hand hygiene
- Garbing
- Cleaning and disinfection
- Calculations, measuring, and mixing
- Aseptic technique
- Achieving and/or maintaining sterility (and apyrogenicity if compounding with nonsterile components)
- Use of equipment
- Documentation of the compounding process (eg, master formulation and compounding records)
- Principles of high-efficiency particulate air (HEPA)-filtered unidirectional airflow within the ISO Class 5 area
- Proper use of primary engineering controls (PECs)
- Principles of movement of materials and personnel within the compounding area

Douglass provides a good review of considerations for training adults in CSP preparation that is still applicable to the modern workplace.[31]

Many technician-specific textbooks on sterile compounding and aseptic technique have been published with authors of varying degrees of authority. Trainers are advised to review the selection carefully, especially with respect to currency and application to the latest USP Chapter <797> and legal standards. Additional resources for training in sterile compounding available from ASHP include the following:

1. Practical Training in Compounding Sterile Preparations Certificate[32]: A 22.25-contact-hour, self-guided, online activity incorporating recorded presentations, readings, video demonstrations, and exercises in curricular modules. The program covers compounding sterile preparation practice standards and regulations, pharmacy calculations, facilities and engineering controls, environmental monitoring, cleanroom personnel behaviors, sterile compounding components and procedures, stability and sterility, beyond-use date assignment, nonsterile to sterile compounding, hazardous drugs, and the overall compounding process from sourcing through final check or disposal. Successful completion of a comprehensive exam and specified practice exercises is required to earn the professional certificate.
2. *Aseptic Compounding Technique: Learning & Mastering the Ritual* by Zachary T. Jordan, CPhT: An in-depth guide to all aspects of aseptic compounding work, designed for pharmacists and technicians at all levels of experience.
3. *Compounding Competency Assessment Center*: This comprehensive training tool allows institutions to customize training based upon specific roles and responsibilities of the staff involved in compounding to comply with the USP standards.

Hazardous Drug Training

The ASHP *Model Curriculum* includes key elements addressing hazardous drug training under Standard 3: Processing and Handling of Medications and Medication Orders.

- 3.9 (entry level): "Use information from Safety Data Sheets (SDS), National Institute of Occupational Safety and Health (NIOSH) Hazardous Drug List, and the United States Pharmacopeia (USP) to identify, handle, dispense, and safely dispose of hazardous medications and materials."[20]
- 3.25 (advanced level): "Prepare or simulate chemotherapy/hazardous drug preparations per applicable, current USP Chapters" along with additional material in Standard 5 Element 5.6. "Describe Occupational Safety and Health Administration (OSHA), National Institute of Occupational Safety and Health (NIOSH), and United States Pharmacopeia (USP) requirements for prevention and treatment of exposure to hazardous substances."[20]

For each of these, direction for didactic, simulated, and experiential learning exercises is provided. While this is by no means a map of comprehensive training in hazardous drug handling, it provides a starting point for the introductory lessons needed in the workplace.

USP Chapter <800>, which details practice standards for handling hazardous drugs in healthcare settings, requires training for all personnel handling HDs "based on their job functions (eg, in the receipt, storage, compounding, repackaging, dispensing, administrating, and disposing of HDs)."[33] This training must include, at a minimum, an overview of the HDs being handled and their risks, institutional standard operating procedures (SOPs) for handling HDs, proper use of PPE, proper use of equipment and devices (such as engineering controls), appropriate response to HD exposure, spill management, and proper disposal. USP Chapter <800> even requires training for personnel (both technicians and pharmacists) who are experienced in handling HDs but are new to an institution or department. The training must be complete, and competency must be demonstrated/documented before an employee independently handles HDs. Employees must be reassessed at least every 12 months. Additional training is required for the introduction of new HDs or equipment and prior to changes in a process or SOP.

ASHP offers several technician-appropriate learning activities relevant to HD handling. Designed for self-guided study, they range from basic and general overviews of USP Chapter <800> to more specific offerings on topics such as engineering controls, containment strategies, and PPE. All activities include ACPE continuing education credit for technicians and pharmacists.[34]

Measuring Performance

Quality management requires the ongoing monitoring of an employee's technique. Therefore, a baseline evaluation of a new technician employee's knowledge and aseptic technique is an important part of orientation (see Chapter 5). Trapskin and colleagues described the development and implementation of a pharmacy department sterile compounding training and evaluation program.[35] They found that pharmacy technicians improved their scores via computer-based learning from a baseline of 78% to 86% for USP Chapter <797> material and from 84% to 92% for aseptic manipulation questions. One out of 43 technicians failed the media fill test. The authors proved that computer-based learning was effective at a statistically significant level. In the years since this study was conducted, many new e-learning programs (see previous sections on focus areas and resources) have been developed and can provide a time- and cost-effective performance improvement.

Competency and Assessment

The Joint Commission describes *competency* as "a combination of observable and measurable knowledge, skills, abilities and personal attributes that constitute an employee's performance" and *assessment* as "the process by which the organization validates, via a defined process, that an individual has the ability to perform a task, consistent with the education and training provided."[36] USP Chapter <797> details the competencies to be assessed and required assessment intervals for each area[30]; technicians with duties related to sterile preparations must be included in this process.

A checklist format is recommended for documenting the satisfactory recall of sterile compounding information. This documentation, with space for the employee's signature and validation by the responsible supervisor, should be placed in the employee's personal record. Checklists may include, for example, forms assessing hand hygiene and garbing, aseptic technique, and cleaning and disinfection procedures.

Technician Regulation

The practice of pharmacy is regulated at the state level, where state legislatures pass laws or statutes and state agencies, such as boards of pharmacy, promulgate rules and regulations to enable the laws to be followed. Most state boards of pharmacy are responsible for maintaining and updating rules and regulations for their respective pharmacy practice act—a set of laws that govern the practice of pharmacy within a state. State boards of pharmacy may register or license pharmacy practitioners (pharmacists and pharmacy technicians). Registration is as simple as listing the practitioner and the licensed pharmacy where the practitioner works. State law may or may not require that a pharmacy technician be certified to be registered or work in that state; it depends on currently enforced laws, rules, and regulations. Licensing implies that the practitioner has passed an examination recognized by the respective board of pharmacy.

Most states regulate the position of a pharmacy technician and permit pharmacy technicians to assist pharmacists.[37] Permissible technician duties and the requirements for personnel performing them, however, vary widely. Many states do not mention sterile compounding by pharmacy technicians, simply including the task in the general category of "assistance to pharmacists." Others, however, have more specific rules and requirements for pharmacy technicians involved in sterile compounding, with qualifications that vary from one state to another. Ohio, for instance, restricts preparation of IV admixture to pharmacists, pharmacy interns, and certified pharmacy technicians.[38] Texas has stricter regulations, requiring pharmacy technicians who engage in sterile compounding to have completed "a course sponsored by an ACPE accredited provider which provides 40 hours of instruction and experience; or a training program which is accredited by the American Society of Health-System Pharmacists" and complete a "structured, on-the-job didactic and experiential training program at the pharmacy, which provides sufficient hours of instruction and experience in the facility's sterile compounding processes and procedures."[39]

In the August 2022 version of the *Model Act*, the National Association of Boards of Pharmacy (NABP) lists compounding as an acceptable activity for a certified pharmacy technician and includes pharmacy technicians among compounding pharmacy personnel who "shall be trained and proficient in the particular operations that are performed by that individual."[40] The act lists the education, training, and certification requirements for certified pharmacy technicians:

- Graduated from a competency-based pharmacy technician education and training program approved by the Board of Pharmacy, and have completed a minimum number of pharmacy technician practice experience hours approved by the NABP
- Have successfully passed an examination developed using nationally recognized and validated psychometric and pharmacy practice standards approved by the NABP

SUMMARY

Pharmacy technicians do not always receive the education and training required to competently compound sterile preparations. Many states recognize pharmacy technicians who have not had formal training and/or have not passed a national certification examination. Even those who are certified and have graduated from an accredited program may not have acquired hands-on experience in sterile compounding and aseptic technique. The enforceability of USP Chapter <797> places the onus on pharmacy managers to orient and train pharmacy technicians properly to compound sterile preparations.

REFERENCES

1. Sanders LH, Mabadeje SA, Avis KE, et al. Evaluation of compounding accuracy and aseptic techniques for intravenous admixtures. *Am J Hosp Pharm*. 1978;35(5):531–536. **https://pubmed.ncbi.nlm.nih.gov/350042/**.
2. ASHP invitational conference on quality assurance for pharmacy-prepared sterile products. *Am J Hosp Pharm*. 1991;48(11):2391–2397. **https://pubmed.ncbi.nlm.nih.gov/1746572/**.
3. Sesquicentennial stepping stone summits—summit two: pharmacy technicians. *J Am Pharm Assoc*. 2003;43:84–92. **https://www.japha.org/article/S1086-5802(15)30082-6/fulltext**.
4. Summary of the final report of the scope of pharmacy practice project. *Am J Hosp Pharm*. 1994;51(17):2179–2182. **https://pubmed.ncbi.nlm.nih.gov/7985698/**.
5. History. Pharmacy Technician Certification Board. **https://www.ptcb.org/history**. Accessed August 18, 2023.
6. White paper on pharmacy technicians. *Am J Health Syst Pharm*. 1996;53(15):1793–1796. doi:10.1093/ajhp/53.15.1793.
7. Muenzen PM, Greenberg S, Murer MM. PTCB task analysis identifies role of certified pharmacy technicians in pharmaceutical care. *J Am Pharm Assoc (Wash)*. 1999;39(6):857–864. **https://pubmed.ncbi.nlm.nih.gov/10609452/**.
8. Model curriculum for pharmacy technician training. 2nd ed. American Society of Health-System Pharmacists; 2001:iv,1.
9. Academy of Managed Care Pharmacy. White paper on pharmacy technicians 2002: needed changes can no longer wait. *Am J Health Syst Pharm*. 2003;60(1):37–51. doi:10.1093/ajhp/60.1.37.
10. Buchanan EC, Schneider PJ, eds. *Compounding Sterile Preparations*. 3rd ed. Bethesda, MD: American Society of Health-System Pharmacists; 2009.
11. Emily's Act, HR 5491, 110th Congress (2008). **https://www.govtrack.us/congress/bills/110/hr5491**. Accessed August 18, 2023.
12. Albanese NP, Rouse MJ. Scope of contemporary pharmacy practice: roles, responsibilities, and functions of pharmacists and pharmacy technicians. *J Am Pharm Assoc*. 2010;50(2):e35–69. doi:10.1331/JAPhA.2010.10510.
13. Council on Credentialing in Pharmacy. Pharmacy technician credentialing framework. Published August 2009. **http://www.pharmacycredentialing.org/Files/CCP%20technician%20framework_08-09.pdf**. Accessed August 8, 2023.
14. Pharmacy practice model summit executive summary. *Am J Health Syst Pharm*. 2011;68(12):1079–1085.
15. ASHP and ACPE announce new commissioners for the pharmacy technician accreditation commission. National Association of Boards of Pharmacy. **https://nabp.pharmacy/news/news-releases/ashp-and-acpe-announce-new-commissioners-for-the-pharmacy-technician-accreditation-commission/**. Published June 11, 2014. Accessed August 8, 2023.
16. American Society of Health-System Pharmacists. Model curriculum for pharmacy technician education and training programs. 4th ed. **https://www.ashp.org/-/media/assets/professional-development/technician-program-accreditation/docs/aso-model-curriculum-for-pharmacy-technician-education-and-training-programs.ashx**. Published 2015. Accessed August 8, 2023.
17. American Society of Health-System Pharmacists. Accreditation standards for pharmacy technician education and training programs. **https://www.ashp.org/professional-development/technician-program-accreditation/accreditation-standards/accreditation-standards-for-pharmacy-technician-education-and-training-programs?loginreturnUrl=SSOCheckOnly**. Effective January 1, 2016. Accessed August 8, 2023.

18. Pharmacy employers cite safety benefits of employing PTCB-certified compounded sterile preparation technicians (CSPTs™). Pharmacy Technician Certification Board. **https://www.ptcb.org/news/pharmacy-employers-cite-safety-benefits-of-employing-ptcb-certified-compounded-sterile-preparation-technicians-cspts**. Published March 28, 2019. Accessed August 8, 2023.

19. American Society of Health-System Pharmacists, Accreditation Council for Pharmacy Education. Accreditation standards for pharmacy technician education and training programs. **https://www.ashp.org/professional-development/technician-program-accreditation/accreditation-standards/accreditation-standards-for-pharmacy-technician-education-and-training-programs**. Effective January 1, 2019. Accessed August 8, 2023.

20. American Society of Health-System Pharmacists, Accreditation Council for Pharmacy Education. Model curriculum for pharmacy technician education and training programs. 5th ed. **https://www.ashp.org/-/media/assets/professional-development/technician-program-accreditation/docs/model-curriculum-for-pharmacy-technician-education-training-programs-final-2018.ashx?la=en&hash=161B697B83DEEF83FE59C893985AFD7975A2764D**. Published 2018. Accessed August 8, 2023.

21. PTCB announces new certificate programs in hazardous drug management and billing and reimbursement. Pharmacy Technician Certification Board. **https://www.ptcb.org/news/ptcb-announces-new-certificate-programs-in-hazardous-drug-management-and-billing-and-reimbursement**. Published July 20, 2020. Accessed August 8, 2023.

22. Technician directory. American Society of Health-System Pharmacists. **https://accreditation.ashp.org/directory/#/program/technician**. Accessed July 24, 2023.

23. About PTEC. Pharmacy Technician Educators Council. **https://www.pharmacytecheducators.com/about**. Accessed June 3, 2023.

24. American Society of Health-System Pharmacists. The value of ASHP/ACPE accreditation for pharmacy technician training programs. **https://www.ashp.org/Professional-Development/Technician-Program-Accreditation/The-Value-of-ASHP-ACPE-Accreditation-for-Pharmacy-Technician-Training-Programs**. Accessed June 3, 2023.

25. About PTCB. Pharmacy Technician Certification Board. **https://www.ptcb.org/about-ptcb**. Accessed August 8, 2023.

26. Certified pharmacy technician (CPhT). National Healthcareer Association. **https://www.nhanow.com/certification/nha-certifications/certified-pharmacy-technician-(cpht)**. Pharmacy Technician Certification Board. Accessed August 10, 2023.

27. Credentials by the Numbers. Pharmacy Technician Certification Board. **https://www.ptcb.org/history/credentials-by-the-numbers**. Updated December 2022. Accessed June 3, 2023.

28. Certified Compounded Sterile Preparation Technician (CSPT). Pharmacy Technician Certification Board. **https://www.ptcb.org/credentials/certified-compounded-sterile-preparation-technician**. Accessed June 3, 2023.

29. Hazardous Drug Management Certificate. Pharmacy Technician Certification Board. **https://www.ptcb.org/credentials/hazardous-drug-management-certificate**. Accessed June 3, 2023.

30. USP <797> Pharmaceutical compounding—sterile preparations. In: *2023: USP Compounding Compendium*. Rockville, MD: The United States Pharmacopeial Convention. doi:10.31003/USPNF_M99925_07_01.

31. Douglass K. Training and competency considerations for pharmacies providing compounded sterile preparations. *Int J Pharm Compd*. 2006;10(4):253–261. **https://pubmed.ncbi.nlm.nih.gov/23974256/**.

32. Practical training in compounding sterile preparations certificate. American Society of Health-System Pharmacists. **https://elearning.ashp.org/products/9298/practical-training-in-compounding-sterile-preparations-certificate**. Accessed June 3, 2023.

33. USP <800> Hazardous drugs—handling in healthcare settings. In: *2023: USP Compounding Compendium*. Rockville, MD: The United States Pharmacopeial Convention. doi:10.31003/USPNF_M7808_07_01.

34. Pharmacy technician activities. American Society of Health-System Pharmacists. **https://elearning.ashp.org/products/10734/practical-training-in-compounding-sterile-preparations-certificate**. Accessed July 19, 2023.

35. Trapskin PJ, Reagan R, Hite K, et al. The implementation of a personnel training and assessment program for new standards in the U.S. Pharmacopeia General Chapter <797> Pharmaceutical Compounding of Sterile Preparations. *Hosp Pharm*. 2006;41:43–48. **https://journals.sagepub.com/doi/abs/10.1310/hpj4101-43?journalCode=hpxa**. Accessed July 24, 2023.

36. Competency assessment vs orientation. The Joint Commission. **https://www.jointcommission.org/standards/standard-faqs/hospital-and-hospital-clinics/human-resources-hr/000002152/**. Accessed June 3, 2023.

37. Occupational outlook handbook: pharmacy technicians. U.S. Bureau of Labor Statistics. **https://www.bls.gov/ooh/healthcare/pharmacy-technicians.htm**. Modified September 2022. Accessed August 8, 2023.

38. Ohio Revised Code 4729.91. **http://codes.ohio.gov/orc/4729.91**. Accessed August 8, 2023.

39. Texas administrative code. §22.14.291.133. Pharmacies Compounding Sterile Preparations. **https://texreg.sos.state.tx.us/public/readtac$ext.TacPage?sl=R&app=9&p_dir=&p_rloc=&p_tloc=&p_ploc=&pg=1&p_tac=&ti=22&pt=15&ch=291&rl=133**. Accessed August 8, 2023.

40. Model state pharmacy act and model rules of the national association of boards of pharmacy. National Association of Boards of Pharmacy. **https://nabp.pharmacy/members/board-resources/model-pharmacy-act-rules/**. Published August 2022. Accessed August 10, 2023.

41. Credentialing guidelines and requirements: a candidate guidebook. Pharmacy Technician Certification Board. **https://www.ptcb.org/guidebook**. Updated May 2023. Accessed August 10, 2023.

5

PERSONNEL TRAINING AND COMPETENCY EVALUATION OF GARBING AND ASEPTIC WORK PRACTICES

Linda F. McElhiney

INTRODUCTION

Contact or touch contamination is the primary cause for microbial contamination of compounded sterile preparations (CSPs).[1;2] USP Chapter <797> recognizes and requires that all compounding personnel must be properly trained and evaluated in their knowledge of USP Chapter <797> standards, proper aseptic manipulation skills (aseptic technique), personnel cleansing and garbing, and cleaning and disinfecting to prevent and minimize the risk of contact contamination of CSPs within and outside of International Organization for Standardization (ISO) Class 5 areas.[3]

PERSONNEL TRAINING

All personnel who prepare CSPs must be trained and knowledgeable in aseptic manipulations and achieving and maintaining ISO Class 5 environmental conditions before compounding sterile preparations for patients. There are several training options to learn these skills and information. However, a combination of written information, audio-visual aids, and hands-on training by expert professionals is preferred.

The first step in the training process is to have the trainee actually read USP Chapter <797> and USP Chapter <800>.[3;4] These chapters are very extensive, and the trainee may need to read them several times in order to understand all of the requirements and principles in them. It is important for personnel to have this knowledge base and understand the theoretical principles before attending a formal training program and learning the practical skills. Most training programs and seminars actually require the participants to read them and pass a written exam prior to attending the live program.

When choosing a professional training program, make sure that the focus is on USP Chapter <797> and USP Chapter <800>. The training program should also be accredited through the Accreditation Council for Pharmacy Education (ACPE). Several professional organizations (eg, American College of Apothecaries), pharmaceutical chemical wholesalers (eg, Letco Medical, Medisca, Fagron, Spectrum Pharmacy Products, Professional Compounding Centers of America), and consultants (eg, Critical Point) offer live training courses for sterile compounding and hazardous compounding with a focus on USP standards. If the facility is a 503B outsourcing facility (see Chapter 34), the training program should focus on the current good manufacturing practice (CGMP) regulations, primarily the Code of Federal Regulations Title 21 Part 210 and Part 211. These regulations are posted on the U.S. Food and Drug Administration website.[5] Although USP standards and CGMP regulations have similarities, they are specific for certain practice settings (503A or 503B), so the appropriate material for the practice setting must be taught.

Many health systems have also developed their own in-house training program in addition to using formal published training programs.[6] In-house training programs can be more cost effective and can be tailored to meet the specific needs of each health system. An expert trainer, such as an education coordinator, manager, or supervisor, should be on site to train the personnel. The site may have one expert trainer for both sterile and hazardous compounding or there may be a specific trainer for each type of compounding.

Personnel must be trained and demonstrate competency in sterile and hazardous compounding before any compounding for patients may occur. Personnel trained in sterile compounding must demonstrate competency in at least the following[3]:

- Hand hygiene
- Garbing
- Cleaning and disinfection
- Calculations, measuring, and mixing
- Aseptic technique

DOI 10.37573/9781585286492.005

- Achieving and maintaining sterility (and apyrogenicity if compounding with nonsterile components)
- Use of equipment
- Documentation of the compounding process (eg, master formulation and compounding records)
- Principles of high-efficiency particulate air (HEPA)-filtered unidirectional airflow within the ISO Class 5 area
- Proper use of primary engineering controls (PECs)
- Principles of movement of materials and personnel within the compounding area

For hazardous drug compounding, each facility or health system must have a designated person who is qualified and trained to be responsible for developing and implementing appropriate procedures, overseeing compliance with USP Chapter <800> standards and applicable regulations, ensuring the competency of personnel, and ensuring environmental control of the storage and compounding areas.[4] The Accreditation Commission for Health Care University (ACHCU), a division of the Accreditation Commission for Health Care (ACHC) offers the Pharmacy Compounding Accreditation Board (PCAB) Hazardous Drug Designated Person Certification, which covers all of the requirements for the designated person.[7]

The expert trainer for handling hazardous drugs (HDs) must understand the following[4]:

- Rationale for risk prevention policies
- Risks to themselves or others
- Risks of noncompliance that may compromise safety
- Responsibility to report potentially hazardous situations to management
- Monitoring the environment
- Maintaining records of testing and sampling and acting on the results

WRITTEN ASSESSMENT OF KNOWLEDGE

After personnel have read the standards and regulations and had didactic training, they must complete written or electronic testing to determine their level of understanding. Although USP does not state what is considered a passing grade on a written exam, this author believes that personnel should pass the exam with an 80% or higher score. The passing score should be determined before the written exam is administered. Personnel who fail the written or electronic exam must immediately be re-instructed and re-evaluated by expert compounding staff to ensure that the person understands the material and corrects all aseptic technique deficiencies.

The written exam should be developed so that it accurately assesses the person's knowledge of sterile compounding, and it should not be riddled with trick questions or double negatives.[8] There should be a clear and concise answer for each question. Avoid answers such as "all of the above," "none of the above," and "both a & b." Make sure that the answers are objective and not subject to interpretation. A good exam reflects the goals of the instruction. Use terms that are used in USP standards or CGMP regulations to be consistent. Fair written assessments should include the following:

- The overall exam should reflect the objectives of the written materials and training.
- Expectations from personnel should be clearly known.
- Each test item should present a clearly formulated task.
- One item should not aide in answering another question.
- Ample time should be allowed for completion of the test.
- Assignment of points should be determined before the test is administered.

All personnel must pass the written or electronic test initially. From then on, personnel must perform a didactic review and pass the written or electronic test for sterile and hazardous compounding annually. These tests should be kept in the personnel file as part of the training and evaluation records.

GARBING AND GLOVING COMPETENCY EVALUATION

Compounding personnel must be visually observed while performing hand hygiene and garbing procedures. To ensure that personnel are actually practicing good garbing and hand hygiene and not putting on a show, the observer may watch personnel without their knowledge. The visual observation must be documented on a form or electronically, and it must be maintained in the employee's permanent record and long-term assessment of competency.

USP Chapter <797> specifies where garb must be donned according to the category of compounding. When preparing Category 1 CSPs, all garb must be donned within the perimeter of the segregated compounding area (SCA). For Category 2 or 3 CSPs, all garb must be donned in a classified area before entering the buffer room. If hand hygiene is performed outside of the classified area, an alcohol-based hand sanitizer must be used prior to garbing. Donning and doffing in these areas should not be done at the same time.

All garb should be low-lint and powder-free. The minimum garbing requirements for Category 1 and 2 include the following[3]:

- Garment with sleeves that fit snugly around the wrists and an enclosed neck
- Shoe covers
- Cover for the head that covers hair and ears
- Cover for facial hair if applicable
- Face mask
- Sterile powder-free gloves

Category 3 includes the above requirements as well as the following additional requirements[3]:

- No exposed skin in the buffer room including face and neck
- Garb must be sterile
- Garb must not be reused (disposable garb is discarded and laundered garb must be laundered and resterilized)

Personnel must be assessed for the following requirements, and it must be documented[3]:

- Presents in clean appropriate attire and manner
- Removes all personal outer garments
- Wears no cosmetics or visible jewelry
- Wears no headphones or earbuds
- Brings no electronic devices that are not essential for compounding
- Brings no food or drinks into ante- or buffer room
- Dons personal protective equipment (PPE; eg, shoe covers, head covers, face mask, etc.) according to facility standard operating procedures (SOPs)
- Wipes eyeglasses, if worn
- Performs proper hand hygiene
- Disinfects hands again with waterless alcohol-based surgical scrub before donning sterile gloves
- Selects proper gloves and inspects them for holes and tears
- Routinely disinfects gloves using sterile 70% isopropyl alcohol (IPA) during compounding process
- Removes PPE in anteroom and properly discards
- Performs hand hygiene after compounding and doffing

All garbing competencies must consist of documented visual observation of the compounder's hand hygiene and garbing process, which is followed by collection of gloved fingertip and thumb samples from both hands.

Gloved Fingertip and Thumb Sampling

All compounding personnel must successfully complete garbing and gloving and the gloved fingertip and thumb sampling at least three consecutive times before being allowed to compound sterile preparations for human use. A passing test means absolutely no growth or zero colony forming units (CFUs) on the appropriate agar plates or paddles. These agar plates or paddles are commercially available and should be sterile so that a false positive does not result. The agar media is usually tryptic soy agar (TSA) with lecithin and polysorbate 80. The agar medium should be conducive to microorganism growth, and the lecithin and polysorbate 80 are added as neutralizing agents.

The procedure for the gloved fingertip sampling is a simple process. Immediately upon completing hand hygiene and garbing procedure, after donning the sterile gloves, and prior to disinfecting with sterile 70% IPA, the evaluator collects two samples, one for each hand. Gloves are not disinfected prior to the sampling to prevent a false negative result. The fingertips and thumb are lightly pressed onto the agar plate or paddle. The plates or paddles are securely covered, inverted, and incubated in house or by a laboratory at 30°C to 35°C for at least 48 hours and then at 20°C to 25°C for at least an additional 5 days. The gloves are discarded and replaced immediately after taking the samples.[3]

Results are documented and kept in the person's profile as a permanent record and for long-term assessment of competency. The report should include the number of CFUs per employee hand. However the CFU action level is based on the number of CFU per both hands. The CFU action level in an ISO Class 5 area is greater than 3. If the action level is exceeded, an immediate re-evaluation should be done to determine the adequacy of that person's work.

The initial three samplings may be done on the same day or done over a period of several days. However, garbing and hand hygiene must be completely performed prior to each sampling. After the initial samplings, personnel compounding Category 1 and 2 CSPs must be re-evaluated with a gowning observation and gloved fingertip and thumb samples at least every 6 months and at least every 3 months for personnel compounding Category 3 CSPs.[3]

Aseptic Manipulation Competency Evaluation via Media Fill Testing

Competency of aseptic manipulation is demonstrated during the media fill test. The test should be designed to represent the most challenging or stressful conditions actually encountered by personnel when compounding sterile preparations. For instance, if nonsterile-to-sterile preparations are being compounded, the culture media should be nonsterile and then sterilized through the testing process to mimic the most complicated similar process. USP Chapter <797> also specifies that the environment, including the number of other personnel in the buffer room or SCA, must also mirror typical conditions encountered by the compounder.

The initial media fill test should be done after successful completion of the initial hand hygiene and garbing competency evaluations. According to USP Chapter <797>, media fill evaluation for personnel compounding Category 1 and 2 must be done at least every 6 months and every 3 months for personnel compounding Category 3 CSPs.[3] Immediately after each media fill test and before gloves are sanitized or the direct compound area (DCA) is cleaned, gloved fingertip and thumb (GFT) sampling must be completed on both hands. Successful completion of a post media fill GFT is defined as no more than 3 CFUs total from both hands. Additionally, a surface sample must be collected from the DCA. In order to pass, the surface sample must also have no more than 3 CFUs per media device.

All of the evaluations should be documented, acknowledged by the evaluator and the person assessed, and maintained as part of their personnel permanent record and long-term assessment of personnel competency. The following items should be assessed and documented:

- Successfully completes hand hygiene and garbing competency
- Performs hand hygiene, garbing, and gloving according to the facility's SOPs
- Properly disinfects environment and components used in sterile compounding
- Introduces only essential materials in the ISO Class 5 area
- Does not disrupt, impede, or divert first-air flow to critical sites
- Ensures that individual packaging remains intact for needles, syringes, and tubing until opened in ISO Class 5 air
- Performs manipulations only in the appropriate DCA of the ISO Class 5 area
- Does not expose critical sites to contact contamination or worse than ISO Class 5 air
- Labels preparations correctly
- Disinfects sterile gloves routinely with sterile 70% IPA throughout the compounding process
- Cleans, sets up, calibrates, and maintains equipment, such as an automated compounding device, according to manufacturer's instructions
- Disposes of sharps and waste according to policy and guidelines

USP Chapter <797> is very specific about how to perform a media fill challenge test.[3] This test uses sterile, fluid bacterial culture media fill verification and assesses the quality of the aseptic skill of compounding personnel. There are commercial kits available to simulate sterile-to-sterile or nonsterile-to-sterile conditions. Some analytical laboratories may also provide these kits. Soybean-Casein Digest Medium is commercially available and suitable for media fill challenge testing because it is able to promote exponential colonization of bacteria that are most likely to contaminate CSPs by compounding personnel or the environment. The media fill test samples must be incubated for a minimum of 7 days at two temperatures (20°C to 25°C and 30°C to 35°C) in order to detect a broad range of microorganisms. The order of incubation temperatures must be delineated in the facility's SOPs. At both temperatures, the samples must be incubated in an incubator to assure temperature control within the specified range. Any visible turbidity during the incubation period indicates failure.

The results of media fill testing and any corrective actions must be documented. The documentation must be maintained to provide a record and long-term assessment of personnel competency. Documentation must include the following at a minimum[3]:

- Name of the person evaluated
- Evaluation date and time
- Media and components used, including manufacturer, expiration date, and lot number
- Starting temperature for each interval of incubation
- Dates of incubation
- Results after incubation
- Identification of the observer and the person who reads and documents the results

Personnel who fail a media fill challenge must be immediately re-instructed and re-evaluated by expert compounding personnel to ensure correction of all aseptic practice deficiencies.

Cleaning and Disinfecting Competency Evaluation

The compounding environment suitable for preparing CSPs can be inadvertently contaminated through touch by compounding personnel. All compounding personnel must maintain a suitable microbially controlled environment for compounding CSPs. Compounding personnel and other personnel responsible for cleaning and disinfecting this environment must be visually observed during the process of cleaning and disinfecting procedures, during the initial personnel training on cleaning procedures, during changes in cleaning staff, and at the completion of any media fill testing.

Training on cleaning and disinfecting procedures and assessment of initial and ongoing competency must be defined in the facility's SOPs. Training and evaluation must support compliance with USP Chapter <797> and the facility's specific SOPs. Evaluations must be documented, acknowledged by the evaluator and the person assessed, and maintained as part of the personnel permanent record and long-term assessment of personnel competency.

See Chapter 14 for a detailed discussion of cleaning and disinfecting requirements.

Additional Requirements for Hazardous Compounding

All of the requirements for sterile compounding also apply to compounding sterile HDs. However, there are additional requirements for hazardous compounding that should be evaluated for competency. All personnel who handle HDs must understand the following:

- Fundamental practices and precautions for handling HDs
- Continuous evaluation and monitoring of the environment, procedures, and quality of final HDs to prevent harm to patients, minimize exposure to personnel, and minimize contamination of the work and patient environment

Personnel who handle HDs must be trained based on their job function. Some personnel may only transport and deliver HDs and may not require training in sterile compounding. However, they still need to be trained in proper use of PPE, know how to respond to known or suspected HD exposure, and spill management. Before personnel are allowed to independently handle HDs, training must occur and competency must be demonstrated. Personnel competency must be re-assessed at least every 12 months. It can coincide with other sterile compounding competencies since some of them may overlap. Personnel must also be trained prior to the introduction of a new hazardous product or equipment used to prepare HDs and prior to a new or significant change in a process or SOP for handling HDs. Training must include the following[4]:

- Overview of the facility or health system's list of HDs and their risks
- Review of the SOPs related to handling HDs
- Proper use of PPE
- Proper use of equipment and devices
- Response to known or suspected HD exposure
- Spill management
- Proper disposal of HDs and trace-contaminated materials

In addition to the applicable requirements for sterile compounding, personnel should be assessed initially and at least every 12 months for the following when handling HDs:

- Proper use of closed system drug-transfer devices (CSTDs) and other devices or equipment used for HDs
- Garbing and gloving with proper disposable gowns; American Society for Testing and Materials (ASTM) standard D6978 gloves (2 pairs); head, hair, shoe, and sleeve covers; eye and face protection; and respiratory protection
- Deactivation, decontamination, cleaning, and disinfection of environment and equipment
- Spill management
- Proper disposal of HDs and contaminated materials

The expert trainer for handling HDs is responsible for developing assessment forms. Again, these assessments should be permanently maintained in personnel files to demonstrate competencies for handling HDs.

Summary

The quality of CSPs relies on the compounder, not just the equipment and environment. Compounding personnel are often the source of contamination for compounded sterile preparations. All personnel responsible for compounding sterile preparations must be properly trained and knowledgeable in USP Chapter <797> and USP Chapter <800> standards, aseptic technique and manipulations, hand hygiene and garbing, maintaining an ISO Class 5 environment, and cleaning and disinfecting. Monitoring these activities through routine and continuous evaluation is an essential part of a good quality assurance program (see Chapter 33 for information on quality assurance programs).

REFERENCES

1. Trissel LA, Gentempo JA, Saenz LM, et al. Effect of two work practice changes on the microbial contamination rates of pharmacy-compounded sterile preparations. *Am J Health Syst Pharm*. 2007;64(8):837–841. doi:10.2146/060199.
2. Thomas M, Sanborn MD, Couldry R. I.V. admixture contamination rates: traditional practice site versus a class 1000 cleanroom. *Am J Health Syst Pharm*. 2005;62(22):2386–2392. doi:10.2146/ajhp050078.
3. USP <797> Pharmaceutical compounding—sterile preparations. In: *2023: USP Compounding Compendium*. Rockville, MD: United States Pharmacopeial Convention; 2023; Issue 1. **https://doi.org/10.31003/USPNF_M99925_07_01**.
4. USP <800> Hazardous drugs—handling in healthcare settings. In: *2020: USP Compounding Compendium*. Rockville, MD: United States Pharmacopeial Convention; July 1, 2020. **https://doi.org/10.31003/USPNF_M7808_07_01**.

5. U.S. Food and Drug Administration (FDA). Current Good Manufacturing Practice (CGMP) regulations. **https://www.fda.gov/drugs/pharmaceutical-quality-resources/current-good-manufacturing-practice-cgmp-regulations**. Accessed August 11, 2023.

6. American Society of Health-System Pharmacists. Compounding Sterile Preparations Competency Library. **https://elearning.ashp.org/subscriptions/1001/ashp-sterile-compounding-competency-library**. Accessed April 14, 2023.

7. Accreditation Commission for Health Care. PCAB hazardous drug designated person certification. ACHCU Website. **https://achcu.com/hdhdp**. Accessed September 5, 2023.

8. Clay B. *Is This a Trick Question? A Short Guide to Writing Effective Test Questions*. Kansas Curriculum Center, October 2001. **www.k-state.edu/ksde/alp/resources/Handout-Module6.pdf**. Accessed September 5, 2023.

SECTION 3: Engineering Controls and Equipment

DOI 10.37573/9781585286492

6

PRIMARY ENGINEERING CONTROLS

Richard C. Capps

INTRODUCTION

A primary engineering control (PEC) is "a device or zone that provides an International Organization for Standardization (ISO) Class 5 air quality environment for sterile compounding."[1] PECs are commonly referred to simply as "hoods." The purpose of the primary engineering controls is to provide protection of the compounded sterile preparation (CSP) from airborne contamination and, in the case of hazardous drugs (HDs), to ensure containment of the hazardous agents for the protection of patients, personnel, and the environment. The concepts of protection and containment must be designed into the engineering controls used for sterile compounding. USP Chapter <797>, Pharmaceutical Compounding—Sterile preparations[1] and USP Chapter <800> Hazardous Drugs—Handling in Healthcare Setting[2] set the requirements for the engineering controls used for sterile compounding.

All PECs used for sterile compounding must provide: 1) ISO Class 5 or better air quality, 2) unidirectional airflow, and 3) maintained, appropriate air pressure relationships relative to the buffer area in which the PEC is placed. Containment primary engineering controls (C-PECs), used when compounding hazardous drugs, have the additional requirements of operating under negative pressure and being externally exhausted. PECs and C-PECs are available in a variety of styles and configurations to meet a facility's needs but all the designs appropriate for sterile compounding must have these characteristics and must meet the standards to maintain the required compounding environment.

HEPA FILTERS

The first characteristic of PECs is that they must provide an ISO Class 5 air quality environment for sterile compounding. This is achieved through high-efficiency particulate air (HEPA) filtration using HEPA filters within the PEC. The Institute of Environmental Sciences and Technology (IEST) defines a HEPA filter as, "An extended-medium, dry-type filter in a rigid frame, having a minimum particle collection efficiency of 99.97% for particles with a mass median diameter of 0.3-μm when tested at a rated airflow in accordance with MIL STD 282 using the Institute of Environmental Sciences and Technology (IEST) Recommended Standard RP-CC0001.5."[2,3] When filter manufacturers efficiency-test their filters, they test at what is referred to as the most penetrating particle size (MPPS). The MPPS is "The particle size at which a given filter has its highest penetration (or lowest efficiency); i.e., the worst-case particle size with respect to filtration efficiency."[3] Particles larger than the most penetrating size are filtered more effectively through impaction, interception, and sieving. Particle collection through diffusion (or Brownian motion) favors particles smaller than the MPPS. When referring to the efficiency of a HEPA filter, it is not accurate to state "down to 0.3 micron" because particles below that size are generally removed at a higher efficiency than the filter rating. (See **Figure 6-1**.)

HEPA filters have been proven effective in removing most particulate contamination. As an example, they are very effective in removing virus particles that are smaller than 0.3 micron. They are not, however, effective at filtering gases and vapors.[4,5] As part of a containment strategy, USP Chapter <800> requires that all C-PECs used for compounding hazardous drugs must be vented to the outside.[2]

The HEPA filter in a PEC must be leak tested to no more than 0.1% penetration. Because a HEPA filter is "at least 99.97% efficient on 0.3-micron particles," this allows for up to 0.03% penetration. Consequently, a HEPA filter does not necessarily have to be leak free if the overall penetration does not exceed the filter rating. An accumulation of multiple leaks in a filter can occur and the overall efficiency still be within 99.97%. Leaks and penetrations of a HEPA filter may be patched. According to CAG-002-2006, "Filter patch size shall not exceed 3% of the effective filter area of the side being patched. The maximum width of any one patch shall not exceed 1.5 inches (3.8cm)."[6]

HEPA filters are available in many filter types with C, J, and K common in pharmacy compounding environments. To ensure a replacement filter meets the required performance

DOI 10.37573/9781585286492.006

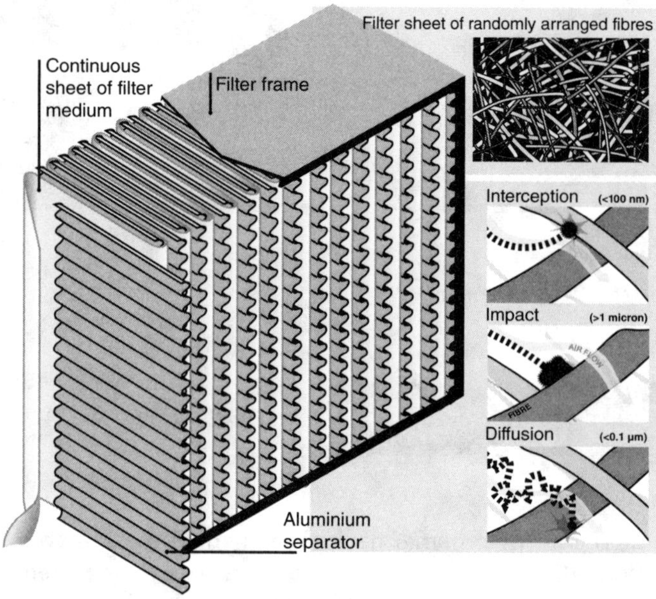

FIGURE 6-1. HEPA filter diagram

Source: Reprinted with permission of LadyofHats (public domain). https://commons.wikimedia.org/w/index.php?curid=4552953. Accessed April 6, 2023.

TABLE 6-1. ISO Classification of Particulate Matter in Room Air

ISO Class	Maximum Particle Count (Particles of 0.5 µm and Larger in Size) per Cubic Meter of Air
3	35.2
4	352
5	3,520
6	35,200
7	352,000
8	3,520,000

Source: Adapted with permission of International Organization for Standardization (ISO). *ISO 14644-1: Cleanroom and associated control environments.* Geneva, Switzerland: International Organization for Standardization; 1999.

expectations (eg, efficiency, frame, airflow, and pressure rating), be certain to consult a qualified certifier and the manufacturer before purchasing a replacement HEPA filter for a PEC or C-PEC.

CLASSIFICATION OF AIR CLEANLINESS

Classification of air cleanliness is described in the international standard ISO 14644-1.[7] This standard replaced the Federal Standard 209E. ISO 14644-1 defines the level of airborne particulate cleanliness applicable to a cleanroom or clean zone, expressed in terms of an ISO Class *N*, which represents the maximum allowable concentrations in particles per cubic meter of air for considered sizes of particles. The concentration of particles defined in Fed. Std. 209E was the same concentration of particles as the current ISO standard, but the volume was based on a cubic foot of air versus a cubic meter of air (see **Table 6-1**). When specifying a cleanliness class, one must specify the appropriate particle size. Clean zones can be classified by particle sizes ranging from 0.1 micron to 5 microns. For the purposes of USP Chapter <797> and USP Chapter <800>, the 0.5-micron particle size is used.[1,2] PECs must meet the ISO Class 5 standard under dynamic operating conditions. No more than 3,520 0.5-micron and larger particles per cubic meter (ie, 100 particles per cubic foot for Fed. Std. 209E) can be counted while using an electronic discrete particle counter. When a test is performed under "dynamic operating conditions" it means that the test occurred when the environment is in use and not under static conditions. "The conditions should reflect the largest number of personnel and highest complexity of compounding expected during routine operation as determined by the designated person(s)."[1]

In addition to particle count sample locations dictated by ISO 1644-1, USP Chapter <797> requires that dynamic airflow smoke pattern tests be taken during dynamic operating conditions in each PEC to "demonstrate unidirectional airflow and sweeping action over and away from the preparation(s)."[1] Particle count classification of the PEC must be performed initially and recertified every six months. Counts must be completed under dynamic operating conditions. It is important that the certifier and designated person(s) work together to accommodate the testing.

UNIDIRECTIONAL AIRFLOW

Unidirectional airflow is the second characteristic of all PECs. USP Chapter <797> states:

> Unidirectional airflow must be maintained in the PEC. HEPA-filtered air must be supplied by the PEC at a velocity sufficient to sweep particles away from critical sites and maintain unidirectional airflow during operations. Proper design, control, and use minimizes turbulence and creation of eddies or stagnant air in the PEC...[1]

Proper design will create and maintain a continuous flow of HEPA-filtered air across the work zone. HEPA-filtered air is often referred to as "clean air." By providing continuous airflow in one direction and using well-placed air returns, PECs can sweep process-generated particulates from the work area and prevent influx of environmental contamination from the surrounding area. **Figure 6-2** demonstrates this air movement. In an enclosed space such as a biological safety cabinet (BSC) or a restricted-access barrier

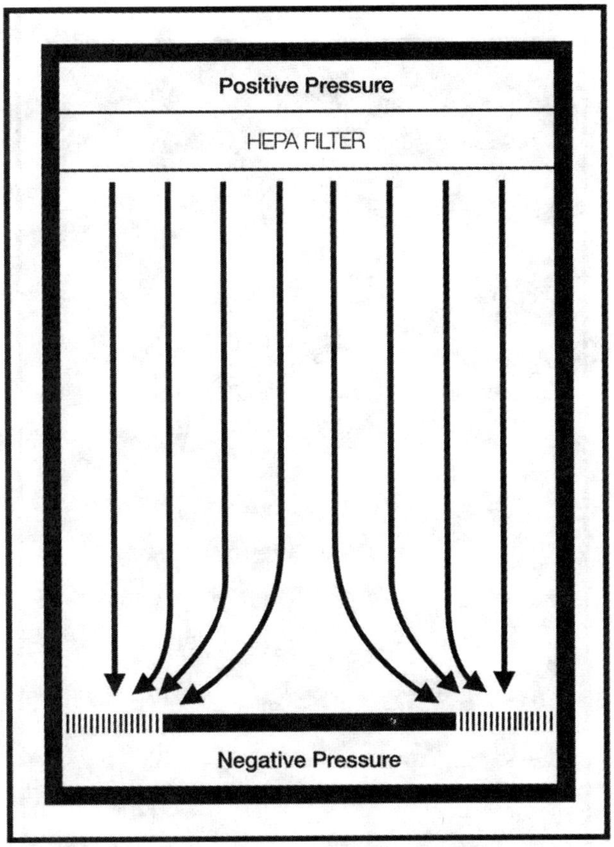

FIGURE 6-2. Unidirectional airflow

Source: Reprinted with permission of Tyler E. Berkey.

system (RABS), the design and placement of the air return or exhaust grilles are as important as the design of the supply air diffusers. Placement of materials within the compounding area and process manipulations must be carefully planned to take advantage of the unidirectional airflow and ensure critical sites are bathed in clean air. The supply HEPA filter pushes the air into the work area and the return grilles pull the air across the work area eliminating turbulence and removing process-generated contaminants. In an open PEC, such as a laminar airflow workbench (LAFW), the velocity of the airflow is important because in addition to pushing particulates out of the LAFW, the airflow also prevents room air from entering the PEC and compromising the air quality of the work area within the device.

DIRECT COMPOUNDING AREA AND FIRST AIR

USP Chapter <797> defines the direct compounding area (DCA) as "A critical area within the ISO Class 5 PEC where critical sites are exposed to unidirectional HEPA-filtered air, also known as first air."[1] Chapter <797> defines first air as "The air exiting the HEPA filter in a unidirectional air stream."[1]

Many of the processes employed during compounding of sterile preparations create particulate contamination. For example, opening and removing the overwrap from sterile syringes and needles creates thousands of particles.[8] The PEC must be designed so that a particle-free stream of HEPA filtered air sweeps across the DCA without re-entrainment, refluxing, or creating dead air zones that prevent the removal of process-generated contamination from the critical area. Open devices, such as LAFWs, push the particles out of the DCA past the operator's body to the room and then eventually to the air returns of the room. Recirculated and exhausted devices with defined and directed airflow such as a BSC or a RABS pull the particles from the DCA to well-placed air grilles positioned at the opposite end of the DCA from the HEPA filter. The DCA is the only portion of the ISO Class 5 work area dedicated to the task of aseptic manipulation. The unidirectional airflow prevents cross-contamination from adjacent areas within the ISO Class work area.

A properly designed PEC will provide ISO Class 5, unidirectional airflow across the DCA. Regardless of the type of PEC used—horizontal versus vertical, open-faced versus RABS—compounders must understand the principles of unidirectional airflow and develop proper work practices to maintain first air in the DCA while compounding. An important role of the designated person is to ensure the standard operating procedures and work practices of compounding personnel utilize these principles to protect CSPs from contamination. An understanding of the principles of unidirectional airflow to maintain first air within the DCA must be part of the initial and ongoing training and competency assessments of all compounding personnel. Observation of smoke studies within the PEC, either directly or via video recording, can be a very useful training tool to help personnel visualize and understand the patterns of air movement.

AIR PRESSURE MANAGEMENT

The third characteristic of all PECs is that they maintain appropriate air pressure relationships relative to the buffer area in which the PEC is placed. Maintaining positive or negative air pressure within the PEC or C-PEC is an important attribute of the device because these pressure differentials aid in the protection of the CSP from contamination by less clean air from outside the PEC or help ensure the containment of hazardous drugs within the C-PEC. A positive pressure PEC maintains a higher pressure than the room in which it is located and therefore prevents room air from entering the device. A negative pressure C-PEC maintains a lower pressure than the room in which it is located and therefore prevents potentially contaminated air from escaping into the room and surrounding environment. The pressure differential between the PEC/C-PEC and the room or the individual compartments within a RABS or pharmaceutical isolator are defined by the manufacturer for optimal results. Confirming the ongoing achievement of the defined pressure differentials is an important component of the semiannual certification process. The compounding staff should have an awareness of the defined pressure differentials and notify the designated person if the pressures fall outside of the correct range.

REQUIREMENTS OF CONTAINMENT PRIMARY ENGINEERING CONTROLS

Containment primary engineering controls must meet the standards set forth in USP Chapter <800>.[2] The standards of USP Chapter <800> include the design and operation of the primary and secondary engineering controls, additional training, and well-defined work practices. The goal of USP Chapter <800> is to protect workers and the environment from harm caused by exposure to hazardous drugs. C-PECs achieve this

> ...by controlling emissions of airborne contaminants through the following:
>
> - The full or partial enclosure of a potential contaminant source
> - The use of airflow capture velocities to trap and remove airborne contaminants near the point of generation
> - The use of air pressure relationships that define the direction of airflow into the cabinet
> - The use of HEPA filtration on all potentially contaminated exhaust streams.[2]

TYPES OF PRIMARY ENGINEERING CONTROLS

USP Chapter <797> describes three types of PECs used for sterile compounding. These include laminar airflow systems (LAFS), restricted-access barrier systems (RABS), and pharmaceutical isolators. Both RABS and pharmaceutical isolators are enclosure devices that separate room air from the compounding environment within the PEC/C-PEC. The configuration and installation of the device will determine if it is suitable for use with hazardous drugs.[1]

LAMINAR AIRFLOW SYSTEMS

A laminar airflow system (LAFS) is a device or zone that provides an ISO Class 5 or better air quality environment for sterile compounding. The system provides unidirectional HEPA-filtered airflow across the compounding area and is designed to minimize the risk of contamination of the compounding area by less clean air. Types of LAFS include laminar airflow workbenches (LAFWs), integrated vertical laminar flow zones (IVLFZs), and biological safety cabinets (BSCs).

LAMINAR AIRFLOW WORKBENCHES

A laminar airflow workbench (LAFW) is the simplest of the primary engineering control devices (see **Figures 6-3**, **6-4**, and **6-5**). Air is drawn through a prefilter into a blower then blown into a plenum where the air finally passes through a HEPA filter and through a partially enclosed work surface.

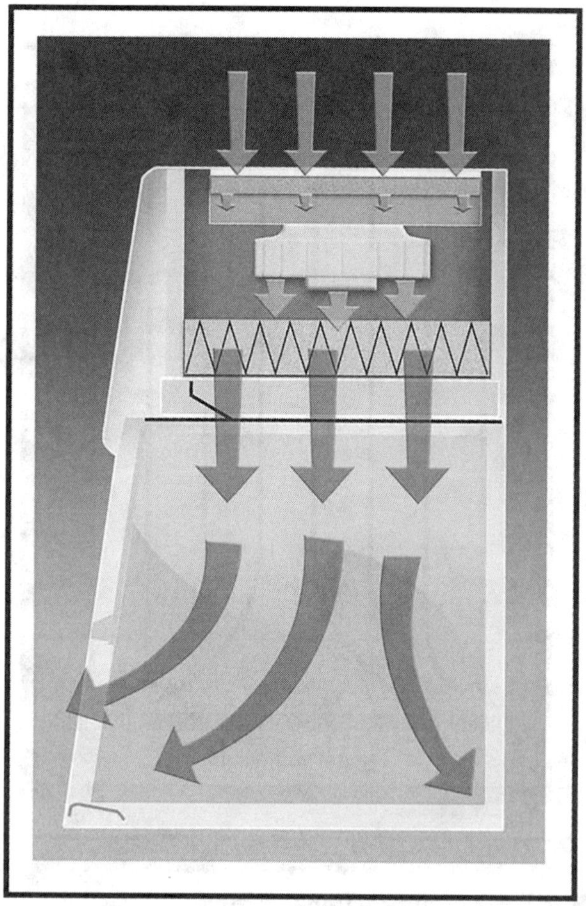

FIGURE 6-3. Vertical laminar airflow

Source: Reprinted with permission of Labconco Corporation.

Using unidirectional airflow, the filtered air sweeps the work area providing an ISO Class 5 environment for sterile compounding. The air washes across the work area and the product, sweeping particulates away, before discharging into the room. This basic design has been the cornerstone of contamination control since the development of the HEPA filter. An LAFW must not be used when compounding hazardous drugs. The airflow typically blows directly into the face of the operator, making it the worst possible choice for compounding anything hazardous.

LAFWs are available as both horizontal and vertical flow devices. The type of operation and equipment used in the compounding process should be considered when deciding if a horizontal or vertical flow device is appropriate for the compounding process. Some automated equipment may work better in one direction of airflow than it does in another. Consider how the aseptic operations or connections (ie, attaching tubing to an automated compounding device) are made and then determine which airflow direction is better for ensuring clean air is maintained across the critical sites when in use.

Regardless of whether a horizontal or vertical LAFW is used, it is imperative that personnel using the LAFW are aware of the direction of airflow and take this into consideration

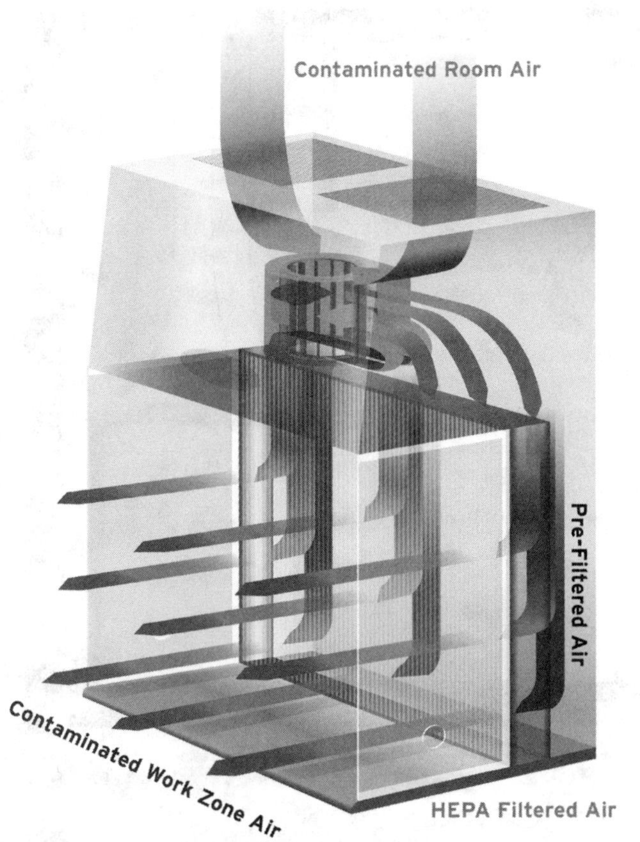

FIGURE 6-4. Blower above horizontal LAFW work surface
Source: Reprinted with permission of Nuaire, Inc.

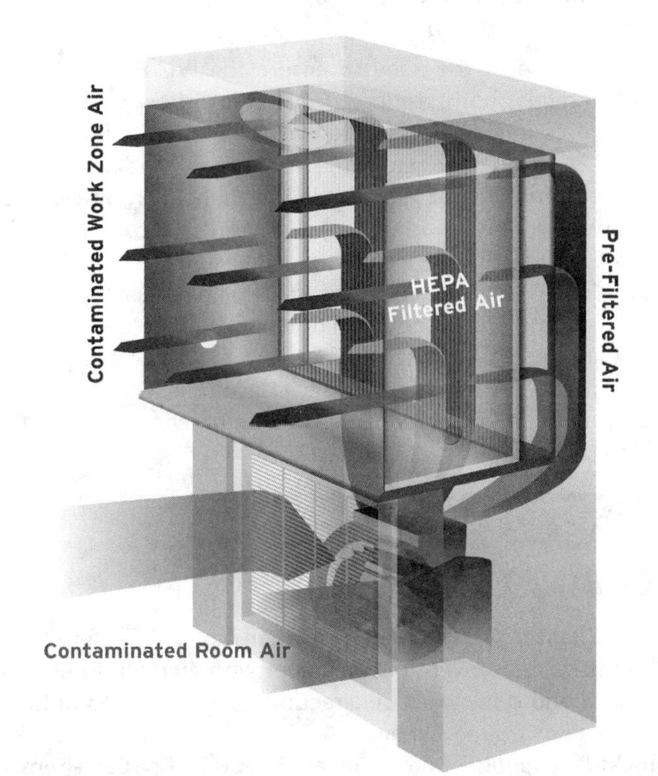

FIGURE 6-5. Blower below horizontal LAFW work surface
Source: Reprinted with permission of Nuaire, Inc.

when setting up their workspace and performing aseptic manipulations. Using airflow visualization techniques such as smoke studies is an excellent way to demonstrate airflow characteristics within a PEC and to optimize routine manipulations and equipment setup. Ensuring compounders have an awareness of the airflow characteristics of the PEC helps prevent contaminated air reaching critical sites caused by improper hand placement and disrupted airflow.

Vertical laminar airflow workbenches (VLFs) are available in a variety of configurations. In all cases, the air is delivered from above the work surface, passes downward through the DCA, splits just before the surface, and exits the work area by flowing either towards the front or rear of the work deck (see Figure 6-3).

Laminar airflow workbenches are available with the blower placed above or below the work surface. Both have benefits and drawbacks that need to be considered.

Blower Above the Work Surface

This setup may be placed on an adjustable table that can be raised or lowered to accommodate different height compounders (see Figure 6-4). Cleaning under an open stand is easier than an enclosed base. Since the blower/motor is placed closer to the operator's ears, they may be slightly louder than units with bottom mounted blowers. Access to the top of the device for changing prefilters may be more difficult with an above the work surface device. Because the device pulls air from higher in the room, it will pull more HEPA supplied air and contribute less to the overall air cleanliness of the SEC.

Blower Below the Work Surface

This setup does not easily accommodate adjustable work surface heights. These LAFWs may, however, be ordered with a variety of base and wheel configurations to customize the final height of the work surface to accommodate staff or the planned use of the device. A device with the motor below the work surface may be slightly quieter to the operator (see Figure 6-5). Access to the prefilters may be simplified with this design. Placement of the air intake under the work surface has the advantage of pulling particulates from close to floor height allowing the PEC to serve as an additional low air return for the room.

INTEGRATED VERTICAL LAMINAR FLOW ZONE

"An integrated vertical laminar flow zone (IVLFZ) is a designated ISO Class 5 area serving as the PEC within an ISO Class 7 or cleaner buffer room. In the IVLFZ, unidirectional airflow is created by placing HEPA filters over the entire surface of the worktables and effective placement of air returns."[1] A ceiling mounted physical barrier separates the HEPA-filtered air of the IVLFZ from the ISO Class 7 air of the buffer room and directs the airflow downward over the work area. For an IVLFZ to be effective, the entire area over the

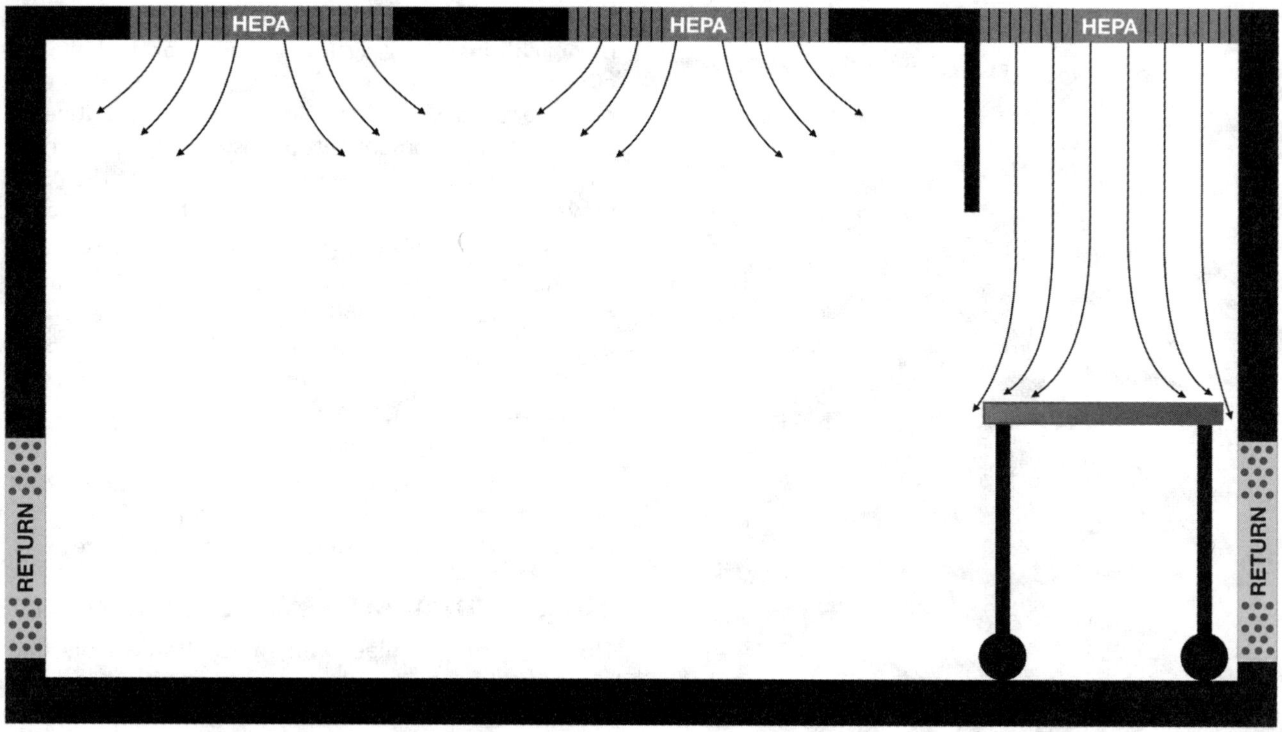

FIGURE 6-6. Diagram of a properly functioning IVLFZ

Source: Reprinted with permission of Tyler E. Berkey.

work surface (ie, the area between the physical barrier and the walls) must be fully covered with HEPA filters and the low air returns behind the work surface must be strategically placed and properly balanced to ensure uninterrupted airflow across the DCA. (See **Figure 6-6**.)

Proper air balancing is critical for the success of an IVLFZ. The HEPA filtered air must bathe the entire work surface in clean air and prevent less clean air from entering the compounding area. Creating proper airflow in an open vertical airflow environment is more difficult than in a closed system such as a CAI or in an open system such as a LAFW. Visualize the challenge created by blowing air downward over the work surface by thinking of moving a cooked spaghetti noodle across a table. If you push the noodle, it will twist and turn and move randomly but not necessarily where you want it to go. If you also pull the noodle, it will be directed to go wherever you want. So, the best way to direct the air in an IVLFZ is to push it from above and use the low air returns in the wall below the work surface to pull the air away. The amount of air passing behind the table must be properly balanced. Too much air may be drawn to the rear of the work surface if the air returns and/or if the gap between the wall and the work surface is too large. This configuration may allow the ISO Class 7 air of the buffer room to be drawn over the DCA. If there is too little air being drawn into the air return and/or the gap between the work surface and the wall is too small, then not enough air will pass behind the work surface. This may result in turbulence, dead air zones, and refluxing of the HEPA-filtered air over the work surface. (See **Figures 6-7** and **6-8**).

Because of the need to ensure the IVLFZ is performing correctly, both static and dynamic airflow smoke pattern tests must be performed verifying a continuous flow of HEPA-filtered air across the entire work area and to the air returns while not allowing any surrounding room air into the work area (eg, with video). Maintaining a consistent air gap between the work surfaces and the wall is critical and there should be a means to ensure the gap remains the same during routine use and cleaning. Smoke studies should be repeated when the work surfaces are moved or equipment within the PEC is changed. Because of the way an IVLFZ operates, it must never be used for the preparation of hazardous drugs.

CLASS II BIOLOGICAL SAFETY CABINETS

USP Chapter <797> defines a Class II biological safety cabinet (BSC) as: "A ventilated cabinet with an open front and inward and downward unidirectional HEPA-filtered airflow and HEPA-filtered exhaust. A BSC used to prepare a CSP must be capable of providing an ISO Class 5 or better environment for preparation of the CSPs."[1]

Figure 6-9 shows how room air is drawn into the front grille of the cabinet preventing the escape of HD

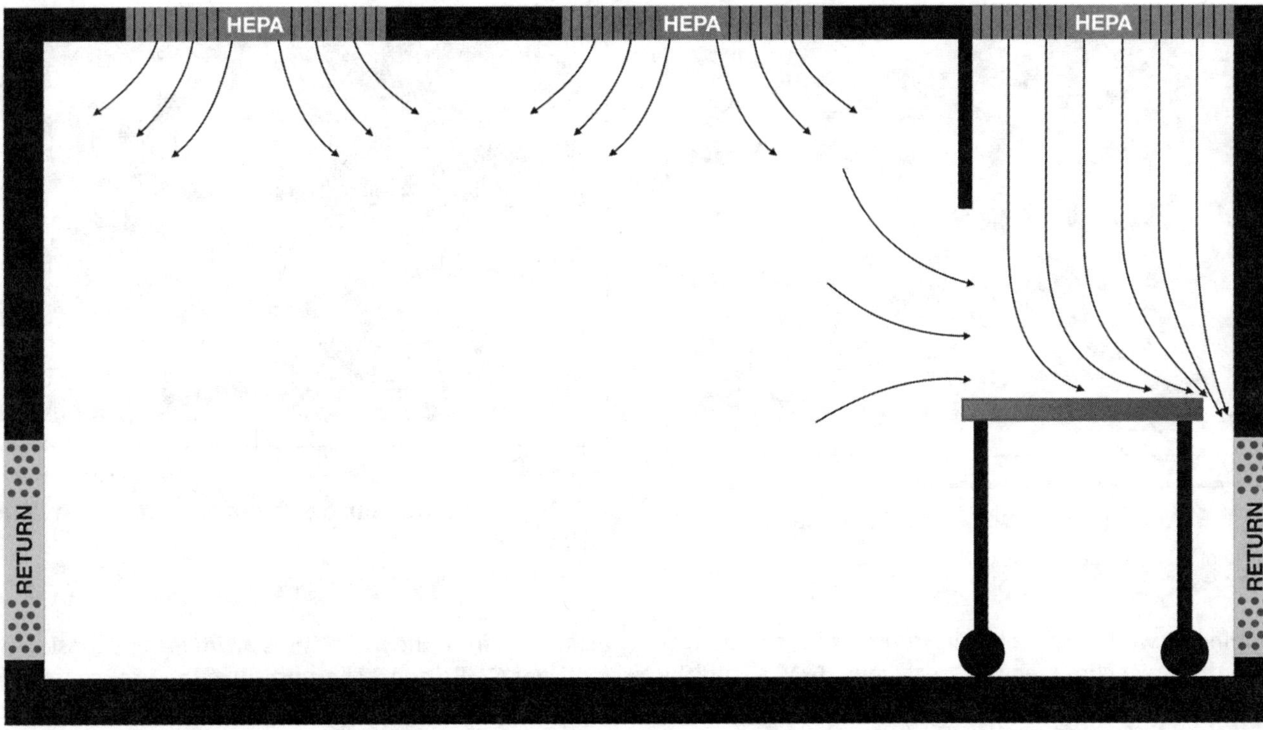

FIGURE 6-7. Diagram of an improperly balanced IVLFZ

Source: Reprinted with permission of Tyler E. Berkey.

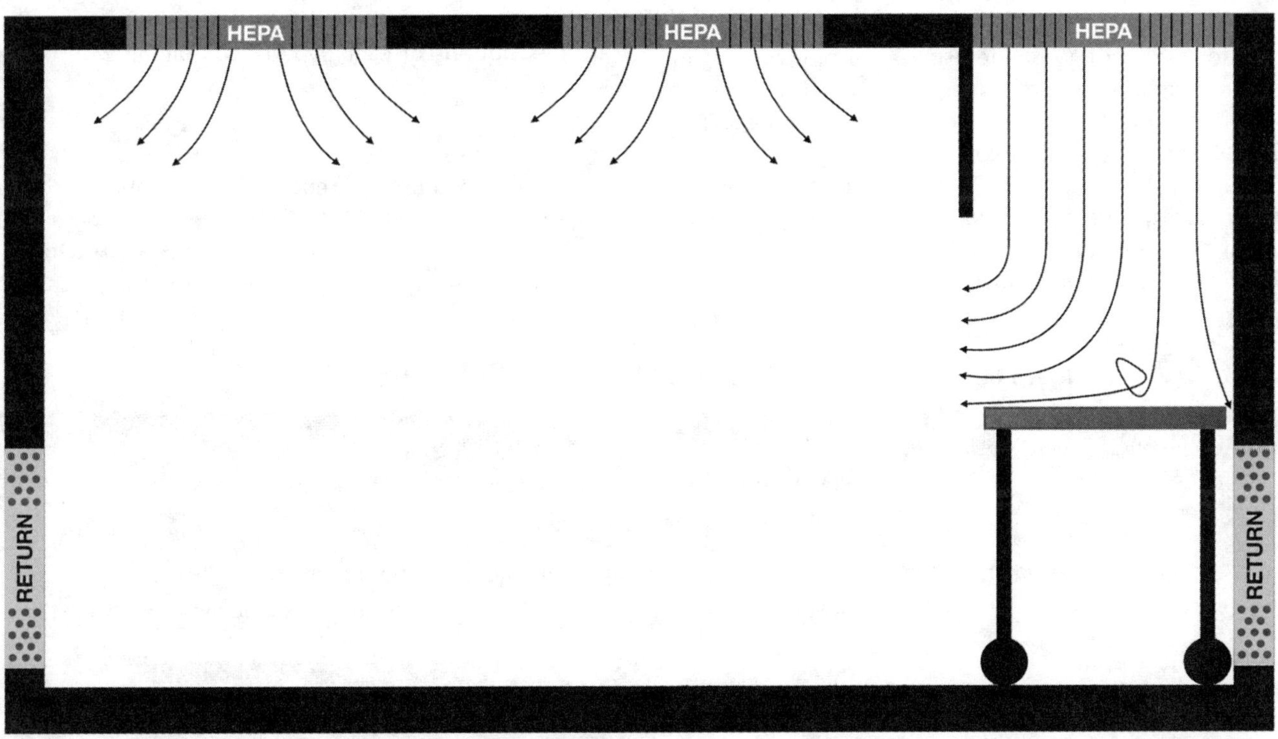

FIGURE 6-8. Diagram of an improperly balanced IVLFZ

Source: Reprinted with permission of Tyler E. Berkey.

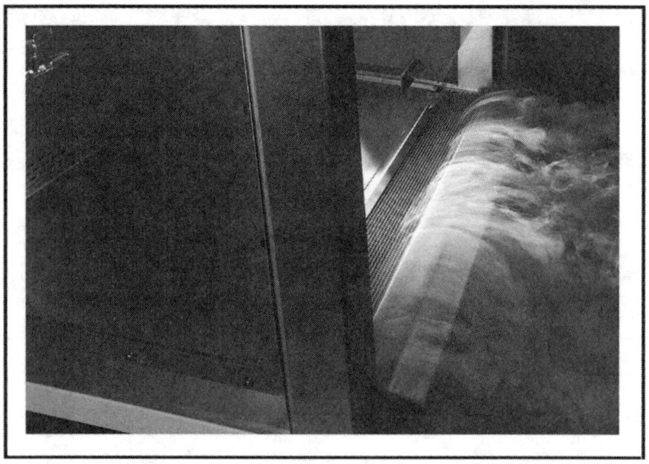

FIGURE 6-9. Demonstration of a BSC air barrier

Source: Reprinted with permission of Nuaire, Inc.

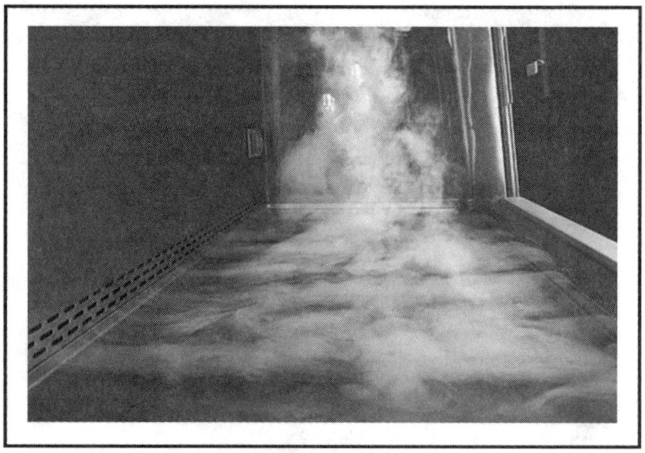

FIGURE 6-10. Demonstration of proper air movement within a BSC

Source: Reprinted with permission of Nuaire, Inc.

contaminants while also preventing room air from encroaching into the direct compounding area. **Figure 6-10** shows the ISO Class 5 air passing vertically from the HEPA filter to the work surface before splitting and exiting through the front and rear grilles.

The industry standard for Class II BSCs is NSF/ANSI Standard 49:2020.[9] Within Class II, there are four types of BSCs listed in USP Chapter <800>. The need for different types is due to limitations of HEPA filters combined with the most energy efficient configuration. Type A BSCs allow for the cabinets to be vented directly into the room but have the option of venting outside using a canopy connection. There are operating cost advantages to venting air back into the room so, when possible, that is a good choice. Type B BSCs must be vented to the outside through a hard connection. Type A1, A2, and B1 BSCs recirculate a percentage of air through the supply HEPA filter back into the workspace of the cabinet before exhausting air from the device. (See **Table 6-2**.) The recirculating air means that less air is exhausted from the BSC. This is an important consideration for Types A2, B1, and B2 because all of the air exhausted from the BSC must be replaced by air from the surrounding room and the building HVAC system. The amount of exhausted air must be accounted for when planning the negative pressure buffer room to ensure the correct negative pressure and ISO air classification of the room are achieved. If the BSC is to be used for preparing HDs, it is classified as a *containment* primary engineering control (C-PEC) and must be externally vented and located in a properly designed containment secondary engineering control (see Chapter 7). The following are descriptions of each type of BSC along with potential applications.

Class II Type A1

This design is mostly intended for recirculation back into the room (see **Figure 6-11**). These are not commonly used in pharmacies but will be found in a lab setting. While an A1 can be exhausted outdoors through a canopy connection,

TABLE 6-2. Comparison of Class II Biological Safety Cabinets

Type	Face Velocity	Acceptable for HDs	Airflow Pattern	Exhaust Connection
A1	75 fpm	No	70% recirculated through HEPA filter 30% exhausted through filter	Into room
A2	100 fpm	Yes (when exhausted outside)	70% recirculated through HEPA filter 30% exhausted through HEPA filter	Into room for non-HDs Through canopy connection to the outdoors for HDs
B1	100 fpm	Yes	30–40% recirculated through HEPA filter 60–70% exhausted through HEPA filter	Through hard connection to the outdoors
B2	100 fpm	Yes	100% exhausted through HEPA filter	Through hard connection to the outdoors

HEPA = high-efficiency particulate air; HDs = hazardous drugs.

Source: Adapted with permission of Chosewood LC, Wilson DE. Appendix A – Primary containment for biohazards: selection, installation and use of biological safety cabinets. In: *Biosafety in Microbiological and Biomedical Laboratories.* 5th ed. Washington, DC: U.S. Department of Health and Human Services; 2009. https://www.cdc.gov/labs/pdf/CDC-BiosafetyMicrobiologicalBiomedicalLaboratories-2009-P.PDF. Accessed April 6, 2023.

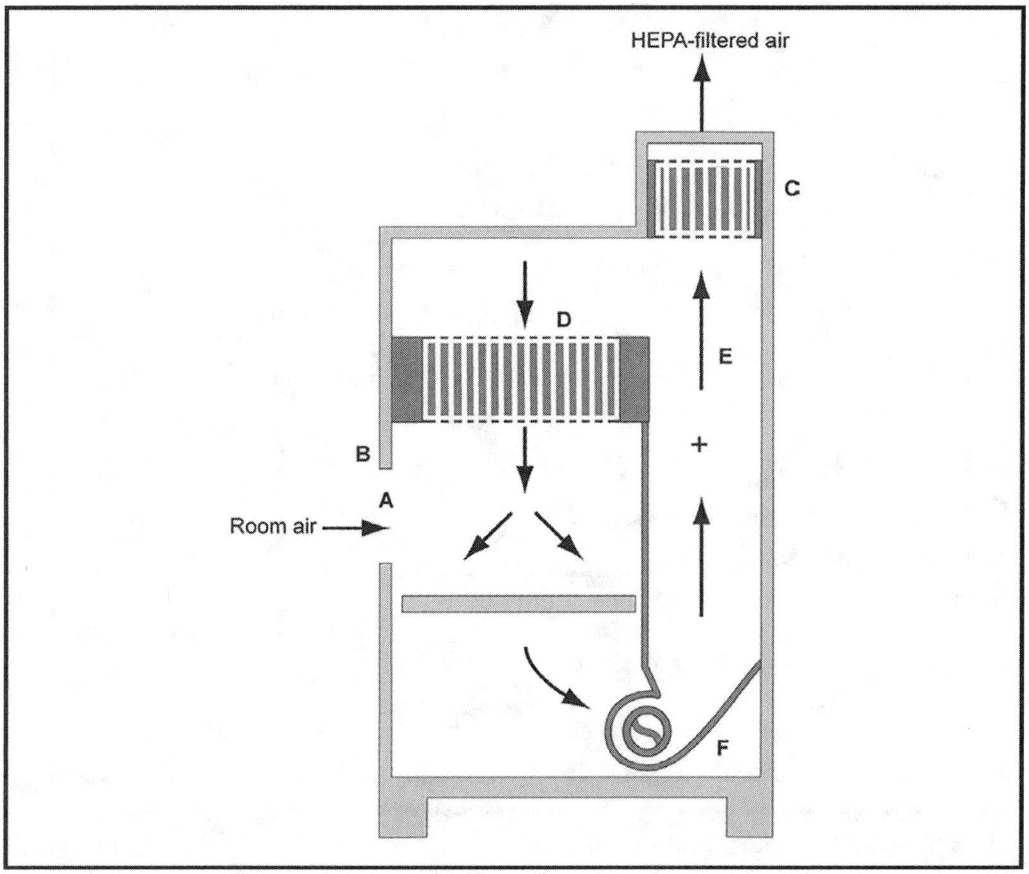

FIGURE 6-11. Class II type A1 biological safety cabinet

A = front opening; B = sash; C = exhaust HEPA filter; D = supply HEPA filter; E = common plenum; F = blower

Source: Reprinted with permission of Chosewood LC, Wilson DE. Appendix A – Primary containment for biohazards: selection, installation and use of biological safety cabinets. In: *Biosafety in Microbiological and Biomedical Laboratories.* 5th ed. Washington, DC: U.S. Department of Health and Human Services; 2009. https://www.cdc.gov/labs/pdf/CDC-BiosafetyMicrobiologicalBiomedicalLaboratories-2009-P.PDF. Accessed April 6, 2023.

it is not to be used with any volatile hazardous materials. This cabinet has HEPA-filtered down-flow air that is a portion of the mixed down-flow and inflow air from a common plenum. This design is not acceptable for hazardous applications because it may have positive pressure contaminated ducts and plenums that are not surrounded by negative pressure plenums. In the event there is a leak in the cabinet itself, it will leak into the room. The minimum intake velocity for this cabinet is 75 feet per minute (fpm) while all cabinets intended for use with toxic or volatile hazardous materials have a minimum intake velocity of 100 fpm. This cabinet design is not recognized by USP Chapter <800> as appropriate for compounding HDs. It works well as a vertical laminar airflow platform for compounding nonhazardous drugs.

Class II Type A2

This design is similar to the A1 design with a few caveats. Like the A1, this cabinet has HEPA-filtered down-flow air that is a portion of the mixed down-flow and inflow air from a common plenum (see **Figure 6-12**). Vendor designs vary but approximately 70% of the air flow is recirculated through the supply HEPA filter and 30% passes through the exhaust HEPA filter. The A2 requires all biologically contaminated ducts and plenums to be under negative pressure or surrounded by negative pressure ducts and plenums. With this design, in the event of a leak in the cabinet itself, it will leak into the cabinet and not escape into the room. The minimum inflow velocity of an A2 is 100 fpm. It may exhaust HEPA-filtered air into the room when used for nonhazardous compounding or to the outside environment through an exhaust canopy when used for HD compounding. All A2 cabinets that exhaust to the outside must have a canopy connection (see **Figure 6-13**) with an exhaust airflow alarm.[9] The building's exhaust must be sufficient to exhaust the air from the C-PEC plus the air drawn in through the gap between the C-PEC and the canopy. The canopy alarm will alert users when the airflow in the canopy connection is insufficient to ensure containment and proper venting of any volatiles that may escape the A2.

When used in conjunction with the ventilation and pressurization requirements of the C-SEC or C-SCA, this cabinet is an acceptable choice for compounding most hazardous drugs. Because the HEPA filters do not remove volatilized materials, these vapors will be recirculated within the cabinet until, through dilution, they are exhausted from the hood.

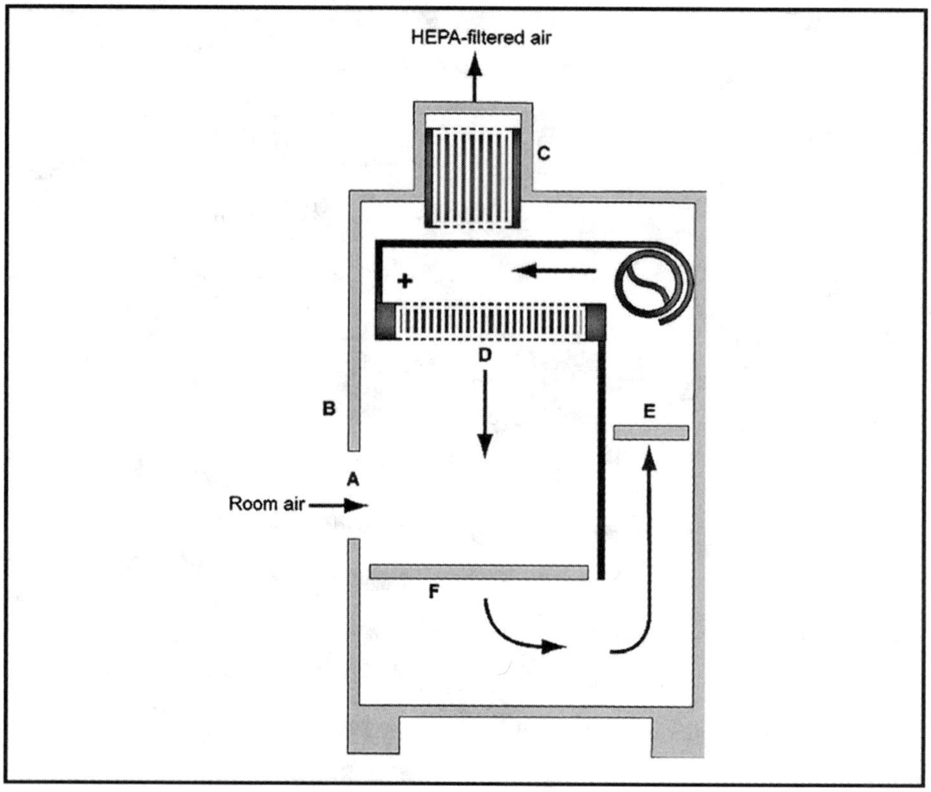

FIGURE 6-12. Class II type A2 biological safety cabinet

A = front opening; B = sash; C = exhaust HEPA filter; D = supply HEPA filter; E = positive pressure common plenum; F = negative pressure plenum

Source: Reprinted with permission of Chosewood LC, Wilson DE. Appendix A – Primary containment for biohazards: selection, installation and use of biological safety cabinets. In: *Biosafety in Microbiological and Biomedical Laboratories.* 5th ed. Washington, DC: U.S. Department of Health and Human Services; 2009. https://www.cdc.gov/labs/pdf/CDC-BiosafetyMicrobiologicalBiomedicalLaboratories-2009-P.PDF. Accessed April 6, 2023.

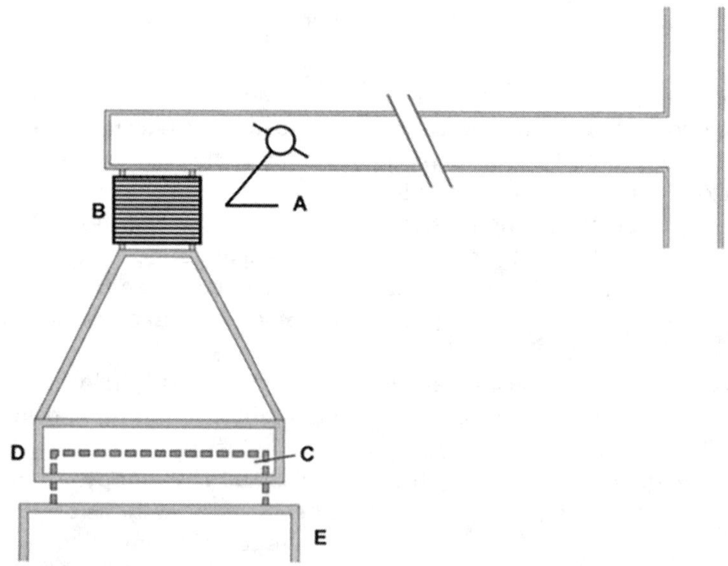

FIGURE 6-13. Canopy (Thimble) unit for ducting a class II, type A1 biological safety cabinet

A = balancing damper; B = flexible connector to exhaust system; C = cabinet exhaust HEPA filter housing; D = canopy unit; E = BSC.

Note: There is a 1 inch gap between the canopy unit D and the exhaust filter housing C, through which room air is exhausted.

Source: Reprinted with permission of Chosewood LC, Wilson DE. Appendix A – Primary containment for biohazards: selection, installation and use of biological safety cabinets. In: *Biosafety in Microbiological and Biomedical Laboratories.* 5th ed. Washington, DC: U.S. Department of Health and Human Services; 2009. https://www.cdc.gov/labs/pdf/CDC-BiosafetyMicrobiologicalBiomedicalLaboratories-2009-P.PDF. Accessed April 6, 2023.

Class II Type B1

This design differs from the A1 and the A2 in that the HEPA-filtered down-flow air is composed mostly of uncontaminated recirculated inflow air. Vendor designs vary but approximately 30% to 40% of the air flow is recirculated through the supply HEPA filter and 60% to 70% passes through the exhaust HEPA filter (see **Figure 6-14**). With this design all the air that passes through the front work surface grille is recirculated (approximately one third of the down-flow air) and all the air that passes through the rear work surface grille (approximately two thirds of the down-flow air) is exhausted to the outside. The intended advantage to this design is that if an operator works in the back of the cabinet, then any escaping volatiles are captured by the rear grille and vented directly to the outside without recirculation.

The Class II Type B1 cabinet must be vented using a hard connection and a dedicated duct to the outside. The exhaust system should have pressure monitors in place to alert operators if the system is not working properly. A B1 cabinet will have a minimum intake velocity of 100 fpm, making it an acceptable choice for most volatile hazardous materials. The B1 cabinet recirculates less air than other Class II designs (except the B2) and it exhausts a higher percentage of the recirculated air than an A2 design, so it is worthy of consideration for most applications.

Class II Type B2

The B2 cabinet is referred to as a total exhaust BSC. A supply blower draws air from the room and passes it through a HEPA filter located on the top of the cabinet. The HEPA-filtered down-flow air is pushed towards the work area of the cabinet. The building's exhaust system draws the HEPA-filtered down-flow air plus the front access inflow air through the cabinet's front and rear grilles. The air intake velocity is at least 100 fpm making it acceptable for HD containment. All the air entering the cabinet (both down-flow and inflow air) is passed through a HEPA filter and exhausted to the outside. No air is recirculated back into the cabinet or returned to the room (see **Figure 6-15**). All contaminated ducts and plenums are under negative pressure

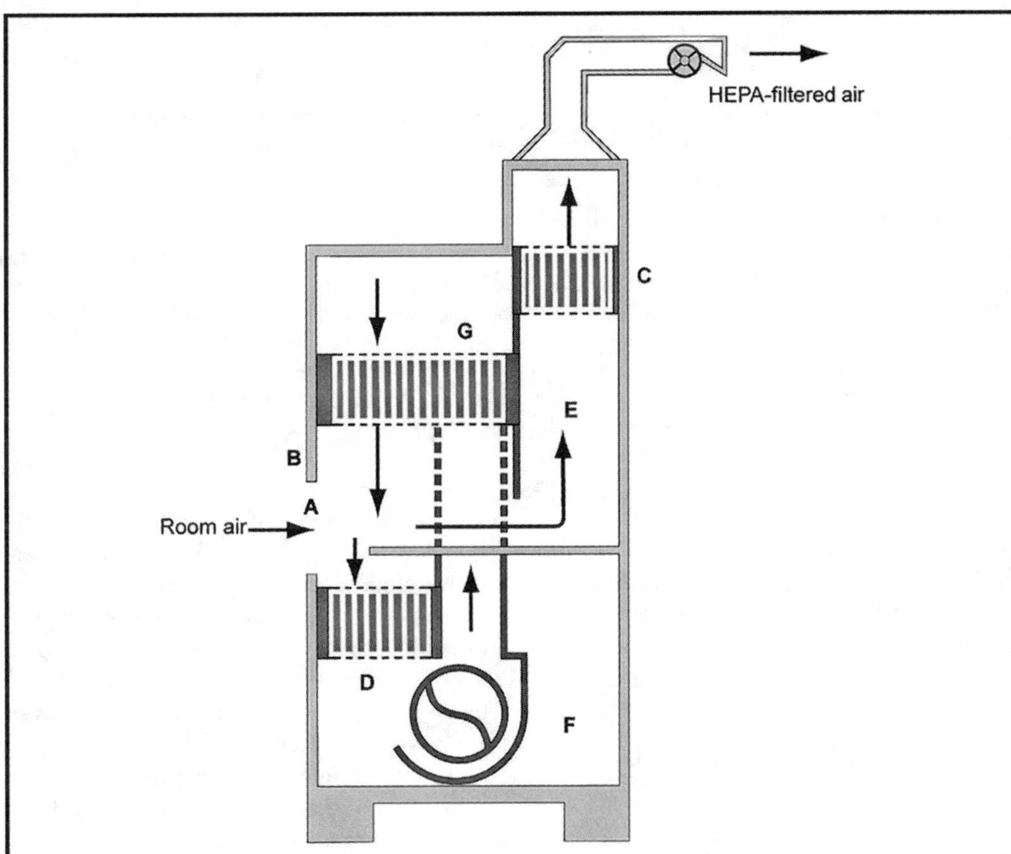

FIGURE 6-14. Class II type B1 biological safety cabinet

A = front opening; B = sash; C = exhaust HEPA filter; D = supply HEPA filter; E = negative pressure dedicated exhaust plenum; F = blower; G = additional HEPA filter for supply air

Source: Reprinted with permission of Chosewood LC, Wilson DE. Appendix A – Primary containment for biohazards: selection, installation and use of biological safety cabinets. In: *Biosafety in Microbiological and Biomedical Laboratories.* 5th ed. Washington, DC: U.S. Department of Health and Human Services; 2009. https://www.cdc.gov/labs/pdf/CDC-BiosafetyMicrobiologicalBiomedicalLaboratories-2009-P.PDF. Accessed April 6, 2023.

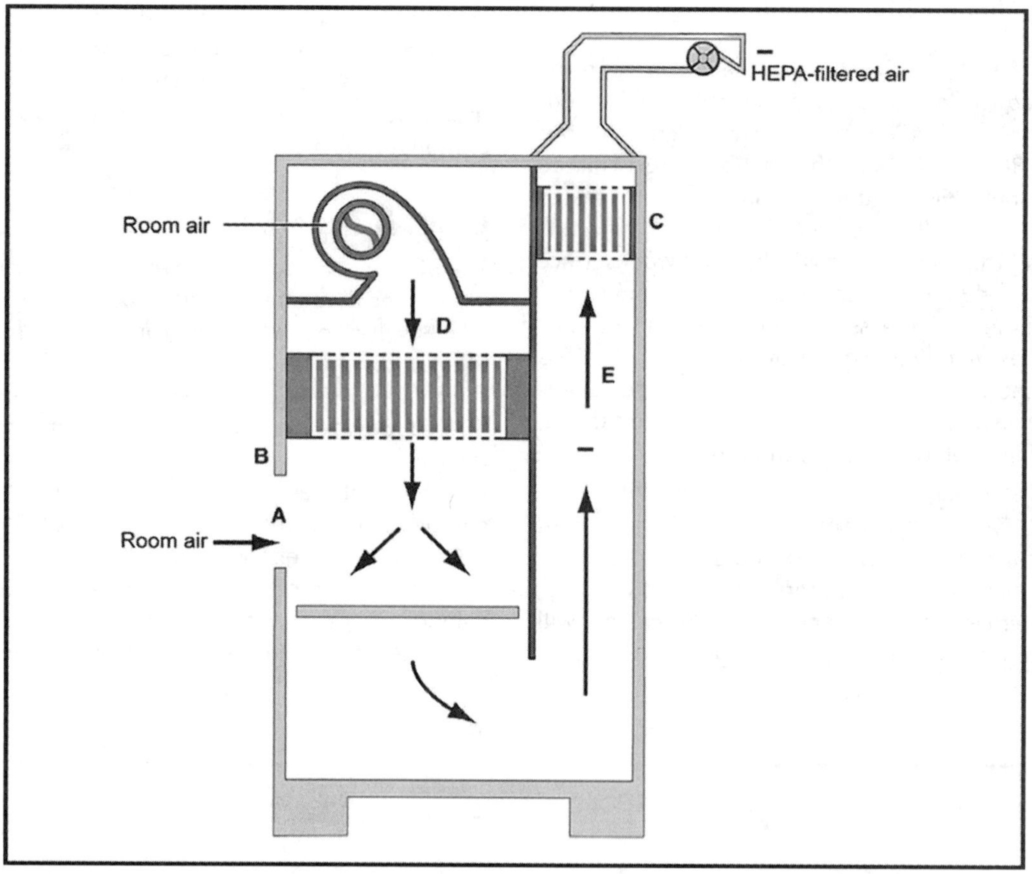

FIGURE 6-15. Class II type B2 biological safety cabinet

A = front opening; B = sash; C = exhaust HEPA filter; D = supply HEPA filter; E = negative pressure dedicated exhaust plenum

Source: Reprinted with permission of Chosewood LC, Wilson DE. Appendix A – Primary containment for biohazards: selection, installation and use of biological safety cabinets. In: *Biosafety in Microbiological and Biomedical Laboratories.* 5th ed. Washington, DC: U.S. Department of Health and Human Services; 2009. https://www.cdc.gov/labs/pdf/CDC-BiosafetyMicrobiologicalBiomedicalLaboratories-2009-P.PDF. Accessed April 6, 2023.

or surrounded by directly exhausted negative pressure ducts and plenums. B2 cabinets are attached to the exhaust system with hard connections and must have pressure monitors installed to prevent the supply blower from operating when the exhaust system fails. Because there is no recirculation, this design is typically reserved for use when there is concern with volatile HDs. The Type of BSC to use when compounding hazardous drugs should be part of an organization's hazardous drug assessment of risk.

Class III

From USP Chapter <800>, Appendix 3: Types of Biological Safety Cabinets:

> The Class III BSC is designed for work with highly infectious microbiological agents and other hazardous operations. It provides maximum protection for the environment and the worker. It is a gas-tight enclosure with a viewing window that is secured with locks and/or requires the use of tools to open. Both supply and exhaust air are HEPA/ULPA filtered. Exhaust air must pass through two HEPA/ULPA filters in series before discharge to the outdoors.[2]

BSC Selection for Compounding Hazardous Drugs

Class II (Types A2, B1, and B2) BSCs meet the USP Chapter <797> requirements for sterile compounding and the additional USP Chapter <800> requirements as C-PECs and are considered acceptable for sterile HD compounding.[1,2] The differences to be considered between these cabinets include how they exhaust to the outside (ie, hard connection versus canopy connection), if they recirculate the airflow (and what percent), and the impact the cabinet has on the secondary environmental controls. (See Table 6-2.) The 2004 NIOSH Alert recommended selecting ventilated cabinets that exhausted 100% to the outside and did not recirculate.[10] This recommendation was made because some hazardous drugs (eg, cyclophosphamide, fluorouracil, cisplatin, and carmustine) that are commonly compounded have demonstrated some degree of volatility and will pass through a HEPA filter into the work environment or cabinet.[4,5] The only BSC to match the 2004 NIOSH recommendation was the B2 cabinet. Unfortunately, the NIOSH recommendation did not consider all aspects associated with purchasing, installing, and maintaining B2 cabinets.

The Class II B2 designs do not offer any additional personnel or environmental protection compared to the other designs. The only advantage offered by the B2 cabinet is that the volatile (gaseous) hazardous materials are immediately evacuated from the work area. The other designs will recirculate air internally prior to exhausting it outside of the cabinet. It should be noted that any aerosols (small droplets) generated during compounding will be trapped on the HEPA filter. There might be a potential for the small volume of volatile hazardous material trapped on the HEPA filter to recirculate after sublimation and cross-contaminate other preparations in the cabinet if adequate purging time between processes does not occur.

The B2 cabinet is difficult to integrate into the air handling system of a facility. Since the B2 (and B1) cabinet depends on a properly installed and operating roof exhaust fan, if the exhaust blower ever fails or the exhaust volume drops below a safe level, the potential exists for the C-PEC's supply fan to pressurize the work area and any hazard present within the cabinet could be blown back directly into the room. Type B cabinets must be equipped with interlocks and alarms to alert the operator of improper operating conditions.

Close to an equal amount of air exhausted by the BSC must be replaced through the building supply air system back into the room. Handling the necessary amount of exhaust air is difficult to achieve and it must be done precisely. A B2 cabinet "exhausts as much as 1200 cubic feet per minute of conditioned room air."[11] The A2 cabinet design, on the other hand, is simple and straightforward. When connected with a canopy connection as shown in Figure 6-13, the A2 BSC offers the distinct advantage of safe operation even in the event of an exhaust failure. The face velocities of the air entering the BSC are maintained at a safe level even without building exhaust. Since all particulate hazards are removed by the exhaust HEPA filter, the only hazard that is released is the small amount of volatile hazardous drug which will be diluted by the large volume of exhaust air from the BSC before being discharged to the room through the canopy gap.

In the final analysis, if a facility decides to use a BSC then it must conduct its own assessment of risk to determine the type of BSC that will meet their safety and operational needs. To aid in the assessment a recent study was conducted by Taylor, Baker, et al. that reviewed the containment effectiveness of A2 and B2 BSCs. The conclusion of the study states:

> The data generated from this study demonstrate that use of an A2 for hazardous compounding can provide a comparable level of safety for the environment, users, and product while having less stringent airflow requirements relative to a B2. The simpler requirements for an A2 make them an appealing alternative as they have the potential to reduce the overall operating costs associated with a compounding pharmacy while maintaining safe levels of containment.[12]

RESTRICTED-ACCESS BARRIER SYSTEMS

Restricted-access barrier systems (RABS) are discussed in USP Chapter <797>:

> A restricted-access barrier system (RABS) is an enclosure that provides HEPA-filtered ISO Class 5 unidirectional air that allows for the ingress and/or egress of materials through defined openings that have been designed and validated to preclude the transfer of environmental air contamination, and that generally are not to be opened during compounding operations. Examples of RABS include CAIs and CACIs.[1]

Glove ports provide physical separation between the surrounding area and the interior of the device, where aseptic compounding occurs.

Material Transfer

When developing standard operating procedures (SOPs), it is important to establish how to move the materials into and out of the RABS. The purpose of a transfer chamber is to isolate the compounding chamber from the less clean room air and maintain and ISO Class 5 environment for compounding. Materials are placed into the transfer chamber from the room through the outer door, which is then sealed. With the product in the transfer chamber, the space is now "contaminated" by the ambient room air and by the outside of the packages that have been introduced. Wiping down the packages and allowing time for the RABS to purge the contaminated transfer chamber with HEPA-filtered airflow prior to opening the interior door reduces the particulate load that is transferred into the compounding chamber. The "recovery time after opening the transfer chamber to achieve ISO Class 5 air quality must be documented (eg, by the manufacture), and internal procedures must be developed to ensure that adequate recovery time is allowed."[1] Planning for the recovery time is important because less clean air enters the transfer chamber whenever the door is opened.

Transfer chambers can utilize unidirectional air, turbulent air, or in some older models, stagnant airflow. Because the passthrough can impact overall product contamination, compounders should consider the quality of room air where the isolator is located, how the materials will be wiped down before placement in the transfer chamber, and how effective the purge cycle is expected to be. Unidirectional transfer chamber designs offer the shortest purge times, afforded by the single pass of HEPA-filtered air. Longer purge times are required for the turbulent flow transfer chambers because contaminants are removed through dilution rather than washed away in a flow of filtered air. Stagnant air transfer chambers offer no purging of contamination prior to transferring products to the isolator. HEPA filter purged transfer chambers are preferred for isolators that are to be used for sterile compounding. Regardless of the type of transfer chamber used, a wipe down of the outside surfaces of all materials with sterile 70% isopropyl alcohol using sterile low-lint wipers must be performed prior to transfer into the isolator. This is done prior to placement in the transfer chamber.

Recovery Time

Recovery time is the amount of time it takes for the air quality inside the RABS to recover to its operating level after an excursion. Transferring materials in and out of the isolator or a surge of process-generated contamination would potentially elevate the particle counts from operational levels.

The recovery time is a function of how often the air within the isolator is replaced with HEPA-filtered air. Air exchange rates in a unidirectional isolator are typically in the range of 1,100 to 1,500 air changes per hour (ACPH). The recovery time should be noted for every isolator and SOPs developed around the actual time to recover from an excursion.

COMPOUNDING ASEPTIC ISOLATOR

A compounding aseptic isolator (CAI) is a type of RABS designed for compounding sterile nonhazardous CSPs. A CAI maintains ISO Class 5 unidirectional air, operates under positive air pressure, and exhausts into the room.

Airflow

Isolation from the room is provided by over pressurization and not a gastight seal. Most CAIs are not gas tight. HEPA-filtered air is typically delivered at the top of the compounding chamber and flows down across the work surface where it splits front to back and is removed by well-placed returns at the work surface (see **Figure 6-16**). The air from the front grille then passes beneath the work surface and is either recirculated or exhausted to the room. Careful planning is required to assure a free path from the DCA to the return grilles for removal of process-generated contamination. There is no mandated airflow velocity to which all isolators are designed. The manufacturer is expected to determine the optimum airflow velocity range for every isolator design they produce.

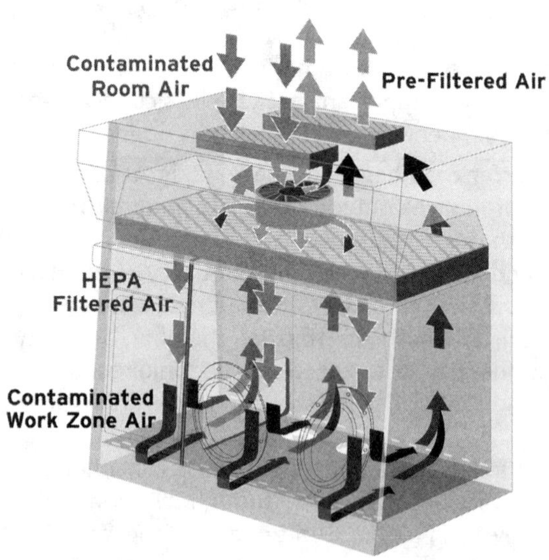

FIGURE 6-16. Airflow within a compounding aseptic isolator

Source: Reprinted with permission of NuAire, Inc.

COMPOUNDING ASEPTIC CONTAINMENT ISOLATORS

USP Chapter <800> defines a compounding aseptic containment isolator (CACI) as: "A specific type of CAI that is designed for the compounding of sterile HDs. The CACI is designed to provide worker protection from exposure to undesirable levels of airborne drugs throughout the compounding and material transfer process and to provide an aseptic environment with unidirectional airflow for compounding sterile preparations."[2]

CACIs are typically used when handling HDs and are classified as C-PECs. In addition to the requirements discussed for CAIs, the following applies to CACIs:

Airflow

As with other C-PECs, a CACI must be externally vented. CACIs are available as total exhaust systems or as systems that recirculate a percentage of the air back through the cabinet before exhausting the air to the outside after passing through a HEPA exhaust filter. CACIs must maintain negative pressure to prevent escape of internally generated hazardous contamination. When combined with unidirectional airflow and a leak-free enclosure, a particle-free DCA can be maintained even under dynamic operating conditions.

Enclosure Integrity

Since CACIs operate under negative pressure relative to the room, they must be airtight. In a negative pressure device, even the smallest of leaks will potentially result in ingress of airborne contamination from the room. This type of contamination is more significant when the CACI is placed in a C-SCA. Care should be taken to inspect gloves and the sleeve assemblies regularly and to replace when needed. It is always a good idea to have a spare set of sleeve assemblies on hand in the event of a torn sleeve.

Disinfection/Decontamination

The RABS design should facilitate cleaning and disinfection and, in the case of CACIs, decontamination of all work surfaces. Interior seams should be shaped and sized to facilitate easy cleaning. All interior surfaces should be easily reached through the gloves to accommodate cleaning. If the interior is designed in a manner that does not permit easy physical disinfection of all surfaces, an alternative gaseous decontamination process may be developed and validated. Most RABS are difficult to disinfect because of the limitations of working through gloves. This may require more frequent opening of the RABS to access areas that are difficult to reach with a cleaning tool or through the glove ports. Many cleaning products and aids are available to make this task easier. Time should be factored into the workflow for adequate daily cleaning and disinfection as well as work surface disinfection between compounding processes.

Ergonomics

RABS present several ergonomic challenges, and they should be fully investigated prior to investing in this technology. In most cases, accommodations to worker comfort create unintended consequences of their own so it is important to weigh each issue carefully.

Proper operating height is important for all primary engineering controls, but possibly more so for isolators than other devices. The compounder works through relatively small openings that must be positioned correctly for all compounders. An adjustable height stand should be considered when purchasing an isolator. The size of the arm openings will affect worker comfort. This is often a tradeoff. In some cases, the size of these openings is limited by the displacement airflow provided to the isolator. One of the performance criteria is a requirement that the isolator maintain a velocity of at least 100 fpm through the glove opening in the event the glove sleeve (gauntlet) becomes dislodged during operation.[6] If the glove opening is too large, the isolator would not meet this criterion. Another limiting factor is the ability to see into the isolator. If too much of the view screen area is given up to the glove openings, lines of sight are sacrificed. In general, the larger the arm opening, the more comfortable it will be for the operator. Some manufacturers have gone to offset elliptical openings to aid in worker comfort.

Plan the process of working in the isolator for the amount of time needed to accomplish all the work your facility needs to accomplish. What may be acceptable worker comfort for one to two hours may not be acceptable for six to eight hours.

PHARMACEUTICAL ISOLATOR

USP Chapter <797> defines a pharmaceutical isolator as, "An enclosure that provides HEPA-filtered ISO Class 5 unidirectional air operated at a continuously higher pressure than its surrounding environment and is decontaminated using an automated system. It uses only decontaminated interfaces or rapid transfer ports for material transfer."[1]

A pharmaceutical isolator is comprised of four components intended to reduce human interaction in the compounding process.

1. Controlled workspace
    a. The controlled workspace is part of the physical barrier that separates the ISO Class 5 environment from human interaction with the materials used in the compounding process.
2. Transfer device(s)
    a. A transfer device is a mechanical process to bring materials into the ISO Class 5 environment (controlled workspace). There is no direct human interaction.
3. Access device(s)
    a. Access devices(s) are used when compounder intervention is required inside the ISO Class 5 environment.
4. Integral decontamination system
    a. The integral decontamination system is used to disinfect all interior surfaces of the controlled workspace further reducing the potential of contamination of any surface within the device. Hydrogen peroxide (H_20_2) vapor is a common product used for this application.

ROBOTIC ENCLOSURES

If a robotic enclosure is used as a PEC, or placed within the PEC, dynamic airflow smoke pattern tests must be performed initially and every 6 months thereafter. Testing ensures the device is properly integrated into the facility, there is no turbulence or refluxing at any critical sites(s), room air does not enter the PEC, and all processes are performed without introducing contamination into the DCA(s). Refer to Chapter 9 for an in-depth review of these automated systems.

EXTERNAL VENTING OF C-PECs

Hazardous drugs are handled by a combination of HEPA filtration for the particulate component and exhausting from the building for the volatile hazardous component. Because HEPA filters do not filter out vapors and gases, USP Chapter <800> requires all C-PECs to be externally vented.[2]

In general, C-PECs that do not have an internal exhaust blower or a blower that pressurizes air through the exhaust filter, require an external exhaust blower to pull air from the unit to create the required airflow and/or negative pressure. The exhaust blower should be located on the roof of the building or in a location that will ensure that air from the C-PEC exhaust cannot reenter the building. The exhaust stack should be directed upward and ideally extend 10 feet above the roof to push the air off the roof. Placing the exhaust blower outside of the building ensures that air is pulled from the C-PEC and the building thereby maintaining negative pressure throughout the entire exhaust system. If there is a leak in the duct, air would be drawn into and not blown out of the duct.

C-PECs that have an internal blower that pressurizes the exhaust still need a roof-mounted external blower, but the building exhaust and the C-PEC exhaust must be isolated from one another in a manner that promotes harmony rather than the potential to work against one another. NSF/ANSI Standard 49 requires all Class II Type A2 cabinets that are externally vented be connected to the exhaust system through a canopy connection.[9] The exhaust volume is adjusted to approximately 20% above the BSC exhaust volume to create a negative pressure at the gap created by the canopy. Variances in the balance between the two blowers will result in lower or higher gap velocities but will not affect the performance of the BSC. The same rules that affect external venting of BSCs should be applied to CACIs.

A means of adjusting the exhaust airflow from the C-PEC must be provided. The exhaust system should be equipped with a balancing damper or a variable air volume exhaust motor. Ideally, each C-PEC would be vented on its own exhaust system. However, this is often not possible especially in larger facilities where exhaust system resources are precious and must be shared. If more than one PEC is connected to an exhaust system, consideration should be given to an automatic constant volume exhaust controller. For safety purposes, a monitoring system should be in place to monitor the exhaust airflow and alert workers of low airflow or a loss of negative pressure.

PLACEMENT OF PRIMARY ENGINEERING CONTROLS

"Proper placement of the PEC is critical to ensuring an ISO Class 5 environment for preparing CSPs. Placement of the PEC must allow for cleaning around the PEC."[1] A LAFS must not be placed where the proper airflow of the device could be affected by the traffic patterns of the compounding personnel or by the air currents within the room. This is potentially of greater significance in a segregated compounding area and should be considered when establishing the boundaries of the SCA.

USP Chapter <797> and USP Chapter <800> have well defined requirements for the placement of PECs and C-PECs that affect the assigned beyond-use dates (BUDs) of compounded sterile preparations (CSPs) and provide additional safety when preparing hazardous drugs. Because the air quality surrounding a PEC is integral for ensuring the ISO Class 5 or better environment required to prepare CSPs, USP distinguishes three categories of CSPs with the primary differentiator being the environmental conditions in which the PEC is located. Category 1 CSPs may be prepared in an unclassified segregated compounding area (SCA) and have a shorter maximum BUD. Category 2 and Category 3 CSPs must be prepared in a PEC located in a cleanroom suite and may have longer BUDs (see Chapter 16). Because IVLFZs must be located within an ISO Class 7 or cleaner buffer room, Category 1 compounding does not apply. When a pharmaceutical isolator is used for Category 2 compounding it must be placed in an ISO Class 8 or better room, but the room does not need an anteroom. **Table 6-3** provides a summary of the minimum requirements for the placement of a PEC for non-hazardous compounding.

A C-PEC must be placed in a negative pressure containment secondary engineering control that is externally vented. The C-SEC may be in the form of an unclassified containment segregated compounding area (C-SCA) or an ISO Class 7 negative pressure buffer room with an ISO Class 7 anteroom. The BUDs of hazardous drug CSPs are determined by the categories described in USP Chapter <797>.

CERTIFICATION AND RECERTIFICATION OF PRIMARY ENGINEERING CONTROLS

USP Chapter <797> states: "Before a compounding area is used to compound either Category 1, Category 2, or

TABLE 6-3. Summary of Minimum Requirements for Placement of PEC for Compounding Non-HD CSPs

PEC Type	Device Type	Placement for Compounding Category 1 CSPs	Placement for Compounding Category 2 and 3 CSPs
LAFS	LAFW	Unclassified SCA	ISO Class 7 positive pressure buffer room with an ISO Class 8 positive pressure anteroom
	IVLZ	N/A	ISO Class 7 positive pressure buffer room with an ISO Class 8 positive pressure anteroom
	BSC	Unclassified SCA	ISO Class 7 positive pressure buffer room with an ISO Class 8 positive pressure anteroom
RABS	CAI or CACI	Unclassified SCA	ISO Class 7 positive pressure buffer room with an ISO Class 8 positive pressure anteroom
Pharmaceutical isolator	Pharmaceutical isolator	Unclassified SCA	ISO Class 8 positive pressure room

Source: Reprinted with permission of USP <797> Pharmaceutical compounding—sterile preparations. In: *2023: USP Compounding Compendium.* Rockville, MD: United States Pharmacopeial Convention; 2023. https://doi.org/10.31003/USPNF_M99925_07_01.

Category 3 CSPs, it must be certified using the requirements in this chapter and when applicable, manufacturer specifications. Certification indicates that the compounding area is meeting its design and air quality specifications."[1]

The certification process is much more than just contracting with a service provider and having them visit every six months to place a sticker on a hood and tell you everything is ok. The purpose of the testing is to confirm that the engineering controls are working correctly and meet air quality specifications. A properly working compounding environment ensures your facility is in the best possible position to safely compound sterile preparations. Where hazardous drug compounding is involved, the testing and certification is also critical for ensuring the safety of personnel and the environment.

One very important consideration is that testing must be conducted under dynamic conditions. This means that pharmacy personnel must be part of the testing process and that testing must be completed under normal working conditions. Be concerned if a certifier requests to conduct the testing during lunch or a quiet period of the day. This may speed up the testing and be less disruptive to the work process, but it will not provide the needed information to assess the operation nor is it compliant with the USP Chapter <797> standard. It is helpful to educate the sterile compounders on the tests being conducted and the best way to interact with the certifiers. It is a good practice to have a written plan for your team to follow when a certifier arrives. The certifier should follow your standards for hand hygiene and proper use of the needed PPE. Discussing your quality procedures with the certifier before they arrive may help things go smoother.

The final, and equally important aspect of the biannual certifications, is for the designated person to thoroughly review and understand the reports, share the information with staff, look for trends, and take actions when needed based on any abnormal findings. If there are questions about the tests or the report, contact the vendor. They should be able to interpret what the findings mean for the facility and advise on corrective actions.

PURCHASING A PRIMARY ENGINEERING CONTROL

There are many decisions that must be made when purchasing a PEC for sterile compounding that go beyond the initial decisions of size and whether it will be used for hazardous or nonhazardous compounding. Even though pharmacies may be familiar with types of PECs they have used in the past, the devices and the regulations concerning the use of the devices have changed over time. If a new PEC is needed, take time to speak with vendors and other pharmacy users to learn about different PECs and the available options. Consider the ergonomics of the designs and features that may benefit your staff immediately as well as in the foreseeable future.

When purchasing a PEC for hazardous drug compounding, acceptable C-PECs include Class II Type A2, Type B1, Type B2 BSCs, and CACIs. A common characteristic of these devices is that they exhaust to the outside environment. They differ in whether they recirculate the air or are total exhaust, and the amount of air they vent. As such, when purchasing a C-PEC, it is advisable to involve your Engineering Department early in the planning process to ensure they understand the environmental and ventilation requirements of the containment engineering controls. Their input may make you aware of any planning limitations from a facilities perspective. USP Chapter <800> treats CACIs and BSCs equally in this regard allowing either device to be used within the same environmental conditions without affecting the maximum assigned BUD. This change is worth considering when researching the purchase of a C-PEC.

Options to investigate when purchasing a PEC or C-PEC include:

- What is the best work surface height for the hood based on the functions that it is intended for? Hoods may be purchased on various height stands, bases, or wheels that will allow you to determine the final work surface height. Some vendors allow for electronically adjustable stands so that the user can change the work height based on each user's preferences.
- Does the design facilitate or hinder routine cleaning, disinfection, and decontamination of the device?
- Understandable gauges and indicators to ensure the staff can easily determine if the PEC is working correctly and within normal limits. These may include airflow and pressure alarms.
- Upgraded wheels and longer power cords to facilitate movement and cleaning around the PEC.
- Electrical outlets inside or outside of the PEC.
- Sharps and waste disposal systems.
- Cable cord passthroughs or sealed data ports for cables and power cords. This is particularly important for isolators that may have electronic equipment installed in them.
- Camera mounts or preinstalled cameras are now available for placement inside or outside of the hood.
- Monitor and keyboard arms mounted to the PEC may work better than a workstation set up on an adjacent table or cart.
- An IVLFZ is not a prefabricated device that can be purchased and installed on site ready to go. They are individually designed and built into a facility's secondary engineering control. Additional time and research should be taken before designing a clean room with an IVLFZ to ensure it is a good fit for your application.

SUMMARY

Primary and secondary engineering controls must work together to "minimize the risk of airborne contamination of the area in which sterile compounding occurs."[1] Primary engineering controls are used to provide the clean, essentially particle free air that is needed for sterile compounding. For PECs to perform in an optimal manner, it is important to select a device that best meets the need, install it in a well-designed compounding area and ensure that all of the needed maintenance and cleaning is performed by competent individuals. This ongoing critical oversight is needed for the safety of our patients and for protection of our staff.

REFERENCES

1. USP <797> Pharmaceutical compounding—sterile preparations. In: *2023: USP Compounding Compendium*. Rockville, MD: United States Pharmacopeial Convention; 2023. **https://doi.org/10.31003/USPNF_M99925_07_01**.
2. USP <800> Hazardous drugs handling in healthcare settings. In: *2020: USP Compounding Compendium*. Rockville, MD: United States Pharmacopeial Convention; July 1, 2020. **https://doi.org/10.31003/USPNF_M7808_07_01**.
3. Institute of Environmental Sciences and Technology (IEST). *IEST-RP-CC001.6: HEPA and ULPA filters*. Arlington Heights, IL: Institute of Environmental Sciences and Technology; 2016.
4. Kiffmeyer TK, Kube C, Opiolka S, et al. Vapour pressures, evaporation behavior and airborne concentrations of hazardous drugs: implications for occupational safety. *Pharma J*. 2002;268:331–337.
5. Conner TH, Shults M, Fraser MP. Determination of the vaporization of solutions of mutagenic antineoplastic agents at 23 and 37° C using a desiccator technique. *Mutat Res*. October 10, 2000;470(1):85–92. doi:10.1016/s1383-5718(00)00105-4.
6. Controlled Environment Testing Association (CETA). *CAG-002: CETA Compounding Isolator Testing Guide*. Raleigh, NC: Controlled Environment Testing Association; 2008.
7. International Organization for Standardization (ISO). *ISO 14644-1: Cleanroom and associated control environments*. Geneva, Switzerland: International Organization for Standardization; 1999.
8. Kastango ES, Wagner JT, Kastango KB, et al. Generation of particulate matter during handling of needle and syringe packaging. *Am J Health-Syst Pharm*. 2008;65:1443–1450.
9. NSF International (NSF) and American National Standards Institute (ANSI). *NSF/ANSI 49–2020: biosafety cabinetry: design, construction, performance, and field certification*. Ann Arbor, MI: NSF and American National Standards Institute; 2019.
10. The National Institute for Occupational Safety and Health (NIOSH). *NIOSH Alert: preventing Occupational Exposure to Antineoplastic and Other Hazardous Drugs in Health Care Settings*. Cincinnati, OH: The National Institute for Occupational Safety and Health; September 2004. **www.cdc.gov/niosh/docs/2004-165/**. Accessed December 2015.
11. Chosewood LC, Wilson DE. Appendix A—primary containment for biohazards: selection, installation and use of biological safety cabinets. In: *Biosafety in microbiological and biomedical laboratories*. 5th ed. Washington, DC: U.S. Department of Health and Human Services; December 2009. **https://www.cdc.gov/labs/pdf/CDC-BiosafetyMicrobiologicalBiomedicalLaboratories-2009-P.PDF**. Accessed April 6, 2023.
12. Taylor AV, Baker N, et al. Evaluating containment effectiveness of A2 and B2 biological safety cabinets. *Am J Health-Syst Pharm*. 2019;76:599–607.

SECONDARY ENGINEERING CONTROLS AND CLEANROOM DESIGN

Elaine Strauss, Chuck Gaziano, and F. Kurt Last

INTRODUCTION

Regulatory standards and professional guidelines require pharmacists and cleanroom designated personnel to evaluate their sterile compounding facilities (see Chapter 2). These standards and guidelines specify that sterile preparations should be compounded in an area separate from other activities unrelated to compounding. The most prominent standards, USP Chapter <797> Pharmaceutical Compounding—Sterile Preparations and USP Chapter <800> Hazardous Drugs—Handling in Healthcare Settings, require that most sterile compounding be done in an International Organization of Standardization (ISO) Class 5 primary engineering control (PEC) that is properly placed in a buffer room, which is supported by an anteroom.[1;2] USP Chapter <797> states that "aseptic techniques, processes, and procedures must be followed for preparing any sterile medication. Processes and procedures must be in place to minimize the potential for contact with nonsterile surfaces, introduction of particulate matter or biological fluids, and mix-ups with other products or CSPs."[1] While acknowledging the importance of aseptic technique, processes, and procedures, the standard goes further by categorizing compounded sterile preparations (CSPs) "primarily based on the state of environmental control under which they are compounded."[1] For PECs to work properly and for personnel to maintain aseptic technique, a very clean and well-maintained compounding area is mandatory. In addition, USP Chapter <800> sets forth standards for handling hazardous drugs (HDs) to protect personnel, patients, and the environment from contamination with these hazardous substances. The American Society of Health-System Pharmacists (ASHP) has promulgated guidelines that supplement USP Chapter <797> and USP Chapter <800>.[3;4]

This chapter explains the functional requirements of engineering controls that establish the environmental control of the sterile compounding areas, how to plan and design new sterile compounding areas or alter existing ones, and how to justify, purchase, validate and certify sterile compounding facilities.

FUNCTIONAL REQUIREMENTS

Functional cleanroom and compounding requirements must be aligned with USP Chapter <797> and USP Chapter <800> because they are the enforceable standards that most pharmacists must abide by. Segregated compounding areas (SCAs) and cleanroom suites, comprised of an anteroom and buffer room, are known collectively as *secondary engineering controls* (SECs) because they provide the controlled environments in which a PEC (eg, laminar airflow system [LAFS], restricted-access barrier system [RABS], or pharmaceutical isolator) is placed. The most commonly used PECs in hospital pharmacy sterile compounding are laminar airflow workbenches (LAFWs), class II biological safety cabinets (BSCs), and compounding aseptic isolators (CAIs), which are explained in Chapter 6. The SCA is type of SEC containing the PEC. The SCA is a designated space, area, or room that is not required to be classified and is defined with a visible perimeter. The SCA must be located away from unsealed windows, doors that connect to the outdoors, traffic flow, and areas where there are environmental control challenges (eg, restrooms, warehouses, food preparation areas) that could negatively affect the air quality within the SCA.[1] For the preparation of non-hazardous CSPs, the SCA is required to have a visible perimeter to establish the boundaries of the SCA as well as clean, smooth, impervious surfaces that are easy to clean and nonshedding. The SCA is not required to have a minimum high-efficiency particulate air (HEPA)-filtered air changes per hour (ACPH). However, facilities may choose to include HEPA filtration to the SCA while maintaining the room as nonclassified. In many compounding and manufacturing settings, this space

Note: The authors would like to acknowledge the contributions of Chuck Gaziano who made significant contributions to this chapter prior to his passing.

DOI 10.37573/9781585286492.007

is considered controlled not classified (CNC) and is only for the preparation of Category 1 CSPs. Additional information on the buffer and anteroom requirements of the cleanroom suite are outlined in this chapter.

Air Cleanliness

In order to ensure compliance with the standards outlined in USP Chapter <797>, pharmacists must understand controlled environment classifications. For nearly 40 years, U.S. Federal Standard 209 (FS 209) defined air cleanliness in contamination control, but FS 209 has been retired by the U.S. General Services Administration in favor of the internationally accepted definitions for cleanrooms and clean zones promulgated by the ISO.[5;6] (**Table 7-1.**)

Compounded Sterile Preparation Microbial Contamination Categories and Primary Engineering Control Placement

Unlike previous versions which set risk levels, the newest version of USP Chapter <797> distinguishes categories of CSPs according to the state of environmental control under which they are compounded, the probability of microbial contamination during the time they are stored, and how soon preparations need to be used.[1] The appropriate category, Category 1, 2, or 3, is assigned according to the corresponding probability of contaminating a CSP with (1) microbial contamination (eg, microbial organisms, spores, and endotoxins); and (2) chemical and physical contamination (eg, foreign chemicals and physical matter).[1] USP Chapter <797> applies more stringent facility requirements to Category 2 and 3 compounding as compared with Category 1 compounding (**Table 7-2**). Category 1, 2, and 3 CSPs must be prepared in a PEC generating an air quality of at least ISO Class 5 classification.[1]

Category 2 and 3 CSP compounding sites are required to have an LAFS, such as an LAFW, integrated vertical laminar flow zone (IVLFZ), or BSC which must be placed in an ISO Class 7 positive pressure buffer room with an ISO Class 8 or better positive pressure anteroom. If the site only compounds Category 1 CSPs, the LAFS can be placed in an unclassified SCA. A IVLFZ may not be used in an unclassified SCA, however, and therefore would not be used for Category 1 compounding.

A RABS, such as a CAI or a compounding aseptic containment isolator (CACI), must be placed within a cleanroom suite with an ISO Class 7 buffer room and an ISO Class 8 anteroom or better if used to prepare Category 2 or 3 CSPs. CAIs or CACIs can only be placed in an unclassified SCA for the preparation of Category 1 CSPs.[1] When using a RABS, the following requirements must be performed:

- The recovery time specified by the manufacturer to achieve ISO Class 5 air quality after opening the transfer chamber must be documented.
- Procedures must be in place to ensure adequate recovery time after opening and closing the RABS throughout compounding operations.
- Dynamic airflow smoke pattern tests must initially be performed in the PEC and retested at least every six months. These tests are necessary to ensure that the RABS is properly integrated into the facility. Additionally, these tests ensure that personnel understand how to properly compound, use the unidirectional airflow, and maintain first air in the direct compounding area (DCA).[1]

Pharmaceutical isolators, which are different than RABS (see Chapter 6), provide isolation from the surrounding area and maintain ISO Class 5 air quality. They can be placed in an unclassified SCA only when preparing Category 1 CSPs. If used for Category 2 or 3 CSPs, the pharmaceutical isolator must be placed in a room meeting ISO 8 classification or better. An anteroom is not required within the cleanroom suite for the preparation of Category 2 or 3 CSPs when a pharmaceutical isolator is used. Dynamic airflow smoke pattern tests must be performed at a minimum of every 6 months. These tests are necessary to ensure that the pharmaceutical isolator is properly integrated into the facility. Additionally, these tests ensure that personnel understand how to properly compound, use the unidirectional airflow, and maintain first air in the DCA.[1]

For sterile hazardous drug (HD) compounding, USP Chapter <800> specifies that a class II BSC or a CACI may be

TABLE 7-1. ISO Classification of Particulate Matter in Room Air as Limits in Particles 0.5 Microns and Larger per Cubic Meter (Current ISO) and Cubic Feet (Former FS 209E)

Class Name		Particle Counts Per	
ISO Class	U.S. FS209E	ISO, m^3	FS209E, ft^3
3	Class 1	35.2	1
4	Class 10	352	10
5	Class 100	3,520	100
6	Class 1,000	35,200	1,000
7	Class 10,000	352,000	10,000
8	Class 100,000	3,520,000	100,000

ISO = International Organization of Standardization.

Source: Adapted with permission of ISO 14644-1, Cleanrooms and associated controlled environments—Part 1: Classification of air cleanliness by particle concentration.

TABLE 7-2. Secondary Engineering Control Requirements by USP Chapter <797> CSP Category

Category 1

- PEC can be located in an unclassified segregated compounding area (SCA).
- SCA is an unclassified space with no anteroom or buffer room.
- The location of the SCA must be away from areas with poor air quality and challenging environmental areas, including exterior doors, unsealed windows, traffic flow, restrooms, food preparation areas, warehouses, air handler, elevator, or pneumatic tube station.
- The SCA used for nonhazardous drug compounding is not required to have a door. However, boundaries must be established with a visible perimeter.
- The sink must be at least 1 meter away from the PEC and outside the perimeter of the SCA.
- The area within 1 meter of the PEC should be dedicated only for sterile compounding.
- Surfaces of ceilings, walls, floors, fixtures, counters, and cabinets in the SCA should be smooth, impervious, free from cracks and crevices, nonshedding, and resistant to damage by disinfectants. Dust collecting overhangs should be minimized. They must be easily cleanable if present.

Category 2

- In a cleanroom suite, the ISO classified anteroom and buffer room must be physically separated from the surrounding unclassified areas of the facility by fixed walls and doors.
- An anteroom is an ISO Class 8 or cleaner area where personnel hand hygiene and garbing procedures, staging of components, and other high-particulate-generating activities are performed. The anteroom must have a line of demarcation to separate the clean side from the dirty side. The anteroom must meet at least ISO Class 7 classification if adjacent to a negative pressure buffer room.
- A buffer room is an ISO Class 7 or cleaner area where the PEC is physically located. Activities that occur in this area include the preparation and staging of the components and supplies used when compounding CSPs.
- Buffer room must be supplied at least 30 ACPH during dynamic operating conditions. At least 15 ACPH must come from the HVAC through ceiling-mounted HEPA filters. If the PEC supplies some of the required ACPH, the PEC must remain on except for during maintenance.
- Anterooms meeting ISO Class 8 classification must be supplied with at least 20 ACPH during dynamic operating conditions. At least 15 of the total air change rate must originate from the HVAC through ceiling-mounted HEPA filters. Anterooms meeting ISO Class 7 standards must meet the minimum required 30 ACPH during dynamic operating conditions.
- Classified rooms must be equipped with a pressure differential monitoring system.
- HEPA-filtered air must be introduced at the ceiling, and air return vents should be mounted low on the walls.
- A temperature of 20°C (68°F) or cooler and a relative humidity of 60% or below should be maintained by the HVAC system to provide comfortable conditions for compounding personnel.
- Surfaces of ceilings, walls, floors, fixtures, counters, and cabinets in the buffer room must be smooth, impervious, free from cracks and crevices, nonshedding, and resistant to damage by disinfectants.
- Sinks must not be located within 1 meter of the entrance to an ISO Class 7 negative pressure buffer room.
- PECs (LAFWs, BSCs, and CAIs) must be certified and maintain ISO Class 5 as described in USP Chapter <797> for exposure of critical sites. They must be in a segregated compounding area (SCA) restricted to sterile compounding activities.

Category 3

- Same facility requirements as Category 2 CSPs

ACPH = air change per hour; BSC = biological safety cabinet; CAI = compounding aseptice isolater; CSPs = compounded sterile preparations; HEPA = high-efficiency particulate air; HVAC = heating, ventilation, and air conditioning; ISO = International Organization of Standardization; LAFW = laminar airflow workbench; PEC = primary engineering control.

Reprinted with permission of USP <797> Pharmaceutical compounding—sterile preparations. In: *2023: USP Compounding Compendium*. Rockville, MD: United States Pharmacopeial Convention; 2023.

placed in either an ISO Class 7 buffer room or a containment segregated compounding area (C-SCA). See **Table 7-3** for a summary of SECs required for each classification of CSPs.

Hazardous Drugs

HDs must be handled under conditions that promote patient safety, worker safety, and environmental protection. This chapter will review the facility requirements for the handling and compounding of HDs. A more comprehensive discussion of HDs can be found in Chapter 27.

Signs designating a hazard must be prominently displayed before the entrance to HD handling areas. Access to areas where HDs are handled must be restricted to authorized personnel to protect persons not involved in HD

TABLE 7-3. Summary of Secondary Engineering Controls Required for Each Classification of Compounded Sterile Preparation

Type of CSP per USP Chapter <797>	ISO Class Requirement		Segregated Compounding Area or Other Designated Compounding Area
	Anteroom	Buffer Room	
Category 1	Not Required	Not Required	Separate, unclassified room with PEC restricted to preparing CSPs with a BUD of 12 hr or less at controlled room temperature or 24 hr or less when refrigerated
Category 2	ISO Class 8 positive pressure to main pharmacy and physically separated from buffer room by a wall	ISO Class 7 positive pressure to anteroom	Not permitted
Category 3	ISO Class 8 positive pressure to main pharmacy and physically separated from buffer room by a wall	ISO Class 7 positive pressure to anteroom	Not permitted
Immediate use with administration beginning within 4 hours after the start of preparation	Not required	Not required	Not required
Hazardous drug per USP Chapter <800>	Separate ISO Class 7 anteroom is positive pressure to buffer room	Separate ISO Class 7 negative pressure buffer room	C-SCA restricted to preparing HD CSPs with a BUD of 12 hr or less at controlled room temperature or 24 hr or less when refrigerated
Radiopharmaceutical	ISO Class 8 anteroom	ISO Class 8 buffer room ISO Class 7 buffer room ISO Class 8 or better for ^{99m}Tc and ^{99}Mo	Dependent on manipulation: Dispensing, repackaging, and preparation with minor deviations can be performed in segregated radiopharmaceutical area (SRPA) Radionuclide generator storage/elution (eg, nondirect infusion system, ^{99m}Tc or ^{68}Ga) requires an ISO Class 8 SRPA
Immediate use radiopharmaceuticals prepared for a single patient	Not required	Not required	Does not require SRPA
Allergen extract appropriately preserved for intradermal or subcutaneous injection	Not required	Not required	ISO Class 5 PEC or in a dedicated allergenic extracts compounding area (AECA)
Docking proprietary bag and vial systems	Required when docking for future activation and administration Not required for activation and immediate administration	Required when docking for future activation and administration Not required for activation and immediate administration	Not required

BUD = beyond-use date; C-SCA = containment segregated compounding area; CSP = compounded sterile preparation; ISO = International Organization of Standardization; USP = *United States Pharmacopeia.*

handling. HD handling areas must be located away from breakrooms and refreshment areas for personnel, patients, or visitors to reduce risk of exposure.[2]

Radiopharmaceuticals

With the publication of USP Chapter <825> Radiopharmaceuticals—Preparation, Compounding, Dispensing, and Repackaging, information on radiopharmaceuticals was removed from USP Chapter <797>. USP Chapter <825> specifies the importance of balancing aseptic handling practices (patient safety) with radiation protection practices (worker safety).[7]

The compounding of sterile radiopharmaceuticals must be performed using appropriately shielded vials and syringes in a properly functioning and certified ISO Class 5 PEC, which is located in an ISO Class 7 or cleaner buffer area with an ISO Class 8 or better anteroom. Differential air controls are a cornerstone of balancing the maintenance of air quality requirements of the SEC with occupational safety concerns, such as radiation exposure. Users must consult their radioactive materials (RAM) license conditions for environmental controls, as the RAM license requirements may supersede the environmental controls outlined in USP Chapter <825>. USP Chapter <825> requires the buffer area to be positive pressure to the anteroom, and the anteroom must be positive pressure compared with unclassified portions of the restricted area. In the presence of volatile or airborne radiopharmaceuticals (eg, I-131 sodium iodide and xenon), the restricted area must be negative pressure compared with unrestricted areas.[7]

When preparing sterile radiopharmaceuticals that only require minor deviations, dispensing, or repackaging, the ISO Class 5 PEC may be placed in a segregated radiopharmaceutical processing area (SRPA). The SRPA is an unclassified area without an anteroom or buffer area. USP Chapter <825> specifies the following must be met for a SRPA:

- Only sterile radiopharmaceutical preparation, preparation with minor deviations, dispensing, and repackaging may be performed in an SRPA.
- If the SRPA meets ISO Class 8 total airborne particle count specifications, it can also be used for storage and elution of nondirect infusion radionuclide generators (eg, ^{99m}Tc).
- The SRPA must be located away from unsealed windows, doors that connect to the outdoors, and traffic flow, which may adversely affect the air quality in the PEC. The impact of activities that will be conducted around or adjacent to the SRPA must be considered carefully when designing such an area.
- A visible perimeter must establish the boundaries of the SRPA.
- Access to the SRPA must be restricted to authorized personnel and required materials.
- An SRPA must not be located adjacent to environmental control challenges.[7]

The SRPA must be negative pressure compared with unrestricted areas when volatile or airborne radiopharmaceuticals are present (eg, I-131 sodium iodide and xenon). Due to the limitations added from the radiation shielding in the direct processing area (DPA), dynamic airflow smoke pattern tests must be performed at least every 6 months to ensure the PEC is properly placed in the facility and personnel understand how to prepare and compound radiopharmaceuticals in the unidirectional airflow and maintain first air. Storage and transport of properly shielded vials of radiopharmaceutical CSPs may occur in a limited access ambient environment without a specific ISO class designation.[7]

Immediate use sterile radiopharmaceuticals for a single patient can be prepared in an ambient environment that lacks primary and secondary engineering controls. This ambient environment should be away from patient care areas and be a functionally separate space, such as a radiopharmaceutical handling space or hot lab in a hospital, clinic, or mobile coach. This ambient space should be clean, free from clutter, and be located away from high traffic areas. However, due to the absence of engineering controls, strict aseptic technique and limited beyond-use dating (BUD) must be applied. Immediate use sterile radiopharmaceuticals do not require a SRPA. These agents must be administered within one hour of the first container puncture or exposure of any critical site exposed to ambient air, whichever is first.[7]

To minimize the risk of microbial proliferation and ensure comfortable conditions for garbed personnel, the classified areas and the SRPA must be maintained at a maximum temperature of 25°C (77°F) and maximum relative humidity of 60%.[7] While the maximum temperature allowed is 25°C (77°F), a lower design temperature may be needed to ensure user comfort when garbed in the personal protective equipment (PPE) required for these spaces. Temperature and humidity must be monitored and either manually recorded each day the facility is used or stored in a continuous recording device. These recording devices must be verified for accuracy at least every 12 months or as required by the manufacturer. Free standing humidifiers, dehumidifiers, and air conditioning units must not be used within the classified areas or the SRPA.[7]

^{99m}Tc/^{99}Mo generator systems must be stored and eluted under conditions recommended by manufacturers and applicable state and federal regulations. Such generator systems must be eluted in an ISO Class 8 or cleaner air environment to permit special handling, shielding, and air flow requirements. For further discussions on radiopharmaceuticals, see Chapter 25.[7]

Allergenic Extracts

When licensed allergenic extracts are mixed and diluted into prescription sets for an individual patient, they must be done so in facilities compliant with USP Chapter <797> requirements. Prescription sets are combinations of allergenic extracts that can be mixed and diluted to provide subcutaneous immunotherapy to an individual patient, even though these allergenic extract combinations are not specified in the approved Biological License Applications (BLAs) for the licensed biological products. Allergen extract compounders must follow specified hand cleansing, garbing, and aseptic techniques, and labeling standards.[1] Therefore, suitable space is required for handwashing, compounding and storage of equipment, supplies, and finished preparations.

USP Chapter <797> Section 21 includes details on the facility requirements for compounding allergenic extracts. Compounding must occur in an ISO Class 5 PEC or in a dedicated allergenic extract compounding area (AECA). Unlike an SCA or C-SCA, the AECA does not contain a PEC. The following outlines requirements for the compounding area containing the PEC or the AECA:

- The room must be located away from areas that will negatively impact air quality, such as unsealed windows, doors that connect to the outside, or areas of high traffic flow.
- The room must be located away from areas with difficult to control environments, such as restrooms, warehouses, and food preparation areas.
- The PEC or work surfaces in the AECA must be located at least one meter away from a sink.
- If a PEC is used, it must be certified every 6 months.[1]

If an AECA is used, a visible perimeter must establish the boundaries, and the following requirements must also be in place for the AECA:

- Access during compounding is restricted to authorized personnel.
- No other activities can take place during compounding in the AECA.
- Surfaces of walls, floors, fixtures, shelving, counters, and cabinets must be cleanable, smooth, impervious, nonshedding, free from cracks and crevices, and resistant to damage by cleaning and sanitizing agents.
- Carpet is not permitted.
- Dust-collecting overhangs should be minimized and must be easily cleanable.
- The design of the AECA must allow for a well-lit working environment, and it must have temperature and humidity controls to ensure the comfort of garbed personnel.[1]

For an expanded discussion of personnel qualifications, hygiene and garbing, cleaning, and disinfecting, compounding, BUDs, labeling, shipping and transport, and documentation, see also Chapter 24, Allergenic Extracts.

Facilities for Immediate-use CSPs and Preparation for Administration

In the most recent version of USP Chapter <797>, the section on immediate use is no longer restricted to emergency situations. The chapter indicates that the compounding of CSPs for direct and immediate administration is not subject to the requirements for Category 1, 2, and 3 when the following seven conditions are met:

1. Aseptic techniques are strictly followed. Policies and procedures are in place to minimize the risk of contamination by nonsterile surfaces, the introduction of particulate matter or biological fluids, or mix-ups with other commercially available or compounded sterile products.
2. Personnel compounding under immediate use have undergone training and demonstrate competency in aseptic processes.
3. The immediate use preparation is conducted in accordance with evidence-based information for physical and chemical compatibility.
4. No more than 3 sterile products are involved in the preparation.
5. Single dose containers must not be used for more than one patient. Any unused starting components must be discarded after preparing each individual patient-specific dose.
6. Administration must begin within 4 hours following the start of the preparation. If 4 or more hours have elapsed since the start of the preparation, the immediate-use CSP must be promptly discarded.
7. Unless administered by the person who prepared it or administration is witnessed by the preparer, the CSP must be labeled with the names and amounts of all active ingredients, name or initials of person preparing, and the exact 4-hour time period in which administration must begin.

USP Chapter <797> does not consider preparation for administration to be compounding, and therefore it is outside the scope of the chapter. *Preparation for administration* is defined as mixing, reconstituting, or other such acts that are performed in accordance with directions contained in approved labeling or supplemental materials provided by the product's manufacturer. A preparation is considered outside the scope of the chapter if it includes the following criteria:

- The product is prepared as a single dose for an individual patient.
- The approved labeling includes information for the diluent, the resultant strength, the container closure system, and storage time.[1]

When the above conditions are met for either immediate use or preparation for administration, none of the engineering controls are applicable. However, USP Chapter <800> requirements should be considered for hazardous drugs.

Regardless of the USP chapter requirements, The Joint Commission (TJC) and other regulatory or accreditation bodies have facility standards for medication preparation. In addition to this chapter, Chapter 21 offers additional discussion on immediate use compounding.

Proprietary Bag and Vial Systems

USP Chapter <797> allows an exemption to facility standards for docking and activation of proprietary bag and vial systems for immediate administration to an individual patient when performed following the manufacturer's labeling. USP Chapter <797> indicates that docking and activation for immediate administration in accordance with manufacturer's labeling is not considered compounding and exemption is therefore allowed to the facility standards. However, when performing docking of proprietary bag and vial systems for future activation and administration it is considered compounding, and must be performed following the requirements of the chapter with the exception of assigning BUDs. Because the vast majority of proprietary bag and vial systems have a manufacturer's specified expiration date beyond the BUD established for Category 1 CSPs, the assembly of these systems for future activation and administration must occur in conditions which meet at least Category 2 CSPs. The assembly must occur in an ISO Class 5 or better PEC within an ISO Class 7 buffer room and adjacent ISO Class 8 anteroom (ie, a cleanroom suite). The sterility, storage, and stability BUDs for docked or docked and activated (where *activated* is defined as allowing contact of the previously separate diluent and drug contents) proprietary bag and vial systems for intravascular administration are to be applied as indicated by the manufacturer.[1]

Other Regulatory or Accrediting Organizations and Certifying Body Requirements for Cleanroom Facilities

In addition to the USP Chapter <797> and USP Chapter <800> standards discussed above, USP has published the informational (nonenforceable) USP Chapter <1066> Physical Environments That Promote Safe Medication Use.[8] This chapter includes detailed discussion about the importance of organizational support and leadership, principles from human-factors research, using lean-production techniques for work processes, simplification and standardization, innovative solutions, forcing functions, and work system elements when considering the design of medication safety zones (MSZs).

USP Chapter <1066> includes specific sections pertinent to cleanroom facilities, including the following:

- Illumination
- Sound and noise
- Odor
- Activities and tasks performed
- Multitasking
- Tools and technologies in the physical environment
- Distractions and distractibility index
- Physical environment elements
- Work system design
    - Evidence-based design
- Challenges in the physical environment
    - Preparation and compounding
- Physical environment factors (see further discussion of these factors below)

As of January 1, 2018, TJC published enhanced details for on-site evaluation of sterile compounding facilities within hospitals, critical access hospitals, and home care organizations.[9] With this update, TJC has a more detailed process for evaluating staff competencies, the compounding facility, the compounding process, and environmental monitoring and certification. Additionally, TJC offers a medication compounding certificate program for pharmacies wishing to validate compliance of their compounding programs with USP compounding standards. While this is optional, some state boards of pharmacy require pharmacies conducting sterile compounding to obtain certification. In a question and answer article, Robert Campbell from TJC discussed the new and revised TJC standards, the top medication management-related noncompliant standards, and red flags involving sterile medication cleanroom facilities. TJC accredited facilities should expect to see a more robust survey for assessing sterile compounding compliance as part of medication management, life safety, infection control, and competency assessment components. TJC requirements for hospital sterile preparation facilities are updated based on the most current version of USP Chapter <797>. TJC suggests the following as areas of focus for a survey of the medication compounding process:

- Ensure sites remain informed with updates and revisions to the compounding standards to ensure compliance with the updated chapters
- Environmental assessment of facility engineering controls and review of testing and certification reports
- Assessment of product preparation
- Competency assessment program for all compounding staff[10]

Outsourcing facilities (503B pharmacies) have more stringent Food and Drug Administration (FDA) regulated cleanroom facility requirements. (See Chapter 34 for a more comprehensive discussion of outsourcing of CSPs.)

In November of 2020, the FDA also issued a final guidance document on insanitary conditions, which provides details on conditions where a drug may be deemed adulterated. The guidance describes instances of unsanitary conditions that the FDA has observed in compounding facilities. The document includes the following specific examples of facility and engineering control unsanitary conditions for nonsterile and sterile compounding[11]:

- Sources of contamination (eg, vermin, bacteria, mold, rust, glass shavings, hair, and paint chips)
- Evidence of environmental control challenges in or near the production areas (eg, construction or areas of standing water or leakage)
- Inadequate engineering controls in place for handling hazardous, highly potent, or sensitizing drugs
- Exposing sterile drugs and materials to lower than ISO 5 quality air
- Lack of engineering controls and monitoring that compromise the ISO classified spaces, including an absence or lack of the following:
    - Scheduled and routine environmental monitoring
    - Personnel sampling
    - Routine certification under dynamic conditions of the ISO 5 areas
    - Proper facility design preventing the influx of lower quality air into an area of higher quality air
- Situations contributing to a loss of environmental control that may impact drug sterility, including the following:
    - A lack of frequent pressure differential monitoring
    - A lack of HEPA-filtered air or inadequate HEPA-filtered airflow over the critical areas and HEPA filters lacking sealing around the perimeter
    - Improper ISO classification of rooms based on the activities performed
    - Areas and design features in classified rooms contributing to dirt and particle generation, such as difficult to clean areas, overhangs and ledges, presence of sinks or water sources in the buffer room or the presence of drains in any ISO classified areas, and equipment within or close to the ISO 5 area that has the potential to compromise the ISO 5 air[11]

Chapter 2 provides a more detailed review of regulatory requirements relevant to compounding sterile preparations.

THE CLEANROOM SUITE: BUFFER ROOM AND ANTEROOM

Background

Writing for the *New York Times*, William Yardley reported the following:

> Half a century ago, as a rapidly changing world sought. . . more sanitary hospital conditions, one of the biggest obstacles to progress was air, and the dust and germs it contains. . . . Unchecked bacteria could quickly infect a patient after a seemingly successful operation. . . . Then in 1962, Willis Whitfield invented the clean room. . . . His clean rooms blew air from the ceiling and sucked it out from the floor. Filters scrubbed the air before it entered the room. . . . Particle detectors in Whitfield's cleanrooms started showing counts so low—a thousand times lower than other methods—that some people did not believe the readings. . . . Whitfield who worked at Sandia from 1954 to 1984 died on November 12, 2012.[12]

Prior to Willis Whitfield's invention of cleanrooms that produce constant laminar airflow, critical environments had turbulent and unpredictable airflow. With a greater recognition of particle levels due to dust and skin cells in the manufacturing and healthcare environments in the 1950s and 1960s, extensive research was conducted on applying principles of HEPA-filtered laminar airflow to complex industrial manufacturing and healthcare environments. This led to the development of a federal cleanroom standard for air cleanliness based on specific concentrations of particles that are 0.5 microns and larger, adoption of cleanroom concepts in pharmaceutical manufacturing in the 1970s, and greater recognition of cleanroom design technology.[13] Isn't it incredible that hospital pharmacies have taken over 50 years to begin to embrace cleanroom technology in CSPs?

Heating, Ventilation, and Air Conditioning Design Considerations

The design of heating, ventilation, and air conditioning (HVAC) systems in cleanrooms requires a thorough understanding of guidelines, air pressurization, temperature, humidity, cleanliness guidelines, codes, and standards. An HVAC system for cleanrooms differs dramatically from systems for other commercial spaces based on their size, system requirements, reliability, and equipment design.[14]

While awareness of compounding standards continues to grow, in 2022 only 72% of hospital pharmacy departments reported *meeting or exceeding* all the requirements of the USP Chapter <797> published in 2008. Only 29% of facilities indicated compliance with *all* of the requirements from the 2019 revised version of the chapter, which, while remanded, was very similar to the final, official version released in 2022. More encouraging is that 50% of hospital pharmacy departments reported to meet *most* of the requirements of the revised USP Chapter <797> version.[15]

To be compliant with USP Chapter <797>, sterile compounding areas must provide a comfortable and well-lit working environment, which typically includes a temperature of 20°C (68°F) or cooler and a relative humidity (RH) less than 60% to minimize the risk of microbial proliferation and maintain comfortable conditions for compounding personnel to perform when wearing the required aseptic compounding garb.[1]

Temperature and Humidity

The combination of temperature and RH (20°C at 55% RH design maximum) requires a supply air source with a maximum dewpoint temperature of 10.72°C (51.3°F), which is significantly lower than the dew point used in other comfort cooling applications. Dew point temperature is a function of how much moisture is in the air, and it is related to the temperature of the air leaving the cooling coil. While a maximum RH of 60% is allowed by USP Chapter <797>, the design basis should have a safety factor of at least 5% below the allowed limit. Allowing for a safety factor accounts for deviations in the performance of the mechanical equipment. A temperature lower than the maximum allowed of 20°C (68°F) is frequently required to maintain a comfortable environment for personnel who work for extended periods wearing the required compounding garb.

Frequently, poorly designed cleanrooms are served by a shared HVAC source that is not capable of providing the low dew point temperature air required for classified spaces. If that is the case, the shared HVAC system must be modified to meet the new dew point requirements. The preferred design is for the classified spaces to be served by a dedicated, low-temperature HVAC system.

Temperature and humidity must be monitored in each room of the cleanroom suite each day that the cleanroom suite is in operation. Monitoring can be done manually or by a continuous recording device. The results of the temperature and humidity readings must be documented at least once daily or stored in the continuous recording device and must be retrievable. Temperature and humidity monitoring devices must be verified for accuracy at least every 12 months or as required by the manufacturer. Free-standing humidifiers/dehumidifiers and air conditioners are prohibited from being placed within classified spaces or within the perimeter of the SCA.[1]

USP Chapter <1066> states that humidity should be monitored and controlled in compounding and storage areas because of its effect on drug stability and integrity. A hygrometer should be placed on an interior wall away from supply air diffusers, heat sources, or door entrance/exits so that it provides a representative reading of the RH in the compounding area or storage facility.[8]

There are no requirements in USP Chapter <797> and USP Chapter <800> to maintain a minimum RH in the classified spaces. The 2020 version of the American Society of Heating, Refrigerating and Air-Conditioning Engineers (ASHRAE) Standard 170 lists no minimum relative humidity requirement for pharmacies.[16] The argument for maintaining some level of minimum relative humidity usually consists of one of the following concerns:

- Reduction of static electricity to protect electronic equipment
- Occupant comfort
- Impact on component compounds (particularly powders)

Static electricity and protection of sensitive electronic components is critical in applications where the internal components, such as the processing chips, are exposed. This is not the case in a typical pharmacy compounding suite, which is more likely to have standard equipment such as desktop, tablet, or touchscreen computers. The storage range for a typical desktop computer is 5% to 85% relative humidity.[17] The ASHRAE Technical Committee 9.9 (TC9.9) also lists this same range of 5% to 85% relative humidity for electronic equipment in data center applications.[18;19]

Regarding occupant comfort, ASHRAE Standard 55-2020 has no lower humidity limit.[19] From a practical standpoint, humidifying the pharmacy compounding suite can only be effective if the adjacent areas are also humidified, due to the migration of vapor from higher to lower pressures. The areas adjacent to most compounding pharmacies are seldom humidified, and adding humidification to these large open areas would entail a major capital expense. The 2020 Controlled Environment Testing Association (CETA) Application Guide 003:2022 recommends relative humidity be maintained below 60%, and certifiers should test a minimum of one location in each room for temperature and humidity.[20]

The ASHRAE Handbook—HVAC Applications states that in pharmaceutical cleanrooms, humidification is usually not needed for the protection of products.[21] Exceptions to this are cases of bulk powder material handling in regard to explosion hazards and hindering bulk transfers of dry materials.

The team must carefully weigh the actual need for humidification relative to the potential risk of bacterial and fungal contamination, capital and operating costs, and increased operational complexity. If a minimum RH option is selected, be advised that great care must be taken in the design, installation, and maintenance of humidifiers installed in the HVAC infrastructure to prevent the growth of mold and mildew in the humidifier and downstream ductwork. Introduction of water into the HVAC system needs to be considered very carefully. Consider the use of a clean steam generator for this application, which uses low bioburden water. The humidifier must be easily accessible to allow frequent environmental monitoring (EM) testing, cleaning, and decontamination.

Air Handler Systems

The preferred system configuration is to provide a dedicated air handling unit for individual classified pharmacy compounding spaces. This design allows for better control of the operating schedules and planned outages by the pharmacy team. The choice of a suitable cooling source is a key discussion point for the entire team, particularly the pharmacists, facility operators, and mechanical designers. Chilled water is the preferred cooling source due to its simplicity, which is subject to the system's ability to provide a reliable source of low temperature (6.67°C [44°F] or lower) water year-round, with emergency power back-up.

If chilled water is not an option, direct-expansion (DX) cooling coils can be used. DX cooling coils are commercial versions of systems found commonly in residential applications. In both cases, the designer should avoid the use of an air-side economizer, as it will impact the ability of the system to maintain the space differential pressures because the amount of outdoor air is varied at the air handler. The designer should calculate the required cooling capacity based on the dehumidification design data for outdoor air rather than cooling design. This will ensure that the cooling system has the capacity needed to remove the correct amount of moisture from the outdoor air to maintain the RH in the compounding areas.

Air Exchange Requirements

Buffer rooms must be designed to maintain at least ISO Class 7 conditions for particles ≥ 0.5 µm under dynamic operating conditions with at least 30 HEPA-filtered ACPH. Since airflow may slowly degrade over time as filters load, the system should be designed to provide more than the prescriptive minimum of 30 ACPH to ensure the buffer room can maintain at least ISO Class 7 conditions for particles ≥ 0.5 µm under dynamic operating conditions. A factor of 20% or a total of 36 ACPH or more can be used (allows for a reasonable amount of time between filter changes) to minimize downtime resulting from filter replacements and rebalancing. The design team should consider several factors, such as the number of personnel and equipment in the work area, the resulting heat gain and dust generation, room pressure, temperature, and frequency of access to the room. Every cleanroom suite is unique. Designing the room to meet only the minimum air exchange requirements may lead a cleanroom to be out of a state of control during dynamic conditions.

The total HEPA-filtered ACPH for ISO Class 7 rooms must meet the following requirements:

- The total HEPA-filtered air change rate must be adequate to maintain ISO Class 7 during dynamic operating conditions considering the factors listed above.
- At least 15 ACPH of the total air change rate in a room must come from the HVAC through HEPA filters located in the ceiling.
- The HEPA-filtered air from the PEC, when added to the HVAC-supplied HEPA-filtered air, increases the total HEPA-filtered ACPH to at least 30 ACPH.
- If the PEC is used to meet the minimum total ACPH requirements, the PEC must not be turned off except for maintenance.
- Rooms where activity levels are high may require more HEPA-filtered ACPH to maintain ISO Class 7 air quality under dynamic operating conditions.
- The ACPH from HVAC, ACPH contributed from the PEC, and the total ACPH must be documented on the certification report.[1]

The anteroom for nonhazardous compounding must be designed to maintain at least ISO Class 8 conditions for 0.5 µm and larger particles under dynamic conditions. The ISO-classified buffer room and anteroom must be separated from the surrounding unclassified areas by fixed walls and doors. Controls must be in place to reduce the risk of contaminants being blown, dragged, or otherwise introduced into the filtered, unidirectional airflow environment. A minimum of 20 HEPA-filtered ACPH must be supplied to ISO 8 rooms to maintain the required air quality during dynamic operating conditions. At least 15 of the total ACPH must come from the HVAC system through ceiling-mounted HEPA filters. Similar to the buffer room, the anteroom is recommended to be designed with higher than the minimum 20 ACPH in order to maintain a microbial state of control and ISO Class 8 air conditions during dynamic operating conditions.[1]

Pressurization and Filtration Concepts

Consistent differential pressure relationships are critical to maintaining the integrity of classified spaces. The supply, return, and exhaust air flows for each classified space must be controlled to maintain constant volumes at all times with no variations due to space temperature control, filter loading, and duct static pressure fluctuations. The use of an air-side economizer, in which the amount of outside air delivered to the space is varied based on outdoor air temperature, is not recommended due to the challenges of maintaining constant space differential pressures while introducing variable amounts of outdoor air to the spaces.

Continuous differential positive pressure is required between each ISO classified area. For each ISO classified area designated for nonhazardous compounding, a minimum differential positive pressure of 0.020-inch water column (WC) is required to minimize airflow from an area of lower air quality classification to an area of higher air-quality classification. The pressure differential between the anteroom and the unclassified area must be at least 0.020-inch WC.[1] While required for classified spaces, no pressure differential is required between the SCA and the surrounding area. In locations where pressure differentials are required, a pressure differential monitoring device must be used to continuously monitor the pressure differential. Results must be reviewed and documented at least daily on days when the facility is in operation.[1]

Air in the classified spaces must be supplied through HEPA filters at the point of delivery into the space (above the ceiling diffusion device), with the air flowing in a unidirectional manner into the buffer rooms and anterooms. The air supply from the HEPA filters in the ceiling should be placed in a way that avoids creating air currents inside any PEC device. Return air grilles must be located low on the walls, with the bottom of the grilles ideally located 6 inches above the floor. The requirements for low-wall grilles must be followed unless the users can provide a visual smoke study that conclusively demonstrates an absence of stagnant airflow where the particulate will accumulate.[1] Low wall returns should be placed near areas of high particle generation, such as where garbing and handwashing occur, to sweep particles from all parts of the room away from any entrance to a cleaner space.

Facility Design and Surface Characteristics

When designing the compounding space, the architects, engineers, and pharmacy team should carefully consider how the location and placement of PECs, doors, and pass-through chambers will impact workflow and airflow within the cleanroom suite. Future volume growth should be included in the design. Any necessary additional electrical and ductwork should be placed in anticipation of future PEC or technology additions to the space.

The design of the cleanroom should be centered around the PECs. PECs must be placed within a buffer room in such a manner as to avoid conditions that could adversely affect their operation. For example, strong air currents from opened doors, personnel traffic, or air streams from the HVAC systems can disrupt the unidirectional air flow in open-faced LAFWs or BSCs.[1] PECs must also be placed in a way that allows for cleaning above, below, and behind them. This becomes a critical consideration when designing a HD compounding space where the C-PEC will be externally exhausted and not easily moved to facilitate routine cleaning activities. A common error that can occur during the design phase is placing the C-PEC adjacent to the wall with no space behind for cleaning.

The anteroom must have a line of demarcation to separate the clean and dirty sides of the anteroom. USP Chapter <797> has language that also allows for flexibility in designing the anteroom with placement of the sink on either the dirty or clean side of the anteroom or use of two separate anterooms. When the two-anteroom design is employed, one anteroom is the dirty or wet anteroom where handwashing and garbing would occur. The second anteroom is the clean or dry anteroom that is adjacent to the ISO class 7 buffer room. Personnel enter from the dirty side or dirty anteroom, perform handwashing and garbing, then enter the clean side or room prior to entering the buffer room.[1] If the clean or dry anteroom is adjacent to the HD buffer room, that anteroom must be designed as an ISO class 7 space. Whichever anteroom design is employed, the order of hand washing and garbing depends on the placement of the sink, so policies and procedures must be considered in the design process. Further discussion on the benefits of a two-anteroom design is continued in this chapter in the containment secondary engineering controls section.

USP Chapter <797> specifies that the surfaces of ceilings, walls, floors, fixtures, shelving, counters, and cabinets in the buffer room must be smooth, impervious, free from cracks and crevices, and nonshedding, thereby promoting ease of cleanability and minimizing spaces in which microorganisms and other contaminants may accumulate. The surfaces must be resistant to damage by disinfectant agents and should not contain wood or other cellulose products like medium-density fiber board.[1]

If ceilings consist of inlaid panels, the panels must be impregnated with a polymer to render them impervious and hydrophobic. Panels must be caulked around each perimeter to seal them to the support frame. Walls may be constructed of flexible material (eg, heavy gauge polymer panels locked together and sealed) or of epoxy-painted gypsum board. While epoxy-painted gypsum board is acceptable, the durability of such a system should be considered when selecting finishes. The cleanroom suite often contains equipment on wheels that can damage gypsum walls and require repairs that may be costly or disruptive to operations. It is preferred for floors to be overlaid with wide sheet vinyl flooring with heat-welded seams. The floors must have coving to the sidewalls or the juncture between the wall, and the floor must be caulked. Dust-collecting overhangs, such as ceiling utility pipes and ledges (eg, windowsill), should be avoided. The exterior lens surface of ceiling lighting fixtures should be smooth, mounted flush, and sealed air tight. Any other penetrations through the ceiling or walls (eg, fire suppression system escutcheons or alarms) must be sealed, preferably with a silicone cleanroom-grade caulk. Ensuring the cleanroom envelope is well sealed is especially critical for negative pressure HD buffer rooms, which constantly pull in contamination from outside the space.[1]

The placement of doors within the sterile compounding facility is essential to maintain proper airflow and differential pressure dynamics. The airflow can be affected by the location of doors, the design of door closures, door surfaces, and the movement of the doors. Doors in ISO classified and CNC areas should be constructed of materials that are specifically manufactured for sterile environments. They must be designed to withstand the application of the aggressive cleaning chemicals used in the facility.

Doors must have a smooth, impervious, and nonshedding surface, and have flush and seamless top and bottom edges. Wood doors are not permitted, as they may shed material in use and do not withstand frequent exposure to cleaning agents. Open channels at top and bottom edges are not permitted. Sweeps, such as brush style sweeps, should not be used on the doors between the anteroom and the buffer room, as these sweeps are known to break down and release particles into the air.[1] Adjustable door gaps can often be deployed to aid the test and balancing firm or commissioning firm in dialing in precise differential pressure relationships between ISO classified spaces.

Doors serving ISO classified and SCA spaces should swing closed with the direction of the designed airflow. Doors serving non-ISO classified spaces may swing closed either with or against the direction of airflow when floor space limitations do not allow for door swings as required for ISO classification spaces. Sliding glass doors are another option commonly used for cleanroom suites. Sliding doors have the advantage of not requiring floor space for the door swing. However, safety features and cleanability requirements of the sliding glass doors should be understood before using this option. Other features of sliding glass doors, such as light current barriers, should be thoroughly reviewed with the vendor to ensure doors close in a timely manner.[22] Touch-free technology (ie, hand wave) should be included for all doors in the cleanroom suite. Touch-free technology actuators should be adjustable to prevent issues with opening. The design team must consider the placement of doors and the surrounding wall corners to ensure sufficient clearance for PECs and other equipment delivery during installation.

All doors in classified areas should ideally be interlocking so that both doors cannot be opened simultaneously. In some jurisdictions, electrically interlocked doors are not permitted due to local fire codes or other life safety regulations. Without interlocking doors, policies must be in place to prevent more than one door being opened simultaneously. To prevent more than one door from opening at a time, consider a user indicator system, which provides an audio-visual indication to staff if a door is opened for passage. This can be accomplished by using a red light and green light door passage system with a piezo style sounding system that uses a high intensity waterproof LED type indicator with a waterproof sounder. If using this type of system, indicators and sensors should be installed on door passages between rooms selected by program management. Visual and audio indicators should be placed on both sides of designated door passages to notify staff when a door is opened.

Pass-through chamber doors should also be interlocked so that both doors cannot be opened simultaneously.[1] While USP Chapter <797> does not require HEPA filtered pass-through chambers, the FDA indicated in the 2020 guidance *Insanitary Conditions at Compounding Facilities Guidance for Industry* that the facility should be designed in a way that prevents the influx of lower air quality into a higher air quality space. The Insanitary Conditions document specifically says that an unclassified pass-through may allow for the influx of lower quality air into a higher quality air space.[11] Therefore, HEPA-filtered pass-through chambers are recommended for use any time there is a change in ISO classification. Roll-up style pass-through chamber doors can introduce challenges to maintaining required pressure differential in classified spaces, and they can introduce multiple environmental monitoring challenges. Therefore, roll-up style pass-through chamber doors are not appropriate for classified spaces and should not be installed.

The buffer room must not contain sources of water (eg, sinks, eye washes) or floor drains. If the institution requires an emergency eye wash in the buffer room, only those that use sealed, sterile eye wash solution marked with an expiration date should be considered.

Work surfaces must be a solid-surface type (nonlaminated) constructed of smooth, impervious materials (eg, stainless steel or molded plastic) without the use of wood as either a backing or a bracing material so they can be easily cleaned and disinfected.[1] It is preferred that stainless carts and racks be made of solid stainless steel versus wire to facilitate easier cleaning.

Placement of Equipment and Supplies

USP Chapter <797> explains that the quality of environmental air improves with movement from the outer boundary of the anteroom to the DCA within PECs. The PEC location within the buffer room or SCA must be away from conditions that increase turbulence and microbial contamination, such as strong air currents, opened doors, and high personnel traffic. To ease and simplify floor cleaning, consider placing equipment on rolling stainless steel tables when possible. Fixed casework, including base and storage cabinets, should be avoided in all ISO classified areas to reduce areas of floors and walls that cannot be visually inspected and easily cleaned. Placement of devices in the anteroom and buffer room is dictated by their effect on the designated environmental quality of atmospheres and surfaces, which must be verified by viable (microbial) and nonviable (particulate) air sampling (see Chapter 31 for more details).[1]

Placement of devices (eg, computers, printers) and objects (eg, carts, rolling cabinets) that are not essential to compounding in buffer rooms is determined by their effect on the required environmental quality of air and surfaces, which must be verified by dynamic viable and nonviable air sampling.[1] Space should be provided in or convenient to the anteroom for storage of garb (gowns, gloves, hair and shoe covers, face masks, and goggles) and for supplies that are needed for compounding (eg, automatic compounder sets and labels). For HD compounding, glove storage space should be increased because each compounder must wear two pairs of chemotherapy gloves that are nonreusable and require frequent changing. PPE for HD handling must be worn for receipt, storage, transport, compounding, deactivation and decontamination, cleaning and disinfecting, spill control, and waste disposal. Sometimes, different types of chemotherapy gloves must be kept on hand due to material compatibility (eg, carmustine can penetrate nitrile gloves). Chapter 8 provides a more detailed discussion of ancillary equipment and supplies used during compounding that should be considered during the design of any SEC.

If preparing Category 2 or 3 CSPs using nonsterile starting components, presterilization procedures, such as weighing and mixing for CSPs, must be completed in no worse than an ISO Class 8 environment (eg, in a separate room with a controlled air environment). Presterilization procedures must be performed in single-use containment glove bags, containment ventilated enclosure (CVE), BSC, or CACI to minimize the risk of airborne contamination.[1]

Microbiological Air and Surface Monitoring

Environmental sampling must occur as part of a comprehensive quality management program and must occur minimally under any of the following conditions:

- As part of the commissioning and certification of new facilities and equipment
- Following any servicing of facilities and equipment
- As part of the recertification of facilities and equipment
- In response to identified problems with end products or staff technique
- In response to issues with CSPs, observed compounding personnel work practices, or patient-related infections (where the CSP is being considered as a potential source of the infection)
- As part of the routine viable air (ie, at least every 6 months for Category 1 and 2, monthly for Category 3) and surface monitoring (ie, at least monthly for Category 1 and 2, weekly for Category 3)

Suitable space must be provided for environmental sampling swabs, agar plates, incubator, and other required materials. Incubators used for growing sample plates must not be installed in the buffer room or anteroom. They should instead be located and used in non-ISO classified general work areas.[1]

USP Chapter <800> recommends that environmental HD sampling be performed routinely (eg, initially as a benchmark and at least every 6 months or more often as needed) to verify containment of HDs. Surface sampling is an important part of a comprehensive HD management program because it ensures the adequacy of workplace engineering controls and administrative controls. For additional information, see Chapter 27.

HD Sterile Compounding

Compounding of Hazardous Drugs and Containment Requirements

USP Chapter <800> requires that containment PECs and containment SECs protect compounding personnel from exposure and hazardous CSPs from cross-contamination and microbial contamination during all phases of the compounding process. The engineering controls used for HD compounding are divided into primary, secondary, and supplemental levels of control. A *containment primary engineering control* (C-PEC) is an externally ventilated device designed to minimize worker and environmental HD exposure. Neither a LAFW or CAI can be used to handle HDs because they do not provide worker or environment protection.[2]

A *containment secondary engineering control* (C-SEC) is the room in which the C-PEC is placed. The preferred configuration of a C-SEC is a negative pressure ISO Class 7 buffer room with an adjacent ISO Class 7 anteroom. Another configuration, the C-SCA, is an unclassified room that serves as a C-SEC and contains the C-PEC. The C-SCA must have fixed walls and doors, a negative pressure between 0.01 and 0.03 inches of WC relative to adjacent areas, a minimum of 12 ACPH, and external ventilation. In prior versions of USP Chapter <797>, a low volume exemption from the requirement of a negative pressure C-SEC was allowed if two tiers of containment were utilized. However, this is no longer valid under USP Chapter <797> and USP Chapter <800>. A C-PEC must now be placed in a C-SEC and never in a neutral pressure or negative pressure room. A *closed system drug-transfer device* (CSTD) is a supplemental engineering control that offers additional levels of protection. CSTDs must not be used as a substitute for a C-PEC or C-SEC when compounding HD CSPs. CSTDs should only be used for compounding HDs and administering antineoplastic HDs when the dosage form allows CSTD use.[2]

Whether a cleanroom suite or a C-SCA, the C-PEC must operate continuously in a C-SEC if the C-PEC supplies negative pressure or supplements the ACPH requirements of the space. A sink must be available for handwashing and as an emergency access to water for removal of hazardous substances from eyes and skin. An eyewash station and other emergency or safety precautions that meet applicable laws and regulations must be readily available. Sinks and eyewashes must be located in areas where their presence will not interfere with required ISO classifications (ie, not within an ISO Class 7 buffer room).[2] When placed in the anteroom, the sink must be at least one meter away from the entrance to the HD buffer room. When placed in a C-SCA, a sink must be at least one meter away from the C-PEC.[2]

For entities that compound both nonsterile and sterile HDs, the respective C-PECs must be placed in separate rooms unless the C-PECs used for nonsterile compounding are sufficiently effective enough at containment to continuously maintain ISO 7 classification throughout the nonsterile compounding activity.[2] If the C-PECs used for sterile and nonsterile HD compounding are placed in the same room, they must be placed at least one meter apart, and nonsterile particle-generating activities must not be performed when sterile compounding is in progress. All C-PECs used for manipulation of sterile HDs must be externally vented to the outside.

ISO Class 7 Buffer Room for HD Sterile Compounding

When operating in a cleanroom suite configuration, the C-PEC must be placed in an ISO Class 7 buffer room that has negative pressure between 0.01 and 0.03 inches WC relative to adjacent spaces, has a minimum of 30 ACPH of HEPA-filtered supply air, is externally vented through the presence of low exhaust grilles, and is physically separate from adjacent areas.[2]

The negative pressure differential should not exceed 0.03 inches because a more negative differential could cause air particles to be drawn into the buffer room. The ISO Class 7 room through which the HD buffer room is entered (ie, anteroom) must be positive pressure relative to the HD buffer room. This provides for inward air migration of equal cleanliness of classified air into the negative pressure buffer room to contain any airborne HD. The C-SEC (negative pressure) for HD sterile compounding must be externally vented.[2]

A line of demarcation must be defined within the negative pressure buffer room for donning and doffing PPE prior to entering and exiting the HD buffer room. There must be a method to transport HDs, HD CSPs, and HD waste into and out of the negative pressure buffer room to minimize the spread of HD contamination. This may be accomplished via a pass-through chamber between the negative pressure buffer room and adjacent space. The pass-through chamber must be included in the facility's certification to ensure that particles do not compromise the air quality of the negative pressure buffer room. A refrigerator pass-through must not be used for HD compounding spaces. Other methods of containment (eg, sealed containers) may be used if the entity can demonstrate HD appropriate containment and environmental control.[2]

HD CSPs prepared in an ISO Class 7 buffer room (**Table 7-4**) may use the BUDs described in USP Chapter <797> based on CSP category, sterility testing, and storage temperature.[1;2]

Anteroom Design for HD Sterile Compounding Areas

When using a cleanroom suite configuration, an ISO Class 7 anteroom with fixed walls adjacent to the ISO Class 7 HD buffer room is required to provide an equal level of classified air into the HD buffer room and to contain any airborne HD. A hand-washing sink in the anteroom must be at least one meter from the entrance to the HD buffer room to avoid contamination migration into the negative pressure HD buffer room.[2]

The anteroom design within the C-SEC should be carefully considered. If cleanroom garb will be donned and doffed in the ISO Class 7 anteroom that connects to a negative pressure HD buffer room or if hand washing will take place in that room, there is a risk that skin debris from garbing and aerosols from hand washing will be mechanically transported into the HD buffer room in the offset balancing airstream. A typical person sheds 10^6 cells per hour, and the rate of skin cell shedding can increase during activities such as walking or garbing.[1] Approximately 10% of these particles carry microorganisms that can lead to concerns for contamination in a cleanroom environment.[23-25] Skin cells with attached viable particles drop to the floor during garbing activities and are transported with the inward air migration into the HD buffer room.

The design team should carefully consider decoupling garbing and handwashing from the HD buffer room by adding an intermediate ISO Class 7 dry anteroom where no garbing or hand washing activity takes place. The revised USP Chapter <797> refers to the double anteroom as having a dirty/wet anteroom and a clean/dry anteroom. The air pressure maintained in the dry anteroom should be approximately 0.02 to 0.05 inches WC positive to the wet anteroom where garbing and hand washing are performed, and between 0.01 and 0.03 inches WC positive to the HD buffer room. In this design, the dry anteroom adjacent to the HD buffer room must meet ISO 7 air quality during dynamic conditions. The wet anteroom should be designed to maintain ISO 8 conditions. This setup stops viable particles generated by garbing and hand washing from entering the HD buffer room. **Figure 7-1** shows a schematic of a cleanroom suite containing a wet anteroom, dry anteroom, HD, and non-HD buffer room design.

Receipt and Storage of Hazardous Drugs

Antineoplastic HDs and all HD active pharmaceutical ingredients (APIs) must be unpacked (ie, removed from external shipping containers) in an area that is neutral/normal or negative pressure relative to the surrounding areas.[2] HDs must be stored in a manner that prevents spillage or breakage if the container falls (eg, cabinets or drawers or shelves with a raised front lip). HDs must not be stored on the floor. In locations prone to specific types of natural disasters (eg, earthquakes) the manner of storage must meet applicable

TABLE 7-4. Engineering Controls for Sterile HD Compounding

Configuration	C-PEC	C-SEC	Maximum BUD
ISO Class 7 buffer room with an ISO Class 7 anteroom	Externally vented (eg, Class II BSC or CACI)	• 30 ACPH • Externally vented • Negative pressure between 0.01 and 0.03 inches WC	As described in USP Chapter <797> See Chapter 16 for more information about BUDs.
Unclassified C-SCA	Externally vented (eg, Class II BSC or CACI)	• 12 ACPH • Externally vented • Negative pressure between 0.01 and 0.03 inches WC	As described in USP Chapter <797> for CSPs prepared in a segregated compounding area

ACPH = air changes per hour; BSC = biological safety cabinet; BUD = beyond-use date; C-PEC = containment primary engineering control; C-SCA = containment segregated compounding area; C-SEC = containment secondary engineering control; CACI = compounding aseptic containment isolator; HD = hazardous drug; WC = water column.

Reprinted with permission of USP <800> Hazardous drugs—handling in healthcare settings. In: *2023: USP Compounding Compendium*. Rockville, MD: United States Pharmacopeial Convention; 2023.

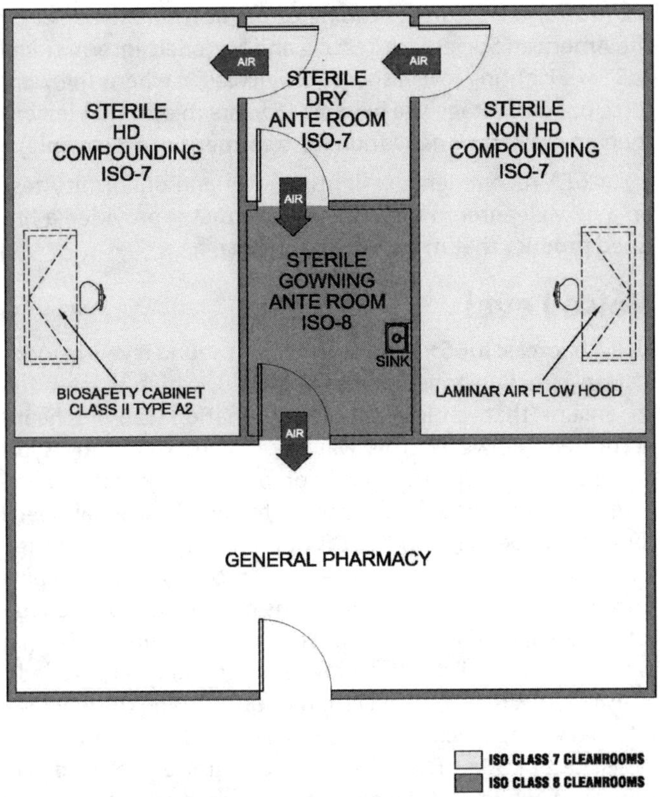

FIGURE 7-1. Cleanroom schematic with dual dirty and clean anteroom design for C-SEC areas

C-SEC = containment secondary engineering control. Image not to scale.

Source: Reprinted with permission of WorkingBuildings.

safety precautions. Antineoplastic HDs requiring manipulation other than counting or repackaging of final dosage forms and any HD API must be stored separately from non-HDs in a manner that prevents environmental contamination and personnel exposure. These HDs must be stored in an externally vented, negative pressure room with at least 12 ACPH.[2]

Refrigerated antineoplastic HDs must be stored in a dedicated refrigerator in a negative pressure area with at least 12 ACPH (eg, storage room, buffer room, or C-SCA). If a refrigerator is placed in a negative pressure-buffer room, an exhaust located adjacent to the refrigerator's compressor and behind the refrigerator should be considered.[2] The presence of refrigerators in cleanrooms can contribute to microbial contamination due to the presence of moisture containing pans. Therefore, placing the HD storage refrigerator in the dedicated HD storage room rather than the buffer room should be considered. If refrigerators must be placed in ISO classified areas, use caution to install and maintain a model that prevents the accumulation of condensation. This typically requires the refrigerator to have a heated condensate pan.

Nonantineoplastic, reproductive risk only, and final dosage forms of antineoplastic HDs may be stored with other inventory if permitted by entity policy. Sterile and nonsterile HDs may be stored together, but HDs used for nonsterile compounding should not be stored in areas designated for sterile compounding in order to minimize traffic into the sterile compounding area.[2] There are no requirements for external venting, pressure differentials, or ACPH for these types of HDs.

Containment Segregated Compounding Area

The C-PEC may be placed in an unclassified C-SCA that has a negative pressure between 0.01 and 0.03 inches WC relative to all adjacent spaces and a minimum of 12 ACPH of HEPA-filtered or non-HEPA filtered supply air. Because of the negative pressure requirement, a C-SCA must be a closed room with walls and doors. Handwashing sinks must be placed at least one meter from the C-PEC and outside the perimeter of the C-SCA. HD CSPs prepared in a C-SCA in accordance with Category 1 requirements meet the BUD of 12 hours or less at controlled room temperature or 24 hours or less when refrigerated.[1,2] See Table 7-4, and Chapter 16 for a summary.

Cleaning and Disinfecting

Because surfaces in classified areas and SCAs are a potential source of microbial contamination of CSPs, cleaning, disinfecting, and the application of sporicidal disinfectants are critical elements of maintaining a state of control.[1] Appropriate space must be provided for important items, such as cleaning supplies, sterile 70% isopropyl alcohol, other detergents and disinfectants, sporicides, and trash containers for all waste streams involved. Cleaning and disinfecting supplies used in classified spaces environments should not be used in other areas of the pharmacy. Equipment should only be taken out of the ISO classified environment for disposal.

USP Chapter <800> states the following:

> All areas where HDs are handled (e.g., such as during receiving, compounding, transport, administering, and disposal) and all reusable equipment and devices (e.g., C-PEC, carts, and trays) must be routinely deactivated/decontaminated and cleaned. Additionally, sterile compounding areas and devices must be subsequently disinfected..... All personnel performing these activities must wear appropriate PPE resistant to the cleaning agents used, including two pairs of ASTM-tested chemotherapy gloves and impermeable disposable gowns..... Additionally, eye protection and face shields must be used if splashing is possible. Respiratory protection must be used if warranted by the activity.[2]

Suitable storage space must be provided for HD cleaning supplies, like deactivation, decontamination, cleaning, and disinfecting agents. Storage for other items, such as gloves, gowns, eye protection, face shields, and respiratory protection, must also be provided. Cleaning solutions are available in a ready to use (RTU) form that includes sterile water as the diluent. If RTU solutions are not purchased and concentrates are instead used, sterile water is the preferred type of water to use as the diluent. Tap water, particularly in large buildings, can harbor high bioburden levels that may compromise the cleaning process. Sinks, drains, and traps under sinks can harbor a biofilm that can spread bacterial and fungal contamination when the sink is used for handwashing. Consider adding the anteroom sink to the environmental monitoring surveillance program and developing a disinfection protocol that will reduce bioburden in the sink, drain, and trap. This also applies to plumbed eye wash units and emergency showers located outside the ISO classified spaces.

Lighting Level and Uniformity

USP Chapter <1066> states the following:

> Lighting, temperature, and ventilation should be optimal to prevent decomposition of active pharmaceutical ingredients (APIs), excipients, and drug products. These measures can also ensure a workplace where personnel are not distracted by physical discomfort.[8]

Proper illumination is necessary because the labels on some containers have very small or lightly colored print. Proper illumination levels can improve accuracy and efficiency of performance. The recommendations described below take into consideration the need to work quickly and accurately during medication handling, the level of task visibility, and the comfort of personnel.[8] These recommendations are made because of evidence that lighting levels are inversely related to medication errors.

LED, fluorescent cool white deluxe lamps, and compact fluorescent lamps are recommended because they have a color rendering index of 80 or more and are highly efficient compared to incandescent lamps. LED lamps have a very long service life that prevents disruption in the pharmacy caused from lamp replacement activity. Providing the recommended color rendering index can help avoid misidentification of medications. If illumination levels are below recommendations, task lighting is required in areas where critical visual tasks are performed. If task lighting is not available, workers might cast shadows on the workspace, further reducing lighting levels.

Examples of critical tasks include reading handwritten prescriptions and small print on labels as well as inspecting medication dosage forms. Because individuals perceive lighting levels differently, adjustable 50-W or LED equivalent high intensity task lights are recommended for situations where personnel encounter difficult-to-read prescriptions and product labels. Lighting levels are important for key healthcare providers involved in computer order entry (eg, technicians or pharmacists), prescription filling, inspection, and patient counseling. Illumination levels for computer order entry areas should be at least 750 lux (75 fc). Higher levels, such as 1,000 lux (100 fc), are recommended when handwritten orders are read. Lighting should be positioned so there is no glare on the computer monitor that may make it difficult to read the screen accurately. Prescription preparation areas, compounding areas, and medication inspection stations (for double-checking) should have illumination levels between 900 and 1500 lux (90 to 150 fc). These standards are all above the minimum of 200 lux (20 fc) for accurate reading of medication labels set by the American Society for Testing and Materials International (ASTM). Lighting levels should be increased where the work force has an average age beyond 45 years to optimize legibility (general recommendation for treatment of presbyopia).[8]

CETA recommends a lighting level and uniformity test on a new cleanroom to verify the contractor provided a finished product that meets design criteria.[26]

Noise Level

USP Chapter <1066> recommends that sound levels in medication handling zones be set at 45 dB, which is intended to ensure that critical verbal information can be heard accurately. However, this will be exceeded in many typical pharmacy dispensing and compounding areas. Healthcare providers should be sensitive to their individual needs for quiet depending on the task being performed, and they should have a quiet area available to promote accurate performance. Accuracy when dispensing medication can be affected by specific characteristics of the sound/noise (ie, whether it is predictable and whether it can be controlled). These factors may mask environmental cues and the worker's internal voice, which is used to rehearse and recall important tasks. Out of 58 studies, 7 showed that noise improved performance, while 29 showed that it impaired performance. In one study, unpredictable but controllable sounds and noise were found to improve prescription filling accuracy, contrary to previous research. This may indicate that some environmental stimuli are needed to maintain proper alertness and attention of workers.[8] CETA recommends a noise level test on a new cleanroom to verify the contractor provided a finished product that meets design criteria.[26]

It is not advisable for compounding personnel working in a buffer room to have or use ear buds, headphones, or similar equipment because the devices can introduce contamination and are difficult to clean without damaging the equipment. However, there are several vendors for cleanroom speakers, but whether to employ them in a buffer room would be an institutional decision. Such speakers must be sealed against air and cleaning solution leakage, tolerate cleaning and disinfection, and, in the case of HD compounding, deactivation chemicals. Controls for such speakers should be outside the cleanroom area. CETA recommends that a noise level test be performed in new cleanrooms.[26]

PLANNING THE STERILE PREPARATION FACILITY

Many health-system pharmacies must build, rebuild, or relocate sterile compounding facilities to remain in compliance with USP Chapter <797> and USP Chapter <800>. In the 2022 State of Pharmacy Compounding Survey, approximately two-thirds of respondents were operating in recently renovated cleanrooms.[27] This demonstrates the industry's focus on facility construction and compliance considering compounding standard revisions and increased scrutiny by regulatory and accrediting bodies.[28] Getting approval for cleanroom renovations remains challenging. Facility size and compounding volumes have a strong impact on the cost of pharmacy cleanroom renovations, which are cited to be at least $500,000 and often over $1 million. So, it is not surprising that over half of pharmacy directors (55%) find it difficult to get budget approval for their renovation.[29] Supply chain disruptions should also be considered when planning for cleanroom construction, as equipment ordering lead times may be increased.

Allan et al. presented a detailed planning process for designing and evaluating a sterile compounding facility.[30] The authors used a strategic functional planning approach. This allowed them to meet hospital goals for efficiency, functionality, and a planned future relocation of the sterile compounding center. The functional program development took them through workflow, workload, equipment, storage, arrangement of work areas, space requirements, floor plan, and evaluation of the facility. They conducted a travel study (ie, how far a person walks in a fixed period of time) that resulted in a reduction in distances traveled to 42% for pharmacists and 29% for technicians, which lead to an improved layout. Not only does the reduction of travel time reduce the amount of non-value-added time spent by pharmacists and technicians, but it also may result in lower levels of worker fatigue.

The functional planning approach includes eight key steps that can be used for large or small construction projects[31]:

1. Strategic master facilities plan: Sets forth the implications of the hospital strategic plan in terms of the facilities needed to accommodate planned activities, and includes a timeline to show when facility needs will occur. The pharmacy department should have its own master facilities plan that is keyed to its strategic plan and congruent with the hospital's strategic plan.
2. Analysis of existing facility: This includes as-built plans; space inventory room by room; equipment list showing age and replacement value; site surveys; assessment of structural, mechanical, and electrical systems; code conformity; and traffic patterns.
3. Functional program: This includes block diagrams that show department components, flow and traffic relationships, phases in development, new versus renovated space, gross cost estimate, and a statement of assumptions and priorities.
4. Architectural schematic plans: These include alternatives that show layout and design of departments and relationships plus workflow of staff, materials, and patients (includes a brief description of fixtures, mechanical and electrical systems, and a cost estimate).
5. Architectural design: It should add all other architectural details including the last review by the users.
6. Construction contract: Includes final drawings for regulatory approval and bidding plus the final cost estimate. Submittal reviews are usually completed during this step. This involves the final review and approval of all equipment, construction materials, and other pertinent fixtures that have been ordered to ensure there has been no inappropriate substitution.
7. Construction: This includes demolition, construction, equipment ordering, and inspection. Oversight of construction quality is a key part of this step to ensure installation occurs correctly, especially in stick-build construction where finish installation errors can lead to downstream issues with the cleanroom envelope. Additionally, if submittal substitutions need to occur due to supply chain issues for items, such as equipment, paint, furniture, or other items, a designated individual should be specified to review any substitutions.
8. Commissioning for occupancy: This includes installation of equipment, orientation of staff, moving, postoccupancy evaluation, commissioning evaluations to ensure engineering controls are operating as indicated (ie, validation, certifications), and follow-up.

Key Players

As a facility embarks on a facility plan, it is critical to understand the roles of the various members of the construction team. Once a pharmacy department is granted approval to begin a construction project, a large construction team is assembled to assist with various aspects of the project. The pharmacy project lead interacts with all members of the team during various stages of the project. The parties involved in creating the facility are the following:

- Health-system facility engineering manager/director: Their role is to ensure alignment of the project and installed systems with the operations and maintenance strategy of the institution. This person is generally responsible for maintenance of the facility and its systems after the construction process ends. They should be continuously involved with the design and construction process.
- Construction project management firm: Their role is to ensure correct sequencing of the project. They also provide construction quality control during the entire project.
- Architecture firm: Their role during the project is to provide a consolidated design process, including all design subcontractors (eg, structural and mechanical engineering), and to publish construction documents to direct the construction contractors. All building code issues, such as local fire codes, are considered and resolved by this team member.
- Commissioning engineering consulting firm: Their responsibilities are to review construction

documents at all progress points to ensure that the systems being commissioned can be constructed as designed, and that they function to meet the intended need. The firm conducts final commissioning of all systems (such as mechanical, plumbing, and electrical) related to the cleanroom. Additional commissioning of electrical and plumbing systems can also be provided by the commissioning firm.

- Cleanroom consultant: Their primary role is to work with the pharmacy program staff to determine exact needs for the planned facility, such as throughput, and to ensure that the facility will comply with the appropriate regulations. This consultant often works with the program manager to select equipment for use in the facility. They can also develop standard operating protocols.

Strategic Master Facilities Plan

The first step, developing a master facilities plan, involves identifying and justifying the need for a new facility.

Identifying Need

Before updated facilities can be justified, the pharmacy department must determine its specific need based on its patient population and anticipated future workload. The following questions can be asked to determine need:

- *What guidelines apply to the patient population?*
    - Many state pharmacy laws or regulations require that USP Chapter <797> and USP Chapter <800> standards be followed, and that compliance is validated through a certification program.
- *What category CSP will be compounded and what corresponding BUD is needed?*
    - A low volume facility or an ambulatory infusion center may be able to operate under the reduced BUDs for Category 1 CSPs, while other facilities need to have longer BUDs corresponding with Category 2 or Category 3 CSPs.
- *Will HDs be compounded?*
    - Compounding HDs will require additional PECs (eg, BSC or CACI) and SECs (eg, C-SEC or C-SCA).
- *Will nonsterile starting ingredients be used?*
    - The use of nonsterile starting components, supplies, and equipment requires additional levels of protection and control to achieve a sterile preparation that is free from excessive bacterial endotoxins.[1]

Justifying Need

Pharmacy directors may face resistance (both from administrators and pharmacy personnel) when justifying the need to improve their facilities. Frequently, hospital administrators or project managers want to know the bare minimum that can be done to achieve compliance with the regulations. After a gap analysis is performed, a recommended approach outlining construction requests can be illustrated in three categories when presenting to administration. The categories are (1) requirements in USP Chapter <797> or USP Chapter <800>, (2) items not directly stated in the chapters that are directly related to meeting ongoing environmental monitoring requirements, and (3) a section on best practices. Some commonly asked questions and their corresponding answers follow.

- *If CSPs are made within a PEC, why does its location matter?*
    - LAFWs do not eliminate 100% of airborne particles. These workbenches have HEPA filters that remove 99.97% of particles over 0.3 µm when operating properly.[32] A significant increase in airborne contamination outside the workbench significantly increases contamination within the workbench. Workbenches cannot prevent microbial contamination introduced by poor aseptic technique downstream from the HEPA filter (eg, from air currents pushing room air into the workbench). Also, high background colony-forming unit (CFU) counts in the room may be mechanically transported into the LAFW on supplies and staff that work in the LAFW as a result of poor aseptic technique.
- *If the PEC is already in a separate room, do you really need a buffer room and anteroom?*
    - A separate room will minimize unnecessary traffic near the PEC, but it will not reduce the contamination already in a room. The primary functions of a well-designed buffer room and anteroom suite are to remove internally generated contamination and to wash it away from the DCA.[31] Consider the following[25]:
        - A person sitting motionless generates about 100,000 particles/cu ft/min.
        - A person sitting down or standing up generates about 2,500,000 particles/cu ft/min.
        - A person walking generates about 10,000,000 particles/cu ft/min.
        - An open nonairlocked door can add billions of particles/cu ft/min.
- *If pharmacy-prepared CSPs at a hospital have never been implicated in nosocomial infections, why should these facilities be upgraded?*
    - Pharmacy-prepared sterile preparations are not commonly implicated because few institutions thoroughly investigate the root causes of nosocomial infections. In fact, pharmacy CSPs have often been traced back to poor pharmacy compounding technique. Furthermore, USP Chapter <797> requires EM testing under dynamic conditions. Therefore, in order to comply with

these new testing requirements under dynamic rather than static conditions, the facility, finishes, equipment, and HVAC engineering controls must all be updated.

- *Isn't good aseptic technique more important than a buffer room in preventing microbial contamination?*
    - One study showed that when sterile preparations are contaminated, touch contamination (as evidenced by skin-type bacteria) is much more common contamination than from the environment.[33] However, well-maintained buffer rooms provide a clean, comfortable, correctly arranged environment for PECs to optimally create an aseptic DCA where critical sites can be exposed. Requiring proper personnel garbing and hand cleansing prior to entering a buffer room also minimizes unnecessary traffic in the area of compounding.
- *Because building an anteroom and buffer room will be expensive, why not return the responsibility for CSP preparation to nurses?*
    - True, in admixtures prepared just prior to administration, accidentally introduced microbes have less time to grow to pathologic levels. But one study showed that 21% of nurse-made admixtures were compounded incorrectly (eg, incorrect ingredients, dosage, unordered admixture, or incompatibility) in nursing units.[34] A meta-analysis of 34 studies showed a significantly higher frequency of microbial contamination in CSPs prepared at the bedside versus in a pharmacy (3.7% versus 0.5%).[35] Furthermore, because many sterile preparations are used for 24 hours or more (eg, total parenteral nutrition and patient-controlled analgesia syringes), microbes can easily grow to pathologic levels at room or body temperatures. USP Chapter <797> does exempt docking and activation of the manufacturer proprietary bag and vial systems for immediate administration from all chapter standards, and this exemption is used in many hospitals for critical patient needs. However, docking of the proprietary bag and vial systems for future activation and administration is considered compounding and must be done in the appropriate facility for the BUD desired.[1]
- *Who is going to force our institution to adopt USP Chapter <797> and USP Chapter <800> sterile compounding facility standards?*
    - The state board of pharmacy is the most powerful agency inspecting pharmacies. As of February 2018, the Pew Charitable Trusts study found that 32 states require direct compliance with USP Chapter <797>. Another 11 have compounding regulations that are in line or stricter than USP Chapter <797>. At the time of the study, an additional 4 states had pending policy changes that, if passed, would require full compliance with USP Chapter <797> or other quality standards.[36] Due to an Office of the Inspector General report, hospital accreditation agencies are training surveyors to investigate compliance with USP Chapters. An increase in accreditors and state boards of pharmacy are reported to be inspecting for USP Chapter <797> compliance. While completing inspection, 74% of state board inspectors ask about USP Chapter <797> compliance, 70% of accreditation surveyors ask about USP Chapter <797> compliance, and 18% of CMS surveyors ask about USP Chapter <797> compliance.[37] Additionally, over the past 5 years, the FDA has increased its scrutiny of hospital compounding pharmacies, especially with the publication of the 2020 Insanitary Conditions Guidance for Industry.[11]

Mark et al. explained how to improve pharmacy services through effective facility planning and design. They address the following issues: (1) matching facility design to departmental services, (2) developing an architectural and business plan, (3) implementing the facility plan, and (4) following case studies.[38] The authors emphasized the importance of having staff input during the planning process. Stevenson and Jorgenson laid out a thorough method for selling a capital project by thinking like a salesperson to demonstrate the need and make the case for the project.[39]

Douglass recommended that pharmacy directors write a 5- to 10-page white paper to justify physical plant changes in order to bring pharmacies into conformance with USP Chapter <797>.[40] To be effective, the white paper must address regulatory standards, patient safety improvement and reduced potential for litigation, fiscal impact in relation to personnel efficiency, capital expenditures and return on investment, competitive advantage in the healthcare market, and alternative solutions and why they were ruled out.[41] It is important to determine the stakeholders who will read the white paper. Use language that is familiar to the stakeholders (eg, patient and employee safety, finances, and regulations). Use tables to present more detailed information, such as alternatives considered, pros and cons, effects on staff efficiency, and building, equipment, and supply costs. Diorio and Thomas also outline a process for justifying and designing a cleanroom project by creating a project plan, presenting the case, deciding on modular versus stick build, and matching design with workflow needs.[42]

Existing Facility

Once the need has been justified, the next step is to determine whether a current sterile compounding area can be updated or whether a new compounding area is needed. Existing room size and environment (eg, ceiling height, electrical supply, water supply, mechanical systems, and adjacent activities) are important considerations. The magazine *Pharmacy, Purchasing and Products* has published several accounts of planning a new pharmacy and cleanroom.[43-46] A plan for how operations will continue without interruption should be devised prior to construction.

Power and Other Utility Interruptions

The facility's emergency management plan should include steps to meet patient care needs during times of utility interruptions, including the need for CSPs. Consideration should be given to providing emergency power for all systems associated with the compounding spaces, including cooling, heating, supply and exhaust air, lighting, receptacles, and the associated building automation system.

In other cases, immediate-use procedures may be safely implemented. Methods to identify and safely meet interim compounding needs or address patient care needs with noncompounded alternatives should be developed, put into standard operating procedures (SOPs), in-serviced to staff, and tested as part of the organization's emergency planning process.[3]

Other service interruptions, such as a flooded cleanroom, a rapid need for service expansion (eg, during the Covid-19 pandemic), or major supply chain disruptions as a result of natural disasters should also be anticipated, discussed, and planned. Siegel described the use of a mobile cleanroom which was used during periods of downtime to handle a variety of causes for service interruptions.[46]

Automated Compounding Technology Space Requirements

In 2022, 6% of hospitals used a standalone robotic device in the pharmacy department for compounding nonhazardous flushes, syringe-based small-volume parenteral preparations, and minibags.[47] The use of a robot to compound products differed significantly by hospital size, with the largest hospitals (400 or more staffed beds) most likely to use such a device. The adoption of IV workflow continues to grow, and many hospitals undergoing or planning future cleanroom renovations are urged to take into consideration the adoption of this technology when discussing cleanroom designs. Many published examples discuss strategies for successful adoption of IV workflow technology.[48] In 2022, 47% of hospitals with more than 400 beds and 47% of hospitals with 200 to 400 beds have planned implementations of IV workflow automation.[49]

There is evidence suggesting some robotic devices that prepare CSPs improve the accuracy and efficiency of medication preparation and reduce potentially harmful staff safety issues in HD compounding.[50-53] Hospitals, especially large hospitals, pediatric hospitals, and cancer hospitals, will want to consider the space needed to install sterile compounding robots. In fact, several robots may be optimal. For example, one for syringes, one for just-in-time CSPs, and one for HD compounding. Many hospitals have pursued implementing IV robotics to insource a variety of CSP agents in a safe and cost-effective manner.[54]

The size and weight of compounding robots can differ considerably. Operating and maintenance space may range from 20 to 180 square feet.[55] Be sure to determine the floor load capacity, the space available (including ceiling height), processed chilled water or compressed air requirements, heat loading requirements, HVAC requirements of machines plus personnel to maintain 20°C or lower during operations, and the workload requirements before deciding which compounding robot(s) to obtain. If sufficient space is available for a larger robot, the increased storage capacity it has may sway the choice.[56] Be aware that sterile compounding robot installation may be as complex as cleanroom installation.

Several publications discuss how IV workflow management systems (IVWMSs) improve the safety, accuracy, and efficiency of IV sterile compounded products.[57-59] Fan and colleagues discuss various options for IV technology-assisted compounding, including bar code scanning, gravimetric measurement, photo images, record of preparation, and minimal to no screen touching.[57] All of these combined should result in minimal to no screen touches and no interference with the unidirectional airflow inside of the PEC. Considerations for cleaning and environmental monitoring should be part of the evaluation and implementation process of IVWMS. Plan the placement of the IVWMS within the PEC using smoke studies so they do not affect the DCA.[59]

Integrated Vertical Laminar Flow Zone

USP Chapter <797> discusses the concept of IVLFZ cleanrooms. The IVLFZ serves as the PEC within the ISO Class 7 or cleaner buffer room. In this design, the ISO Class 5 DCA is created through unidirectional, vertical airflow with HEPA filters placed over the entire surface of the work tables and effective placement of air returns. Cleanrooms with IVLFZ design cannot be used for HD compounding because the DCA is positive air pressure to surrounding areas, and it would therefore spread rather than contain HDs (see **Figure 7-2**).[1]

Because of the extraordinary operating burden of IVLFZ cleanrooms, these rooms should only be used after a critical evaluation of every other alternative. These cleanrooms are extremely expensive to build and operate, and they suffer very frequent environmental monitoring failures caused by human movement in the room. There are exceedingly few conditions that require the consideration of an ISO Class 5 room.

The following are advantages to ISO Class 5 cleanrooms that studies have noted[60-62]:

- Larger DCA than available with LAFWs (thus, larger production capacity in the same floor space; note that the need remains to separate work from different medication orders or medication batches to prevent mix-ups)
- Larger area to place equipment like ACDs for parenteral nutrition
- Greater freedom of personnel movement (note the need remains to limit traffic near DCAs)
- Easier flow of material

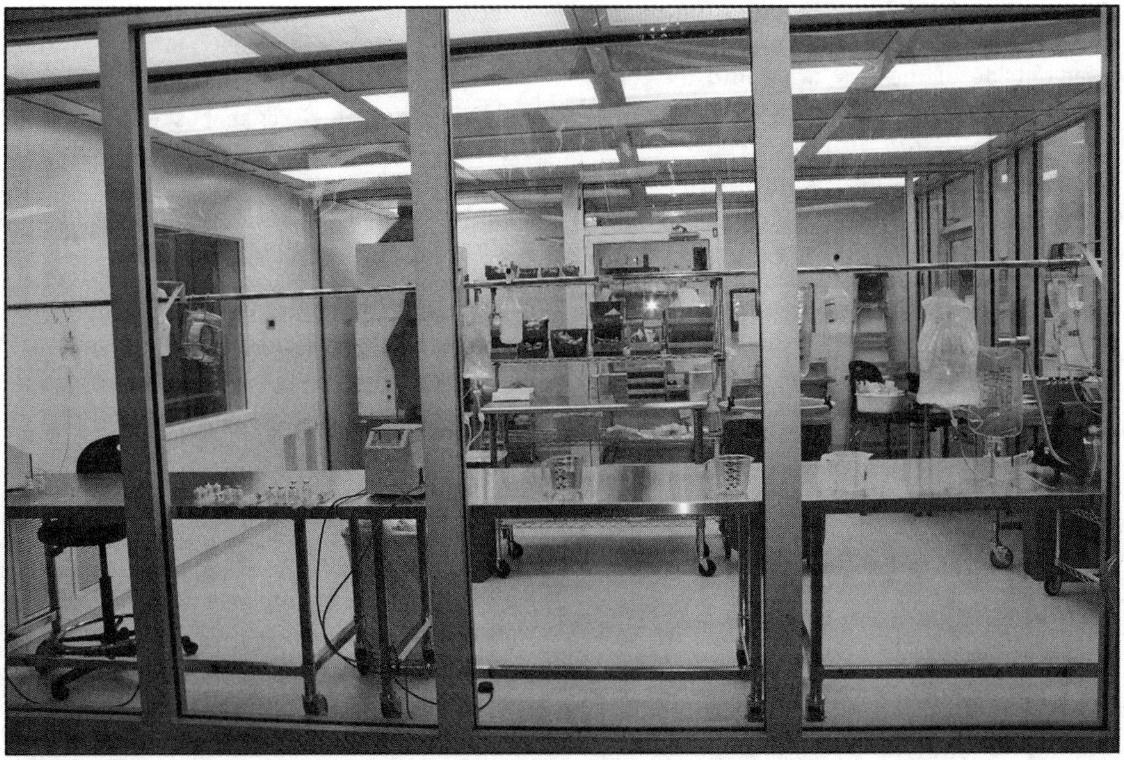

FIGURE 7-2. Cleanroom featuring IVLFZ PEC work tables that are direct compounding areas

IVLFZ = integrated vertical laminar flow zone; PEC = primary engineering control.

Source: Reprinted with permission of the American Society of Health-System Pharmacists.

- Easier cleaning access to the compounding area (ie, the stainless-steel table, walls, and air foils)
- Clearer sight lines for supervisors, video cameras, electronic data capture systems, etc.

However, the following are some disadvantages to ISO Class 5 cleanrooms[61;62]:

- The ISO 5 cleanroom is unsuitable for handling HDs.
- Space is needed for height clearances (slab to slab) for HEPA filter accommodation and HVAC lines.
- Space is needed for a suitable cleanroom width for more low-wall air returns.
- Extra ceiling support is needed for the air foil.
- A knowledgeable team of consultants must be hired (eg, independent cleanroom design and construction engineer, certification person, construction material supplier, and experienced cleanroom certifiers).
- There is a lengthy period of design, construction, and certification.
- Larger air handling capability, versus a traditional ISO Class 7 cleanroom, might be necessary (eg, 90 ACPH or more rather than the minimum 30 ACPH in a traditional ISO 7 cleanroom).[63;64]
- Personnel training specific to working in an IVLFZ cleanroom is necessary (eg, material transfer, traffic control, aseptic technique in vertical air, garbing, handwashing, and cleaning).
- Walls and ceiling inside the ISO 5 clean bench area must be cleaned and disinfected daily because this area serves as the PEC.

Wagner described some mandatory IVLFZ cleanroom design features[62]:

- Position low-wall air return vents for proper performance of a unidirectional airflow system. Unidirectional airflow must proceed down from ceiling HEPA filters and split across the work bench with a portion traveling behind the work table and the remainder moving in front of the work table.
- Perform a smoke pattern test to determine the exact height of the air curtain (air foil). The air curtain can be fabricated from several materials, but the first smoke test can be done with cardboard to save costs.
- Make sure there are no gaps between the HEPA filter media, the walls, and the air curtain (ie, no horizontal surfaces to interrupt the unidirectional flow of air from the HEPA filter).

- Position the steel work table to ensure it extends 2 to 3 inches from the wall, and so it does not extend too far outside of the air curtain into the room. Consider adding cleanable space bumpers between the wall and the back of the work table.
- Make sure there is easy access to the HEPA filter intake areas for integrity testing every 6 months. Gilmore installed special mounting tracks to facilitate removal of HEPA filters from the work area for maintenance.[60]
- Ensure that the delivery velocity of unidirectional air from the ceiling HEPA filters is in the range of 90 to 105 ft/min as measured 6 inches from the face of the HEPA filter. Diorio and Thomas mandate an in-situ smoke testing video during the initial certification process.[61]

Functional Program Document

The functional programming document, also referred to as the design narrative or basis of design, is a large volume of detailed performance specifications to provide the designer or architect with room-specific details for all sterile compounding and related activities, such as work flows; workloads; numbers of personnel to be accommodated; required finishes, fixtures, and equipment; storage needs; transportation and communications; services; utilities; environmental controls; security considerations; etc.[38] This document is usually assembled by the cleanroom consultant, and it serves to identify every specific function along with the required methods, equipment, and systems to be employed in the facility.

Hansen et al. describe best practice approaches for designing an inpatient pharmacy cleanroom. Planning for a construction project should also include accounting for any potential future increases in volume and growth in technology requirements within the cleanroom. Operational pharmacy staff should consider data ports near each PEC that may be needed for future IV workflow technology implementation, and additional HVAC ductwork may be needed for future PECs added to the room.[65]

Anterooms and Buffer Rooms

A highly clean anteroom reduces the number of particles in the buffer room. Appropriate activities for the anteroom include but are not limited to handwashing, gowning and gloving, removal of packaging, and cleaning and disinfecting of hard surface containers and supplies before they are placed in the buffer room.[1]

Figure 7-3, which can also be found in the 2004 first official edition of USP Chapter <797>, shows the important parts and spatial relationship of a buffer room to an anteroom.[66] With the recent revision to USP Chapter <797>, this configuration is no longer allowed for Category 2 or Category 3 CSPs. This design is actually considered a segregated classified area because it does not meet the requirement of the anteroom and buffer room being separated by walls and doors, and therefore it is only permitted for Category 1 CSPs.[1,2]

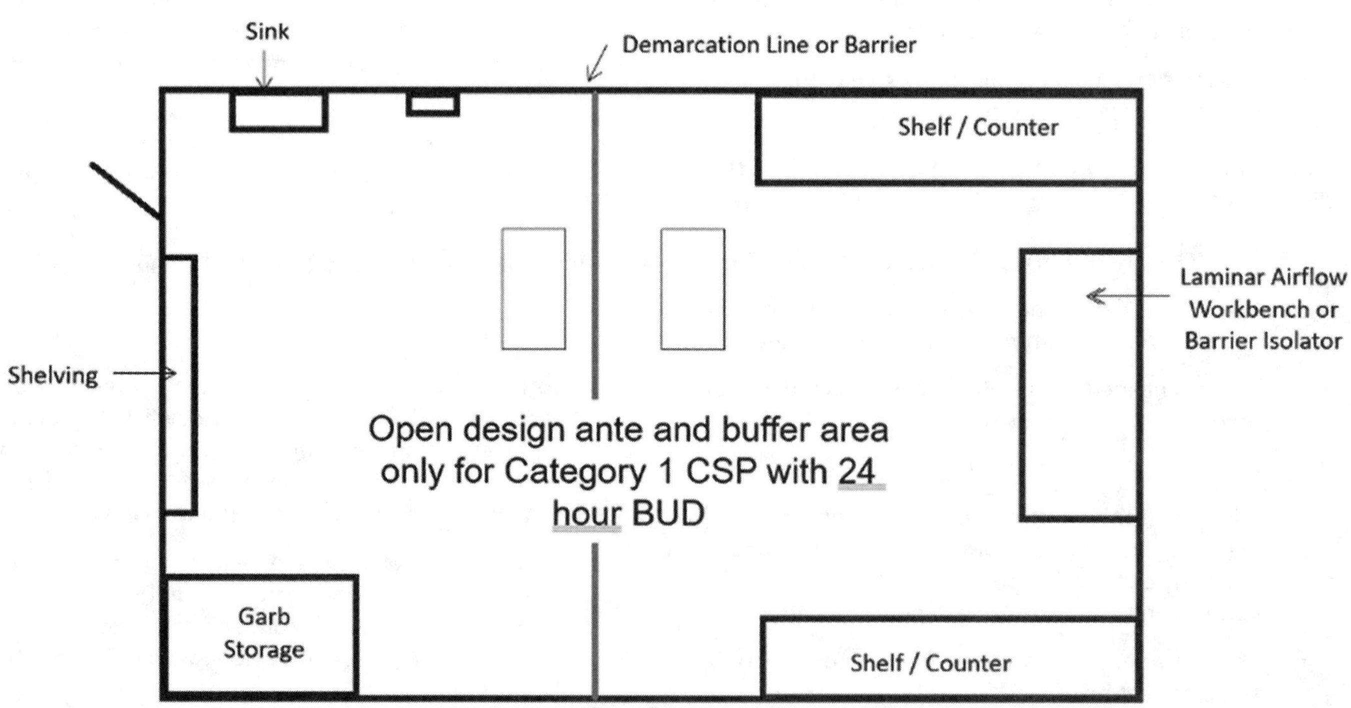

FIGURE 7-3. Schematic drawing of a segregated compounding area for category 1 compounding

Image not to scale.

Source: Reprinted with permission of the American Society of Health-System Pharmacists' Certificate Program.

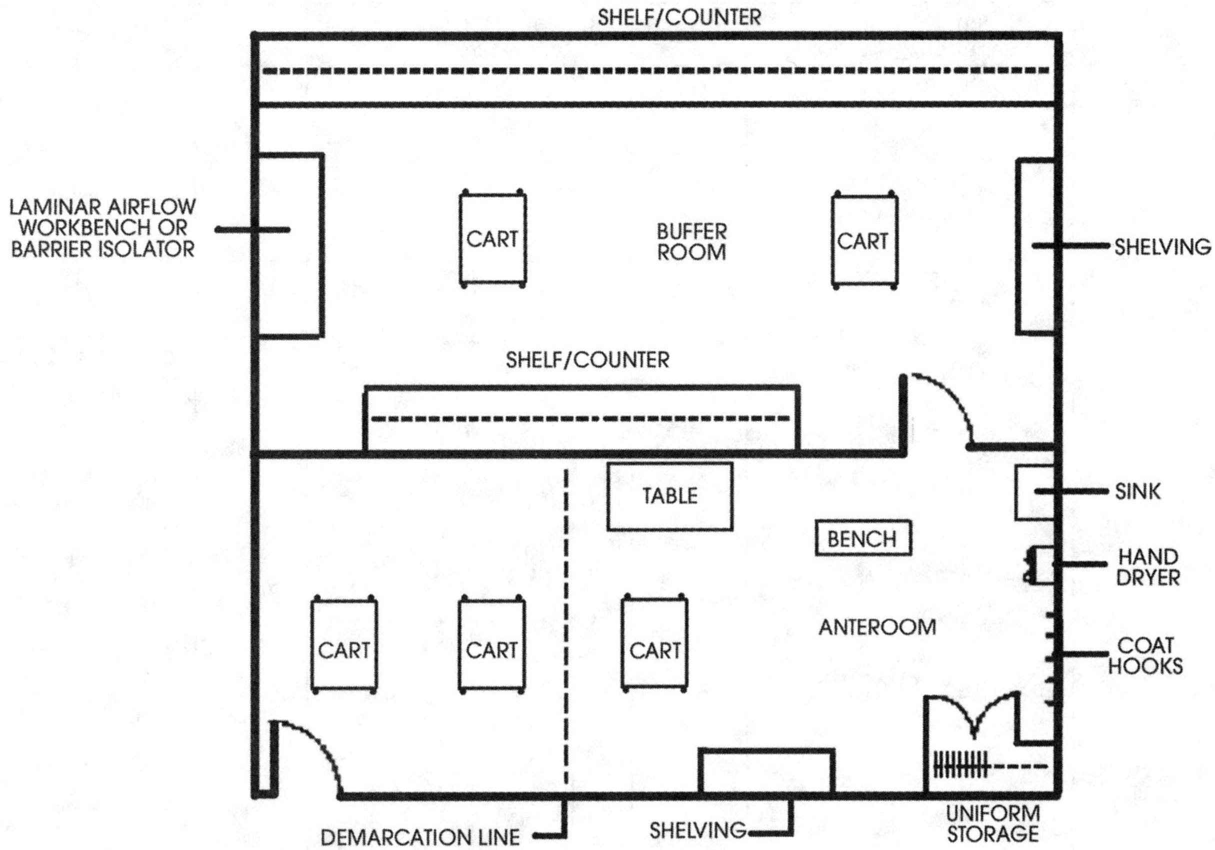

FIGURE 7-4. Schematic drawing of an anteroom and buffer room

Image not to scale.

Source: Reprinted with permission of Ridgewood Medical Media, LLC. Douglas K. Best practices for garbing in HD sterile compounding. *Pharmacy Purchasing & Products.* 2016;13(11):56-64. https://www.pppmag.com/article/1968/. Accessed March 1, 2023.

Figure 7-4 represents a schematic floor plan for a sterile compounding facility designed for Category 2 or Category 3 CSPs. Access to the buffer room for personnel is via the anteroom door and via an airlock pass-through chamber for most supplies. As supplies are moved from the anteroom into the buffer room and then into the PEC, there are a series of cleaning steps that should be followed prior to transferring supplies into areas of higher air quality.

Figures 7-5 and **7-6** illustrates USP Chapter <800> approved schematic floor plans for HD compounding areas.[2] Another recommended schematic design for HD compounding areas is to have a double anteroom design with an ISO 7 dry/clean anteroom directly adjacent to the HD buffer room. In addition, it includes a separate ISO 8 wet/dirty anteroom. HDs must be handled under conditions that promote patient safety, worker safety, environmental protection, and freedom from microbial contamination. Although it is not a recommended design, if a negative pressure HD buffer room is entered through a positive pressure non-HD buffer room, a line of demarcation must be defined immediately inside the negative pressure buffer room for doffing PPE.[2] Regardless of facility design, a doffing area should be present just before the exit of any C-SEC or C-SCA to prevent tracking HD residue outside those rooms. Two pairs of shoe covers must be donned at the line of demarcation when entering the C-SEC or C-SCA.[66]

After existing facilities have been analyzed, one primary question should be asked. Should a custom built (ie, stick-built) anteroom and buffer room be planned, or should a modular cleanroom suite be purchased?

When designing buffer rooms, facility planners must consider workflow patterns, such as how personnel performing double checks will affect air quality and environmental monitoring. If supervisory personnel are not located in the buffer room, movement in and out of the buffer room is likely to increase airflow interruption and may contribute to the introduction of contamination. Communication devices may be used to minimize traffic between areas, and cameras may be installed to supplement supervision of staff or to check compounding accuracy, if permitted by state regulations.[3]

Modular Cleanrooms

Hardwall modular anteroom and buffer rooms feature rigid panels attached to a frame. Modular anteroom and buffer rooms (as opposed to a custom-built cleanroom) have several advantages:

Use	Optimal Primary and Secondary Control[a]	Minimum ACPH	Limitations Primary and Secondary Control[a]	Minimum ACPH	Notes for Limitations
Nonsterile HD compounding	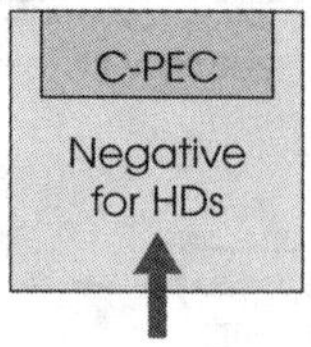	12			
Sterile HD compounding	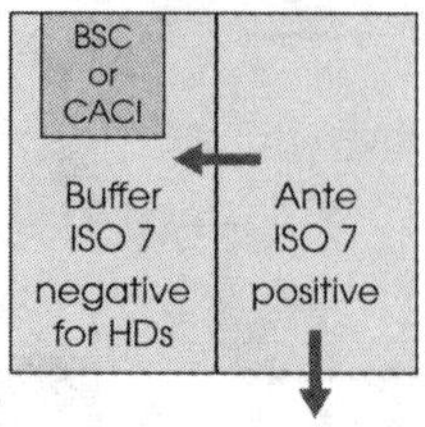 OR 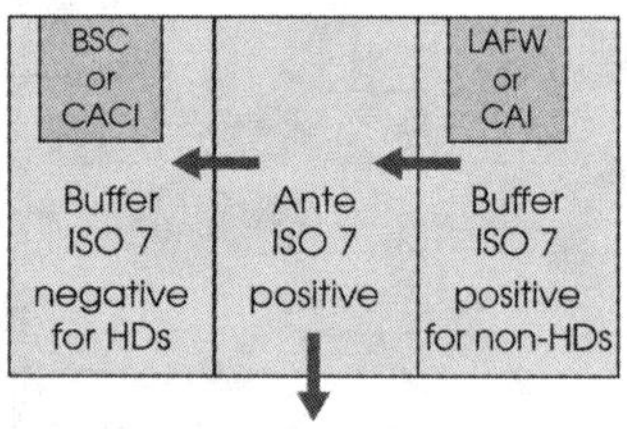	30	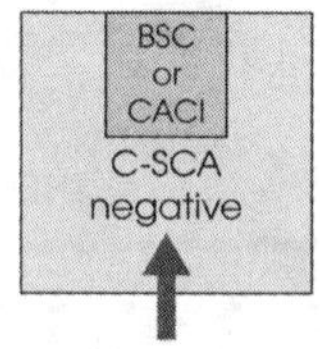 OR 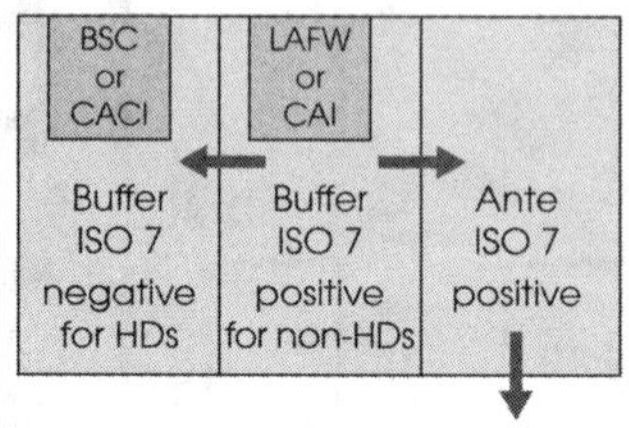 This design is not recommended OR 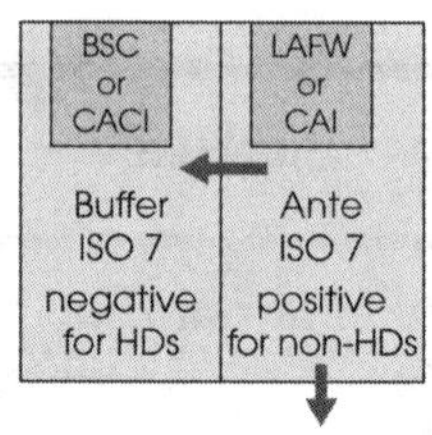	12 30 30	Maximum BUD as described in <797> for segregated compounding area If this design is in place, measures must be taken to avoid contamination of the positive-pressure buffer room Maximum BUD as described in <797>
Both sterile HD and nonsterile HD compounding	A separate room for sterile and nonsterile compounding is recommended		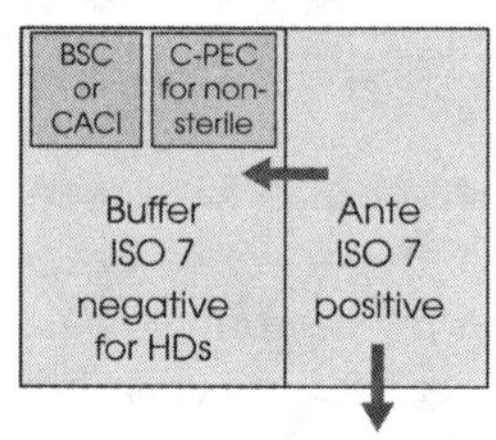 OR 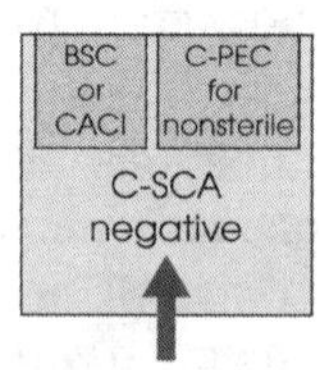 OR 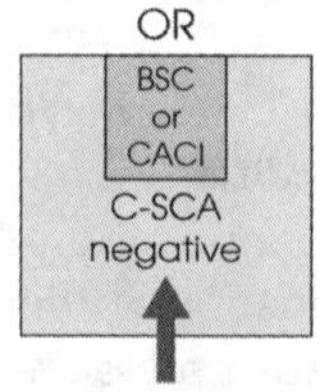	30 12 12	For rooms used for both sterile and nonsterile compounding, particle-generating activity must not be performed when sterile compounding is in process; C-PECs must be at least 1 meter apart Maximum BUD as described in <797> for segregated compounding area Maximum BUD as described in <797> for segregated compounding area

[a]The arrows indicate direction of airflow.

FIGURE 7-5. Examples of designs for hazardous drug compounding areas

Source: Reprinted with permission of USP <800> Hazardous drugs—handling in healthcare settings. In: *2020: USP Compounding Compendium.* Rockville, MD: The United States Pharmacopeial Convention. doi:10.31003/USPNF_M7808_07_01.

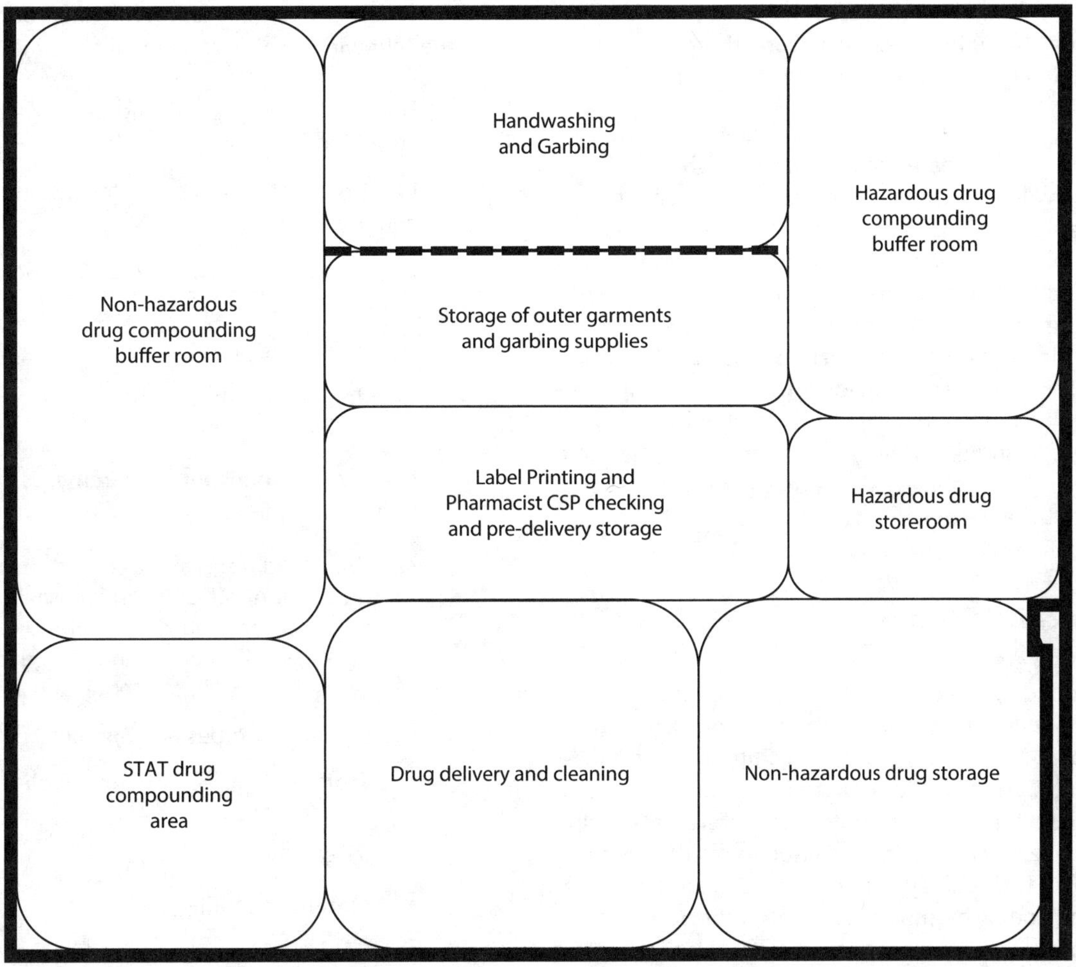

FIGURE 7-6. Example bubble diagram for a pharmacy sterile compounding suite

Source: Reprinted with permission of E. Clyde Buchanan.

- No sanding, spackling, or painting of walls is necessary, which leaves a cleaner startup environment. Modular panels are constructed in a very clean and highly controlled environment.
- Modular design facilitates future modifications if changes are anticipated in aseptic processes and volume or relocation to another site.
- Modular anteroom and buffer rooms are more rapidly installed, reducing construction time.
- Modular systems use standard components that are often available from multiple suppliers.
- Installation may cost less because the vendor will do most of the installation, except for electrical, water, and HVAC connections.
- Some modular vendors offer flush seam wall, window, and door construction, which makes for easy cleaning according to USP Chapter <797> requirements.
- Most modular vendors offer a variety of materials and accessories (eg, pass-through chambers and automatic doors).
- Modular cleanrooms can be bought or leased, as opposed to being a capitalized construction project. This may be a financial advantage because cleanrooms can depreciate at a faster rate than construction.

Compared with custom-built anteroom and buffer room construction, modular cleanrooms have some disadvantages as well:

- Some modular cleanroom vendors just supply the "box" (only walls and ceilings), which requires other vendors to supply the remaining components, such as flooring, HVAC, and electrical and plumbing fixtures, in addition to the utility connections.
- Modular cleanrooms usually cost more for the initial build-out process.
- Some hospital engineers prefer to deal with just one general contractor who does all the subcontracting. Having one contractor may offer more accountability for custom construction work.

- Some modular cleanrooms have continuous flat ledges throughout the structure that can collect dust and create a significant cleaning burden.

When considering custom and stick-built construction, the pharmacy and design teams must consider whether local contractors have expertise and experience with constructing these highly specialized facilities. Whether a modular or custom-built cleanroom, pharmacy management and staff must find a vendor with the required expertise. This may involve hiring an independent cleanroom design consultant or visiting sites where the vendor has installed prior cleanrooms. It is important to involve the hospital engineer in reviewing and determining HVAC and electrical capacity, plumbing, fire sprinkling systems, overhead utilities and pipes (in use and abandoned), and exhaust options for HD compounding. Because of this, installing a certifiable cleanroom is complex work.

Minimal Facility Change

Pharmacy managers find it tempting to convert an existing sterile compounding space that is acceptable for Category 1 sterile compounding to a separate anteroom and buffer room space that allows for greater flexibility in compounding Category 2, Category 3, or HD sterile preparations. This is difficult for several reasons. Adding an anteroom usually takes more space. There may not be enough overhead space for adding HEPA filters and grills. Low wall air returns can be a problem, and adding plumbing for a sink in the anteroom is tough if the pharmacy is on the bottom floor. Also, exhausting a BSC or CACI to the outside for compounding HDs may be difficult. Finally, remodeling existing spaces also poses the difficulty of finding an alternative space for sterile compounding during weeks or months of construction.

In lower volume facilities or for pharmacy night shift or satellite operations, consideration should be given to installing or maintaining a PEC in a separate room with unclassified air supply (SCA or C-SCA) for the preparation of Category 1 CSPs. If a C-SCA is utilized during construction for HD CSP preparation, it must be a negative pressure room with a minimum of 12 ACPH. For any Category 2 or Category 3 sterile preparations, alternatives (eg, centralized compounding within the hospital or health system, outsourcing, etc.) may be considered.

Architectural Schematic Plan

Pharmacists should prepare plans with a hospital designer or architect that is in line with the detailed specifications in the functional programming document. Select an architect that is very knowledgeable with the design and construction requirements for cleanroom facilities as specified in ISO Standard 14644-4.[67] This standard is intended for use by purchasers, suppliers, and designers of cleanroom installations. It also provides a checklist of important parameters of performance. Construction guidance is provided, including requirements for qualification and startup activities. Discuss the requirements in advance, and, ideally, visit or communicate with sites that the architect has previously designed.

The pharmacy project lead and cleanroom consultant have the following roles in functional planning[38]:

- Derive pharmacy goals and objectives as to sterile compounding.
- Identify functions to be performed in the anteroom and buffer room.
- Determine workflow in the anteroom and buffer room.
- Determine the physical environment needed.
- Decide how to handle workload during the renovation process.
- Specify the following requirements for the anteroom and buffer room:
    - Workload (eg, average and maximum daily numbers of all CSPs and specialty items, such as parenteral nutrition solutions, batches of syringes, HD compounding, peritoneal dialysates, nonsterile to sterile, and stat CSPs)
    - Equipment types and numbers
    - Storage requirements for supplies and finished preparations
    - Personnel types and numbers
    - Material handling
    - Communication systems (eg, intercom, email, telephones, and overhead paging)
    - Services expected from other departments (eg, IV solution deliveries and housekeeping)
    - Security (eg, locked doors, access control systems, and video cameras)
    - Utilities (eg, lighting, electrical outlets, plumbing, and computer lines)
    - Environmental quality control (ie, ISO Class 5, 7, or 8)
    - Housekeeping and cleaning routines
    - Environmental sampling routines (eg, PEC testing, air and surface microbial counts, and air particulate counts)
    - Routine certification and maintenance requirements (eg, location of injection ports for HEPA testing and HVAC valve locations, which may also require maintenance access)

Together, the pharmacist and designer or architect find optimal arrangements for work areas, find the best location, calculate space, and develop trial schematics. The architect's role is to translate all of this into architectural plans (ie, determining how much square footage is needed, designing the layout of the space, specifying construction materials, developing project budgets, producing blueprints, and issuing change orders). The architect may be on the hospital staff, may be hired by the construction project, or may be supplied by the construction company. Throughout the design phase, the pharmacy project lead should consider having the commissioning firm or pharmaceutical consultant review the plans to ensure compliance with regulatory requirements.

Construction Contract

Preparing the Request for Information

Before asking a vendor to bid on building a cleanroom suite, evaluate potential vendors by preparing a request for information about their abilities and resources, solicit financials or Dun and Bradstreet reports, and ask for a listing of recently completed projects for similar facilities. Call references and visit some of these facilities. Ask the vendor to submit a set of design plans for a similar project and resumes for the proposed project team. Select three to five vendors to which you will submit a request for proposal (RFP).

Handling the Request for Proposal

Together, the pharmacy project lead and hospital engineer or architect should prepare the RFP and select the potential vendors most likely to serve the facility's needs. Purchasing department personnel can be helpful also. The request for proposal can follow these guidelines[67;68]:

- Supply potential vendors with pertinent information to meet the requirements. Be careful not to make it so detailed that it stifles their creativity.
- Provide a general overview of the facility and its requirements (eg, the type of work to be done and hours of operation).
- Present the scope of work to be provided by the vendor (eg, design, construction, electrical, HVAC, institutional or vendor-supplied connections for electrical, ventilation, and gases). Include key details that will impact the scope of the project. For example, one cleanroom consultant specified that Type C HEPA filters should be used in pharmacy anteroom and buffer room air supplies.[69]
- Ask for a proposed project schedule, floor plan, ceiling plan, elevations, equipment location plan, and air balance schematic, as well as details and catalog cuts of preparations and materials used as the basis of the design. Ask for heat load calculations and rough power requirements. Determine if construction and service personnel should be union members. Use all this information to compare proposals and for interviews with potential vendors.
- Show taxable status of the project so the vendor knows what to include or not to include (eg, permits, stamps, and fees).
- Specify that your compounding area is to be a cleanroom suite with an ISO 7 buffer room and an ISO Class 8 anteroom (or ISO Class 7 anteroom if adjacent to HD buffer room) for airborne particles, temperature (eg, 20°C), humidity (eg, 45% to 60% relative humidity), air pressure gradients between the buffer room and anteroom and the anteroom and surrounding space and ACPH (ie, 30 ACPH in the buffer room or ISO 7 anteroom; 20 in ISO 8 anteroom). HVAC control is the biggest issue in design because garb, workbenches, and refrigerators increase warmth for people in the cleanroom suite. The number of people in the compounding area will also add heat and moisture to the environment.
- Supply a schematic floor plan or bubble diagram (see Figure 7-6 for an example), equipment list, material pathways, ceiling height (slab to slab), current floor construction, and any seismic or structural issues so the vendor can accurately assess construction requirements. What cleaning agents will be used on ceilings, walls, and floors? Are windows or viewing panels required? If so, where should they be? Are pass-through chambers required? If so, where and what size should they be in the anteroom and buffer room? Do they need to be HEPA-powered? Where are doors to be located in the anteroom and buffer room? What type of door (eg, swing or sliding, automatic or manual opening) should be installed? Do perimeter walls require fire rating? If so, identify rating in hours for the anteroom and buffer room. Are temperature recording and monitoring devices to be built within the anteroom and buffer room?
- Present a utility plan. Will additional electrical power be needed? Hospital engineering personnel can usually bring the power source to a single point of connection at a lower cost than having the anteroom and buffer room vendor arrange the power source. What lighting levels are needed (in foot-candles) at 30 inches from the floor in the buffer room (eg, 140) and anteroom (eg, 100)?
- Requirements for a sprinkler system in the anteroom are dependent on the occupancy code and use as well as local building codes. Sprinkler heads should be flush with the ceiling and have gasketed trim plates that prevent air leakage around the sprinkler head. How far away is the tie-in point for sprinkler water supply? Will the water supply be shut down or will it need to operate during the tie-in process? What are the insurance policy requirements for the sprinkler system? Will smoke or fire alarms be needed in the anteroom and buffer room? Are hot and cold water available for the anteroom? Can a sink drain be installed in the anteroom? Who will remove waste material? How will hazardous and nonhazardous waste be handled?
- Require the vendor to do an onsite inspection of your facility before developing a quotation.
- Ask for the vendor to train personnel who will use and maintain the anteroom and buffer room (eg, engineers, housekeeping, and pharmacy personnel).

- Ask for a price breakdown, per building trade, allowing you to evaluate where there are differences in proposals. Is payment or performance bonding required?
- Develop an evaluation matrix to compare proposals. Interview the two or three vendors who look most promising based on criteria that you have set for your institution. Discuss architecture, mechanical systems, heat load calculations (including wall insulation), and electrical and lighting systems.
- Arrange to have the completed anteroom or buffer room evaluated by an independent company based on your RFP performance criteria. Determine who will pay for the final evaluation.
- Negotiate the schedule that protects both parties from unforeseen delays and costs.
- Ask what you, as the owner, will have to do to operate the anteroom or buffer room after the vendor's work is complete.
- Finally, have the institution's pharmacy project lead, engineer, administrator, and lawyer select the best cleanroom vendor. Lawyers for the vendor and institution will finalize the contract for the administrator's approval.

Construction and Construction Quality Control

Whether planning custom-built or modular construction, everyone involved in constructing the cleanroom suite should understand that this is no ordinary building project. The microbial contamination potential of all activities should be reviewed before they are begun. Institutional staff should monitor vendor personnel to ensure that they follow proper techniques so as not to introduce further contamination into the cleanroom suite or its surroundings during the construction phase. Specifically, a designated individual should be assigned to monitor construction quality, installation of materials and equipment per specifications, and adherence to cleaning and garbing protocols throughout the construction phases. Construction quality control (CQC) is a key part of ensuring quality and accurate application of materials and finishes. Errors in paint, sealant, specification of finishes, and more can be mitigated by deploying CQC. Issues identified during construction should be resolved with the vendor on site, not after construction is complete. Diorio and Thomas published an article describing the use of a cleanroom construction checklist.[70] Their generic cleanroom construction checklist is also available online.[71]

A clean construction protocol (CCP) should be developed to direct and guide the contractor and subcontractors on the level of staff garbing, bioburden, and particle control required during each phase of the construction process. As each phase of construction commences, progressively cleaner standards for material handling and garbing are required. This is required because construction debris left behind in wall cavities and similar areas can be blown or vibrated out. This is particularly problematic in negative pressure HD buffer rooms where contamination will constantly try to find any means possible to enter into the spaces under negative pressure through cracks and crevices.

Materials for walls, floors, and ceilings should never be stored outdoors. Packaging materials (usually double wrapped) cannot be torn or removed until the anteroom or buffer room vendor is ready for installation. A general wipe down of building materials with clean wipes is recommended before and after installation.[72] After any cutting or drilling operation, resealing should be completed as soon as possible to prevent oxidation or deep contamination of building materials.

Once the floor is laid, construction workers should wear gowns and shoe covers to reduce contamination and prevent damage to the floor. No eating, smoking, chewing, etc. should be allowed in the area. All spills and filings should be cleaned up immediately. After walls and ceilings are in place (even before the air supply is turned on), the area should be restricted to authorized personnel. Finally, once the air supply is on, construction workers should be gowned like the operators will be.[67]

After construction is complete, all dirt should be cleaned until it is no longer visible. While the PECs may already be in the buffer room, it is advisable to avoid bringing in any additional new equipment prior to completing a triple cleaning process. Clean all surfaces of the room, furniture, and PECs one time with a nonsporicidal disinfectant cleaner, and then clean two times with a sporicidal disinfectant cleaner.[67] See Chapter 14 for further discussion on cleaning and disinfecting.

Commissioning for Occupancy

Final steps include inspecting and approving the new facility, installing and evaluating equipment, moving supplies, assessing workflow, and following up on needed changes (which are inevitable). Use of a qualified independent testing agency (ie, CETA-certified) is recommended to ensure unbiased test results.[74] The sterile compounding supervisor must be sure that air quality (ie, pressure differentials and particle levels), surface conditions, environmental requirements (ie, temperature and humidity), and working conditions (eg, space, sound, and lighting levels) are as specified in the original bidding and contracting process. These requirements must be satisfied before any equipment or supplies are moved into the anteroom or buffer room. The vendor should supply an operation and maintenance manual that will help identify problems and possible solutions. This manual should also provide scheduling for maintenance and part replacements. Furthermore, the institution's facilities management personnel must check that all policies regarding electrical fixtures, heating, ventilation, fire control, and emergency management have been met. An agreement must be reached with the vendor to rectify deficiencies before the contract can be considered satisfied.

The cleanroom suite construction vendor should be required to pay to have independent facility certification and validation. This may involve three phases of certification.[67;73;74]

1. Installation qualification: For as-built testing or construction approval, this proves the environment was correctly installed and that it meets functional design specifications.
2. Operational qualification: For at-rest testing or functional approval, this testing is performed with all the equipment present and operating but without personnel present. It is necessary to see that PECs and SECs work together properly.
3. Performance qualification: Also called *dynamic operational testing*, it is a series of tests or certifications that determine whether the completed installation achieves the functional standards during routine operations. USP Chapter <797> and USP Chapter <800> require that SECs meet standards during dynamic operations like those in the CETA *Certification Guide for Sterile Compounding Facilities*.[27] The CETA guide covers tests for airflow testing, which includes smoke patterns, room pressurization, airflow displacement, HEPA filter installation leaks, air particle counts, and optional tests for lighting and noise levels, temperature, and humidity controls.

Another recommended series of tests to perform before occupying the space include establishing baseline and excursion levels, also known as performing an Environmental Monitoring Performance Qualification (EMPQ). An EMPQ is a mainstay in CGMP pharmaceutical manufacturing facilities. It assesses the current state of environmental control in the cleanroom suite and determines the recovery time of the cleanroom environment during a planned or unplanned downtime. It is a best practice and recommended to have a previously established baseline and excursion level for temperature, humidity, and nonviable particle counts before beginning to operate a facility. The qualification determines the time after which the controlled environments exceed defined limits for temperature, humidity, differential air pressure, and particles.

When performing the baseline assessment, the pharmacy team works with their facilities department, cleanroom consultant, and certification vendor to design a study examining the engineering controls in the space and determine testing locations. During the baseline excursion testing, tests performed at various time points include the following:

- Static EM sampling (include viable air, total particulates, and viable surface)
- Dynamic EM sampling (viable air, passive air [settle plates], total particulate counts, and viable surface)
- Room recovery testing (determine capability of cleanroom suites to return to specified particulate level after nonroutine exposure events)
- Measure differential pressure, room temperature, and humidity throughout downtime

The experience gained from this baseline excursion level testing allows the pharmacy team to put an action plan in place for responding to planned and unplanned downtime. An SOP should be created outlining appropriate actions for conducting an investigation, cleaning, environmental monitoring, and sampling prior to resuming routine operations.[3]

FACILITY MAINTENANCE

Planning, building, and implementing a cleanroom suite is a detailed process. Because of this, all the preparation must be preserved with proper maintenance. Preventive maintenance of anteroom and buffer room prefilters, HEPA filters, and ducts should be arranged with appropriate maintenance personnel or a service vendor. Similarly, lighting should be checked periodically, and bulbs should be changed. A facility SOP detailing downtime and planned preventive maintenance (PM) activities should be outlined. Cleanroom managers and facility directors must understand the life cycle of key equipment (PECs, refrigerators, HEPA filters) and create a planned downtime PM schedule.

Cleaning and Disinfecting

Each day, work surfaces near the PECs (eg, counter tops and carts) should be cleaned with a freshly prepared mild detergent solution followed by an approved disinfectant. An exception to this is a one-step combination disinfectant cleaner that is registered by the Environmental Protection Agency or equivalent. Sufficient time must be allowed for the agent to exert its antimicrobial effect when cleaning. Additionally, storage shelving should be emptied of all supplies, cleaned, and disinfected at least monthly. Recleaning should be performed if spillage or other events indicate the need.[1] During and after cleaning, surfaces of the SEC and the equipment should be inspected to ensure their integrity and ability to function as expected. Any material breakdown caused by routine cleaning and disinfecting of the SEC and equipment may be considered an insanitary condition (eg, rust, exposed gypsum).[11]

When no aseptic operations are in progress, floors should be cleaned at least once daily by trained and supervised personnel. Floors should not be waxed because dried, worn wax adds to airborne particulates. All cleaning and sanitizing agents should be approved (eg, by the infection control committee), with careful consideration of compatibilities, effectiveness, and inappropriate or toxic residues. In addition, all cleaning tools (eg, wipers, sponges, and mops) should be nonshedding and dedicated to the ISO classified or SCA areas. There should be separate, dedicated tools for the HD areas. Dedicated cleaning supplies should be used in the cleanest areas first (buffer room) then in the dirtier areas (anteroom).[1]

Wipes, pads, and mop heads should be disposable and discarded after one use. If cleaning tools are reused, they must be cleaned and disinfected before and after each use, and they must not be removed from these dedicated areas. Ceilings and walls should be cleaned monthly with a mild detergent solution followed by an approved sporicidal disinfectant agent.[1] Sporicidal agents should be applied to all surfaces on a monthly basis for entities compounding Category 1 or Category 2 CSPs. For entities compounding Category 3 CSPs, all surfaces inside and outside the PEC must be cleaned with a sporicidal disinfectant on a weekly basis with the exception of walls, doors, door frames, ceilings, and storage shelving and bins, which remain monthly. Trash should be collected in suitable plastic bags and removed with minimal agitation.

Recertification

USP Chapter <797> requires that recertification procedures, such as those in the CETA *Certification Guide for Sterile Compounding Facilities*, be performed by a qualified individual at least every 6 months and whenever a PEC or other major equipment is relocated within the SEC, the SEC is altered, or major service to the facility is performed.[1;26]

Environmental Sampling and Testing

In addition to recertification, USP Chapter <797> stipulates that routine monitoring and testing of SECs, such as air microbial and surface microbial testing, air pressure differential monitoring in anteroom and buffer rooms, and temperature and humidity controls, be conducted under dynamic operating conditions.[1] A pressure differential monitoring system that operates continually must be used. Ideally, this system should give staff an audible warning when pressure differentials are outside limits.

For hazardous drugs, additional wipe sampling on surfaces of the C-SEC should be considered. USP Chapter <800> states the following:

> Environmental wipe sampling for HD surface residue should be performed routinely (e.g., initially as a benchmark and at least every 6 months, or more often as needed, to verify containment).[2]

See Chapter 27 for more information on HD handling procedures and Chapter 31 for environmental monitoring.

Corrective Actions and Excursions

Whenever monitoring and testing fall outside acceptable ranges, corrective actions are required. If colony-forming unit counts are too high in microbial air or surface testing, a review of personnel garbing, traffic patterns, and cleaning and disinfecting is required. A formal corrective and preventative action (CAPA) program should be implemented to oversee the testing and investigation program. The isolates identified on the EM test report should be carefully reviewed to determine the likely source and to determine which agents should be used for cleaning and disinfecting. The identification of isolates should also initiate a root cause investigation to prevent a repeat of the failed test.

If air pressure differential, airflow velocity monitoring, temperature, or humidity are outside the normal range, the HVAC system must be inspected by a qualified engineer and corrections must be made.

SUMMARY

Facilities used for sterile compounding play an integral role in guaranteeing sterility, as does proper garbing, hand hygiene, and aseptic technique. Proper design of the compounding facility, SECs, and finishes are crucial for maintaining safe and efficient operations. Furthermore, initial cleanroom design is paramount for sustaining a successful environmental monitoring program. Therefore, pharmacy departments should assess their current facilities, and, if needed, upgrade or replace them in order to maintain and surpass compounding standards. Once facilities have been brought up to the standards of USP Chapter <797> and USP Chapter <800>, a proper maintenance program for the anteroom and buffer room must be followed.

REFERENCES

1. USP <797> Pharmaceutical compounding—sterile preparations. In: *2023: USP Compounding Compendium*. Rockville, MD: The United States Pharmacopeial Convention. doi:10.31003/USPNF_M99925_07_01.
2. USP <800> Hazardous drugs—handling in healthcare settings. In: *2020: USP Compounding Compendium*. Rockville, MD: The United States Pharmacopeial Convention. doi:10.31003/USPNF_M7808_07_01.
3. American Society of Health-System Pharmacists. ASHP guidelines on compounding sterile preparations. *Am J Health Syst Pharm*. 2014;71(2):145–166. doi:10.2146/sp140001
4. Power LA, Coyne JW. ASHP guidelines on handling hazardous drugs. *Am J Health Syst Pharm*. 2018;75(24):1996–2031. doi:10.2146/ajhp180564
5. U.S. General Services Administration. *Federal Standard Airborne Particulate Cleanliness Classes in Cleanrooms and Clean Zones*. Washington, DC: U.S. General Services Administration; 1992:1–48.
6. Notice of Cancellation of FED-STD-209E Notice 1: November 29, 2001 [news release]. Schaumburg, IL: Institute of Environmental Sciences and Technology (IEST); 2001. **https://www.iest.org/Standards-RPs/ISO-Standards/FED-STD-209E**. Accessed January 23, 2023.
7. USP <825> Radiopharmaceuticals—preparation, compounding, dispensing, and repackaging. In: *2020: USP Compounding Compendium*. Rockville, MD: The United States Pharmacopeial Convention. doi:10.31003/USPNF_M11915_04_01

8. USP <1066> Physical environments that promote safe medication use. In: 2015: *USP Compounding Compendium.* Rockville, MD: The United States Pharmacopeial Convention. doi: **https://doi.org/10.31003/USPNF_M3367_01_01.**

9. Blum K. JC survey has pharmacists feeling the pain. *Pharmacy Practice News*. July 11, 2018. **https://www.pharmacypracticenews.com/PrintArticle/50165**. Accessed August 18, 2023.

10. Campbell R. The Joint Commission Updates. *Pharmacy Purchasing & Products*. November 2022;19(11):14. **https://www.pppmag.com/article/3007**. Accessed August 18, 2023.

11. U.S. Food and Drug Administration. Insanitary conditions at compounding facilities guidance for industry. November 2020 **https://www.fda.gov/regulatory-information/search-fda-guidance-documents/insanitary-conditions-compounding-facilities-guidance-industry**. Accessed August 18, 2023.

12. Yardley W. Willis Whitfield, inventor of clean room that purges tiny particles, dies at 92. *New York Times.* December 5, 2012:B17.

13. Naughton P. History of cleanrooms. *ASHRAE J*. November 2019:38–54.

14. Bhatia A. PDHonline course M331 (5 PDH): HVAC design for cleanroom facilities. Online continuing education course at: PDH Online. 2020. **https://pdhonline.com/courses/m331/m331content.pdf**. Accessed August 18, 2023.

15. <797> Compliance. *Pharmacy Purchasing & Products*. 2022;19(4):S16. **https://www.pppmag.com/article/2901**. Accessed August 18, 2023.

16. American Society of Heating, Refrigerating and Air-Conditioning Engineers. *Ventilation of Health Care Facilities: ANSI/ASHRAE/ASHE Addenda to ANSI/ASHRAE/ASHE Standard 170-2017*. Peachtree Corners, GA: ASHRAE; 2020.

17. Dell EMC. *Dell PowerEdge C6320 Owner's Manual.* **https://dl.dell.com/topicspdf/poweredge-c6320_owners-manual_en-us.pdf**. August 2017. Accessed August 18, 2023.

18. American Society of Heating, Refrigerating and Air-Conditioning Engineers. ASHRAE TC9.9: data center networking equipment – thermal guidelines, issues, and best practices. 2015. **https://www.ashrae.org/file%20library/technical%20resources/bookstore/ashrae_storage_white_paper_2015.pdf**. Accessed August 18, 2023.

19. American Society of Heating, Refrigerating and Air-Conditioning Engineers. *Standard 55 – Thermal Environmental Conditions for Human Occupancy*. Peachtree Corners, GA: ASHRAE; 2020.

20. Controlled Environment Testing Association. CETA certification matrix for sterile compounding facilities. (Secondary Engineering Controls) CAG-008-20. March 22, 2022. **http://www.cetainternational.org**.

21. Clean spaces (TC9.11, clean spaces). In: Kennedy HE, ed. *ASHRAE Handbook – HVAC Applications.* **https://www.ashrae.org/technical-resources/ashrae-handbook/description-2019-ashrae-handbook-hvac-applications**. Accessed August 18, 2023.

22. Jensen B. Minimizing environmental risk factors to CSPs. *Pharmacy Purchasing & Production*. 2015;12(12):14–18. **https://www.pppmag.com/article/1807**. Accessed August 18, 2023.

23. Sandle T. Sanitization of pharmaceutical facilities. *J GXP Compliance*. 2014;18(4):1–5.

24. Sandle T. A review of cleanroom microflora: types, trends, and patterns. *PDA J Pharm Sci Technol*. 2011;65(4):392–403.

25. Sandle T. People in cleanrooms: understanding and monitoring the personnel factor. *J GXP Compliance*. 2014;18:1–5.

26. Controlled Environment Testing Association. CETA application guide for sterile compounding facilities: CAG-003-2022. **www.cetainternational.org**. Accessed February 8, 2023.

27. Cleanrooms. *Pharmacy Purchasing & Products*. 2022:19(11):16. **https://www.pppmag.com/article/3009**. Accessed January 1, 2023.

28. Halvorsen D. Prepare for intense inspections. *Pharmacy Purchasing & Products*. 2019;16(4):4. **https://www.pppmag.com/article/2373**. Accessed August 18, 2023.

29. Budgeting & Renovations. *Pharmacy Purchasing & Products*. 2022;19(4):S8. **https://www.pppmag.com/article/2898**. Accessed January 1, 2023.

30. Allan EL, Barker KN, Severson RW, et al. Design and evaluation of a sterile compounding facility. *Am J Health Syst Pharm*. 1995;52(13):1421–1427.

31. Barker KN, Allan EL, Kvancz DA. Facility planning and design. Brown TR, ed. *Handbook of institutional pharmacy practice*. 4th ed. Bethesda, MD: American Society of Hospital Pharmacists; 2006:519–541.

32. United States Environmental Protection Agency. What is a HEPA filter. Updated April 26, 2022. **https://www.epa.gov/indoor-air-quality-iaq/what-hepa-filter**. Accessed March 1, 2023.

33. Thomas M, Sanborn MD, Couldry R. I.V. admixture contamination rates: traditional practice site versus a class 1000 cleanroom. *Am J Health Syst Pharm*. 2005;62(22):2386–2392.

34. Thur MP, Miller WA, Latiolais CJ. Medication errors in a nurse-controlled parenteral admixture program. *Am J Hosp Pharm*. 1972;29(4):298–304.

35. Austin PD, Hand KS, Elia M. Systematic review and meta-analysis of the risk of microbial contamination of parenteral doses prepared under aseptic techniques in clinical and pharmaceutical environments: an update. *J Hosp Infect*. 2015;91(4):306–318.

36. The Pew Charitable Trusts. State oversight of drug compounding. **https://www.pewtrusts.org/en/research-and-analysis/reports/2018/02/state-oversight-of-drug-compounding**. Published February 26, 2018. Accessed August 18, 2023.

37. Regulatory inspections. *Pharmacy Purchasing & Products*. 2022;19(4):S18. **https://www.pppmag.com/article/2902**. Accessed January 1, 2023.

38. Mark SM, Kirschling T, Weber RJ. Promoting patient-centered pharmacy services through effective facility planning and design. *Hosp Pharm*. 2008;43:762–769.

39. Stevenson J, Jorgenson J. The quest for capital: selling your automation project. *Pharmacy Purchasing & Products*. 2014;11(10):14–17. **https://www.pppmag.com/article/1578**. Accessed August 18, 2023.

40. Douglass K. Effective strategies for cleanroom budget approval. *Pharm Purch Prod*. 2006;3(4):8–10.

41. Douglass K. Design your cleanroom to ensure easier use, cleaning and maintenance, part 1. *Pharmacy Purchasing & Products*. 2006;3(2):10–14. **https://www.pppmag.com/article/259**. Accessed August 18, 2023.

42. Diorio L, Thomas DL. Tips for designing a new cleanroom. *Pharmacy Purchasing & Products*. 2013;10(5):24, 27. **https://www.pppmag.com/article/1320**. Accessed August 18, 2023.

43. Shepard S. Communication drives renovation success. *Pharmacy Purchasing & Products*. 2022;19(5):22–23. **https://www.pppmag.com/article/2926**. Accessed August 18, 2023.

44. Strauss E, Smith L. EM solutions within cleanroom design. *Pharmacy Purchasing & Products*. 2022;19(4):10–15. **https://www.pppmag.com/article/2914**. Accessed August 18, 2023.

45. Marin C. Key considerations for cleanroom design. *Pharmacy Purchasing & Products*. 2021;18(7):12–15. **https://www.pppmag.com/article/2765**. Accessed August 18, 2023.

46. Siegel J. Three case studies in cleanroom renovation. *Pharmacy Purchasing & Products*. 2015;12(7):2–4. **https://www.pppmag.com/article/1716**. Accessed August 18, 2023.

47. Compounding robots IV. *Pharmacy Purchasing & Products*. 2022;19(8):30–32. **https://www.pppmag.com/article/2966**. Accessed January 1, 2023.

48. McCoy A. An IV workflow management system implementation journey. *Pharmacy Purchasing & Products*. 2019;16(6):6–16. **https://www.pppmag.com/article/2405**. Accessed August 27, 2023.

49. Workflow Management IV. State of pharmacy automation 2022 survey. *Pharmacy Purchasing & Products*. 2022;19(8):34. **https://www.pppmag.com/article/2967**. Accessed January 1, 2023.

50. Urbine TF, Schneider PJ. Estimated cost savings from reducing errors in the preparation of sterile doses of medications. *Hosp Pharm*. 2014;49(8):731–739.

51. Seger AC, Churchill WW, Keohane CA, et al. Impact of robotic antineoplastic preparation on safety, workflow, and costs. *J Oncol Pract*. 2012;8(6):344–349, 1, 349.

52. Bhakta SB, Colaveccia AC, Coffey W, Curlee DR, Garey KW. Implementation and evaluation of sterile compounding robot. *Am J Health-Syst Pharm*. 2018; 5:11(2)S51–S57.

53. Bekri S, Dupart P. Insourcing IV safety compounding with robots. *Pharmacy Purchasing & Products*. 2017; 14(3):S1–S2. **https://www.pppmag.com/article/2015**. Accessed August 18, 2023.

54. Hansen KN, Kang K. Insourcing RTA syringes with IV robotics. *Pharmacy Purchasing & Products*. 2018;15(11):52–60. **https://www.pppmag.com/article/2319**. Accessed August 18, 2023.

55. Franzel S. A tale of two IV robots. *Pharm Pract News*. 2013;40(5):24–25. **https://www.pharmacypracticenews.com/Pharmacy-Technology-Report/Article/05-13/A-Tale-of-Two-IV-Robots/23209**. Accessed August 18, 2023.

56. Ciullo SJ, Pustovalova I, Zahra J. Making the switch to robotic IV preparation. *Pharmacy Purchasing & Products* 2013;10(9):6–12. **https://www.pppmag.com/article/1385**. Accessed August 18, 2023.

57. Fan M, Yang D, Ng B, et al. Impact of technology-assisted versus manual sterile compounding on safety and efficiency in a Canadian community hospital. *Am J Health Syst Pharm*. 2022;79(19):1685–1696.

58. Leary MH, Eckel SF. The selection process for IV workflow technology. *Pharmacy Purchasing & Products*. 2018;15(1):4–10. **https://www.pppmag.com/article/2159**. Accessed August 18, 2023.

59. Brasher C, Smith K, Daniels CC. Implementing IV Workflow Management systems. *Pharmacy Purchasing & Products*. 2022;19(4):2, 4, 7. **https://www.ppmag.com/article/2913**. Accessed March 1, 2023.

60. Gilmore NM. Designing a cleanroom with integrated vertical laminar airflow. *Pharmacy Purchasing & Products*. 2010;7(6):4–7. **https://www.pppmag.com/article/713**. Accessed August 18, 2023.

61. Diorio L, Thomas D. Open architecture design considerations in the cleanroom. *Pharmacy Purchasing & Products*. 2014;11(5):40–42. **https://www.pppmag.com/article/1509**. Accessed August 18, 2023.

62. Wagner J. Integrated Vertical Laminar Airflow design considerations. In: Designing a cleanroom with integrated vertical laminar airflow design considerations. *Pharmacy Purchasing & Products*. 2010;7(6):4-7. **https://www.pppmag.com/article/713**. Accessed August 18, 2023.

63. Lipeles C. HVAC cleanroom design calculation explained. Cleanroom Technology. **https://www.cleanroomtechnology.com/news/article_page/HVAC_cleanroom_design_calculation_explained/156934**. Published August 6, 2019. Accessed August 18, 2023.

64. ISO 4-9 Cleanrooms. Total clean air. **https://www.modular-cleanroom.net/cleanrooms/iso-4-9/**. Accessed August 18, 2023.

65. Hansen KM, Mehta A, O'Neil DP, Wolf M. Designing the pharmacy cleanroom of the future. *Pharmacy Purchasing & Products*. 2019;16(7):10–23. **https://www.pppmag.com/article/2411**. Accessed August 18, 2023.

66. Douglass K. Best practices for garbing in HD sterile compounding. *Pharmacy Purchasing & Products*. 2016;13(11):56–64. **https://www.pppmag.com/article/1968/**. Accessed March 1, 2023.

67. International Organization for Standardization. *International Standard 14644-4:2022. Cleanrooms and associated controlled environments—Part 4: Design, construction and start-up*. 2nd ed. Geneva, Switzerland: International Organization for Standardization; 2022.

68. Loughran T, Burton J. How to write a specification for and evaluate a design/build cleanroom proposal. *IQS Newsroom*. **https://blog.iqsdirectory.com/how-to-write-a-specification-for-and-evaluate-a-designbuild-cleanroom-proposal/**. January 22, 2009. Accessed March 19, 2023.

69. Thompson CA. Revisions continue on USP sterile compounding chapter. *Am J Health-Syst Pharm*. 2005;62:1856, 1858, 1861-2.

70. Diorio L, Thomas D. Tips for planning a pharmacy cleanroom renovation. *Pharmacy Purchasing & Products*. 2014;11(7):18–23.

71. Diorio L, Thomas D. Generic cleanroom construction checklist. *Pharmacy Purchasing & Products*. 2014;11(7):18. **https://www.pppmag.com/documents/V11N7/pdfs/ldt_cleanroom_renovation_checklist.pdf**. Accessed August 18, 2023.

72. Kozicki M, Hoenig S, Robinson P. *Cleanrooms facilities and practices*. New York, NY: Van Nostrand Reinhold;1991:49–79.

73. Controlled Environment Testing Association. CETA national board of testing (CNBT). **https://www.cetainternational.org/cnbtinfo**. Accessed August 18, 2023.

74. Von Holtz K. Preparing for cleanroom certification and validation. *Cleanrooms*. 2006;20(5):34–36.

ANCILLARY EQUIPMENT AND SUPPLIES

Ashley Duty

INTRODUCTION

This chapter focuses on the equipment and supplies used in compounding sterile preparations, which must be in compliance with the requirements of USP Chapter <797> Pharmaceutical Compounding—Sterile Preparations and USP Chapter <800> Hazardous Drugs—Handling in Healthcare Settings.[1;2] Since items on the market are constantly changing, this chapter cannot cover all of the available options for equipment and supplies. For timely information on equipment and supplies covered in this chapter, please refer to *The Pharmacy Purchasing & Products Magazine* at www.pppmag.com.

It can be helpful to visit the exhibit hall of large pharmacy conferences to meet new vendor representatives and see products and equipment in person. Research can also be conducted online. Readers will also find useful information from their group purchasing organization and from other departments within their organizations, such as infection control, housekeeping, surgery, and, of course, purchasing.

This chapter does not cover the selection of primary engineering controls (PECs), such as laminar airflow workbenches, biological safety cabinets, and compounding isolators (see Chapter 6); use of automated compounding devices and robotic compounders (see Chapter 9); or choices for sterile compounding educational equipment and supplies (see Chapters 3 and 4).

Equipment

Equipment decisions often drive the layout of the anterooms and buffer rooms for sterile compounding. The sizing, layout, and overall design of spaces should take into consideration the equipment that is required to perform the work, appropriately store products and preparations, and maintain access to the room. Compiling an equipment list should be the first step of assessing and designing any sterile preparation compounding space.

Carts

Carts can be thought of in two different capacities. The first purpose is for storage of supplies and drugs used for compounded sterile preparations (CSPs). The second is for use as a mechanism that transports necessary supplies into the buffer room and final preparations outside of the buffer room. Regardless of the function of the cart (storage or transport), USP Chapter <797> requires carts "be constructed from nonporous materials with cleanable casters and wheels to promote mobility and ensure ease of cleaning and disinfection."[1]

Carts serve many functions in and around pharmacy anterooms and buffer rooms (eg, work carts, supply carts, transfer carts, etc.).[3] Work carts are usually made of stainless steel and can be used to organize and stage drugs and other components for compounding in the buffer room. When planning a compounding area, work carts are often used with each PEC. Supply carts can be used in the buffer room to hold the ancillary supplies needed for the shift's compounding. Supply carts should have a solid bottom shelf or a liner on the bottom shelf (if made of wire) for infection control purposes and regulatory compliance. Although supply carts may be made of various materials, stainless steel is preferred due to its durability when exposed to the cleaning agents used in the buffer and anteroom. Healthcare plastic shelving made with durable polymers and epoxy coating is also an option. These plastics are generally lighter and may have antimicrobial protective coating options. Wire carts were previously recommended over solid shelving because they do not accumulate dust and debris. However, each individual wire on a wire shelf has to be cleaned monthly, which is tedious. Purchasing solid shelving makes it easier to visualize if the surface has been cleaned thoroughly.

Note: The author acknowledges Ryan A. Forrey who authored this chapter in the previous edition.

DOI 10.37573/9781585286492.008

Supply carts usually remain stationary between floor cleanings, whereas work carts are moved frequently between the anteroom and buffer room.

Transfer carts are used to deliver drugs and components from storage to the anteroom, but they are not introduced into the buffer room. Components and CSPs should be moved in and out of anterooms and buffer rooms on suitable carts (see Chapter 19). Transfer carts may be of molded, nonporous plastic, wire, or sheet metal as long as their construction can bear heavier loads. Wheels must be made of material that does not scuff floors and is cleanable. Carts that have been to patient care areas should never enter the clean side of the anteroom. If the cart does need to cross the line of demarcation in the ante room, the entire cart must be cleaned and disinfected, including the casters.[1]

Casework and Millwork

Casework is a general term that refers to assembled cabinets and storage units. Casework can either be mobile (eg, on casters), freestanding modular, or built in. A familiar example of casework is the laboratory bench from a high school science class. *Millwork* refers specifically to the wooden cabinetry that is built into the space and attached to the walls and floors. Kitchen cabinets and counters found in residences are familiar examples of millwork. When designing a cleanroom, the use of millwork should be avoided if possible, and any casework used should be mobile to facilitate cleaning of the space. Any casework used should be impervious and able to withstand the harsh cleaning chemicals used in the cleanroom.

Benches, Chairs, Tables, and Other Cleanroom Furniture

Stainless steel furniture should be the standard for cleanrooms because it can easily be cleaned and does not generate particles. For comfort, chairs may be covered with a cleanable, durable vinyl. Benches, chairs, stools, tables, and other furniture should have smooth, cleanable wheels so they can easily be moved to clean and disinfect the floor. A bench in the anteroom can be used for seating while personnel put on cleanroom garb. As dedicated shoes or booties are donned, personnel can swing their feet to the clean side of the bench to complete the garbing process. Hooks or hangers should be present in ante rooms when facilities choose to reuse gowns during a single shift. Outside clothing should be kept in a break room or locker room area that is separate from any cleanroom suite.

Chairs and stools used in the buffer room must not have permeable coverings, synthetic foam, or oil-filled hydraulic pistons.[3] Buffer room seating must be comfortable (for long periods of sitting), cleanable, and durable (resistant to frequent disinfectant applications without deterioration). Taller chairs may be easier to use with armrests for shorter employees. Sterile compounding supervisors should consider the height of the PEC, space in the buffer room, and whether they would like to teach employees to compound while standing or sitting. Long periods of standing may cause employees to lean on the PEC for relief. Adding chairs or stools to a cleanroom increases the number of items that need regular, thorough cleaning and disinfection.

In the anteroom and buffer room, having mobile worktables (or workstations) may be advantageous. Their use is more flexible than fixed casework and they are easy to move and clean. Mobile worktables should be made of stainless steel with nonshedding wheels. Although only a few sizes of worktables may be available from a particular manufacturer, almost infinite configurations can be made by utilizing components from mobile shelving manufacturers. For example, a mobile shelf that is 36 inches wide,14 inches deep, and 34 inches high on casters with solid bottom and top shelves makes a perfect work height table when placed under a pass through in the cleanroom. Wheels should have a lockable option. Good quality cleanroom furniture is expensive, so it is important to budget accordingly.

Preferences for drug storage vary by institution and the design and intended use of the cleanroom. Minimizing available storage in the buffer room can help discourage accumulation of excess supplies, which in turn helps to maintain the sterile environment.

Environmental Monitoring

Environmental monitoring (EM) is important to conduct as an early detection of contamination from sources such as personnel, equipment, supplies, the surrounding environment, and primary and secondary engineering controls. EM equipment falls into three categories, which are automatic counters for air particulates, volumetric air samplers, and controls for room pressure, temperature, and humidity.

Air Particulate Counters

Air particulate counters are used to count particles larger than 0.5 μm in a given volume of air to ensure the air quality meets standards (eg, ISO Class 5, 7, or 8). Air particulate counting is only required every 6 months, so compounding personnel usually have semiannual air particulate testing done by qualified certifiers who use current, state-of-the-art electronic equipment.

Volumetric Air Samplers

Volumetric air samples are used to impact a specific volume of air (1000 L per sample) through a device and onto a growth medium plate. USP discusses general types of and has standards for air microbial sampling devices.[4] USP Chapter <797> only requires microbial air sampling every 6 months for Category 1 and 2 compounding, so most compounding personnel have qualified certifiers handle these tests along with air particulate sampling.[1] Facilities engaged in Category 3 compounding are required to collect volumetric air samples at least monthly, which can be insourced or managed by qualified certifiers. In all scenarios, owning a volumetric air sampler can be beneficial when classified areas need quick resampling after positive or actionable results.

When purchasing a volumetric air sampler, several considerations should be made in the selection process. The device should have the following:

- High enough air flow rate to take in the required quantity of air without drying the microbial growth media[5]
- Air volume and air intake rate selector
- Device that does not interfere with unidirectional air flow within PECs
- Design that is portable, easily disinfected, sturdy, and manageable
- An easy way to put growth media in place without contaminating the media
- Available calibration services
- Maintenance that is easy and cost-effective
- Available accessories

Pressure Differential Monitoring

USP Chapter <797> requires pressure differentials to be monitored continuously and be reviewed and documented at least once daily on days that compounding occurs.[1] Technology for monitoring varies greatly from simple Magnehelic gauges to remotely monitored and alarmed systems that can send electronic notifications of deviations. Although the continuous monitoring systems may seem like less ongoing work with fewer documentation requirements for the compounding staff, careful review of the sensitivity, alarming protocols, and maintenance of these devices should be conducted. Regardless of which system is used, compounding personnel should be educated on how to read the device and the protocol to follow if appropriate pressure differentials are not maintained. This process should be confirmed during annual competency testing. Staff should not only rely on set alarms. They must understand what the numbers on the display are confirming. Installing duplicate pressure display monitors outside the cleanroom suite is helpful for monitoring and troubleshooting.

Temperature and Humidity Controls

USP Chapter <797> strongly recommends that anteroom and buffer room temperatures be maintained at 20°C (68°F) or cooler.[1] Because of the need for constant cleanroom conditions, it is wise to continuously monitor the heating, ventilation, and air conditioning (HVAC) and install alarms for out-of-normal temperature variations. The same is true of humidity. USP Chapter <797> recommends humidity be maintained at less than 60%.[1] The Controlled Environment Testing Association recommends that cleanroom humidity be in the range of 35% to 60% relative humidity.[6] Humidity that is too high can cause workers to sweat, while low humidity can cause static electricity, which can cause particles to stick to surfaces. Work with facility engineers to find and install good HVAC systems with appropriate temperature and humidity controls. The HVAC system should be able to maintain temperature and humidity control throughout the year, including in climates that experience large fluctuations of outside weather conditions.

Incubators

An incubator is required for processing microbial tests for air and surface samples, fingertip glove tests, and sterility test samples. The size of incubator needed can be determined based on the number and size of the controlled areas (anteroom and buffer room), the number of personnel, the risk level of CSPs prepared, and an estimate of the maximum number of air, surface, and touch plates available at any one time. It is recommended that pharmacies purchase their own laboratory-grade incubators, since microbiology departments may not have the proper certification or space for pharmacy media samples. Two incubators are needed so that one can be kept at 20-25°C and the other at 30-35°C temperature required for media testing incubation. Incubator temperatures must be monitored to ensure they are within USP Chapter <797> specified temperature ranges. Temperatures within each incubator must be documented daily. Incubators should be calibrated and certified annually according to the manufacturer's instructions. Follow the institution's process for ensuring incubator preventative maintenance. Myles published an introductory review on selecting an incubator for pharmacy use.[7] In addition to what is listed in the review, consider finding an incubator with a digital temperature display.

Refrigerators and Freezers

Many drugs and CSPs require refrigeration to maintain stability. The choice of a refrigerator or freezer is best determined by its intended location, volume of ingredients, and finished preparations to be contained. Only laboratory and pharmaceutical grade refrigerators should be used to store pharmaceuticals.

Commercial, laboratory-grade pharmaceutical refrigerators and freezers are often more durable and have valuable features. They can be designed to be vertical, pass-through, undercounter, or walk-in. Pass-through refrigerators should never be used for hazardous drug (HD) compounding buffer rooms because they cannot maintain the appropriate negative pressure differentials and are not permitted per USP Chapter <800>.[2] Compressors can be located in the unit or off site to reduce noise and heat production. Solid state refrigeration units are newer to the pharmaceutical storage market, and they may offer a compressor-free solution for some applications. Currently, this technology only offers small capacity refrigerators, but as it develops it may provide a viable option on a larger scale.

Other features to consider when choosing refrigerators and freezers include the following:

- Cleanability: Refrigerators and freezers are dust collectors and particle generators, so placement is most ideal outside of the buffer room. It might be convenient to have a refrigerator or freezer in the anteroom as an alternative. Placing the refrigerator on the clean side of the line of demarcation can allow for compounding staff to access refrigerated drugs. According to USP Chapter <800>, refrigerated HD storage may occur in the hazardous buffer room, but the compressor should be located near an exhaust vent. If a pass-through design from anteroom to the outside pharmacy is selected, it should have interlocking doors to help prevent ingression of air from the uncontrolled environment.[1] Stainless steel and glass (interior or exterior construction materials) are the most cleanable and durable.

- Location and space: Refrigerators and freezers are available with different door configurations (eg, hinged glass, hinged stainless steel, sliding glass, or stainless steel). There may be undercounter models that allow more counter workspace. Refrigerators and freezers should be installed and leveled on a floor that will hold the weight plus contents. Do not place a refrigerator or freezer near an oven, radiator, or other heat source.
- Temperature control: Refrigerators and freezers must maintain temperature ranges that meet USP standards for cold (2°C to 8°C) or frozen (–25°C to –10°C) temperature ranges.[1;8] This temperature range should be listed in the specification sheet of the device. Although all pharmacy commercial refrigerators and freezers have a thermometer, a more convenient feature is to have a continuous temperature recording device and alarm to alert users when the required temperature ranges are exceeded for too long a period of time.
- Backup/emergency power: All pharmaceutical refrigerators should be connected to an emergency power (generator backup supply) outlet due to the high dollar value of pharmaceuticals. With emergency power outlets, an automatic transfer switch on the units connects them to alternate electric generators if the power goes out. If emergency power is not available, an uninterruptible power supply (UPS) backup may be considered. It is important for the UPS to accommodate the peak load of the refrigerator (eg, when the compressor starts) and have at least 1 hour of run time to allow alternative storage plans to be enacted. The UPS should have an alarm to notify appropriate personnel of the power failure so that recovery can begin.
- Security: Depending on location relative to nonpharmacy personnel or controlled drug contents (eg, epidural injectable preparations), refrigerators and freezers may need to be lockable and alarmed. Locked storage boxes can also be installed inside refrigerators to allow for controlled substance storage.
- Certification and warranty: Refrigerators and freezers should be Energy Star efficient and meet National Science Foundation (NSF), Underwriter's Laboratory, and National Institute of Standards and Technology (NIST) certifications. Warranties should cover parts, labor, and compressors for 2 to 5 years. Refrigerators and freezers should be calibrated and certified annually.

Refrigerator and Freezer Size and Maintenance

Because refrigerators come in many sizes, proper selection depends on the volume of drugs and final preparations to be stored. Having several smaller units instead of one large unit may be desirable because multiple units provide a safeguard and a backup if one unit fails, and they permit segregation of drugs and final preparations for safety purposes (ie, HDs must be stored separately from non-HDs, and investigational drugs often require segregated storage).

The simplest method to determine the refrigerator and freezer size needed is to add the space required for the maximum inventory of drug supplies and final preparations during the busiest season, plus additional capacity for future growth. Then possible storage areas must be identified so the decision can be made between one large or several smaller refrigerators. If the facility is already built, the maximum size refrigerator or freezer that can be moved through the door and ceiling limitations must be considered. Many refrigerator units will not fit through standard 32-inch doors (due to the unit depth) or make tight turns (due to unit length) in the ante room to get into the HD buffer room. Obtain the exact measurements for the exterior of the unit prior to purchase. Power requirements should be checked against institutional policies before any unit is purchased. Working with the department that assists with preventative maintenance for the device is helpful prior to purchasing. The maintenance staff may have recommendations for brands and models that are preferred, as they may keep parts on hand for quicker repair. Medication refrigerators must be clearly labeled as such with required temperatures for quick reference. If the institution has a preferred maintenance vendor, place contact information on the unit, including an emergency after-hours number. Food and drink must never be stored in a cleanroom refrigerator.

Shelving

USP Chapter <797> makes the following statement about shelving:

> The surfaces of ceilings, walls, floors, doors, door frames, fixtures, shelving, work surfaces, counters, and cabinets in the classified area must be smooth, impervious, free from cracks and crevices, and non-shedding so they can be cleaned and disinfected and to minimize spaces in which microorganisms and other contaminants can accumulate. Surfaces should be resistant to damage by cleaning agents, disinfectants, sporicidal agents, and tools used to clean.[1]

Because personnel compounding sterile preparations are required to wear special garb (gowns, gloves, masks, etc.), they need a place to change clothing and/or don personal protective equipment (PPE) before entering the buffer room. Personal items, such as jackets, coats, and purses, should not enter the anteroom and should be stored in a separate breakroom or locker room. Shelving with bins should be placed in the ante room for storing the appropriate PPE.

Miscellaneous Equipment

Other items that may be considered in sterile compounding facilities include the following:

- Antifatigue floor mats: These floor mats are not recommended for use in a buffer room because they accumulate hair and dust. At a minimum, mats must be moved during floor cleaning, and the mats themselves must be cleaned on both sides and allowed to dry before the mat is replaced.[9;10] An alternative to fatigue mats is wearing soft-soled shoes. Rubber flooring can also provide relief to joints and feet, but the flooring and seams must be compatible with sporicidal, germicidal, and other cleaning products.
- Wireless refrigerator monitoring systems: Because of the high cost of refrigerated and frozen drug inventory, larger pharmacy refrigerators and freezers often have audible temperature alarms, chart monitors, or hardwired monitoring systems. There are several wireless temperature monitoring systems on the market. Such systems can be comprised of monitoring software, a wireless receiver, and a temperature probe attached within a refrigerator or freezer. Users can view the temperature of multiple units, respond to alarms, document follow-up actions, and create summary reports via a centralized website.[11] Refer to USP Chapter <1118> Monitoring Devices—Time, Temperature, and Humidity standards for devices used to monitor time, temperature, and humidity.[12]
- Bubble point tester: If CSPs are made from one or more nonsterile ingredient, they are often sterilized by cold filtration through a 0.22-micron filter. After each sterilization process, filter units used to sterilize CSPs must be subjected to a manufacturer's recommended integrity test, such as the bubble point test (see Chapter 12).[1]

Supplies

Cleaning and Disinfecting Supplies

According to USP Chapter <797>, environmental contact is a major source of microbial contamination of CSPs. Consequently, scrupulous attention to cleaning and disinfecting sterile compounding areas is required to minimize this as a source of CSP contamination.[1] Further, USP Chapter <800> differentiates between disinfection, deactivation, and decontamination as it relates to HDs.[2]

Disinfectant and Sporicidal Agents

USP Chapter <797> says, "Cleaning and disinfecting agents must be selected and used with careful consideration of compatibilities, effectiveness, and user safety. Considerations when selecting and using disinfectants include their antimicrobial activity, inactivation by organic matter, residue, shelf life, preparation requirements of the agent, and suitability for surfaces being disinfected."[1] In general, highly toxic disinfectants, such as glutaraldehyde, are not used on housekeeping surfaces (eg, floors, countertops).[1] Many disinfectants registered by the U.S. Environmental Protection Agency have been formulated to be effective in the presence of light to moderate soiling without a precleaning step. These are known as *one-step agents*. Sporicidal agents are found in some one-step disinfectants.[1] A sporicidal agent must be used at least once monthly for entities compounding Category 1 and 2 CSPs and at least weekly for entities compounding Category 3 CSPs.[1]

Sterile 70% isopropyl alcohol (IPA) is designated as the primary disinfectant for cleaning PECs and frequently used work surfaces, such as counter tops and worktables. Also, sterile 70% IPA is used regularly to disinfect sterile gloves, vial stoppers, ampule necks, and injection ports on containers.[1;13]

Other disinfectants are intended for use primarily on work surfaces, storage shelves, floors, walls, and ceilings. Representatives of pharmacy and infection prevention and control departments should have input on an organization's selection of disinfectants. If an agent is chosen that must be diluted, it is important to follow the instructions for use and to use sterile diluents. Employees must be trained and demonstrate competency for any cleaning and disinfecting agents.

Deactivation and Decontamination Agents

USP Chapter <800> states the following:

> Deactivation renders a compound inert or inactive. Residue from deactivation must be removed by decontaminating the surface. There is no one proven method for deactivating all compounds. The ultimate goal should be complete surface decontamination.[2]

This presents a challenge for the compounder when selecting an agent to deactivate HD preparation areas. Currently, strong oxidizers like sodium hypochlorite, hydrogen peroxide, and potassium permanganate have been shown to deactivate some HDs. A common deactivation process includes using a 2% sodium hypochlorite solution followed by sodium thiosulfate to inactivate excess hypochlorite residue, which is corrosive to stainless steel. Deactivation should be performed before disinfection, and the use of the germicidal disinfection agent serves a further purpose to remove any HD residue.[2]

Cleaning Supplies

USP Chapter <797> requires that all cleaning materials, such as wipers and sponges, be nonshedding, preferably composed of synthetic microfibers, and dedicated to use in the buffer room, anteroom, or segregated compounding area. They must not be removed from these areas except for disposal.[1] Any cleaning supplies used inside the PEC (except tool handles and holders) must be sterile.[1] Devices used in a HD compounding area should be dedicated to that area to prevent contamination of non-HD areas.

Mops and Mop Systems

USP Chapter <797> requires that all cleaning materials, such as mops, be nonshedding and preferably composed of synthetic microfibers. Mops, handles, mop buckets, or other components of mopping systems must be dedicated to use in the buffer room, anteroom, or segregated compounding area. They must not be removed from these areas except for disposal.[1] It is important to have separate labeled mops for HD and non-HD areas to prevent contamination. Bucketless mopping systems are preferred because they eliminate a source of standing liquid and debris accumulation. Mop heads or covers should be single-use only and should not be laundered and reused.[1]

Cleanroom Garb

Sterile compounding personnel should participate in the selection of cleanroom garb to ensure their satisfaction, comfort, and compliance with standard operating procedures (SOPs). Hospital operating room personnel may be able to offer samples and personal experience with products and suppliers.

There are additional garbing requirements for Category 3 buffer rooms. All skin must be covered (including face and neck), all outer garb must be sterile (including sterile sleeves in a restricted-access barrier system), and disposable garb items must not be reused unless they are laundered and resterilized.[1]

Shoe Covers

Consideration should be given to purchase the largest size possible to accommodate the variety of shoe sizes of compounding personnel. There are two important considerations when selecting shoe covers, whether they are low-shedding and the type of tread. It is important that employees are not subject to slips and falls on cleanroom floors, especially during cleaning activities. The surface of the cleanroom floor may impact which shoe cover is chosen. Shoe covers are required even when dedicated cleanroom shoes are used. There are devices that can be purchased to help employees don shoe covers.

Hair Covers

It can be difficult to find hair covers that contain hair around the base of the head where it meets the neck. Some facilities may select whole head covers to assist with this, but keep in mind they may be warmer and cause staff to sweat. If a fabric hair cover or head scarf is worn, it should be laundered daily, and a disposable hair cover should be worn over it to minimize introduction of environmental contamination into the buffer room.

Face Masks and Eye Coverings

Surgical face masks should be fitted to the nose and chin. Options with elastic ear loops or masks with ties are available. Elastic ear loops may help ensure that face masks continuously stay in place. Goggles are optional for compounding Category 1 and 2 CSPs, but they may be needed when working with irritants, such as germicidal disinfecting agents, or when spills or splashes of HDs occur.[1,2] Eyeglasses or eyeglasses with side shields and face shields alone are not considered adequate protection against splashing of HDs. Full facepiece respirators provide both eye and face protection, but they may not be easy for compounding personnel to use or to clean and disinfect between use.[2] Facility SOPs must describe proper disinfection procedures for items that are reused.[1]

Respirators

A fit-tested, National Institute of Occupational Safety and Health (NIOSH)–certified N95 respirator can be used for most activities requiring respiratory protection when gases and vapors or splashing are not anticipated. For unpacking of HDs not contained in plastic, an elastomeric half mask with a multigas cartridge and P-100 filter should be used.[2] Powered air purifying respirators (PAPR) should also be considered in facilities that do not provide fit testing.[2] Either an N95 respirator or PAPR should be on hand for cleaning HD spills and the spill tray of the biological safety cabinet (BSC).[2] Facility SOPs must describe proper disinfection procedures for items that are reused.[1]

Gowns

USP Chapter <797> requires personnel to wear a nonshedding gown with sleeves that fit snugly around the wrists and is enclosed at the neck.[1] Gowns designated for buffer room use must be worn, and they should be disposable. Gown breathability is an important feature to prevent sweating.

When Category 1 and 2 compounding personnel exit the compounding area during a work shift, the exterior gown may be removed and retained in the compounding area if not visibly soiled, and only redonned during that same work shift.[1] Gowns must never be reused for Category 3 compounding.[1] However, shoe covers, hair and facial hair covers, face masks and eye shields, and gloves must be replaced with new ones before compounding begins.[1]

USP Chapter <800> requires disposable gowns that have been tested for permeability against the HDs being compounded. Gowns for HD compounding must also be closed in the back, have long sleeves, elastic or knit cuffs, and have no seams that would allow HD penetration.[2] Refer to the American Society for Testing and Materials (ASTM) standard F3267 to review types of HD gown materials (also Chapters 13 and 27).[14]

Gloves

Gloves are essential for protecting the environment from the shedding of human skin microbes and for protecting people's hands from HDs and other toxic substances. Gloves are the last of the cleanroom attire to be donned. USP Chapter <797> requires that gloves must be sterile and powder-free.[1] Gloves for non-HD compounding may be made of latex, vinyl, nitrile, neoprene, or other materials.

Latex allergies present problems for healthcare professionals and patients and many healthcare organizations have eliminated the use of latex gloves.

Natural rubber latex, neoprene (chloroprene), nitrile, butyl, and polyurethane gloves add protection for compounders of HDs. ASTM has developed standard D6978 (or its successor) for the resistance of gloves to HDs, calling acceptable gloves "chemotherapy gloves." In addition to the composition material, duration of contact, the drug itself, and other solvents contacted affect glove permeability. Wearing two pairs of chemotherapy gloves is required for compounding HDs.[2;15]

Closed-system Drug-transfer Devices

Closed-system drug-transfer devices (CSTDs) are engineered to allow the transfer of hazardous drugs from one container to another without ventilation, while greatly reducing exposure to the healthcare worker. USP Chapter <800> says that CSTDs are supplemental engineering controls and, when used in HD compounding, must be used within a BSC or compounding aseptic containment isolator.[2] The use of CSTDs is preferred for compounding because of their inherent closed system process. Administering antineoplastic HDs requires the use of a CSTD if it is functional for the dosage form.[2] The NIOSH published a draft performance standard for CSTD performance in 2015.[16] Once finalized, this performance standard will allow easy differentiation of devices that meet the NIOSH definition of a CSTD. Halloush et al. demonstrated that not all CSTDs meet the proposed NIOSH performance standards.[17] It is important to ask for validation information from the CSTD manufacturer.

Other HD dispensing and reconstitution devices are available, but they do not have the extensive research available to prove their equality to CSTDs. Refer to Chapter 27 for a detailed discussion of CSTDs.

Microbial Testing Growth Media

Growth media can be general, selective, or differential in type. For most applications, general growth media is adequate because it will support the growth of a variety of bacterial, yeast, and mold species. The manufacturer should provide a certificate of analysis or certificate of performance for each lot of growth media purchased. These certificates should be filed for a reasonable period of time or as long as required by a state board of pharmacy.

Gloved Fingertip and Thumb Testing Kits and Media

Keeping gloves disinfected is key to aseptic technique. USP Chapter <797> requires contact agar plates or paddles be used to sample gloved fingertips and thumbs of compounding personnel after garbing to assess garbing competency and after completing the media fill preparation (without applying sterile 70% IPA) to assess the adequacy of aseptic work practices.[1] All compounding personnel must successfully complete an initial gloved fingertip and thumb sampling procedure (zero colony-forming units) no less than three successive times before they are allowed to compound CSPs for human use.[1] Subsequent gloved fingertip and thumb testing must be completed at least semiannually for Category 1 and 2 and at least every 3 months for Category 3.[1]

Media Fill Testing Kits and Media

USP Chapter <797> defines a *media fill test* as a test used to qualify aseptic technique of compounding personnel or processes and to ensure that the processes used are able to produce sterile preparations without microbial contamination. During this test, sterile soybean-casein digest medium is substituted for all components to simulate admixture compounding.[1] Media fill testing must be done initially and at least semiannually thereafter for each employee that compounds Category 1 and 2 sterile preparations and at least every 3 months for Category 3 sterile preparations.[1] The test must simulate the most complex compounding procedures performed by each compounder.[1] Kits are available to purchase to simulate preparation conditions, although it may be easier to purchase bags and vials of media if testing scenarios are complex. Purchased testing media must be accompanied by a certificate of analysis.[1]

Microbiological Surface Testing Kits and Media

USP Chapter <797> states that surface sampling must be performed in all ISO classified areas and pass-through chambers monthly and after a completed media fill test for Category 1 and 2 preparations.[1] There are additional requirements for Category 3 (see Chapter 31). Sampling can be accomplished using contact plates or swabs.[1] The size of the plate to be used for each sampled location usually ranges from 24 to 30 cm^2. Contact plates are filled with general solid agar growth medium and neutralizing agents above the rim of the plate, and they are used for sampling regular or flat surfaces. Swabs may be used for sampling irregular surfaces, especially for equipment. The chemical neutralizer must be formulated in surface sampling media to neutralize any disinfectant residue left behind that may inhibit microbial growth. Using different media for bacterial and fungal growth will shorten the overall incubation time. Otherwise, a media, such as trypticase soy agar (TSA), can be incubated at separate temperatures for surface sampling.[1]

Hazardous Drug Surface Sampling

USP Chapter <800> states that sampling of HD surface residue should be performed routinely with an initial benchmark sample and follow-up samples every 6 months.[2] Several vendors provide kits to sample surfaces for contamination, and each has a variety of marker HDs.[17] The test kits require a specific size of surface area to be wiped to ensure accurate quantitative measurement.

USP Chapter <800> recommends the following locations for HD wipe sampling[2]:

- Interior of the containment-PEC (C-PEC) and equipment contained in it
- Pass-through chambers

- Surfaces in staging or work areas near the C-PEC
- Areas adjacent to C-PECs (eg, floors directly under C-PEC, staging, and dispensing area)
- Areas immediately outside the HD buffer room or the containment segregated compounding area
- Patient administration areas

Most of the currently available HD surface contamination sampling kits require the samples to be shipped to a vendor for analysis, although some newer testing machines can provide immediate, nonquantitative results above a standard threshold. If using an outside lab, it is important that all samples are labeled appropriately and that the laboratory doing the analysis runs a positive and negative control to ensure accuracy of the testing. Vendors may also vary in limit of quantitation for the same HD, which means that one test may show no contamination while another more sensitive test would show the presence of the HD. There is no standard of an acceptable level of HD surface contamination.[2;18]

Tacky Mats

The purpose of tacky mats is to remove large particles from the soles of street shoes before the compounder puts on dedicated shoes or shoe covers. Therefore, tacky mats can only be placed at the entrance to the anteroom and never inside classified areas. Because the value of tacky mats has not been established for sterile compounding, USP Chapter <797> does not otherwise address them. Tacky mats should be changed frequently to maintain effectiveness at trapping dust and dirt. The minimum frequency should be established in policy, and each change should be documented. An alternative to tacky mats is polymeric contamination control flooring. This flooring is cleanable and reduces particles and contamination from shoes and wheels. It is important to study the appropriate cleaning agents for this specialized flooring to ensure it meets USP Chapter <797> standards.

SUMMARY

The maintenance of sterility depends more on technique than any other single factor. Therefore, having the appropriate equipment and supplies should not give personnel a false sense of security. There is no substitute for good aseptic technique. Appropriate equipment and supplies can minimize the risk of contamination of sterile preparations by minimizing contaminants in the environment.

REFERENCES

1. General chapter <797> pharmaceutical compounding—sterile preparations. In: *2019: USP Compounding Compendium*. Rockville, MD: The United States Pharmacopeial Convention; November 1, 2022. **https://doi.org/10.31003/USPNF_M99925_07_01**.
2. General chapter, <800> hazardous drugs – handling in healthcare settings. In: *2019: USP Compounding Compendium.* Rockville, MD: The United States Pharmacopeial Convention; July 1, 2020. **https://doi.org/10.31003/USPNF_M7808_07_01**.
3. Diorio L. Selecting cleanroom storage fixtures, casework and cleaning equipment. *Pharmacy Purchasing & Products.* **www.pppmag.com/documents/V4N1/PPPMAG/10_11_12_14.pdf**. Published January 2007. Accessed August 18, 2023.
4. General chapter <116> microbiological control and monitoring of aseptic processing environments. In: *USP Compounding Compendium.* Rockville, MD: The United States Pharmacopeial Convention; Prior to 2013. **https://doi.org/10.31003/USPNF_M99835_01_01**.
5. Faylor K, Kastango ES. Getting it under control: products and procedures for environmental monitoring. *Pharmacy Purchasing & Products.* **www.pppmag.com/documents/V3N2/PPP_V3N2_pp8-9_enviroMonitoring.pdf**. Accessed January 22 2023.
6. Controlled Environment Testing Association. *CETA application guide CAG-003: certification of sterile compounding facilities for USP compliance.* Raleigh, NC: Controlled Environment Testing Association; October 2022.
7. Myles L. Selecting an incubator for your health-system pharmacy. *Pharmacy Purchasing & Products.* **www.pppmag.com/documents/V3N8/P24-26.pdf**. November 2006. Accessed January 22, 2023.
8. General chapter <659> packaging and storage requirements. In: *USP Compounding Compendium.* Rockville, MD: The United States Pharmacopeial Convention; April 1, 2021. **https://doi.org/10.31003/USPNF_M2773_06_01**.
9. Douglass K. Design your cleanroom to ensure easier cleaning and maintenance. *Pharmacy Purchasing & Products.* **https://www.pppmag.com/doclibrary/cleanroom.pdf**. Accessed 2023 Jan 22, 2023.
10. Kilgore KM. Cover story: designing a cleanroom. *Pharmacy Purchasing & Products.* **www.pppmag.com/article/367**. Published April 2008. Accessed January 23, 2023.
11. McGregory ME. Wireless refrigerator temperature monitoring systems: selection, implementation and quality assurance. *Pharmacy Purchasing & Products.* **www.pppmag.com/documents/V4N6/p20_22_24_25.pdf**. Published June 2007. Accessed January 22, 2023.
12. General chapter <1118> monitoring devices—time, temperature, and humidity. In: *2013: USP Compounding Compendium.* Rockville, MD: The United States Pharmacopeial Convention; August 1, 2013. **https://doi.org/10.31003/USPNF_M99837_01_01**.

13. Douglass K. Establishing sound practices for cleaning your cleanroom: cleaning products and procedures for USP <797> compliance. *Pharmacy Purchasing & Products.* **www.pppmag.com/documents/V2N5/v2n5pp16_cleancleanroom2.pdf**. Accessed January 22, 2023.

14. ASTM International. ASTM F3267-22: standard specifications for protective clothing for use against liquid chemotherapy and other liquid hazardous drugs. Updated December 20, 2022. doi:10.1520/F3267-22

15. ASTM International. ASTM D6978-05(2019): standard practice for assessment of resistance of medical gloves to permeation by chemotherapy drugs. Updated June 10, 2019. doi:10.1520/D6978-05R19

16. Hirst DVL, Mead KR, Power L, et al. A vapor containment performance protocol for closed system transfer devices used during pharmacy compounding and administration of hazardous drugs; request for comment. *Fed Regist.* 2015;80:53802–53803.

17. Halloush S, Reveles IA, Koeller J. Evaluating six commercially available closed-system drug-transfer devices against NIOSH's 2015 draft vapor protocol. *Hosp Pharm.* 2020;55(6):391–399. doi:10.1177/0018578719848730

18. Massoomi F, Knolla KL. Identifying hazardous drug residue via wipe analysis. *Pharmacy Purchasing & Products.* **www.pppmag.com/article/1358**. Published July 2013. Accessed January 22, 2023.

STERILE COMPOUNDING TECHNOLOGY

9

Craig A. Boyce and Bruce A. Erickson

INTRODUCTION

> *As we continue our journey to excellence in patient safety, transformation of the compounding of sterile preparations is essential to complement the life-saving technologies for prescribing and administration of medications that have been adopted across the health system.*
>
> Michael C. Ganio and Daniel J. Cobaugh[1]

This chapter discusses why automation of the sterile compounding process is important and how these systems impact the safety, efficiency, and productivity value of the pharmacy sterile compounding service. The term *systems* in this context is used to mean the combination of hardware and software that provides safety mechanisms for the sterile compounding processes. Because of the continuous changes and new product introductions in this technology sector, this chapter will not individually describe every system available. Instead, it focuses on the general adoption and use of these systems, the advantages and limitations of the different system types, and the considerations for adding automated compounding technologies based on the compounding processes and workload volume. Some sections of this chapter may not be applicable to all types of sterile compounding technology. At the time of this publication, the *United States Pharmacopeia* (USP) does not yet contain explicit guidance on the types of automated technologies discussed within this chapter. References to USP chapters that may be applicable are included where appropriate.

The goal of sterile compounding technology is to provide a controlled sterile compounding process with an electronic record for each finished dose. The process controls can be system-directed work instructions performed by a human, automated systems that perform the sterile compounding process, or a combination of both. The electronic record should include all ingredients and consumables used in preparation, the lot number and expiration date of each ingredient entered by the user or captured from a barcode scan, the finished dose amount and diluent volume, positive identification of the personnel performing the compounding activities, all patient and order details received through an interface, and a date and time stamp showing when each activity occurred. This chapter will elaborate on these goals and how automation can help achieve them.

Implementing sterile compounding technology requires knowledge and understanding of the chapters in Section IV: Principles and Work Practices of Sterile Compounding and Section VI: Quality Management. These sections should be read before beginning this chapter. This Chapter will not cover the technologies used for compounding parenteral nutrition and radiopharmaceuticals (see Chapters 22 and 25, respectively).

EVOLUTION OF AUTOMATION

The application of automation to repetitive and complex tasks has a well-established history. Mechanization of manufacturing began in the late 1800s and early 1900s using simple devices to perform repetitive tasks. In the 1930s and 1940s, more complex programming and control systems enabled true automation by allowing these mechanized systems to adjust output without human involvement. Introduction of the industrial multi-axis robotic arm in the 1970s coupled with computerized programming advanced automation meant that humans could be removed from many manufacturing processes. Using automation in error-prone or dangerous processes enables improvements in the quality of the manufacturing output by eliminating human error and it allows employers to protect the work force from harm. Over the last three decades, these same principles have been recognized as needs in the healthcare sector as well. These needs have been the driving force behind automating the pharmacy compounding service.

DOI 10.37573/9781585286492.009

The evolution of automated compounding began in 1988 with the introduction of a manually controlled peristaltic fluid transfer pump designed specifically for pharmacy use.[2] The next major step forward in automation of sterile compounding occurred in the early 1990s with software control of the pump and integration of a scale to check the weight of each ingredient after the addition of the compounding product.[3] The connection of multiple fluid sources joined by a valved transfer set that is controlled by the compounding recipe software has become the generally accepted standard for compounding complex admixtures, such as parenteral nutrition or cardioplegia solutions.

By the early 2000s, the first automated syringe fillers became available.[4] These devices combined a peristaltic pump with actuator controllers to move a bandolier of syringes through a filling and capping station, then to a labeler, cutter, and output trough. These systems were the first truly automated sterile compounding systems that were available to hospitals. The devices allowed doses to be prepared without human intervention after the source container was connected to the peristaltic pump tubing. A limitation for some of these systems is the ability to prepare only specific syringe sizes due to the available proprietary disposables.

In the late 2000s, systems that automated most or all of the manual compounding processes for both syringes and bags became available. They are now referred to as compounding robots or automated compounding systems (ACSs).[5;6] These systems differ from other automated compounding devices in design and intended use. ACSs incorporate software control of multiple mechanical manipulators and six-axis robotic arms, racks for holding bags and vials, precision balances for gravimetric validation during the compounding processes, and barcode readers or imaging systems to inspect raw materials and finished products. ACSs enclose the compounding area within a high-efficiency particulate air (HEPA)-filtered air chamber. They may also have dedicated material loading bays to separate the compounding area from the location where compounding materials are placed into the storage racks. The airflow in some systems can be configured to operate under positive or negative pressure, making these systems applicable for use in compounding hazardous drugs. ACSs represent a significant advancement for sterile compounding because they introduced the capability for highly accurate compounding of syringe and bag doses in batch mode (compounding many doses of the same preparation) or patient-specific mode (making a specific dose for a specific patient through an interface to the pharmacy information system).

Another technology adapted from manufacturing to the sterile compounding process is the use of software to manage workflow and guide manual processes. These systems are variously referred to as sterile compounding, IV compounding, or technology-assisted workflow systems (TAWFs). TAWFs may be stand-alone systems or integrated into the pharmacy information systems. One of the first TAWF systems was installed in 2008 to improve sterile compounding safety by guiding workflow and capturing images of the process for later review by the pharmacist.[7] Although TAWF systems have continued to rapidly evolve in the last decade, adoption has not become widespread. A 2022 survey found that 42% of respondents have implemented some form of TAWF.[8]

TAWFs allow orders, standardized preparation methods, ingredient verification, and the manual compounding process to be tied together to increase safety and efficiency within the sterile compounding area. Workflow management within these systems allows for automated sorting of incoming orders to the appropriate manual compounding area or to an ACS. Some workflow management systems can automatically prioritize the order of compounding sequences based on the urgency or due time for the orders in the compounding queue. Such features assist the pharmacy staff by prioritizing compounding activities, stopping wrong drug or diluent errors before they occur, checking the in-process compound for accuracy of dose, and allowing a pharmacist outside the immediate compounding area to see each step in the compounding process. However, these systems do not have the capability to ensure proper aseptic technique, and they may not have adequate image resolution to detect tiny flaws, such as coring.

The need for patient safety in the compounding process is a driving force behind the adoption of technology-assisted workflow and robotic compounding systems. The Institute for Safe Medication Practices (ISMP) has been a strong and persistent advocate for the adoption of technology for sterile compounding processes. The 2016 revision of the ISMP Guidelines for Safe Preparation of Compounded Sterile Preparations (based on the 2013 ISMP Sterile Preparation Compounding Safety Summit) recommends that "barcode scanning of base solutions and ingredients should now be considered the minimum requirement for pharmacy IV admixture services."[9] The ISMP guidelines further recommended that both barcoding and gravimetric analysis be used when preparing chemotherapy and pediatric doses. Similar recommendations are included in the ISMP 2022–2023 *Targeted Medication Safety Best Practice for Hospitals*. The guidelines recommend to "[u]se technology to assist in the verification process (e.g., machine-readable coding [e.g., barcoding scanning, radio frequency identification] of ingredients, gravimetric verification, robotics, intravenous [IV] workflow software) to augment the manual processes."[10] As these technologies become more widely adopted, thought leaders are beginning to put forth recommendations for best practices and suggestions for improvements to the technology. Two recent publications include the summary of an international summit on IV robotics and guidelines from ISMP on sterile compounding technology.[11;12] The increasing acceptance of ACS and TAWF systems as best practice represents one of the most important changes occurring in the evolution of sterile compounding. Using these technologies as the minimum standard in compounding is the next stage in bringing these benefits to every patient.[13]

REASONS TO AUTOMATE

Human beings, in all lines of work, make errors. Errors can be prevented by designing systems that make it hard for people to do the wrong thing and easy for people to do the right thing.

—The Institute of Medicine and the Committee on Quality of Health Care in America[14]

Patient Safety: Prevention of Harm

Preventing errors that lead to patient harm is the key reason to automate the sterile compounding process. Literature and U.S. Food and Drug Administration (FDA) reports contain many occurrences that document errors or contamination of manually compounded products. The Pew Charitable Trust compiled data from 2001 to 2019 and found 73 reported sterile compounding errors or potential errors associated with more than 1,562 adverse events, including at least 116 deaths.[15] Although the majority of these cases and deaths were associated with the 2012 New England Compounding Center tragedy (793 cases and 76 deaths), there has been a reported significant error or contamination event associated with sterile compounding almost every year between 2001 and 2019.

There are a number of commonly used safety measures that help prevent errors for oral medications, such as unit-dose packaging, barcode-based dispensing, and barcode-based verification of patient, medication, and dose at the point of administration. Technology in the oral dispensing and administration process has been widely adopted and demonstrated to have a significant impact on lowering medication errors.[16-18] However, the more risk-prone process of sterile compounding has not yet seen the same degree of safety technology adoption to prevent errors or contamination during the compounding process.

Compounding errors have been shown to occur in all geographical regions in the United States with a mean range from 6% to 10% and a combined error rate of 9%.[19] Studies conducted in pediatric, chemotherapy, and nonhazardous sterile compounding services as part of the adoption of sterile compounding technology found error detection and capture rates less than 0.5% prior to adoption. These rates increased dramatically after implementation, ranging from 0.74% up to 41.48%.[20-25] One study also concluded that use of gravimetrics allowed the pharmacy to prepare a highly consistent dose, with more than 99% of all doses gravimetrically verified to be within 5% of the ordered dose.[26] The increased adoptions of TAWF and ACS systems has provided more published data supporting evidence of the positive impact these systems have on error capture and prevention.[27;28] One study interestingly found that TAWF with gravimetrics had fewer accuracy errors than the ACS gravimetric process, and that the TAWF system can be significantly faster than current ACS throughput.[29] This is an important trend to watch as ACS systems enter their second generation. Can robots become self-correcting when the gravimetric validation is out of acceptance limits? Can they become more productive than humans using guided manual preparation? Both are needed for sterile compounding robotics adoption to progress.

The sterile compounding room setting is a technically demanding work area that can require staff members to compound sterile preparations in a fast-paced and rapidly changing environment. Interruptions (stopping one activity to conduct another unrelated task) and distractions (momentary lapses of attention to the task in progress) occur when orders are added, changed, discontinued, and in-process status requests are made to the compounding technician. Although the literature is lacking a specific study on the impact of interruptions and distractions on sterile compounding errors, other studies have examined the impact of distractions on medication errors. USP in 2008 reviewed MEDMARX data and found that roughly 45% of medication errors cited distractions as a causative factor.[30] Based on these studies, it can be assumed that interruptions and distractions have some degree of impact on the sterile compounding process, and systems that can prevent or mitigate compounding errors caused by interruptions and distractions are desirable.

The quality of manually compounded sterile preparations (CSPs) is primarily determined by visual inspection. Although accuracy of the dose can be checked with some degree of confidence when the pharmacist is directly observing each step in the compounding process, it is impossible to use visual inspection to validate sterility. A high degree of trust is placed in staff members performing the aseptic manipulations during manual compounding that the actions are performed identically each time. However, humans cannot perform a function identically every time. Each human action has a degree of variability, and the cumulative error probability must be considered. This human variability includes the accuracy or precision of calculations and measurements, the likelihood of introducing a contaminant during each manipulation, and failure to follow standard operating procedures (SOPs).

Accuracy

The accuracy of a finished dose depends on the accuracy of each step in the compounding process. Each of the following compounding steps contains many subprocesses, any one of which is a potential source of error that could be cumulative when the error occurs in an early step in the process:

- Selection of drug and diluent
- Performing reconstitution and dilution
- Drawing the dose amount from the vial
- Injecting the dose into the ordered diluent of the correct volume
- Labeling the finished dose
- Visual inspection of the finished dose

Volumetric and gravimetric measurements are the two methods utilized to determine the amount of medication in a prepared dose. Volumetric preparation accuracy depends on the size of the syringe used for the dose, calibration accuracy on the syringe, and the visual acuity of the technician pulling the syringe plunger to the appropriate calibration mark on the syringe. Gravimetric measurement requires the weight measurement of the empty syringe or the intended diluent bag, and then reweighing the syringe or bag after transferring the drug into the container. The change in weight divided by the density of the source drug fluid yields the volume of drug added. Multiplying this volume by the concentration of the source vial provides the exact drug amount in the finished dose.

The accuracy of the delivered dose also depends on using the most appropriate syringe size for the dose being measured (see the section on syringes in Chapter 15). Although syringes are the principal measurement device for compounding, both the accuracy and resolution of syringes have an inherent degree of error. The International Organization for Standardization (ISO) 7886-1 standard for single-use syringes permits tolerances for the syringe's graduated capacity.[31] Because of this allowable manufacturing tolerance, there is always a degree of uncertainty in the accuracy of the prepared dose, and that uncertainty varies with the volume drawn into the syringe. For example, using a 3 mL syringe and drawing up a 2 mL dose, the tolerance is plus or minus 5%, which means the actual deliverable volume in the syringe is somewhere between 1.9 mL and 2.1 mL. For a single dose, this may be within an acceptable dose range. However, if the compound being prepared is a dilution or reconstitution step, the variability in the initial preparation step added to the variability in drawing of the actual dose (another plus or minus 5%) could result in a dose that is outside the acceptable range. A second consideration is drawing doses that fall between graduation marks on the syringe. Compounding personnel must estimate the piston position when drawing the fluid, so the accuracy can be stated only to be within a range and not a precise value. These variances in the actual volume versus the measured volume cannot be detected by visual inspection and may have a clinical impact depending on the drug, the concentration of the fluid, and the patient's condition.

The intrinsic characteristics of the compounding supplies are beyond the control of the pharmacy personnel, which further impacts the accuracy of the finished dose. Some of these characteristics of compounding supplies include the following:

- Syringe graduation accuracy tolerances
- Barrel diameter variance
- Plunger and dead space shape variances
- Deformation of cylinder uniformity
- Needle sharpness, shape, and volume
- Actual fill volume of bags and vials

The fill volume of vials and sterile fluid containers is permitted to be variable within certain standards according to USP and the FDA.[32;33] A visual inspection is not able to definitively detect when a vial or bag falls outside the acceptable fill volume. This variance can have a significant impact on the accuracy of the compounded dose when a specific concentration for the finished solution is needed. The actual volume in the finished container also impacts administration flow rate (mL/hr) for pump programming to deliver the entire contents in a specified period of time or at a controlled drug delivery rate. Although precise control of infusion rate is not needed in every instance, it is vitally important for some continuous infusions, such as insulin, chemotherapy, and vasoactive medications, because a small difference in the infusion rate can have profound clinical impact.

Historically, the pharmacist's inspection of the finished dose has relied on the syringe pullback method. For this method the technician preparing the dose draws the plunger of the used syringe back to the graduation mark indicating the drug volume added, and then pairs the syringe with the used vial. The pullback method for checking shows the intended dose, but it does not definitively show the actual drug and amount added to the finished dose. A study comparing volumetric measurement versus gravimetric measurement in the preparation of injectable oncology medications was conducted. The study found that only 71.7% of volumetrically prepared doses were within plus or minus 5% of ordered doses, and 87.4% of the doses were within plus or minus 10% of the ordered dose.[34] Small volume doses and doses delivered in a syringe had the greatest variances. If plus or minus 10% is considered the outer limit of acceptability, then this study could be interpreted to show that 12.6% of the prepared doses were unacceptable. Another type of error not detected by syringe pullback checking occurs when preparing multi-ingredient admixtures. In this case, the amounts of each ingredient added to the admixture are reversed, but the visual inspection fails to catch the dosing error.[35]

It is particularly critical to have dosing accuracy for certain patient populations and high-risk medications. Neonatal and pediatric patients can be adversely impacted by dosing inaccuracy because the margin of error between a safe and unsafe dose in these patients is small. Critically ill patients may be stabilized by medications delivered at a controlled infusion rate or potent antibiotics, and they can have a lower physiologic capability to tolerate variations in the medication dose.[36] High-risk medication categories that can have adverse effects with small dose changes include drugs with narrow therapeutic ranges, cytotoxic medications, and blood-level sensitive medications. The 2016 revision of the ISMP Guidelines for Safe Preparation of Compounded Sterile Preparations and the ISMP 2022-2023 Targeted Medication Safety Best Practices advocate that syringe pullback should never be used, and that an independent double check of ingredients and labels for high-risk medications should be performed prior to drug addition to the final container when TAWF software is not in use.[9;10]

Sterility

Other quality concerns when compounding sterile preparations are loss of control over the environmental conditions and poor aseptic technique, which results in contamination of the dose with viable microorganisms or spores. Visual inspection cannot detect contamination, so strict adherence to aseptic technique is critical to prevent contamination. Flawless aseptic technique is expected 100% of the time, but that is unrealistic. The number of known contamination events has shown 100% perfection to be impossible.[15] Although scrupulously following USP Chapter <797> Pharmaceutical Compounding—Sterile Preparations standards can reduce the likelihood of a contamination event, even under ideal conditions there is still a nonzero probability of a potentially harmful contamination occurring. One study looked at pharmacists and technicians performing medium-risk compounding activities and found a contamination rate of 0.34% under controlled conditions.[37] Even if only a small fraction of these contaminated doses cause an actual patient infection, there is still some degree of patient harm and increased cost of care.

Both the compounding environment and the expertise of the personnel performing the compounding have an influence on the risk of contamination. A study comparing the contamination rate of growth media syringes prepared within ISO Class 5, ISO Class 7, and an uncontrolled environment showed that contacting the sterile syringe tip to a nonsterile finger or object presented the highest incidence of contamination.[38] Another study found differences in media fill contamination rates for technicians and pharmacists (4.4% and 6.2%, respectively), as well as between personnel who routinely compounded versus those who did not.[39] In the data subset looking only at pharmacist compounding, pharmacists with more compounding experience counterintuitively exhibited higher contamination rates (6.3% versus 3.9%, respectively).

Under aseptic processing conditions with a high degree of quality control, the lowest achievable contamination probability is 10^{-3} (1:1,000).[40;41] This means that it is statistically likely under ideal conditions that 99.9% of the doses are sterile and 0.1% are potentially contaminated with a viable microorganism. It is important to keep in mind that these ideal conditions must be continuously maintained or the risk of contamination will increase. Based on this statistical likelihood, **Table 9-1** shows the number of potentially contaminated doses each year based on the facility bed size and average number of compounded doses administered each day per bed.

The actual contamination rate for CSPs that reach the patient is unknown because there is no method of monitoring for viable organisms or spores as the fluid is administered. Even if this were possible, it would only show that personnel failed to prevent contamination during the compounding process. The dose would then need to be remixed, which delays timeliness of therapy. Furthermore, it is difficult to definitively identify a contaminated CSP as the cause of an apparent infection in a patient. From a sterility quality perspective, it must be accepted that some degree of contamination occurs with manual compounding, and action must be taken to prevent this whenever possible.

TABLE 9-1. Annual Potentially Contaminated Doses with 99.9% Sterility Rate

	Doses per Bed per Day				
Bed Size	1	2	3	4	5
100	37	73	110	146	183
200	73	146	219	292	365
300	110	219	329	438	548
400	146	292	438	584	730
500	183	365	548	730	913
600	219	438	657	876	1,095
700	256	511	767	1,022	1,278
800	292	584	876	1,168	1,460
900	329	657	986	1,314	1,643
1,000	365	730	1,095	1,460	1,825

Manual compounding is dependent on the scrupulous aseptic technique of the individual and the quality of the compounding environment to ensure the sterility of the finished dose. If either the environment or the technique fails, the likelihood of contamination increases. A properly designed, implemented, and enclosed ACS can increase the likelihood of ensuring sterility with a high degree of confidence because it eliminates the two most common sources of contamination, which are airborne or surface contamination from the environment and touch contamination from the human performing the compounding.

Employee Safety

In addition to increasing the safety of CSPs, ACSs can also increase employee safety and satisfaction by doing the following:

- Reducing the risk of hazardous drug exposure
- Reducing other acute or chronic work-related injuries
- Advancing the skill level of pharmacy technicians
- Increasing job satisfaction and pride
- Increasing worker confidence that their tasks are being performed accurately

Although these are often considered soft dollars in the value of automation, the real impact from a financial perspective can be estimated based on historical data for workers' compensation claims, lost productivity due to injuries, and costs of training new employees when existing personnel leave their position due to dissatisfaction with repetitive tasks or lack of growth opportunities. The latter is particularly important to consider with the changing views toward work–life balance and career advancement opportunities in the younger work force entering the market today.[42]

A strong argument for automating any work is eliminating the risk of worker harm. Although the pharmacy sterile compounding room may not be viewed as a particularly hazardous job, there are still a number of possible risks to worker health that should be considered. Beyond the well-recognized hazards of acute sharps injuries (needle sticks and broken glass), chronic work-related injuries and health conditions as well as exposure to allergenic or hazardous materials must be considered.[43]

Typical sharps injuries include finger sticks during the recapping of used syringes or when inserting the needle into a fluid container and cuts during cleanup of broken glass. Although precise statistics on the specific rate for sterile compounding room-related sharps injuries have not been found in literature, it can be assumed to be a nonzero incidence with some injury-related costs.

Work-related health hazards include musculoskeletal injury and conditions related to scrubbing, garbing, and isolation. Repetitive motion injuries (RMI) caused by the repeated manipulation of syringes were found to represent 45% of reported pharmacy injuries in one study.[44] Any common sterile compounding task that requires repeated twisting motions of the wrists or fingers can increase the risk of RMI. Examples of these activities include the assembly of vial-to-bag systems, attachment of needles to syringes, pulling and pushing syringes (especially repeated large volume draws), and attachment and use of closed-system transfer devices (CSTDs). Working within a compounding aseptic isolator or compounding aseptic containment isolator may magnify the potential for fatigue and shoulder, hand, or finger strain. Some potential causes of increased fatigue and strain include the nonergonomic nature of the sleeve-glove systems, the need to wear sterile gloves over the barrier gloves, and the increased hand and finger strength needed to perform manipulations while wearing multiple gloves. Posture while sitting or standing at the ISO Class 5 workbench, lack of proper seating that supports the lumbar region, and standing for long hours on hard cleanroom floors can all contribute to ergonomic work injuries. Heat stress and dehydration are also concerns when working fully garbed in cleanrooms with low humidity and inadequate cooling to maintain a comfortable working temperature.[43]

Allergenic and hazardous drug exposures have immediate and long-term health risks. Some of the common immediate reactions include reactions to latex in gloves or garb (8% to 12% of healthcare workers), reactions to handwashing or environmental disinfection chemicals, and allergic reactions to the drugs being compounded.[45;46] Each of these can be conservatively managed by avoidance of the irritant, but this adds complexity and cost to the cleanroom supply budget by requiring special cleansers, gloves, and other supplies. Workers with allergies to drugs being compounded must also be considered in scheduling the cleanroom staff.

Exposure to hazardous drugs has been shown to have long-term health risks. Working with these medications requires careful attention to the compounding (see Chapter 27). ACSs may reduce exposure to hazardous drugs because they fully enclose the compounding process and are externally exhausted. Several studies outside the U.S. have shown very low environmental contamination levels and no cross-contamination with the use of ACS systems in the preparation of hazardous drugs.[47;48] Another study, however, did find the presence of hazardous drug within the ACS after compounding.[49] Further research using wipe studies conducted before and after implementation of ACSs is needed to demonstrate the effectiveness of these systems in reducing long-term hazardous drug exposure.

Employee Satisfaction

As the level of automation within pharmacy increases, the skills needed to understand and operate automation systems are becoming an important consideration in the hiring and retention process. For employees with an aptitude for this type of work, a new pharmacy practice role and career path is emerging. Some facilities have created new job roles specific to cleanrooms and automation that include a pharmacist as system administrator and pharmacy technicians as advanced system operators or system supervisors.

The employees involved in the daily activities of the sterile compounding room operation have first-hand knowledge of how sterile compounding occurs today. They can make significant contributions by identifying problems and implementing change in the complex compounding process (see the section Assessment of Manual Processes and Automation Future State). While some employees may suspect that automation will eliminate jobs, open communication creates a healthy work environment, and it reduces the fear of change that can accompany implementation of an automated workflow process. When employees have a sense of ownership, engagement, and pride in a workplace, the success of automation implementation and quality of work can be greatly increased.[50;51]

Increase Efficiency and Decrease Waste

As previously discussed, automation of error-prone and hazardous tasks is not a new concept. In addition to error reduction and safety enhancements, automation can also enable increased efficiency and reduction in wastes through the application of a structured improvement program as part of the automation project. One such method is Lean Six Sigma, which relies on a collaborative team to improve performance by combining Lean Manufacturing principles with Six Sigma to improve quality and eliminate waste.[52] Lean Six Sigma has identified eight types of waste, which include defects, overproduction, waiting, nonutilized talent, transportation, inventory, motion, and extra processing (the acronym DOWNTIME is used to represent this).[53] **Table 9-2** provides a short description of each waste type and how automation can reduce the impact of them.

TABLE 9-2. Lean Six Sigma DOWNTIME: Waste Types, Impact on Facility, and Automation Benefit in Reducing Waste

Type of Waste	Impact of Waste	Automation Benefit
Defects: Product that is unsuitable for dispensing or harmful when administered	Direct costs: Consumables and labor Indirect costs: Delayed therapy, treatment costs of adverse drug event, legal costs for errors that cause harm, decreased reimbursement, public relation costs, performance improvement costs to preventing future occurrences	Prepare dose correctly the first time by eliminating human from compounding process
Overproduction: Preparing a quantity of sterile preparations in excess of projected demand	Direct costs: Consumables and labor thrown away, time required for tracking down or remaking missing doses when patient moved Indirect costs: Less operating cash available for other programs	Enables more frequent batching based on shorter term demand without increasing labor for preparing doses
Waiting: Nonproductive time that could be spent on other tasks	Visual inspection takes staff members away from tasks that have higher intrinsic value Compounding staff may be nonproductive while waiting for in-process visual checks to occur	Eliminates most visual inspection by using automated processes to eliminate the types of errors usually caught by visual inspection
Nonutilized talent: Using personnel to perform tasks that could be performed safely by an individual with less experience or training	Employee dissatisfaction with repetitive tasks and lost opportunities to use talent for value added programs	Automation reduces total labor required to prepare same number of doses Reclaimed time can be shifted to tasks which yield most value for time invested
Transportation: Movement of excess materials into cleanroom, deliveries to nursing units, retrieving unused doses; tied closely to defects and overproduction	Increased labor costs to process materials for doses and handling unused doses	Coupled with reduced defects and reduced overproduction, net transportation spend is reduced because only the immediately needed and consumed materials moved
Inventory: Maintaining higher than necessary consumable or finished dose stock ties up available capital	Capital tied up in standing inventory cannot be used for other programs Cost of cash on hand to cover purchases may be increased Increased waste if finished doses not used before expiry	Just-in-time production reduces inventory required on hand, freeing cash for other uses Lower stock of finished doses increase inventory turns, reduces storage space requirements, perpetual counting labor, and decreased potency of stored solution
Motion: Movement is not necessarily productive work and eliminating wasted motion can increase the value of the process[54]	Each step in a process that does not directly increase the value of that product wastes labor Many small motion wastes per day add up to significant nonproductive time	Automation hones the process to a set of standardized steps that eliminate non-value added motions The net gain is reclaimed working hours that can be redirected in tasks with a higher value
Extra processing: Any work that is not needed to produce a high quality finished product that meets the design specifications[55]	Labor and time is increased in double- and triple-checks because human processes cannot be reliably error-proofed Manual documentation does not increase the intrinsic value of the dose, but serves to prove it was prepared according to the SOPs	Automation is engineered to only perform those tasks needed to yield an accurate dose on the first try Documentation is real-time, electronic, auditable, and reportable

DOWNTIME = defects, overproduction, waiting, nonutilized talent, transportation, inventory, motion, and extra processing; SOPs = standard operating procedures.

Decrease Error-related Costs

TAWF and ACS can reduce the risks of accuracy and sterility errors. The costs associated with these types of errors include direct costs (wastes of consumables and time) and indirect costs (extended length of stay, increased acuity of care, increased costs of care, lost productivity), and both can be used to build the business case for automation. TAWF and ACS vendors can typically provide examples of studies from literature or software tools that can estimate the direct and indirect value of their automation solution.

An example of the TAWF benefit was demonstrated in a study at a pediatric hospital. The system detected 2,900 errors (0.68%) during preparation of 425,683 doses.[56] Evaluation of these errors found that 23% were undetectable under the pharmacy's previous verification practice, and that 167 of the errors evaluated had the potential for adverse reactions causing moderate or severe harm. Bates et al. estimated that an adverse drug event increases the cost of that hospital stay by $4,685.[57] Using the Bates et al. dollar-per-event estimate, the TAWF described in the study potentially prevented over $780,000 of additional costs during the 13 month period evaluated.

Probability pathway modeling is another method used to estimate the cost impact that an ACS could have by preventing potential errors in manual compounding. One such model varied the incidence and severity of adverse outcomes associated with errors in 11 compounding steps. The study predicted that 5,420 errors could be prevented in a 250-bed hospital with an associated annual cost avoidance of $288,350.[58] Although predictive modeling alone cannot be used in building a business case, it can be used to demonstrate the possible range of cost avoidance associated with automation systems.

TECHNOLOGY-ASSISTED WORKFLOW SYSTEMS

> *One of the advantages of technology is that it can enhance human performance to the extent that the human plus technology is more powerful than either is alone. Good machines can question the actions of operators, offer advice, and examine a range of factors that humans cannot possibly remember.*[14]

TAWF systems utilize software to direct and document the manual compounding process. Remotely accessible image capture and data logging systems allow the pharmacist to observe the compounding process, inspect the appearance of finished doses, and review data captured during the compounding process. In general, the TAWF system consists of software that manages the formulary and the queue of in-process orders, standardized processes, and recordkeeping. It also includes hardware, such as touchscreen PCs, barcode readers, cameras, and precision balances, and an interface to the pharmacy information system.

TAWFs automate the sequencing and grouping of orders to be prepared, and then guides the pharmacy personnel step-by-step through the compounding process. The software in combination with the hardware that resides within the compounding area checks the selection of consumables, performs calculations, and guides the compounding process. Most systems also have functionality for inspection, verification, in-process tracking, and documentation for each dose compounded. This method ensures that all personnel use the same standardized compounding procedure. Because the system documents the compounding process as it occurs, the pharmacist can inspect and verify the accuracy of each compounding step. Systems that include gravimetric verification add an additional safeguard to prevent dosing errors.

The software is the main functional component of the TAWF, and it ties together orders, workflow, processes, and documentation. The available systems offer different types of interfaces to the pharmacy information system, including flat file, Health Level Seven (HL7), and print stream. The functionality, advantages, and disadvantages of each type of interface is beyond the scope of this chapter. Additional information on pharmacy interfaces is available from sources listed in this chapter's references.[59-61] Most systems also permit direct entry of orders into the workflow queue for managing batch compounding that is not entered into the pharmacy system. The design of the compounding process should be considered when looking at the type of interface offerings and the robustness of the TAWF software. Depending on your goals, it could require interfacing between the pharmacy system and TAWF, and then further interfacing to total parental nutrition (TPN) compounders, ACS, or inventory management systems. If remote verification of compounding is desired, then the connection method (web-based, local PC software, mobile app) to the TAWF must also be considered. A discussion between the vendor and the information technology (IT) department on your goals for the automation system will direct the best choice for the interfaces and determine the amount of effort required to create and manage the interface.

In addition to the software, TAWF uses a variety of hardware to present orders to the compounding personnel, check the materials, and record the compounding process. The hardware varies by vendor but generally includes a touchscreen control PC, barcode scanner and imager, camera system, touch or foot pedal activators for hardware, precision balance, and a printer. The proper placement of this equipment within the primary engineering control (PEC) is essential. Diagramming the workflow in the hood after placement of the equipment will identify the areas for potential airflow contamination, keeping in mind that all manipulations should be performed at least 6 inches from the [front edge of the] PEC. A smoke study should be performed to identify zones of turbulence and blockage of first air created by the placement of equipment in an ISO Class 5 compounding area.

Because touch is generally accepted as the most common source of contamination within the sterile compounding area (see Chapter 13 and Stucki et al. for further discussion.[38]), the workflow process diagram should also include an assessment of occurrences when the compounder's sterile gloves leave the ISO Class 5 area or touch a nonsterile object during interaction with the TAWF. If the system requires the user to touch the screen repeatedly during compounding and the screen is located outside the ISO Class 5 area, then gloves must be resanitized after each touch. Some software can automatically advance to the next instruction after each step is successfully recorded. Alternatively, the touch screen and other equipment requiring user contact can be sanitized and placed inside the ISO Class 5 area. The vendor should provide certification of equipment compatibility (especially touch screens and camera lenses) with common disinfectants. If used within a hazardous drug compounding enclosure, consideration for decontamination should also be given because the equipment may periodically require calibration or servicing.

The vision system of the TAWF consists of a high resolution camera and barcode scanner or imager that records the visual detail of the prepared consumables and products. The vision system sometimes combines the camera, barcode scanner, and balance into a single piece of hardware, which reduces the number of items inside the PEC that can impede airflow. The clarity of the pictures is vital. The system, especially for remote checking, should have zoom, rotation, and inversion features that allow the viewer a more detailed or enhanced image of the item being examined. Some systems utilize a foot pedal to activate the camera or automatically capture the image during a barcode or weight check. The number of images stored per compound and where the data are stored needs to be determined by working with the IT department. The number of image captures will determine the amount of storage space needed. The immediately accessible retention time and archiving period for images should be determined during the system set up.

Most systems also include a printer to produce an interim or final label and for printing labels to affix to partial or reconstituted vials. The printer's placement is a critical consideration because it is a high particle generator, and neither the printer nor the labels can be sanitized easily. The printer must be near the PEC but not in a location where the particles generated can be pulled into the PEC by hand movement or air currents. Ideally, a low wall air return is located behind the printer location to sweep particles away from ISO Class 7 buffer areas surrounding the PEC.

Figure 9-1 describes the steps for preparing a finished patient-specific dose for a medication requiring

Orders are created from interface
↓
System prioritizes orders
↓
Operator selects order to prepare
↓
System prompts operator to ID/weigh/image diluent vial
↓
System prompts operator to weigh empty syringe
↓
System prompts operator to draw a specific amount of diluent into syringe
↓
System prompts operator to weigh/image syringe to verify accuracy
↓
System prompts operator to ID/weigh/image medication vial to be reconstituted
↓
System prompts operator to inject diluent into medication vial
↓
System prompts operator to weigh reconstituted medication vial
↓
System prompts operator to agitate medication vial according to instructions
↓
System prompts operator to visually inspect/image vial to assure dissolution of medication
↓
System prompts operator to ID/weigh/image infusion bag
↓
System prompts operator to weigh syringe to be used for transfer of medication to infusion bag
↓
System prompts operator to withdraw amount of medication from vial into syringe
↓
System prompts operator to weigh/image syringe to verify accuracy
↓
System prompts operator to inject medication into infusion bag
↓
System prompts operator to weigh infusion bag
↓
System prints label when weight is verified and instructs operator to attach to infusion bag
↓
System prints label for medication vial if volume remaining can be used as a stock vial
↓
System retrieves next order per operator selection

FIGURE 9-1. Technology-assisted workflow software process

reconstitution and injection into an infusion bag. The steps are linear in fashion and are repeated for each dose prepared. The process outlined describes a system that uses both imaging systems and gravimetric measurement. The process varies for each TAWF vendor depending on sequencing and the type of hardware.

Because the sterile compounding workflow process varies for different locations within a facility, the TAWF should be flexible enough to handle different processes depending on the location. For example, an oncology infusion center will process chemotherapy medication as patient-specific doses, and they may prepare some of the doses once the patient is at the facility and the blood work has been approved. This just-in-time compounding may be used in conjunction with compounding of previously scheduled orders, and the system should be able to prioritize the compounding process based on the time the order is due for administration. A technician might also utilize a TAWF to guide and document the batch compounding process of doses intended for storage and subsequent dispensing on a patient-specific basis. Some of the considerations for these workflow scenarios when looking at TAWF functionality include the following:

- Can the system prioritize orders based on urgency or due time?
- Can the system handle patient-specific and batch compounding?
- Can the label content and layout be customized depending on the type of order?
- Can the system be used to document assembly of binary bag and vial systems?
- Can the system use previously assembled binary (vial and bag) systems or manufacturer premixed containers that require only a label to be affixed without any actual compounding?
- Can the system be used to make manual additives to a compounded TPN bag?
- Are there any limits on the number of ingredients that can be added to a compounding base solution?
- How are compounds that require a large number of vials per dose handled, and what is the impact on compounding time?
- How does the system know if the technician barcode-scanned one vial multiple times or scanned each vial individually?

The intended use and workflow should be mapped out for each of the different compounding scenarios. Additionally, the differences in compounding processes should be considered in the selection and design of a TAWF system.

AUTOMATED COMPOUNDING SYSTEMS

An ACS goes beyond the guided manual preparation provided by a TAWF in that mechanical systems perform the manipulations required to compound the sterile preparation. These systems range in size from small bench top devices that fit into a PEC to large systems with extensive cleanroom footprints. The smaller devices require more human intervention and have limited capacity, while the larger devices have the ability to perform multiple functions simultaneously and can hold a large supply of consumable inventory. Another difference between the devices is the degree of automation provided. Some devices require more human invention, such as connecting tubing to fluid containers and manually executing some compounding steps, such as verification of source containers. In general, as the size of the device increases, so too does the capacity and degree of manual processes that are replaced by mechanical systems.

Small Automated Compounding Systems

A small ACS generally consists of a fluid drug source connected by tubing to a peristaltic pump that transfers fluid into the final container. These devices have a usage footprint in the range of 2 to 4 square feet. Because they are not enclosed by a dedicated HEPA air filtration system, these ACS are intended for placement in an existing ISO Class 5 PEC. The small size enables automation within a space-constrained sterile compounding area. These systems can be used to compound patient-specific doses and batches of identical doses. The design of each system is unique and requires varying degrees of human interaction to prepare the dose. Small ACSs can be divided into two main categories, single-channel and multichannel.

Single-channel devices accept one drug source or one diluent source. Some systems allow the connection of multiple, identical source vials in a series. Output of the drug and diluent may be connected to a single, dedicated output port or multiple output ports that allow for the connection of infusion bags, devices (eg, infusion cassettes or elastomeric pumps), or syringes. Multichannel devices allow the connection of disparate drug source containers through a special tubing set that allows pumping of each channel separately into a common output container. Multichannel devices are commonly used for compounding parenteral nutrition or other complex multi-ingredient admixtures, such as cardioplegic solutions.

A small ACS further differs on the amount of human interaction needed during the compounding process. Some of the points to consider when selecting a small ACS include the following:

- How is the source container positively identified?
- For multichannel systems, is there a method to check that the source container is connected to the correct tubing channel?

- Does the system have a preconfigured formula to ensure the output volume and container type based on the source container that is attached?
- Does the system automatically attach a cap to syringe doses?
- Does the system automatically label the output dose?

Because smaller ACSs require more human interaction and are not fully enclosed, operator performance according to SOPs is vital to ensure accuracy and sterility. The main advantages of a small ACS are the smaller size, lower cost compared to larger systems, increased throughput over one-at-a-time manual compounding, and automation of simple, repetitive compounding tasks.

Large Automated Compounding Systems

A large ACS consists of an enclosed compounding area that is supplied with ISO Class 5 or better quality HEPA-filtered air, and it can be considered for practical purposes to be a PEC of the restricted access barrier system (RABS) type under USP Chapter <797> standards.[62] The enclosure operates under a positive pressure differential relative to the ambient cleanroom pressure. The ACS enclosure may also be operable under negative pressure for compounding of hazardous drugs. Adequate sealing of the enclosure should be tested to ensure that the negative pressure is not drawing in airborne particulates from the surrounding area. Some systems also have externally accessible chambers for connecting fluid source containers to tubing that carries the fluids into the compounding area. Air quality in these areas should be checked as part of the certification procedure because the fluid connection must be made under ISO Class 5 or better conditions to prevent inadvertent contamination of the bulk solution.

Inventory is loaded into the ACS through access doors that open to a carousel or rack system. Depending on the specific system, the holding location is oriented horizontally or vertically, and inventory may be secured through the use of compression clips or slots within the rack (**Figure 9-2** and **Figure 9-3**). The loading area should be protected by an air curtain or positive pressure clean air source because this is a potential route for viable particulate to enter into the ISO Class 5 area of the enclosure. The software instructs the operator which item to load in a specified location, and then presents that location to the operator. The operator places the item into the designated location, and then uses the software interface to indicate that loading has been completed. Note that in current systems, vial caps must be removed and the port sanitized prior to loading. After loading, the system may check that the item has been loaded correctly and prompt the operator if an error in loading has occurred.

It is important to note that loading consumables into the ACS requires the same degree of scrupulous aseptic

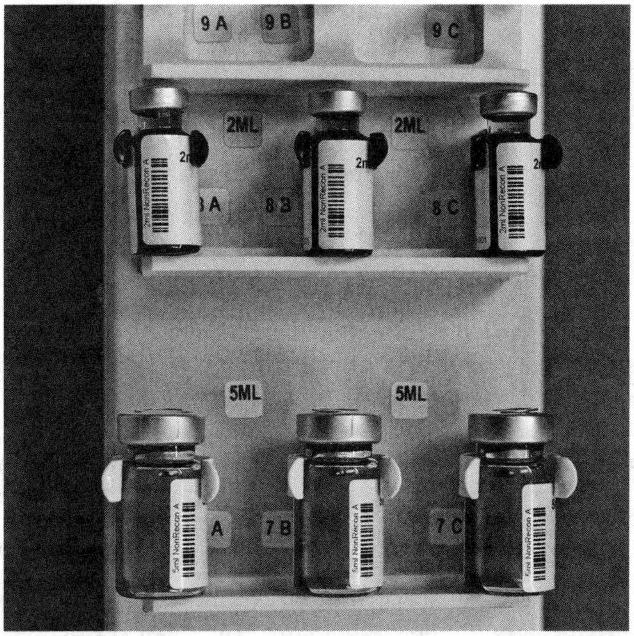

FIGURE 9-2. Vertical vial rack

Source: Reprinted with permission of ARxIUM, Inc.

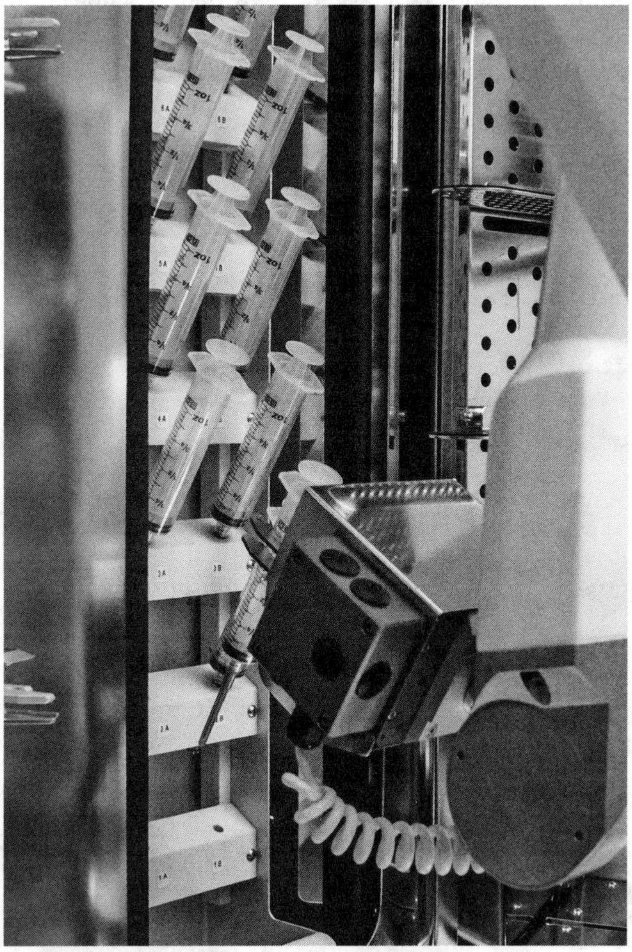

FIGURE 9-3. Vertical syringe rack

Source: Reprinted with permission of ARxIUM, Inc.

technique that is used when bringing items into the PEC's ISO Class 5 compounding area. The introduction of viable and nonviable particulate into the ACS must be vigilantly prevented at all times. Hands and consumables must be sanitized prior to penetrating the ISO Class 5 containment area and after touching a nonsterile surface, such as the ACS control screen or door handles. The system operator must exercise due caution to ensure that the consumables are free of material defects, such as cracks, leaks, or manufacturing imperfections, which the ACS is usually not capable of detecting with the current level of technology. Automated systems are particularly dependent on the uniformity of consumable characteristics, such as size, shape, weight, and label or barcode print quality. In particular, the consistency of the vial and neck diameter is critical so that the vial is not crushed while held in the robot grippers (see **Figure 9-4**).

There are automated components within the enclosure that perform manipulations of the compounding materials. The six-axis robot arm is the most visible feature, and some systems have multiple robot arms. The robot is essentially the transport mechanism, gripping and moving consumables from station to station within the enclosure, and it performs only limited actions in the actual compounding process.

Some systems also use the robot arm to perform complex reconstitution motions, such as a swirling action needed for some products. An important consideration for the robot arm is movement within the compounding area. Just as a human should never break the flow of first air across an exposed critical site, the robot motions should also follow this standard. Exposed needles, syringe tips, syringe caps, and bag and vial ports that have been sanitized should be protected by first air at all times. Smoke studies, as described in USP Chapter <797>, should be used to demonstrate that the ACS enclosure and robotic manipulators do not create unacceptable breaks in the unidirectional airflow within the enclosure during operation. USP Chapter <797> states the following:

> *If a robotic enclosure is used as the PEC, a dynamic airflow smoke pattern test must be performed initially and every 6 months thereafter to ensure 1) that it is properly integrated into the facility, 2) that there is no turbulence or refluxing at any critical site, 3) that room air does not enter the PEC where sterile products and/or preparations may be exposed, and 4) that all processes can be performed without introducing contamination to the DCA(s).*[62]

Highly sensitive scales are another component present in a larger ACS. The scale is used to check incoming consumables for proper weight to detect possible underfilled or overfilled containers, and also to check the in-process compound and the finished dose. Because ACSs use weight differentials to determine if the dose has been correctly prepared, the calibration and sensitivity of the scale for a particular weight range must be considered in the acceptable variance of the finished dose. Scales should be regularly checked for accuracy using both internal calibration (the scale checks itself) and external calibration (checking a known precision mass against the scale reading).

An ACS uses several types of imaging systems to check the incoming consumable items. Barcode scanners read the barcode on an item to confirm the identity of the drug

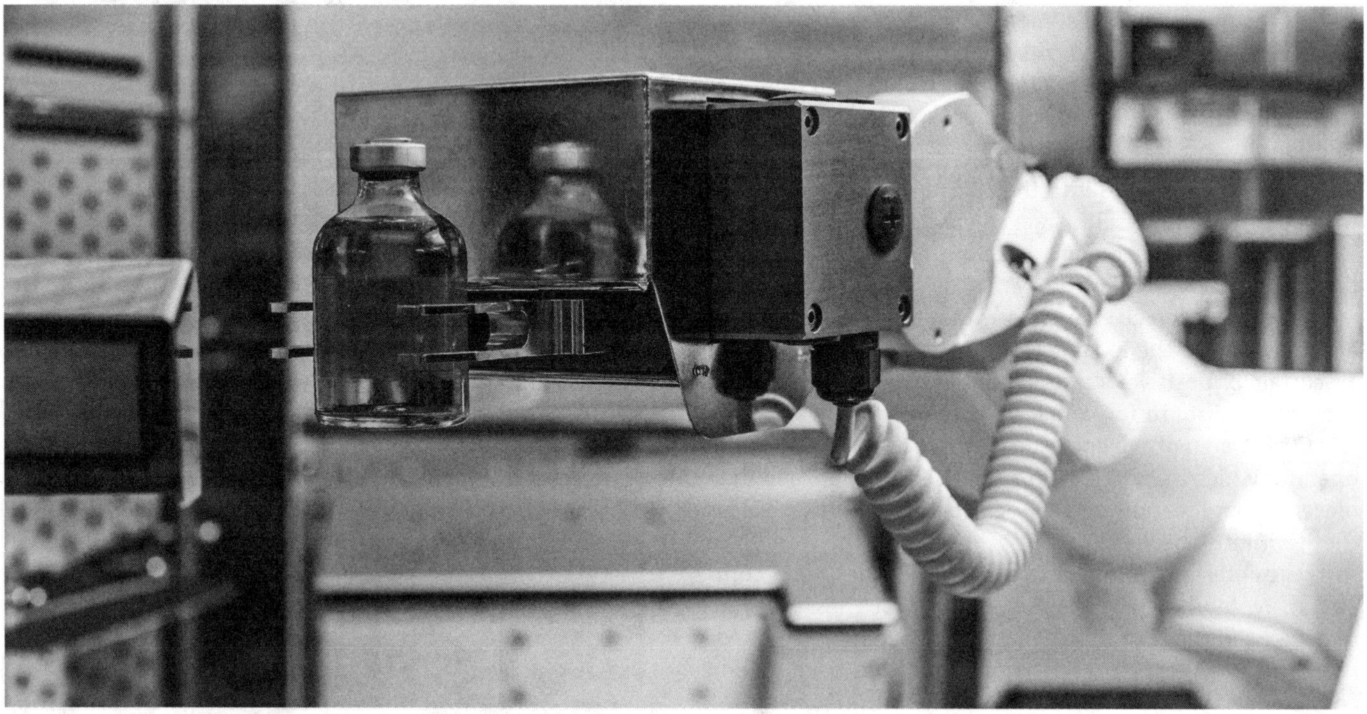

FIGURE 9-4. Robot holding vial body

Source: Reprinted with permission of ARxIUM, Inc.

source and diluent container. Imagers and software can use pattern recognition to confirm the presence, identity, and orientation of other items, such as syringes and caps. This is also beneficial when a drug vial or bag does not have a barcode on the container. Pattern recognition captures one or many images of the item, stitches the images together if needed and compares the captured image(s) to a standard image within the system database. Based on the image match threshold, the item is accepted or rejected for use in the ACS. The captured images can be stored as part of the electronic audit trail, allowing visual inspection of the actual item used. These various camera systems may also be used to capture the finished product's images for the system documentation processes.

Syringe transfer is the main method of compounding for the ACSs currently on the market. The process of getting the medication dose into a transfer syringe can be performed in several ways. One method is connecting the syringe to a tubing set, and then pumping the dose into the syringe with a calibrated peristaltic pump. A second method uses a needled syringe and multiple robot grippers to manipulate the syringe, needle, and vial (see **Figure 9-5**). One gripper holds the syringe barrel while another gripper secures the plunger button, and the system then moves either the vial or syringe so that the needle enters the vial. The plunger gripper then pulls back a specified distance to pull the dose into the syringe. After the fluid is transferred into the syringe, the weight change in the syringe or the vial is checked to ensure that the correct dose has been drawn into the syringe. Some systems use pressure management algorithms to maintain a slight negative pressure inside the vial to prevent drips during the draw process and when the needle is withdrawn from the vial.

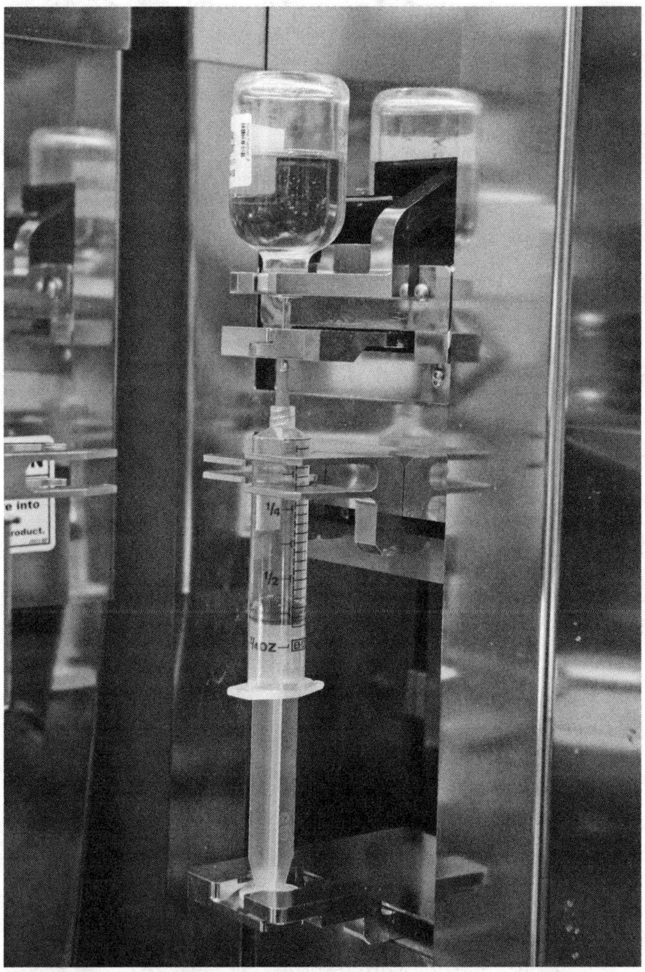

FIGURE 9-5. Syringe draw station

Source: Reprinted with permission of ARxIUM, Inc.

Some components are system-specific and include features such as washing stations, parking shelves for in-process materials, and variable speed vial shakers. Other features include the ability to attach Luer-lock or tamper-evident caps, configurable labeling systems, secured storage of finished doses within the ACS until an operator requests removal of the dose, and segregated waste handling. Ultraviolet (UV) light is used in several ways to maintain sterility of the ACS enclosure and consumables. Some systems employ UV lamps inside the compounding area to disinfect the system's surfaces and mechanical components. This type of UV disinfection system requires an extended exposure to the UV light, so the system may be out of service for several hours while the disinfection is in process. However, UV exposure does not clean the compounding area. Manual wiping to remove particulate or drug residue is still required and must be conducted prior to the UV disinfection cycle. Another type of system uses pulsed high intensity UV light that is applied directly to the vial or bag port. Direct UV disinfection adds an additional safeguard that the critical puncture site is sterile. However, it cannot remove physical particulate present on the critical site. The system vendor should provide documentation that supports claims for a UV disinfection system. Periodic validation of UV disinfection effectiveness should be considered as part of the automation system quality control process.

Workflow for Automated Compounding Systems

Workflow associated with an ACS differs depending on the type of device and the specific functions performed. **Figure 9-6** shows the general workflow for a large-scale ACS. The figure describes the steps in preparation of a finished patient-specific dose for a medication requiring reconstitution and dilution. Although the steps are described in a linear fashion, the system may perform actions in parallel. Each system performs these steps in a slightly different manner and may offer additional capabilities for specific compounding actions.

Some of the differences between compounding system types include the following:

- Inventory loading: Some systems have adaptable loading mechanisms that accommodate especially small or large vials, or they have special bag-loading clips to allow use of multiple fluid container sizes, shapes, or port configurations.

Orders created from interface or compounding template

↓

System calculates consumable inventory requirements

↓

Operator prints list and gathers inventory

↓

Operator sanitizes consumables

↓

Operator follows device prompts to load inventory into device and attach tubing

↓

Operator starts compounding run execution

↓

System reads database for preparation recipe

↓

System retrieves each item needed for compounding from its loading location

↓

System validates each item using barcode, vision system, weight, and or shape

↓

System draws up reconstitution diluent and adds to vial

↓

Reconstitution volume checked by weighing vial after fluid added

↓

System shakes vial for required time period then parks for settling

↓

System prepares dose diluent fluid bag

↓

System draws up dose needed and adds to bag

↓

Dose addition checked by weighing bag

↓

Label printed and system affixes label to bag

↓

System moves dose to output location

FIGURE 9-6. Automated compounding process

- Sanitizing systems: Some systems include integrated compounding cell, vial port, or bag port disinfection systems that mitigate contamination risks.
- Reconstitution profiles: Some systems support medications that require diluent to be directed to the vial wall or added in multiple aliquots. Some systems also use pressure management algorithms to keep vials slightly negative for vapor or fluid containment.
- Mixing profiles: Some systems have the capability of varying the mixing speed and mixing force depending on the medication.
- Serial dilution: Some systems can prepare a serially diluted solution from stock vials, and then draw doses directly from that dilution bag.
- Container closure: Some systems can attach a tamper-evident cap to syringes or have heat-sealing systems to allow the additive port to be closed and clipped off.

These systems have certain limitations because the automated technology has not yet solved certain special considerations that humans can easily accommodate. Some of these limitations include the following:

- Ampules: No current system can open ampules.
- Vial and bag sizes: Very small and very large vials and bags may be outside the handling capabilities of the system, or they may not fit into the storage racks or mechanical manipulators.
- Suspensions: These are generally not usable with automation if they require constant agitation during the draw process because the automation system holds the vial and needle in a stationary position, allowing the suspension to settle.
- Gas-producers: Vials that require venting during the reconstitution or handling process may not be compatible depending on the degree of pressure generated and the type of withdrawal device used.
- Very small and large volumes: The sensitivity of the scale within the system will determine the smallest volume change that can be detected within the accuracy limits of the scale, so very small volumes may not be compatible.
- Custom reconstitution diluents or process: Complex reconstitution processes or using special diluents may not be supported by all systems.
- Visual inspection required after reconstitution to ensure complete dissolution: At this time, no system reviewed has a vision system that is capable of inspecting vials to ensure complete dissolution of drug cake.
- Multiple ingredients: Some systems have a limited capability to prepare compounds with more than one active medication added to the diluent bag.

ASSESSMENT OF MANUAL PROCESSES AND AUTOMATION FUTURE STATE

> *Ideally, health organizations should have a systematic process both to gather relevant scientific information about a technology's safety and effectiveness and to decide whether the technology is suitable for the local setting.*
>
> Paul Poulin, Lea Austen, Catherine M. Scott, et al.[63]

Gathering and analyzing data on the current compounding process must be part of the decision-making processes when considering sterile compounding automation. By determining where risks and waste occur in the current state, personnel are better prepared to assess the applicability of available technologies for solving these problems. There are two main areas in which assessments should be performed: the compounding processes and workload.

Compounding Processes

By obtaining detailed workflow maps, steps that can be improved with automation and steps that require other changes to mitigate risks in that process can be identified. Automating a bad process will amplify the flaws within that process, so the end result could be making errors faster rather than eliminating errors. Because part of the value proposition with sterile compounding automation is also increased labor efficiency and productivity, process maps show the potential time savings that can be utilized for other tasks.

The data gathering process consists of mapping the current workflow that begins when a pharmacist verifies the order, then records each step from receipt of the order in the compounding area through the sterile compounding process, checks the products, and, finally, delivers the product to the nursing care unit. Because the steps involved in compounding an accurate sterile product are numerous with multiple opportunities for an error to occur, each step should be examined to identify possible risks and wastes within the process. An organization's quality department may be able to assist with workflow mapping and analysis. After the process is mapped and potential risks or wastes are identified, what can be mitigated by automation and what still requires human intervention can be determined. It is important to understand that every problem cannot be fixed by automation. For example, TAWF software does not ensure aseptic technique, and sterile compounding automation systems cannot inspect the finished product for particulate matter. Using the data gathered, a matrix of the problems for which solutions are needed can be created. This matrix should be used for evaluating the technology platforms under consideration to determine which automation solution is the best fit for the identified problems.

Figure 9-7 is an example of a generalized process diagram that shows the actions required to manually compound a preparation after the pharmacist has generated a label for that order. The symbols on the process map represent steps with potential errors or risks, such as contamination with viable or nonviable particulate, risks to staff members (eg, exposure to hazardous drugs or RMI), cognitive processes, visual inspection, documentation, and wait states.

Workload

Collecting information on the specific compounds being prepared and the timing of the daily batches is the second element in data gathering. Even if automation technology is not justified in a facility, the information on doses prepared each hour of the day along with the number and timing of returned doses can allow for other process changes that improve efficiency or decrease waste. Data obtained from the pharmacy IT system on doses dispensed or administered may not include everything that is compounded, such as doses prepared and administered in procedural areas

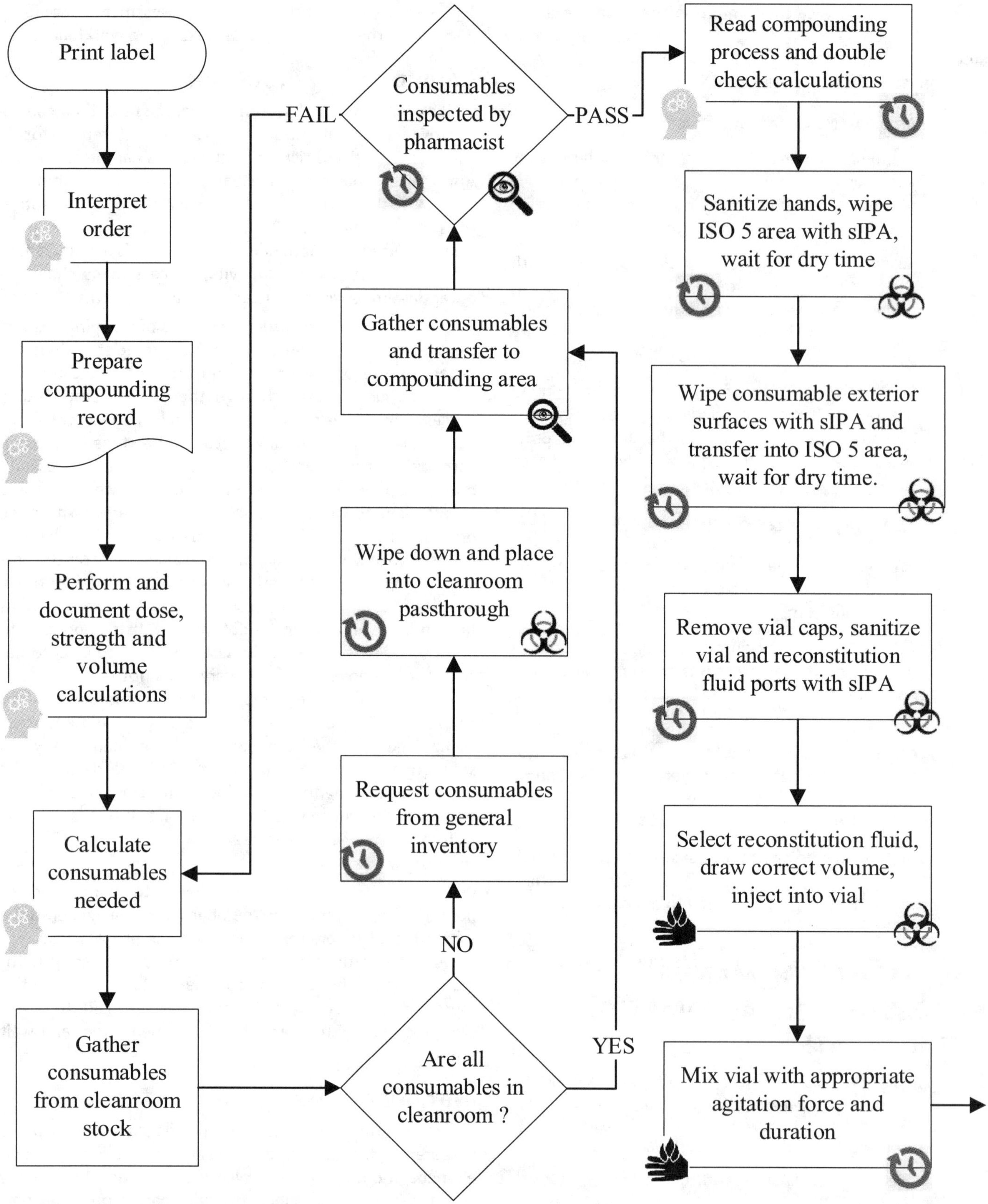

FIGURE 9-7. Manual compounding process and potential risks for errors

ISO 5 = ISO Class 5; sIPA = sterile 70% isopropyl alcohol.

Source: Adapted with permission of ARxIUM, Inc.

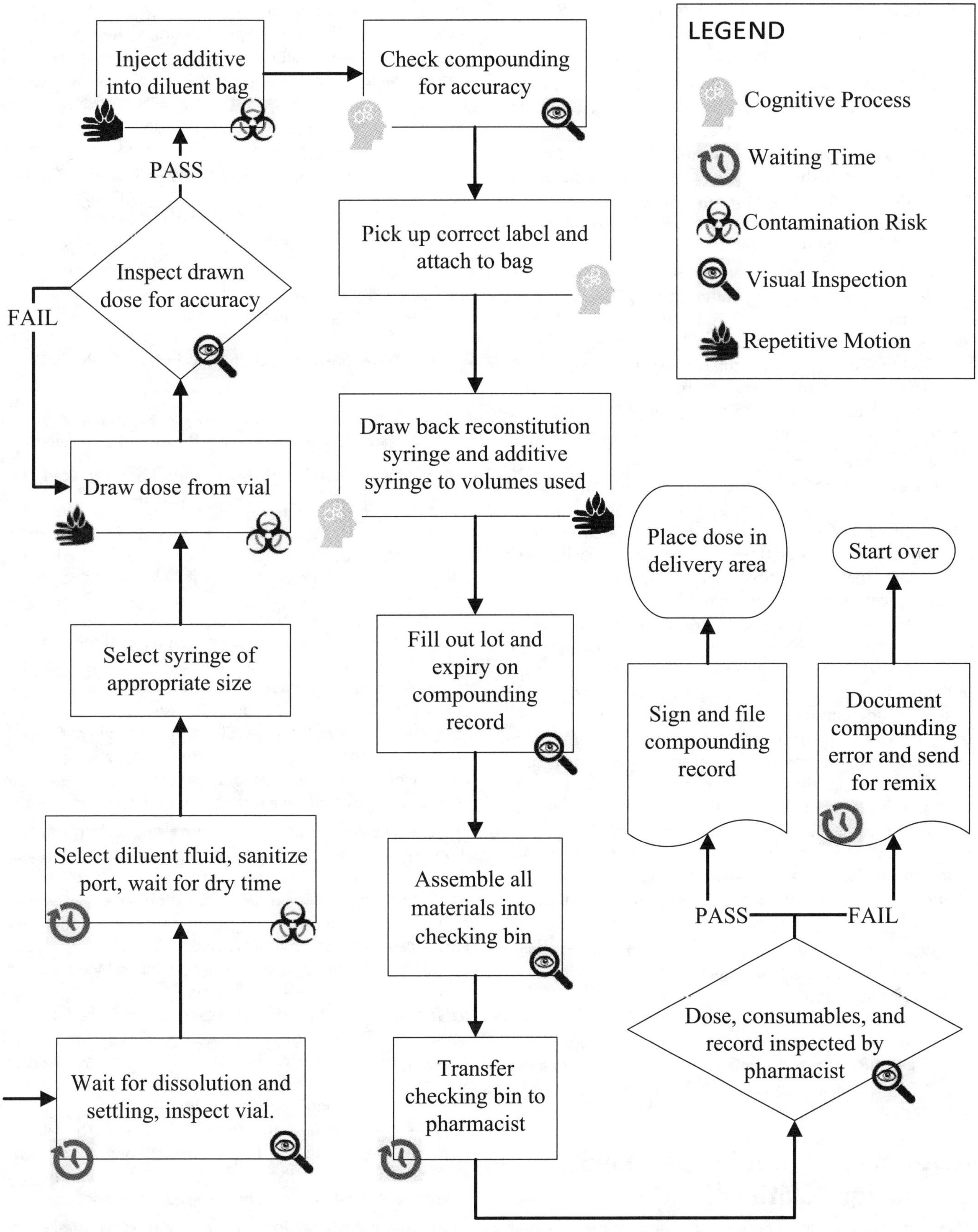

FIGURE 9-7. (Continued)

using a different documentation system. **Appendix 9-1** provides information on data gathering and **Appendix 9-2** gives examples regarding data analysis.

Once the data are collected, patterns throughout the day can be observed. This will be important for determining how much ACS capacity is needed, the amount of time that the system will need to prepare the scheduled doses, and when to send orders from the pharmacy computer system to the automated system. For a TAWF, the number of new and stat doses that will be interspersed with the routine scheduled doses should be considered.

Another point of analysis from the collected data are the utilization of staff. By looking at the workload over the entire day, periods of high intensity and other periods when no work is occurring may be discovered. Periods of high demand in a short time period may contribute to staff members working faster to complete the work on time, which could cause less attention to detail or skipping steps in an SOP, leading to an increased risk of error in a complex preparation.

Because the traditional manual compounding process is dependent on pharmacist inspection of the in-process or finished doses, it is necessary to staff the sterile compounding room continuously. Part of the data collection should quantify the amount of time that the pharmacists spend on activities that have a direct value or legal requirement in the sterile compounding process. With the advent of remote observation systems integrated into TAWF, it is possible, when permitted by pharmacy regulations, for the pharmacist to provide clinical services outside the pharmacy and still visually inspect the compounding process and finished dose. A study comparing local versus remote verification using TAWF demonstrated that error detection was identical, and that the remote process enables workload sharing and generates significant garbing cost savings.[64] Even a small reinvestment of pharmacist time can have significant returns. In a 2011 report to the Surgeon General, the U.S. Public Health Service detailed a number of studies and reported "medication management services demonstrated a return on investment of as high as 12:1 and an average of 3:1 to 5:1."[65]

When completed, the workload examination should help determine an ideal workload per hour, quantify what work might be shifted to an ACS, identify the manual workload that a TAWF can support, what tasks with greater value to the patient and the organization underutilized talent should be shifted to, and identify complex preparations that require greater attention to detail that are not suitable for automation.

Assessment of Sterile Compounding Technology Solutions

Selection of a sterile compounding automation system depends on the risks and wastes identified during the assessment process and the value that the system will return to the hospital. The perfect system would eliminate all possible dose preparation errors; ensure sterility of every dose; work with every bag, vial, syringe, cap, and CSTD on the market; require minimal human intervention; have zero downtime; require no database build or maintenance; and cost less than the manual labor that the system replaces. Because the perfect system does not exist yet, the selection criteria should be based on risk mitigation goals and desirable features in the system. Examples of these goals include assurance of accuracy in the finished dose, improvement of workflow processes, and isolation of the sterile compounding environment. TAWF can provide the first two of these three criteria, and ACS can provide all three.

The selection of sterile compounding automation technology is dependent on how well the system(s) meet each of following considerations:

- What are the risks that automation will eliminate or reduce?
- What are the features of the automation system that will mitigate each of the identified risks?
- What percent of doses could be automated, and what is the associated risk reduction?
- What is the long-term value (cost of system versus risk reduction and labor savings benefit) that the system will provide?

Utilizing an assessment of risk and mitigation tools is a useful method to compare the potential solutions against risk-based criteria. These tools allow an informed decision to be made on the benefits that the solution will bring in eliminating or reducing risks in the sterile compounding process. The outcome of the risk mitigation assessment for each solution can then be coupled to the capital and operating costs, which can be used to develop a value proposition to support the business case for the automation investment.

Because automation can be disruptive technology that dramatically changes how pharmacy personnel perform their duties, understanding current and future workflow is essential for helping staff members transition to an automated environment. Diagrams that compare current and future states can help staff members understand the weaknesses in the current state that are being eliminated by the change to automation. Future state diagrams assist the staff members in understanding the new expectations for work processes. It is likely that many processes will be substantially changed to meet the requirements of how the automation system operates. For example, in a manual compounding process, it is not unusual to group identical doses for simultaneous compounding and then affix labels after all the doses are finished. In an automated workflow environment, each dose is compounded and labeled before starting the next dose, even if the content in the bags is identical.

Future state workflow with automation can define the ideal sterile compounding process and provide an opportunity to eliminate poor processes, even when all doses are not prepared in an automated system. Automating poor current state processes leads to reliably consistent poor processes.

Additionally, the future state diagram can be scrutinized to identify where new types of errors might be introduced and how those risks will be mitigated. The use of failure modes and effects analysis is another tool that can help reduce risk associated with new technology implementation.[66] Some of the new types of errors that automation can introduce include the following:

- Data entry errors during programming: This is a human process. It should have safeguards to ensure each data element is accurate.
- Uncontrolled changes of critical data: These can cause doses to be prepared inaccurately. Particularly critical are reconstitution data (diluent volume significantly changed but vial concentration left unchanged) and fluid density.
- Untested changes in the pharmacy system order structure: The order system could send the wrong information to the automated system, resulting in orders that are compounded according to the data sent, not as the order was intended.
- Network disruptions that cause orders to be lost or delayed: Because there is no paper label generated, the lost order(s) may not be prepared and dispensed in a timely manner.
- Incorrect loading processes: These could cause mechanical damage to the system.

Using future state diagrams can help prepare for the known and unexpected problems that may occur when converting from manual to automated compounding technology.

PROJECT AND CAPITAL PLANNING FOR STERILE COMPOUNDING AUTOMATION

> *Any large-scale, multisystem-dependent automation initiative will require that you take a broad view of the current and projected impact of that system on all other systems in the facility. Creating a comprehensive plan, staying the course, and maintaining proper communication throughout will best ensure success.*
>
> Tom Van Hassel[67]

Each year, most organizations can undertake only a limited number of projects within the available capital budget, and all automation projects are in competition with the organization's other services for the available capital resources. A project plan and business case for automation should present a compelling value to an organization. The project charter and plan should present a clear set of goals, an implementation timeline, and the financial and operational measures of success for the project. The business plan should demonstrate that the capital and operating costs of automation are offset by the reduction in costs associated with errors that lead to patient harm, the costs of waste associated with manual compounding, and increased efficiencies and productivity that allow staff members to perform other tasks with a higher intrinsic value to the patient and the organization.

Project Planning

Because capital requests may only be available at certain times in the fiscal calendar, project planning should be started well in advance because the business case development can take several months to complete. Pharmacy leaders and members of the proposed sterile compounding automation project team should consider the following elements in the project planning phase:

- Development of project charter and project plan
- Project budget
- Regulatory considerations

A project charter approved by leadership is a systematic approach that identifies the problems, determines the goals and objectives, team members, scope, resources needed, potential solutions, performance measurements, and metrics to assess improvement goals.[68] A project plan describes the detailed steps to meet the goals described in the project charter. Together, the project plan and charter will serve as a basis for evaluation of the available systems to determine which will meet the project's goals. All stakeholders should approve the project charter and project plan.

The project budget should include all expenses related to the new automation system. The pharmacy administrator team member should ask the system vendor upfront, during the system consideration phase, for a list of all equipment and consumables needed to operate the system and meet the goals outlined in the project charter. The vendor should provide costs for any custom components and sole-source consumables, such as labels, consumable clips, and regularly replaced system parts. For example, if the system will be used for batch production, have the costs for stability and sterility testing been considered? Have additional refrigerators, freezers, incubators, and quarantine storage spaces been included? Is additional digital storage space for workflow images and database backups needed that may require new hardware in the data center? Preventative maintenance, parts, and airflow certification costs for the ACS or TAWF should be included in the operating budget because these will be ongoing expenses. Future state workflow process diagrams are also useful in forming this list. Working through each step in the new process may identify equipment or supplies not yet budgeted.

Because sterile compounding automation is relatively new to pharmacy practice, it may not be covered in current pharmacy regulations. A board of pharmacy or similar regulatory body is charged primarily with protecting public health. State laws, rules, or regulations may require that the regulatory board review new technology prior to its use to ensure that the technology is safe and effective for its intended use. Additionally, board review allows the inspectors to become familiar with a particular technology prior to inspection of the pharmacy in which it is installed. For these reasons, facilities considering sterile compounding automation technology should plan to present an informational discussion or formal request to a regulatory body. This presentation should cover any specific elements required by the regulatory body. At a minimum, it should also explain how the system works and the benefits to patient safety and efficiency that can be gained by use of the technology. If possible, a video demonstration is often helpful because the board representatives may not have any degree of familiarity with the new technology.

There may be other regulatory considerations depending on local, state, and federal requirements for a facility. These include service marks for electrical or mechanical safety, certification of compliance with FDA or USP standards, medical device clearance or the FDA's granted exemption from clearance, and any required seals such as Underwriters Laboratories (UL Listed) or Conformité Européenne (CE Marked).

Engage Stakeholders

Sterile compounding automation project team members should include representatives from the areas that will be impacted by the change and that need to have input into the evaluation, purchasing, and implementation processes. In addition to pharmacy, other departments to consider including on the project team are nursing, administration, leadership, finance, risk management, quality improvement, facilities management, IT, and, in some facilities, the pharmacy union.

Project charter members are responsible for ensuring that all stakeholders give input on the project. Each stakeholder will provide a different perspective and concern for this project, and the project's outcome will be measured by how well each perspective is addressed. The front-line staff members that use the system on a daily basis must be included in project planning because their engagement will strongly influence the project success. Stakeholders also need to consider the logistic and human factors involved in the transition from manual to automated compounding processes plus the time frame for ramp up to full production. Many facilities have experienced project managers, and as a valuable resource, they should be included on the project team if available. Organizations such as The Project Management Institute can provide a wealth of materials on engaging stakeholders for project success.[69]

Building the Business Case for Automation

A business case should establish the financial reasons for automating the compounding process, and also reflect the key value drivers of the organization and the pharmacy department. Building a business case for technology is one of the more challenging steps in the sterile compounding automation process because the known and estimated harm rates must be determined, and a dollar value must be assigned to these incidents. This requires acknowledgement that errors occur and lead to patient harm, which is a difficult emotional barrier to break down. Tools, such as value stream mapping and business process mapping, can be used to determine how an automation system can benefit pharmacy processes by identifying current risks and wastes in the process. Value drivers can include broad performance metrics, such as safety through error reduction, regulatory compliance (automation may aid in meeting USP Chapter <797> quality and documentation standards), and financial performance (for example, total cost of sterile compounding services, waste reduction, new revenue opportunities).

A large part of the value proposition for using automation within the sterile compounding process is based on the premise that human error cannot be completely eliminated from manual processes. Human error leads to quality issues that could cause patient harm as well as waste, reduced efficiency, and lower productivity. Both TAWF and ACS provide a means to intercept or eliminate human error during the compounding process. Additionally, using ACS can help reduce worker fatigue and repetitive motion injuries. By using facility-specific and published studies on compounding error rates and the cost of harm associated with compounding errors, it is possible to calculate the potential cost of harm and waste associated with manual compounding processes.

One method for preparing a business case is to provide background on how the current manual compounding processes impact each value driver, the financial risk associated with maintaining the status quo, how automation can reduce risks and improve financial performance, and a financial analysis that demonstrates a positive return on the technology investment. Stevenson and Jorgenson outline a method to identify and address the likely value considerations for each committee member.[70] **Table 9-3** shows the common capital committee areas of focus and metrics needed to support the value proposition.

A positive return may be generated through a combination of previously described factors. System vendors can assist in providing data, references, financial modeling, and success stories from other institutions. Pharmacy leadership should work with the system vendor and finance department project team member to develop the business case and prepare the finished document in the facility's preferred format.

Implementation

> *Many implementation efforts fail because someone underestimated the scope or importance of such preparation. Indeed, the organizational hills are full of managers who believe that an innovation's technical superiority and strategic importance will guarantee acceptance.... Experience suggests, however, that successful implementation requires not only heavy investment by developers early in the project but also a sustained level of investment in the resources of user organizations.*
>
> Dorothy Leonard-Barton and William A. Kraus[71]

Bringing an automation system to a live state requires a careful investment of time and effort before the first patient dose is produced. The implementation timeline, goals, expected benefits, and potential barriers to success for the

TABLE 9-3. Capital Expenditure Value Considerations

Decision Maker	Focus	Value Metric	Data Needed (Current State Versus Automated State)
A	Safety	Reduce medication error potential	Medication error rates/types
		Reduce employee exposure to hazardous drugs	Number of employees compounding hazardous drugs
		Reduce employee injuries	Incidence of injuries, needle sticks, carpal tunnel
B	Efficiency	Streamline process	Number of IV runs per day
		Improve personnel utilization	Time pharmacists spend checking
			Time needed to deliver new order to nurse
			Reduce returns/waste
C	Finance	Cost of an error	Cost of error at a specific facility or use national data
			Cost of adverse event associated with medication errors
		Decreases expenses	Cost of personnel time saved
			Cost of purchasing outsourced medications versus automated compounding technology
			Cost of rework in remaking a medication dose
			Waste from expired dating
			Waste from returns
			Decrease in expenses by reducing labor allocated to compounding
		Increase revenue	Revenue opportunities from redeployment of pharmacists
D	Compliance	Meet a legal or regulatory requirement	Check IV preparation electronically
E	Status	Improve technical superiority for the organization	Public relations opportunity around robotic accuracy
F	Convenience	Improve nursing convenience and patient access	Reduced nursing IV preparation Reduced turnaround time for first doses
G	History	Support or align with a historical organizational position	Complement organizational digital strategy, support point of care
H	Security	Reduce organizational risk potential	Reduce risk of purchasing IV medication from outsourced companies
			Reduce risk of IV preparations errors
I	Peer pressure	What is the competition doing?	Any competitors with similar technology?
			Is this now the standard-of-care model for similarly sized organizations?
J	Architecture	Fits with established and future informatics structure	Complement overall technology architecture

IV[a] = intravenous.

[a] When used in this chart, IV also includes sterile compounding intended for other routes of administration.

Source: Adapted with permission of Stevenson JG, Jorgenson JA. The quest for capital: selling your automation project. *Pharmacy Purchasing & Products.* 2014;11:14–17. Accessed July 30, 2023.

system should be clearly defined so that all stakeholders understand and can support the implementation process.

The implementation team should include representatives from pharmacy administration, pharmacy staff, nursing staff, IT, facilities management, and the system vendor. Each of these areas have a role to play in the success of the implementation process. All of them should be involved as early as possible so that resources can be adequately allocated as the project moves forward. The specific steps and sequences of implementation vary depending on the facility's prior experience, whether the installation is occurring in an existing or new cleanroom, and the type of automation being installed (TAWF and or ACS).

The system administrator is usually the main contact for communication with the system vendor. During the design and implementation phase, the system administrator should have regular contact with the vendor to ensure that the project is proceeding according to plan. After the system go-live, regular meetings to review issues or problems and plan the system ramp-up should be held. The system administrator is usually responsible for coordinating these meetings and keeping track of the issues being worked for resolution. Over the long term, these meetings will likely decrease in frequency as the system issues are resolved and the facility achieves independence of daily vendor support.

General Considerations for Implementation

Interface Design and Parallel Testing

The interface between the pharmacy information system and the automated compounding or workflow software is one of the most critical elements in the automation system. The patient and order data must be carefully audited to ensure absolute accuracy in all information being transmitted between systems because the dose compounding will be driven by the information received. In addition to the accuracy of each order, the completeness of the patient-specific batch compounding order list should be checked. It is possible for errors to occur in the interface code that result in orders being dropped or duplicated, which results in missing doses or extra doses, both of which are undesirable. Running the existing system in parallel with the automation system demonstrates that the interface is working properly and identifies flaws that must be corrected prior to the automation system go-live date.

System Installation and Commissioning

The installation and commissioning of the automation system(s) will likely occur in parallel with other parts of the project. The impact on existing operations must be considered during the install process. If the system is installed into an existing cleanroom, staging space for the equipment must be allocated and the vendor must understand and comply with cleanroom requirements, such as scrubbing, gowning, and sanitizing all tools and system components prior to bringing them into the cleanroom. The TAWF or ACS may require penetration of the cleanroom walls or ceiling to install equipment mounts, cameras, or to make additional electrical or network connections. Because TAWF equipment located within the ISO Class 5 compounding area will change airflow, smoke studies may be needed to define the new unidirectional airflow area within the working space. If the ACS is intended for hazardous drug compounding and integrated into the external venting controls, the building automation system engineers must be available to connect, configure, and test the airflow controls.

Commissioning of the system demonstrates that the system performs according to the design specifications. The commissioning stage should include a series of acceptance tests that demonstrate that all functions work properly, and that the system is capable of meeting the goals outlined in the project charter. Designing the acceptance test protocol or adapting a vendor-supplied acceptance test protocol should be performed well in advance of the actual testing with the test documents approved and signed by all participants in the commissioning.

Communication to Stakeholders

Communication is a critical element of the implementation process. Because the implementation requires coordination of multiple resources, regular team meetings to review progress and update the project plan are imperative. Goals for each period should be clearly outlined and barriers to meeting these goals defined. One of the leadership roles in the implementation process is management of expectations and aiding the implementation by removing barriers to the project progress. A member of the implementation team should be assigned responsibility for keeping project minutes and sending updates to the project stakeholders. By keeping everyone informed of the project status, especially reasons for delays impacting the go-live date, negative perceptions regarding the potential success of the project can be avoided.

Training and Practice Leading to Documentation of Competency

Staff members must understand both the automation system user interface (ie, how the software works and presents information or instructions) as well as what they are expected to do to make the automation system perform its task. For pharmacy personnel accustomed to manual and paper-based processes, which are flexible and can be customized to each person's habits, the change to following a software-controlled sequence of events may be a difficult transition. By providing detailed training that incorporates the reasons for the new process into the training, personnel can better understand how the new process benefits the patient, the worker, and the organization. System users should be afforded adequate time to practice using the new system so that they develop proficiency and understand the normal operations so they can identify when the system is not working properly. Documentation of competency for the administrators and operators of an automated system should be conducted after the initial training and periodically repeated, especially following a software update that introduces new functionality or changes to existing functionality.

Support and Issue Resolution

Despite the best efforts of developers, system manufacturers, and installers, automated systems are not without hardware and software issues. Mechanical issues will occur, especially during the initial phase of go-live. During the go-live, the system works through the entire range of possible mechanical actions, which may not have been tested during commissioning. With training and practice, the system users should become familiar with what is normal performance for the system so they can notify the system vendor when the system does not appear to be performing as expected. Part of the contract should clearly specify the expected turnaround and resolution time for service issues. The pharmacy administrator should monitor service calls to ensure that the vendor is meeting these expectations. Once the automation system becomes integrated into the pharmacy workflow processes, it becomes a mission-critical element in meeting patient care expectations, and the vendor should be held to contractual obligations when hardware or software issues impact patient care.

Go-live and Ramp-up Schedule

Selecting the go-live date and ramp-up schedule for the automation system depends on the scope of the project. It should account for staffing requirements, impact on current operations, confidence of the pharmacy staff in operating the new system, and support responsiveness. Some of the key factors that can impact the success of the go-live include the degree of parallel testing conducted (systems extensively tested over longer periods will likely have more system bugs worked out), staff acceptance of the process changes needed, and presence of dedicated system champions that can quickly respond to cries for help.

A common approach for ramping up automated systems is to start with several drugs that demonstrate the entire scope of system performance, such as requiring reconstitution and transfers between vials, syringes, and bags. For systems performing patient-specific dose preparation, selecting several of the most commonly prescribed drugs is a reasonable approach to capture a wide variety of doses and validate that the production interface is working as designed. The system administrator or delegate should inspect each prepared dose using system reports to check the system-recorded accuracy of compounding and verifying the dose data against the pharmacy information system patient profile.

Database Build and Administration

Automation systems require some degree of database build and customization. The amount of build is dependent on how the system will be used. The database consists of system setting options, creating users and drug data, configuring labels, and testing the system functionality.

Automated compounding and workflow systems generally have multiple levels of user privilege, but they can be broadly separated into operators and administrators. *Operators* are responsible for routine compounding activities, such as loading inventory and consumables, executing the automated compounding runs, cleaning, basic troubleshooting, and running reports. *Administrators* are responsible for creating, editing, and testing the system compounding databases; adding or editing users; setting system options; advanced troubleshooting; and evaluating system performance. Because the pharmacist is responsible for oversight of all compounding activities, the senior system administrator should be a pharmacist with expertise in sterile compounding and have a high degree of comfort working with computers and automation systems. The system administrator has two key roles that can be generally grouped into system management and system performance monitoring.

As part of the system implementation process, the system administrator should request a list of configurable system options with explanations of each option from the vendor. After reviewing each option to determine which are essential or optional and what benefits each option can provide, the administrator should set and document the option selection. After the entries are made into the system, they should be compared with the design decisions to ensure accuracy. The options document should be signed off by the administrator and filed for future reference.

User privileges vary with each system, and the system administrator must understand what privileges are required for the responsibilities assigned to each user. Only the privileges needed to conduct the assigned compounding activities should be activated. Most systems provide user group templates that grant the required privileges automatically. If experienced compounding personnel also serve as system administrators, it may be desirable to assign two distinct system access codes. One code should be used during system administration, and a second code should be used during system operation. This approach allows auditing reports to run against user groups, and it also prevents access to system administration tools in the event that the operator or administrator inadvertently neglects to log off during routine operations.

The drug database is the fundamental and most critical element of the sterile compounding technology. A flaw in setting up the drug database could result in every dose being compounded with some degree of inaccuracy. The entry of new drug or consumable data and compounding recipes into the system should follow a controlled process with multiple independent checks of the data prior to activating that item for use in automated compounding. Because the accuracy of data entered into the system is critical for accuracy of the automated compounding process, a multipoint, independent data collection and validation system helps mitigate the possibility of errors during the drug library creation process. **Figure 9-8** shows one method for collecting, entering, and validating the data needed in the automated system.

Each data collector independently gathers the parameters on a standard form. Another person compares the data collected, reconciles any differences, creates a master record,

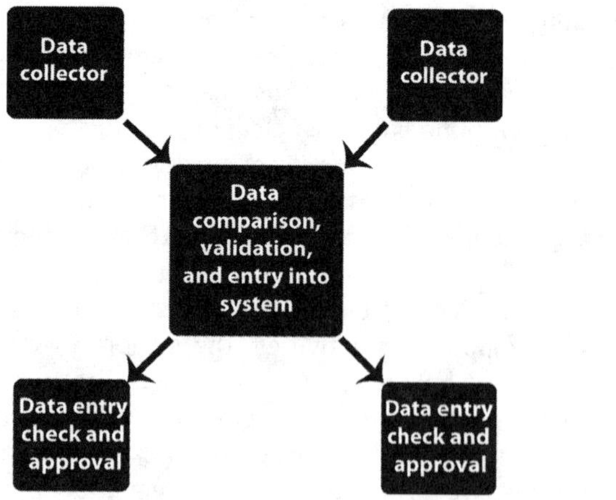

FIGURE 9-8. Data collection and verification

and enters the data into the system. Two people then verify the data entered into the system against the original data collection forms and the master record to detect transcription errors. The same people then independently approve the data entry for use. Ideally, the people performing final review and approval should be pharmacists. The decision should be based on facility policy and regulatory requirements. After creation of a new or modified consumable in the system, testing must be performed to ensure that the system works as designed.

TAWF that rely on visual verification should be tested to ensure that the images are clear and provide adequate resolution under magnification for the verifying pharmacist to read labels and syringe graduations. Image retrieval time is very important for efficiency and user satisfaction. If verification will be conducted on mobile devices, the connection speed and retrieval time over wireless connections should be tested in a variety of locations. TAWF that use gravimetric verification should have the scale tested for accuracy across a range of syringe, vial, and bag sizes to demonstrate that the system is capable of measuring the weight change within the acceptable margin of error for a particular dose size. Both an ACS and TAWF rely on barcode validation or image recognition of the bags and vials used, and some systems also verify weights and shapes of syringes or syringe caps. The test protocol should include checking that the system can distinguish when the wrong item is presented for validation.

For an ACS, the administrator should create a controlled test protocol using the new data, and then the operators should execute the test run in accordance with the protocol. The system administrator should observe the ACS test run for proper robotic handling of the product and note any problems on the test protocol form. The system should produce the correct number of doses within the acceptable accuracy range for the size and type of dose being compounded. The final dose may be confirmed by visual inspection, weight-based checks, or chemical analysis. Any discrepancies in the accuracy of the finished doses must be investigated and corrected before releasing the new programming for use in compounding patient doses.

Copies of all data collection and approval forms should be signed and dated, then filed with the system documentation. If modifications are later needed, the change form, testing results, and approval should be appended to the original records so that a historical record is maintained in sequential order.

The system administrator should be involved in the design, testing, and approval of the labels that will be affixed to the finished doses. Label content and layout may differ depending on whether the system is preparing patient-specific doses or batches of identical compounds. The system administrator should work with the system vendor to determine the data source for each field on the label as well as the label content's formatting and layout. Labels should meet hospital policy and relevant recommendations for safety, such as tall man lettering, presence of leading zeroes and absence of trailing zeroes, and acceptable use of abbreviations for units of measure. For patient-specific labels, all order-specific data should be present along with patient identification information. Once the label design is completed, each type of label must be tested to ensure all data are accurate and complete. Errors must be corrected and the labels retested until perfected. The system administrator should approve label specifications, generate examples of labels during test runs, and retain these samples with system documentation.

It is inevitable that changes will be necessary to the system. New drugs will need to be added or parameters of existing items tweaked to improve performance, and user privileges and options may need to be changed. Change control is an essential part of the system administrator's role to ensure that changes are made with due consideration of the impact and documentation of when the change was implemented. Because seemingly inconsequential changes can dramatically impact compounding accuracy or system performance, only authorized administrators should be permitted to make system changes after following a defined change control process. At a minimum, the proposed change should be documented on a standardized change control form, reviewed by the system administrator(s), and tested successfully prior to using the system to compound doses for patient administration.

Validation of System Performance

Although the automation system demonstrates its capabilities during the commissioning and acceptance testing phase of the implementation, validation of performance is needed to ensure that the system actually performs to the designed specifications under normal operating conditions. This can be conducted by stress testing the system prior to go-live using simulations of the actual compounding load. The consumable and labor expense for system validation needs to be included in the project budget and timeline. During simulation testing, it may be desirable to use surrogates, such as saline or sterile water, instead of active drug vials to avoid wasting products that may be expensive or in short supply. Two types of validation can be conducted prior to go-live: throughput validation and sterility assurance validation.

Throughput validation of ACS and TAWF determines if the number of orders expected from the system can be compounded within the time constraints for the batch and if any special functions, such as order prioritization (eg, stat orders, first doses, time-critical orders), are working properly. The expected throughput is often specified within the performance agreement with the system vendor and should be used as the benchmark during throughput testing. This is particularly critical if the compounding system will be preparing patient-specific doses because the time to prepare the batch is limited by the time at which the finished doses must leave the pharmacy for delivery to the nursing unit. Validation testing should show that all doses in the worst case scenario for the batch can be completed within the time limit. If not, then the batch will need to be smaller or more time will be needed to prepare the batch. If the variance for actual throughput is significantly different than the throughput claimed by the system vendor, the system administrator or pharmacy leadership should work with the vendor to determine why the system is not performing as expected and determine the necessary steps to remedy the difference in throughput.

Sterility assurance validation can be conducted using growth media surrogates for actual drug products if the ACS system vendor claims a particular sterility assurance level with the system. The specific design of a sterility assurance validation protocol is beyond the scope of this chapter because it involves accounting for each of the risk variables in both the manual and automated processes for the particular preparations being compounded. These variables differ for each facility, each automated system, and each compound. The protocol must be designed to demonstrate with statistical significance that the likelihood of contamination does not exceed an accepted standard. It may be beneficial to consult an expert in the field of sterility assurance validation due to the complexities of performing this assessment.

MONITORING AUTOMATED COMPOUNDING SYSTEM PERFORMANCE

After an ACS is installed, validated, and operating, the system administrator should establish a process for monitoring system performance. Because the types of ACS discussed in this chapter are relatively new in practice, no specific standards for these devices currently exist for routine monitoring. However, USP Chapter <797> contains accuracy standards applicable to automated compounding devices (ACDs) used for preparation of parenteral nutrition admixtures, and these standards may be used as a guide in developing specific monitoring parameters for the ACS.[62] USP Chapter <797> standards state the following:

> *Before using ACDs or other similar equipment, compounding personnel must conduct an accuracy assessment before the first use and again each day the equipment is used to compound CSPs. The precision of the equipment can be monitored based on an assessment of day-to-day variations in its accuracy measures. Compounding personnel must maintain a daily record of the accuracy measurements on the days the equipment is in use. Corrective actions must be implemented if accuracy measurements are outside the manufacturer's specification.*

Additionally, although the ACSs are not technically manufacturing equipment, the principles and guidance that the FDA uses for current good manufacturing practices should be considered when developing a system monitoring program. Some of the most important monitoring parameters include the trends for fluid transfer accuracy and precision, dose reject rate, scale calibration deviations, environmental monitoring, and hardware and software issues.

Accuracy and Repeatability Monitoring

Accuracy, precision, and repeatability are prime advantages of automated systems, but they are dependent on the complex workings of the mechanical parts within the system. Each of these requires a separate assessment and is best explained using the bull's-eye analogy shown in **Figure 9-9**.

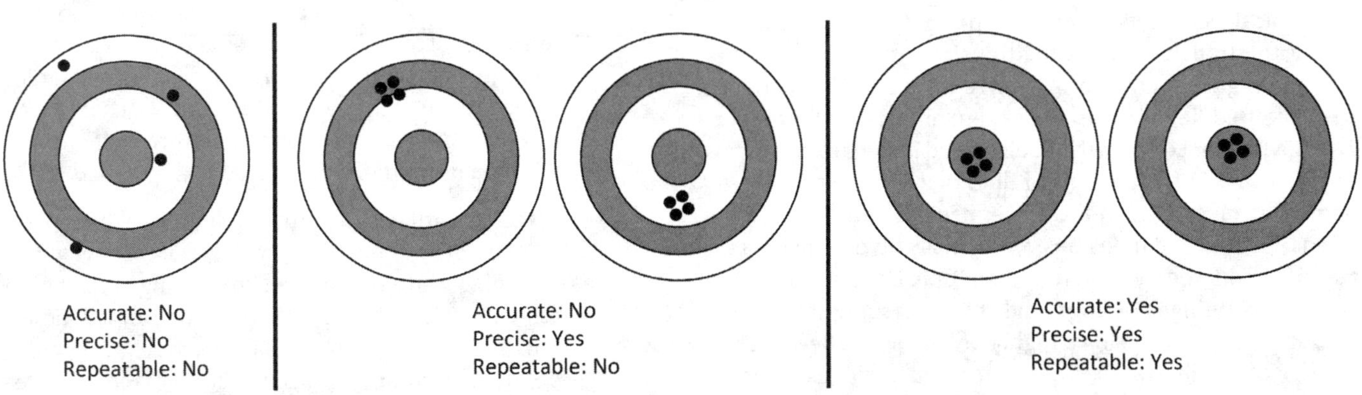

FIGURE 9-9. Accuracy, precision, and repeatability

Accuracy measures performance against a specific expected true value (hitting the bull's eye). *Precision* assesses the aggregate variance between multiple measurements of the same value (clustering of multiple shots). *Repeatability* measures whether the same degree of accuracy and precision are obtained during multiple executions of the same process (ie, hitting the same location every time with the same variance between shots).

System accuracy, precision, and repeatability should be checked initially and routinely during operations to ensure that fluid transfers are being performed properly and are within acceptable variances. The range of acceptability varies depending on the size of the dose, the size of syringe used to transfer fluid, and the sensitivity of the scale. The system vendor should be able to provide the methods used to determine the acceptance limits based on the cumulative measurement errors encountered during the automated compounding process. As part of system commissioning and acceptance testing, the accuracy, precision, and repeatability of each system component that performs weight measurements and fluid draws should be assessed at the performance limit for that component. Once the system is operating, the same tests should be performed to demonstrate that the system remains within the design specifications because, over time, system components may develop wear, alignment, and calibration drifts that require adjustment.

Scale sensitivity is a critical feature to assess because it ultimately determines if a dose is prepared accurately. Because gravimetric systems use both absolute weight and the change in weight (delta weight) during the compounding processes, the scale should be able to measure both of these weight types within its sensitivity limit. For example, if the sensitivity of the scale is accurate to 100 mg plus or minus 10 mg, then a change of 5 mg would not be detected because that is outside the sensitivity limit. This is an important parameter to test, especially if highly accurate small doses will be prepared.

Fluid transfers should be tested for accuracy at the low extreme, in the middle, and at the high extreme for each component performing a fluid transfer action. The reason for multiple tests is that the draw accuracy varies due to performance differences in syringes, elastomeric tubing, and mechanical actuators at the beginning of a fluid transfer, during the transfer, and as the transfer ends. Generally, the low and high extremes of a syringe have a higher variance than the middle, but they must remain within the acceptable tolerance. Elastomeric tubing used in peristaltic pumps can also vary in the amount of fluid delivered depending on numerous factors, such as temperature, pressure, and variations in tubing dimensions.[72] A typical fluid transfer test can be conducted by performing multiple transfers of sterile water into syringes or bags, and then measuring the actual amount transferred using a highly precise scale. Because the density of sterile water at ambient temperature is a known value that is available online or in reference texts, the actual amount transferred can be calculated and compared with the expected transfer volume and the transfer weight reported by the scale system. Plotting the actual weights against the expected volumes allows for the determination of accuracy and precision. The plot should have the values tightly clustered to demonstrate high precision, and all values should be within the acceptable accuracy tolerance (expected mL plus or minus acceptable percent variance). The system vendor should have the capability to adjust the system if the accuracy is not within acceptable limits.

During operation, the system may reject finished doses that fall outside the acceptable limits for accuracy. A system administrator should review each rejected dose to determine cause (eg, air bubble in dose, underdrawn or overdrawn by system, wrong fluid density programming) and the trend as a means of proactively monitoring for slow drifts in system performance. Mechanical systems undergo wear over time and require periodic adjustment. By monitoring the dose reject rate, the system administrator can work with the system vendor to make adjustments before they result in unacceptable failure rates. Additionally, a sudden increase in rejected doses may indicate a change in the consumable physical parameters, such as barrel size in syringes, flexibility of peristaltic pump tubing, or the amount of overfill in vials and bags.

Environmental Monitoring

Another area for routine monitoring is the environmental conditions within fully enclosed compounding systems. The design of these systems is intended to separate the compounding area from the external environment. The design also provides a means of demonstrating a higher level of control over the sterile compounding environment.

Typical measurements that the system should perform, and which the administrator should monitor, include the following:

- Temperature within the compounding area: Mechanical systems generate heat, so the interior temperature should remain within the acceptable range for compounding. This can be especially important if compounding medications are sensitive to temperature.
- Humidity within the compounding area: The performance of system components and consumables can change at extremes of humidity. At low humidity, static electricity buildup and discharge can have a negative impact on the sensitive electronics within automated systems.
- Pressure within the compounding area: The pressure gradient between the interior of the compounding system and the surrounding area should remain within the acceptable range at all times. This is especially critical for hazardous drug compounding systems to ensure that workers are protected from airborne hazardous drug particles or vapors by a continuous negative pressure gradient,

and that the pressure gradient is not excessively high, causing environmental contaminants to be drawn into the compounding system.

- Airflow within the loading and compounding areas: Unidirectional high velocity HEPA-filtered airflow is essential to protect the exposed critical sites on bags, vials, and needles. The velocity and particle counts within each critical area should be continuously monitored, and the system should actively alert the operators when these conditions are not met. The administrator should routinely check system reports for exceptions and trends of the environmental controls within the compounding and loading areas.

Surface Contamination Sampling and Assessment

An enclosed ACS offers the distinct advantage of removing airborne and human contamination risk from the compounding process. But unlike a PEC that is disinfected between each compounding operation, enclosed systems might be cleaned and disinfected less frequently. The effectiveness of less frequent disinfection must be routinely evaluated to demonstrate that the compounding area is remaining in a state of control. The system vendor should provide specific protocols for evaluating the effectiveness of cleaning and disinfection processes and for monitoring the sterility of the compounding environment. Typically, two methods are employed in these protocols: surface sampling and media fill challenges.

Surface sampling should be conducted at each product contact location, such as robot grippers, and at locations likely to be exposed to airborne viable particulate shedding during the loading process or during product manipulation. Examples of the latter include portals opening directly into the ISO Class 5 compounding area and racks or shelves where in-process compounds are temporarily parked. These two testing methods can be considered analogous to gloved fingertip sampling and surface sampling within the ISO Class 5 compounding area.

Media fill challenges of the ACS help demonstrate that the sterility of the system is remaining in a state of control at critical product contact locations throughout the entire period between cleaning cycles. Because USP Chapter <797> does not have explicit requirements for ACS media fill challenges, the compounding supervisor, quality manager, and regulatory expert should apply the principles outlined in USP Chapter <1116> Microbiological Control and Monitoring of Aseptic Processing Environments for developing protocols that can be used for the ACS.[73] The media fill challenge protocol should simulate the most complex compounding activity, and it should be designed so that at least one manipulation is performed at each mechanical component. Facilities operating under CGMP guidance must conduct full-scale production media fill challenges semiannually and when there is a significant change to the compounding process.[74] Facilities operating under USP and state regulations should establish a media fill challenge frequency that allows them to demonstrate a state of control based on the contamination control processes in place at that facility. The protocol should be executed when the system is at its worst state, typically just before cleaning and disinfection.

The detection of viable contaminants during surface sampling or media fill challenges indicates that the processes used for operating and maintaining the system are inadequate for maintaining sterility. A root cause analysis should be conducted to determine the probable causes of the sterility containment failure, and then new processes should be designed and validated to ensure that similar failures do not occur in the future. It is important to point out that using a stronger disinfectant more frequently is not a good response to a positive surface sample or media fill challenge because it does not eliminate the source of the viable contaminant. Thorough cleaning and disinfection may eliminate the immediate problem, but without discovering the root cause, it is likely to recur in the future. The risk is that it will cause product contamination without being detected by the sampling process.

Monitoring System Hardware and Software Performance

Because an ACS is a mechanical device run by software, issues occur that cause downtime. Part of the system monitoring program should include tracking of software and hardware issues and the amount of downtime that these issues cause. Some contracts include system performance guarantees, so a tracking system is critical for documentation of whether the performance guarantee is met.

Although an ACS offers certain advantages over manual processes, it also increases the monitoring requirements because it repeatedly performs the same automated process regardless of whether that process meets the established accuracy and sterility standards. A system administrator must establish processes that continuously monitor system performance and have procedures in place to make corrections when needed.

ACS CLEANING, DISINFECTION, AND MAINTENANCE

Cleaning and routine preventative maintenance (PM) of ACSs should be considered as part of the entire workflow and system costs. Just as the PEC must be routinely cleaned and disinfected, an ACS requires the same periodic inspection, cleaning, and disinfection. It is important to keep in mind that the principal means of contaminant transfer is human interaction inside the sterile compounding environment. Because some automated systems are fully enclosed cabinets that incorporate HEPA filtration and special transfer chambers to prevent ingress of environmental or human-borne contaminants, the vendor may have determined that cleaning between each batch introduces more contamination risk than it eliminates. The system vendor should provide a general cleaning and disinfection process and the recommended methods for deactivation and decontamination if compounding hazardous drugs. The cleaning protocol should be validated during the system commissioning period, and then followed carefully by the pharmacy staff.

Some ACSs contain features that provide integrated cleaning or disinfection of the consumables or the system components. Examples of these features include UV lights within the compounding area to disinfect the mechanical components, high intensity UV port disinfection systems, and automated cabinet washing. Pharmacy leadership should request that the system manufacturer provide documentation of the effectiveness for cleaning (ie, removal of particulates and drug residues) and disinfection (ie, elimination of viable particulate) because both are essential components in the maintenance of a sterile compounding environment.

The time period between each cleaning and disinfection cycle and the disinfecting agents used should be based on the manufacturer's recommendation and results of environmental monitoring studies conducted during the commissioning or early implementation phase of the ACS. Because it is difficult, if not impossible, with current technology to detect residual contamination within the compounding area, the effectiveness of the cleaning and disinfection process should be periodically validated. Systems providing UV disinfection processes should be tested routinely to ensure that the light intensity, duration, and spread are delivering an effective kill dose within the manufacturer's specifications. This can be done through calibrated UV detectors or by using biological indicator strips during a disinfection cycle. Surface wipe studies for hazardous drug residues should be performed periodically to demonstrate that the deactivation and decontamination protocol is effective.

PM is a critical component of keeping an automation system properly performing. If the PM requires entry into the enclosed area of the compounding system, then the time needed to clean and disinfect after PM is completed must be considered in the scheduling. PM should be performed according to a set schedule based on the vendor's risk assessment that identifies which components of the system need regular inspection and adjustment. The system vendor should provide a written PM schedule that includes the amount of system downtime required to accommodate performance of the maintenance tasks. The PM schedule should detail what maintenance will be performed on a daily, weekly, monthly, quarterly, and annual basis. The schedules should also include the time required for each PM event and the additional costs for labor or parts. Some PM checks may be integrated into the system software and hardware. The most common example of this is internal calibration of system scales or fluid pumps. The vendor should provide a list of what system checks are integrated, and reports should be run regularly on these automated PM checks. The amount of time needed for PM must be considered in the compounding schedule because the system will not be available while PM is being performed. Establishing a set day and time that PM will be performed should be part of the system design and implementation processes.

Safety features of the automated system should be routinely tested. This includes components such as emergency stop buttons, building automation sensors that control exhaust air flow, particle sensors built into the system, and door locks or sensors that prevent entry into the compounding cell during active operation. The latter is particularly important for fully enclosed systems with robotic arms. Entry into the compounding area during active compounding could potentially introduce contaminants or allow the operator to move an in-process bag or vial from the location at which the robot parked that item. Additionally, permitting entry into the compounding area during operation exposes staff members to the risk of the moving robotic arm hitting and seriously injuring them. Other safety features that prevent mechanical errors should be tested. Examples of these features include sensors in the robot grippers that prevent excessive gripping pressure that could shatter or puncture bags and vials, sensors that detect when the needle has not been removed from the dose prior to capping, and sensors that detect when the mechanical systems drop a bag, vial, or syringe.

Periodic air certification is part of the PM process and should be done no less frequently than every 6 months, typically on the same cycle as other HEPA filters within the pharmacy.[62] Air certification should include smoke testing to demonstrate that the air within the compounding area moves in a unidirectional fashion from top to bottom. Smoke testing should also be done to ensure that the system's mechanical components are not blocking first air at the critical site during compounding. Because air certification is an invasive process during the airflow measurements and smoke testing, plan on the system being down for an extended period of time for the actual testing, and then thoroughly clean and disinfect the system prior to using it for compounding. The cleaning process should be adequately robust to ensure that residual particulate from the smoke test and any human entry into the compounding area is completely removed from the system. The goal is to suspend and remove particulate residues using a compatible detergent, followed by a high level sporicidal disinfectant, and a final wipe down with sterile 70% isopropyl alcohol to remove residue from the cleaning and disinfecting agents.

DOWNTIME

Downtime is an expected occurrence with any automated system and may be planned or unplanned. At some point, the automation system will need to be offline for service, maintenance, and system updates. A carefully developed downtime plan is essential to maintain the safety and continuity of compounding services. The plan should include detailed procedures to follow prior to, during, and after planned and unplanned downtime. If the automation system has been performing or guiding the compounding of risk-prone medications, reversion to manual compounding could result in human error because staff members are less familiar with compounding these particular preparations.

The two most common types of planned downtime are PM and software updates of the automation system or the hospital information system that sends the orders to the TAWF or ACS. Because these are known events, they should be scheduled at a time that presents the least amount of interruption to compounding services. Based on historical data, the system administrator can determine what day of week and time of day is best suited for the system to be down. Routine service hours of the system vendor must also be considered. Some vendors only perform software updates during normal business hours so that all essential personnel can be available in the event that the update has unintended negative impacts on the system.

The two most common approaches to covering planned downtime periods include preparing expected doses prior to the downtime and reverting to manual compounding. Examples of these processes include the following:

- Temporarily changing the batch compounding schedule so that the needed doses are completed prior to the downtime
- Running the batch compounding cycle from the hospital information system early or from an offline data repository
- Preparing extra bags in advance if the ACS or TAWF is used to prepare stock solutions of diluted medications (an error in the dilution step carries the greatest risk for harm to multiple patients)
- Preparing extra doses in advance for the most commonly needed preparations so that these need only have a patient-specific label applied
- Adding an additional pharmacy technician or pharmacist to cover the additional manual compounding load during the downtime period
- Reverting to paper SOPs and documentation and visual inspection during the compounding process

Unplanned downtime due to hardware, software, or host information system problems will occur. This downtime is one of the poorly controllable risks associated with all types of automation. By accepting that unplanned downtime will occur and preparing for its eventuality, it will be easier to navigate the downtime period with a lower risk of an error occurring during the downtime.

Hardware Failure

A robust PM program is the best method to prevent hardware issues. However, in the event of hardware failure, replacement of the failed part in a timely fashion is critical. The parts most likely to fail should be kept on site when possible. The system vendor should provide these parts within the scope of the service agreement. Parts that are very expensive and rarely fail (eg, a robotic arm) should be maintained in one or more central depots with immediate, year-round access to same day express shipment facilities. During the system evaluation phase, potential vendors should be closely questioned about hardware failure history, replacement frequency, and the location and delivery period for parts that are not kept on site. The adage "anything that can go wrong, will go wrong" should be kept in mind. A critical part is most likely to fail on the evening before an extended holiday weekend during inclement weather! Another consideration is which parts on the system are off-the-shelf components and which are custom made. Although off-the-shelf components may be readily available in the event of failure, a custom component could take weeks or months to manufacture. Knowing which parts are readily available and which require a significant lead time can assist in planning spare part inventory.

Software and Network Failure

Software issues that occur within the automation system can be divided into two categories: intermittent and reproducible. Intermittent issues occur rarely, and a definitive cause cannot be readily identified. Reproducible issues occur every time a certain automation action is attempted. Either type can prevent the system from compounding some or all doses. The system should have logging capabilities, and any software issues should be reported to the system vendor promptly so that the logs can be examined. Based on the type of issue, the system vendor should provide a solution or workaround in a timely manner. The expected resolution time frame should be defined within the service agreement.

Unplanned network and hospital information system issues or downtime are numerous and beyond the scope of this chapter to examine. For systems compounding patient-specific doses, this type of downtime will result in the system being inoperable because no order data are received. Some automation systems have the capability for users to manually enter compounding orders or retrieve previously compounded orders and prepare them again. Most hospital information systems also have some type of downtime redundancy system that gives access to current orders. Additionally, some systems can continuously write future orders to a file in an offline data repository. The order data in the host's downtime system could then be manipulated into the format that the automation system requires and uploaded manually into the automated compounding queue. The system administrator and the hospital's information services department should consider a downtime order repository as part of the implementation process and regularly test the system to ensure that it is available when needed.

Infrastructure Failure

Infrastructure failures should be considered in the automation system downtime and disaster plans. Automation systems are dependent on power; heating, ventilation, and air conditioning; building automation; the internal order processing network; the external network for support connectivity; and possibly telephone and cellular service. Failure in any of these utilities can render the system inoperable and must be considered in the downtime plan. Equipment should be connected to uninterruptible power supplies and plugged into the facility's emergency power circuit. This protects sensitive electronics from power fluctuations and sudden shutdowns during switchovers from regular to emergency power. In regions prone to severe weather emergencies (eg, hurricanes, blizzards, floods) that periodically cause power failures, installation of a dedicated generator for the pharmacy cleanroom and automation system should be considered. The facility and department disaster plan must also include the automation system. Once the system is fully implemented and part of the daily pharmacy operations, any disaster that impacts the pharmacy can also impact the automation system. If the pharmacy location is rendered unusable (eg, flooding, water or sewer line leakage, electrical failure, or fire), the automation system may not be available in a temporary pharmacy location. As part of the automation planning phases, it is beneficial to revisit the disaster plan and ensure the doses prepared by automation are included in the backup plan.

Downtime Plan and Recovery

A downtime plan should include the foreseeable issues that can prevent operation of the system. A printed copy of the downtime plan should be maintained in the compounding area so that is accessible in the event of network failure. The plan should be organized so that the types of issue and the steps to take in response to the issue are well documented. The plan should include a description of the issue, who should be notified of the downtime, how to communicate the downtime, the steps to take during the downtime, and the steps to take after the downtime issue is resolved.

Even with the best planning, the likelihood of orders that require manual compounding during the downtime is high. For this reason, conducting periodic mock downtimes is beneficial so that all staff members on every shift become familiar with the downtime procedures required to compound doses that the automation system routinely handles. Standard compounding procedures and documentation forms for each preparation normally handled by the automation system should be included in the downtime plan.

Following the downtime, a review of the downtime plan and its execution should be conducted. Participants should include the compounding personnel that worked the downtime period, as their input into the effectiveness of the plan is essential to understand. Adjustments to the plan should be implemented promptly after the downtime review, and the printed copies of the plan should be updated to reflect the changes.

SUMMARY

Failures of accuracy and sterility are the two main risks to patient safety in manual compounding. Both depend on the skill and consistency of compounding personnel. Mitigating these known risks should be the primary driver to consider in automating the sterile compounding process. Employee safety, particularly protection from hazardous drugs and workplace injuries, as well as employee satisfaction and engagement are additional considerations. Finally, reducing or eliminating the costs associated with waste and errors provides a strong financial incentive to use automation.

Selection of the automation system or systems should be based on the risks identified in current workflows and the business case that supports the decision to automate. The broadest sterile compounding automation solution is a combination of an ACS and TAWF. An ACS is used for preparing doses that represent the largest compounding volumes and for medications that have the highest risk of harm if a compounding error occurs. A TAWF is used to guide manual compounding of lower volume doses and products that the ACS cannot handle. It is important to involve compounding staff members in the decision-making process because they will ultimately be the daily users of the system.

Implementation, monitoring, and maintenance of the system should be considered as part of a project plan. A structured change control process should be used to mitigate risks of errors in the system data entry. Adequate testing during the install process and after changes to the system is essential to prevent compounding errors caused by flawed data or bad configuration entries. Regular monitoring and PM of the system can help ensure reliability and accuracy during the life of the technology. The system requires periodic updates of software and may experience unplanned downtime, so a carefully designed and regularly rehearsed downtime plan is needed.

Technology changes will occur, but the principles and processes in this chapter can be used and adapted for new technology solutions. Always remember that automation by itself cannot prevent every error. The capabilities of the automation system and how humans interact with the system should be considered when implementing automated sterile compounding technology.

REFERENCES

1. Ganio MC, Cobaugh DJ. Taking a culture of patient safety to the next level: Improving the quality and safety of sterile preparations. *Am J Health Syst Pharm*. 2018;75(16):1182–1183. doi:10.2146/ajhp180500
2. Robinson M. Baxa corporate milestones. 2009. **https://img.pr.com/press_kit/0904/1526/presskit_1526_1239741674.pdf**. Accessed February 1, 2023.
3. Baxa Corporation. Company overview, company history. **www.pr.com/company-profile/overview/1526**. Accessed February 1, 2023.
4. Fox BI, Felkey BG. Automated intravenous preparation: robots for the pharmacy. *Hosp Pharm*. 2009;44:255–257.
5. Pratt MK. A robot in the pharmacy. **https://www.computerworld.com/article/2550632/a-robot-in-the-pharmacy.html?page=3**. Published May 10, 2010. Accessed February 1, 2023.

6. Health Robotics announces IV Station. *Robotic Magazine.* **http://www.roboticmagazine.com/military-medical-vehicles/health-robotics-announces-iv-station**. Published June 5, 2008. Accessed February 1, 2023.
7. Software strategies: new technology catches mistakes on camera. **https://www.reliasmedia.com/articles/15726-software-strategies-new-technology-catches-mistakes-on-camera**. Published November 1, 2008. Accessed February 1, 2023.
8. Halvorsen D, ed. State of pharmacy compounding 2022. *Pharmacy Purchasing & Products*. 2022; 19(4) Supplement:S46.
9. Institute for Safe Medication Practices (ISMP). ISMP guidelines for safe preparation of compounded sterile preparations. **https://www.ismp.org/sites/default/files/attachments/2017-11/Guidelines%20for%20Safe%20Preparation%20of%20Compounded%20Sterile%20Preperations_%20revised%202016.pdf**. Published 2013. Revised 2016. Accessed February 1, 2023.
10. Institute for Safe Medication Practices (ISMP). Targeted medication safety best practices for hospitals. **https://www.ismp.org/guidelines/best-practices-hospitals**. Published February 9, 2022. Accessed February 1, 2023.
11. Long J, Calabrese S, Al-Jedai A, et al. Cleveland Clinic International IV Robotics Summit. *Am J Health Syst Pharm*. 2021;78(9):800–805. doi:10.1093/ajhp/zxab050.
12. Institute for Safe Medication Practices (ISMP). ISMP Guidelines for Sterile Compounding and the Safe Use of Sterile Compounding Technology. ISMP; 2022. **https://www.ismp.org/resources/guidelines-sterile-compounding-and-safe-use-sterile-compounding-technology**. Accessed July 29, 2023.
13. Pates AA, Hansen KN, Boiallis CJ. The state of sterile compounding technology. *Pharmacy Purchasing &Products*. 2022;19(3)(suppl):S2–S11.
14. Kohn LT, Corrigan JM, Donaldson MS, eds. *To err is human: building a safer health system*. Washington, DC: National Academy Press; 2000:ix, 62.
15. The Pew Charitable Trusts. U.S. illnesses and deaths associated with compounded medications or repackaged medications 2001-2019. **https://www.pewtrusts.org/en/research-and-analysis/data-visualizations/2020/us-illnesses-and-deaths-associated-with-compounded-or-repackaged-medications-2001-19**. Published March 2, 2020. Accessed February 1, 2023.
16. Halvorsen D, ed. Trends in BCMA and CPOE adoption over time. *Pharmacy Purchasing and Products: 17th annual state of pharmacy automation*. 2022;19(8):15.
17. Poon EG, Keohane CA, Yoon CS, et al. Effect of bar-code technology on the safety of medication administration. *N Engl J Med*. 2010;362(18):1698–1707. doi:10.1056/NEJMsa0907115.
18. Bonkowski J, Carnes C, Melucci J, et al. Effect of barcode-assisted medication administration on emergency department medication errors. *Acad Emerg Med*. 2013;20(8):801–806. doi:10.1111/acem.12189.
19. Flynn EA, Pearson RE, Barker KN. Observational study of accuracy in compounding i.v. admixtures at five hospitals. *Am J Health Syst Pharm*. 1997;54(8):904–912. doi:10.1093/ajhp/54.8.904.
20. Reece KM, Lozano MA, Roux R, Spivey SM. Implementation and evaluation of a gravimetric i.v. workflow software system in an oncology ambulatory care pharmacy. *Am J Health Syst Pharm*. 2016;73(3):165–173. doi:10.2146/ajhp150169.
21. Deng Y, Lin AC, Hingl J, et al. Risk factors for i.v. compounding errors when using an automated workflow management system. *Am J Health Syst Pharm*. 2016;73(12):887–893. doi:10.2146/ajhp150278.
22. Eckel SF, Higgins JP, Hess E, et al. Multicenter study to evaluate the benefits of technology-assisted workflow on i.v. room efficiency, costs, and safety. *Am J Health Syst Pharm*. 2019;76(12):895–901. doi:10.1093/ajhp/zxz067.
23. Higgins JP, Hardt S, Cowan D, et al. Multicenter study to evaluate the benefits of technology-assisted workflow on i.v. room efficiency, costs, and safety in small community hospitals. *Am J Health Syst Pharm*. 2019;76(13):964–969. doi:10.1093/ajhp/zxz080.
24. Bucci TG, Hedrick TL, Roberts PA, et al. Evaluation of gravimetric-based technology-assisted workflow for nonhazardous sterile product preparation. *Am J Health Syst Pharm*. 2019;76(14):1071–1077. doi:10.1093/ajhp/zxz097.
25. Pugliese S, Nigri N, Moriconi L, D'Arpino A. PP-047 Automated intravenous chemotherapy workflow: the added benefit to reduce potential medication errors. *Eur J Hosp Pharm Sci Pract*. 2017;24:A222.
26. Roberts PA, Willoughby IR, Barnes N, et al. Evaluation of a gravimetric-based technology-assisted workflow system on hazardous sterile product preparation. *Am J Health Syst Pharm*. 2018;75(17):1286–1292. doi:10.2146/ajhp170564.
27. Flanagin CM, Little J, Brookins L, Wills M. Implementation and evaluation of an IV room technology-assisted workflow system integrated within the electronic medical record at oncology infusion center pharmacies. *Am J Health Syst Pharm*. 2021;78(13):1244–1251. doi:10.1093/ajhp/zxab149.

28. Moss A, Kang S, Morbitzer KA, et al. Evaluation of chemotherapy preparation processes: Volumetric method reliability and gravimetric method utility within 5 US hospitals. *Am J Health Syst Pharm*. 2022;79(4):230–238. doi:10.1093/ajhp/zxab414.

29. Pang B, Earl M, Knoer S, et al. Comparison of IV oncology infusions compounded via robotics and gravimetrics-assisted workflow processes. *Am J Health Syst Pharm*. 2021;78(2):122–134. doi:10.1093/ajhp/zxaa366.

30. Hicks RW, Becker SC, and Cousins DD, eds. *MEDMARX data report: a report on the relationship of drug names and medication errors in response to the Institute of Medicine's call for action*. Rockville, MD: USP Center for the Advancement of Patient Safety; 2008.

31. International Organization for Standardization (ISO). *ISO International Standard ISO/IEC 7886-1:2017. Sterile hypodermic syringes for single use—part 1: syringes for manual use*. Geneva, Switzerland: ISO; 2017.

32. Food and Drug Administration. *Allowable excess volume and labeled vial fill size in injectable drug and biological products: guidance for industry*. **https://www.fda.gov/media/88138/download**. Published June 2015. Accessed February 1, 2023.

33. USP <1151> Pharmaceutical dosage forms. In: *2022: USP Compounding Compendium*. Rockville, MD: United States Pharmacopeial Convention; May 1, 2022. **https://doi.org/10.31003/USPNF_M99860_08_01**.

34. Poppe LB, Savage SW, Eckel SF. Assessment of final product dosing accuracy when using volumetric technique in the preparation of chemotherapy. *J Oncol Pharm Pract*. 2016;22(1):3–9. doi:10.1177/1078155214549489.

35. Cohen MR, Metzer JL. ISMP medication error report analysis: syringe pull-back method of verifying IV admixtures is unreliable. *Hosp Pharm*. 2013;48:803–806.

36. Moyen E, Camiré E, Stelfox HT. Clinical review: medication errors in critical care. *Crit Care*. 2008;12(2):208–214. doi:10.1186/cc6813.

37. Trissel LA, Gentempo JA, Saenz LM, et al. Effect of two work practice changes on the microbial contamination rates of pharmacy-compounded sterile preparations. *Am J Health Syst Pharm*. 2007;64(8):837–841. doi:10.2146/060199.

38. Stucki C, Sautter AM, Favet J, Bonnabry P. Microbial contamination of syringes during preparation: the direct influence of environmental cleanliness and risk manipulations on end-product quality. *Am J Health Syst Pharm*. 2009;66(22):2032–2036. doi:10.2146/ajhp070681.

39. Trissel LA, Gentempo JA, Anderson RW, Lajeunesse JD. Using a medium-fill simulation to evaluate the microbial contamination rate for USP medium-risk-level compounding. *Am J Health Syst Pharm*. 2005;62(3):285–288. doi:10.1093/ajhp/62.3.285.

40. Von Woedtke T, Kramer A. The limits of sterility assurance. *GMS Krankenhhyg Interdiszip*. 2008;3(3):Doc19. PMID: 20204091.

41. Trissel LA, Ogundele AB, Ingram DS, et al. Using medium-fill simulation to establish a benchmark microbiological contamination rate for low-risk-level compounding. *Am J Health Syst Pharm*. 2003;60(18):1853–1855. doi:10.1093/ajhp/60.18.1853.

42. Stahl A. Four ways to satisfy (and retain) millenial employees. **https://www.forbes.com/sites/ashleystahl/2015/10/08/four-ways-to-satisfy-and-retain-millennial-employees/#598fb9d45e4f**. Published October 8, 2015. Accessed February 1, 2023.

43. Jackson CA, Wilson DA. World at work: hospital pharmacy clean-rooms. *Occup Environ Med*. 2006;63(1):68–70. doi:10.1136/oem.2005.020719.

44. Occupational Health & Safety Agency for Healthcare (OHSAH). *Reducing repetitive strain injuries in Vancouver/Richmond regional hospital pharmacies*. Vancouver, BC: OHSAH; 2004.

45. Centers for Disease Control and Prevention. NIOSH Alert: preventing allergic reactions to natural rubber latex in the workplace. **https://www.cdc.gov/niosh/docs/97-135/pdfs/97-135.pdf?id=10.26616/NIOSHPUB97135**. Published August 1998. Accessed February 1, 2023.

46. Zilinskaite L, Tamasauskas D, Kvedariene V, Sitkauskiene B. Self-reported drug allergy in health care workers in conservative and surgical medicine departments. *J Investig Allergol Clin Immunol*. 2012;22(5):357–362.

47. Schierl R, Masini C, Groeneveld S, et al. Environmental contamination by cyclophosphamide preparation: Comparison of conventional manual production in biological safety cabinet and robot-assisted production by APOTECAchemo. *J Oncol Pharm Pract*. 2016;22(1):37–45. doi:10.1177/1078155214551316.

48. Iwamoto T, Morikawa T, Hioki M, et al. Performance evaluation of the compounding robot, APOTECAchemo, for injectable anticancer drugs in a Japanese hospital. *J Pharm Health Care Sci*. 2017;3:12. doi:10.1186/s40780-017-0081-z.

49. Sessink PJ, Leclercq GM, Wouters DM, et al. Environmental contamination, product contamination and workers exposure using a robotic system for antineoplastic drug preparation. *J Oncol Pharm Pract*. 2015;21(2):118–127. doi:10.1177/1078155214522840.

50. Avey J, Wernsing T, Luthans F. Can positive employees help positive organizational change? Impact of psychological capital and emotions

on relevant attitudes and behaviors. **http://digitalcommons.unl.edu/cgi/viewcontent.cgi?article=1031&context=managementfacpub**. Published March 2008. Accessed February 1, 2023.

51. Konrad AM. Engaging employees through high-involvement work practices. *Ivey Business Journal*. 2006;26:11–14.

52. Lean Six Sigma. Wikipedia: the Free Encyclopedia. Edited July 18, 2023. **https://en.wikipedia.org/wiki/Lean_Six_Sigma**. Accessed February 1, 2023.

53. 8 wastes.GoLeanSixSigma.com. **https://goleansixsigma.com/8-wastes/**. Accessed February 1, 2023.

54. The waste of motion; causes, symptoms, solutions, examples. Lean Manufacturing Tools website. **http://leanmanufacturingtools.org/96/the-waste-of-motion-causes-symptoms-solutions**. Accessed February 1, 2023.

55. The waste of Overprocessing; causes, symptoms, examples and solutions. Lean Manufacturing Tools website. **http://leanmanufacturingtools.org/121/waste-of-overprocessing-causes-symptoms-examples-and-solutions**. Accessed February 1, 2023.

56. Moniz TT, Chu S, Tom C, et al. Sterile product compounding using an i.v. compounding workflow management system at a pediatric hospital. *Am J Health Syst Pharm*. 2014;71(15):1311–1317. doi:10.2146/ajhp130649.

57. Bates DW, Spell N, Cullen DJ, et al. The costs of adverse drug events in hospitalized patients. *JAMA*. 1997;277(4):307–311.

58. Urbine TF, Schneider PJ. Estimated cost savings from reducing errors in the preparation of sterile doses of medications. *Hosp Pharm*. 2014;49(8):731–739. doi:10.1310/hpj4908-731.

59. Dumitru D. *The pharmacy informatics primer*. Bethesda, MD: American Society of Health-System Pharmacists; 2008.

60. Tribble DA. Print-stream interfaces. *Am J Health Syst Pharm*. 2009;66(11):990–991. doi:10.2146/ajhp070593.

61. Peters M. HL7 Essentials. Confluence HL7 website. **https://confluence.hl7.org/display/HE/HL7+Essentials**. Edited December 28, 2022. Accessed February 1, 2023.

62. USP <797> Pharmaceutical compounding—sterile preparations. In: *2023: USP Compounding Compendium*. Rockville, MD: United States Pharmacopeial Convention; 2023; Issue 1. **https://doi.org/10.31003/USPNF_M99925_07_**.

63. Poulin P, Austen L, Scott CM, et al. Introduction of new technologies and decision making processes: a framework to adapt a Local Health Technology Decision Support Program for other local settings. *Med Devices (Auckl)*. 2013;6:185–193. doi:10.2147/MDER.S51384.

64. Jean SJ, Francart SJ, Eckel SF, et al. Evaluation of telepharmacy and the use of a gravimetric technology-assisted workflow system for remote sterile product pharmacist checks. *Am J Health Syst Pharm*. 2020;77(7):560–567. doi:10.1093/ajhp/zxaa015.

65. Giberson S, Yoder S, Lee MP. *Improving patient and health system outcomes through advanced pharmacy practice—a report to the U.S. Surgeon General*. Rockville, MD: U.S. Public Health Service; 2011.

66. Feemster AA, Augustino M, Duncan R, et al. Use of failure modes and effects analysis to mitigate potential risks prior to implementation of an intravenous compounding technology. *Am J Health Syst Pharm*. 2021;78(14):1323–1329. doi:10.1093/ajhp/zxab179.

67. Van Hassel T. Long-term budgeting for pharmacy automation. *Pharmacy Purchasing & Products*. 2011;8:21.

68. Wiegers KE. Toolkit for using the AHRQ quality indicators: project charter. **https://www.ahrq.gov/sites/default/files/wysiwyg/professionals/systems/hospital/qitoolkit/combined/d2_combo_projectcharter.pdf**. Accessed February 1, 2023.

69. Miller D, Oliver M. Engaging stakeholders for project success. Project Management Institute White Paper. **https://www.pmi.org/learning/library/engaging-stakeholders-project-success-11199**. Published January 1, 2015. Accessed February 1, 2023.

70. Stevenson JG, Jorgenson JA. The quest for capital: selling your automation project. *Pharmacy Purchasing & Products*. 2014;11:14–17.

71. Leonard-Barton D, Kraus WA. Implementing new technology. *Harv Bus Rev*. 1985;63:102–111.

72. Avantor. Peristaltic Pump Tubing and Chemical Compatibility. **https://us.vwr.com/cms/tech-article-matching-the-tubing-to-the-fluid**. Accessed July 29, 2023.

73. USP <1116> Microbiological control and monitoring of aseptic processing environments. In: *USP Compounding Compendium*. Rockville, MD: United States Pharmacopeial Convention; 2013. doi:10.31003/USPNF_M99835_01_01.

74. Food and Drug Administration (FDA). Current good manufacturing practice—guidance for human drug compounding outsourcing facilities under Section 503B of the FD&C Act: guidance for industry. Draft guidance, Revision 2. **https://www.fda.gov/media/88905/download**. Published January 2020. Accessed February 1, 2023.

APPENDIX 9-1. WORKLOAD DATA COLLECTION QUESTIONS

The following data elements assist in determining how the sterile compounding workload occurs throughout the day. Both TAWF and ACSs will need the data to identify which compounds can be made within the limits of the system, for workload assignments, and to determine the formulary build effort.

Daily Quantities by Medication

- Products dispensed daily (in syringes, minibags, and large volume bags)
- Preparations compounded daily (in syringes, minibags, and large volume bags)
- Doses ready to label at time of dispensing (commercial premix, binary systems, frozen, or outsourced compounds)
- Preparations rejected and remade
- Doses returned; Why; Rescheduling
- Doses wasted; Why (eg, change in order, discontinuation, short stability)

Hourly Quantities by Time of Day

- Scheduled doses compounded (standard administration times)
- New, stat, or now orders
- Missing doses
- Discontinued orders (how is this removed from production or delivery queue)

Workload per Shift

- Determine from data above
- Delivery runs to patient care areas; time of runs for doses due at a specific time

APPENDIX 9-2. WORKLOAD DATA COLLECTION EXAMPLES

Volume by Medication Type

The 80/20 rule usually applies to sterile compounding. Eighty percent of the doses needed comprise 20% of the total compounded line items. Identifying which medications make up these high volume drugs assists in determining where and how these products will be prepared. Depending on volume and the type of automation purchased, these 20% may be prepared in specific hoods with a TAWF or ACS.

New Orders or Discontinued Orders

Table 9-4A illustrates the percent of new, change, and discontinued orders by time of day. In this scenario, 65% of new orders are written between 1000 and 1800, and 50% of discontinued orders occur between 0801 and 1200, then another 25% between 1601 and 2000. Using this information assists in determining the optimum times to prepare patient-specific doses to avoid waste.

Standardized Medication Administration Times

Understanding when the doses are needed for administration helps identify workload volume by time of day. Many hospitals have standard administration times. **Table 9-4B** shows that when standard administration times are used, the majority of doses are administered between 0900 and 2100, which allows for better pharmacy planning in the compounding processes. Used in conjunction with the new and discontinued time of day distribution, the compounding and delivery cycle can be refined to ensure doses are available for the nursing unit when needed and determine the compounding time needed during a particular cycle.

Batch Schedules

Table 9-4C illustrates the time lag needed to prepare the sterile compounding run for two batches per day. The labels are printed at 0600 for doses due at 1100. This is a 5 hour window for preparation and delivery. During this 5 hour window, approximately 20% of new orders or discontinued orders occurred when reviewing the data on new orders. However, 70% of all new orders or discontinued orders are written during the time doses are due (between 1100 and 2259).

Table 9-4D is an example of a batch reconciliation data collection form. This tabulation shows whether prepared doses were actually administered and the disposition of a dose if not administered. This allows for determination of the cost associated with wasted doses. Order changes, returns, and rework are a waste of time and product. Using these data can identify the benefits of increasing the number of batches, determining if a staffing pattern change is needed and reducing the number of wasted doses.

TABLE 9-4A. Discontinued and New Orders: Percent by Time of Day Distribution

Time of Day	0001–0800	0801–1000	1001–1200	1201–1400	1401–1600	1601–1800	1801–2000	2001–2200	2201–2400
Discontinued orders	5	30	20	5	5	10	15	5	5
New orders	5	5	10	15	20	20	10	5	10

TABLE 9-4B. Count of Orders per Standard Administration Time

Time/Frequency	Daily	EVERY 12 HR	EVERY 8 HR	EVERY 6 HR
0500			30	5
0900	40	20		
1100				5
1300			30	
1700				5
2100		20	30	
2300				5

TABLE 9-4C. Batch Times for Preparing and Delivering Doses to the Nursing Unit

Doses due: 1100 to 2259	Print labels: 0600	Prepare doses: 0630 to 0900	Deliver doses: 0900 to 1000 (on nurse unit 1 hr prior due time of 1100)
Doses due: 2300 to 1059	Print labels: 1800	Prepare doses: 1830 to 2100	Deliver doses: 2100 to 2200 (on nurse unit 1 hr prior due time of 2300)

TABLE 9-4D. Reconciliation of Doses Prepared to Determine Waste

Batch Period	Number of Doses Prepared	Number of Doses Returned for Credit	Number of Returned Doses Recycled	Number of Returned Doses Wasted	Number of Doses Charted as Administered	Number of Doses Missing
1100 to 2259	515	95	22	37	398	22
2300 to 1059	375	58	16	42	302	15

SECTION 4: Principles and Work Practices of Sterile Compounding

DOI 10.37573/9781585286492

18 FINISHED PREPARATION RELEASE CHECKS AND TESTS

Angela W. Yaniv

19 RECEIPT, STORAGE, MOVEMENT, AND DISPOSAL OF COMPOUNDED STERILE PREPARATION COMPONENTS AND FINISHED PREPARATIONS IN THE PHARMACY

Joshua S. Ilenin

20 MAINTAINING STERILITY, PURITY, AND STABILITY OF DISPENSED AND DISTRIBUTED CSPs

Kevin N. Hansen

10

STERILE PREPARATION FORMULATION

Paul M. Baker

INTRODUCTION

This chapter discusses formulation when applied to a compounded sterile preparation (CSP) using nonsterile and sterile starting components. It is important that care is made in each step to ensure the CSP maintains its safety, quality, identity, potency, and purity throughout the entire process.

COMPOUNDING DRUG REGULATIONS

The Drug Quality and Security Act (DQSA) was signed into law on November 27, 2013. This legislation spells out certain provisions related to the oversight of compounded drugs. The DQSA clearly delineates between traditional compounding and outsourcing. Title I of the DQSA removes certain provisions from section 503A of the Federal Food, Drug, and Cosmetic Act (FDCA) that were found to be unconstitutional by the Supreme Court in 2002. Section 503A describes the conditions under which traditionally compounded drugs for humans are exempt from the three sections of the FDCA. The requirements are as follows[1]:

- Compliance with current good manufacturing practices (CGMPs) (section 501(a)(2)(B))
- Labeling with adequate directions for use (section 502(f)(1))
- U.S. Food and Drug Administration (FDA) approval prior to marketing (section 505)

For further reading on 503A, please refer to Chapter 2.

The new law also created the new section 503B in the FDCA. Under section 503B, a compounder can become an outsourcing facility. An outsourcing facility is able to qualify for exemptions from the FDA approval requirements and the requirement to label products with adequate directions for use, but not exemptions from CGMP requirements. Outsourcing facilities must adhere to the following requirements:

- Comply with CGMP requirements
- Be inspected by the FDA according to a risk-based schedule
- Must meet other specific conditions, such as reporting adverse events and providing the FDA with certain information about the products they compound.[1]

When formulating and compounding sterile preparations, pharmacists must follow state laws and federal regulations. State pharmacy practice acts and board of pharmacy regulations cover these activities. The FDA also regulates formulation and compounding under adulteration, misbranding, and new drug provisions of the FDCA.

Since 1980, in the FDA Field Regulatory Guidance chapter Hospital Pharmacies: Status as Drug Manufacturer, the FDA states that "a physician may prescribe an unusual preparation that requires compounding by a pharmacist from drugs readily available for other uses and which is not generally regarded as safe and effective for the intended use."[2] With the establishment of 503A and 503B pharmacies, the FDA drafted further guidance on how hospitals can compound to meet the needs of patients within their own health system. This is intended to address not only the triad of patient, physician, and pharmacist for specific compounds but also compounds required in areas of emergent use (eg, operating rooms, emergency departments, intensive care areas) where any delay in ordering or preparation of a compound may cause patient harm.[3]

Compounding Phase I investigational drugs does not require full compliance with CGMPs because of the low volume of patients. Compounding medications for Phase II and

Note: The author acknowledges Mark G. Klang who authored this chapter in the previous edition.

DOI 10.37573/9781585286492.010

III trials requires complete adherence to CGMPs, and products prepared for Phase I cannot be used for the subsequent phases if not prepared under full CGMPs.[4]

Pharmacists' Roles

503A Pharmacist

A 503A pharmacist is responsible for compounding and dispensing finished preparations for prescribed therapy. They are also responsible for compounding and preparing those preparations in compliance with established state and federal regulations. These requirements vary from state to state.

503B Pharmacist

A 503B facility must follow CGMP, which requires a complete separation of responsibilities between operational and quality roles, including within the reporting structure. A 503B pharmacist works in research and development, establishing product lines, drugs and diluent to be used, final containers, and stability profiles. Pharmacists also provide a valuable role by establishing the correct processes needed to prepare a formulation on a consistent basis. On the operational or production side of a 503B facility, pharmacists lead a team or are valuable members in oversight of compounding operations, establishing safe workflows, label development, scheduling, facilities oversight, and custodians of controlled substances.

If a 503B pharmacist is employed within the quality department, they oversee incoming materials inspection, label development and approval, or batch record review. They are also responsible for development and implementation of training programs for staff. Training programs include topics such as good documentation practices, aseptic technique, and visual inspection.

PROFESSIONAL STANDARDS

The 503A pharmacist must follow *United States Pharmacopeia* (USP) chapters related to compounding and their respective state boards of pharmacy rules, which are discussed more thoroughly in Chapter 2. A 503B facility must follow the latest guidance from the FDA, including *Current Good Manufacturing Practice–Guidance for Human Drug Compounding Outsourcing Facilities Under Section 503B of the FD&C Act.*[5]

Formulating, compounding, and sterilizing a pharmaceutical from nonsterile ingredients or in nonsterile containers is the most difficult type of sterile compounding.[6] CSPs are classified as either Category 1, Category 2, or Category 3 depending on the conditions in which they are made (see Chapter 16). Master Formulation Records (MFRs) should include anticipated yields, sterilization methods, complete preparation instructions, quality control, and validation of procedures to be used. Presterilized sealed containers should be used when feasible. Final containers must be sterile and capable of maintaining product integrity through the beyond-use date (BUD).[7]

The sterilization method must be based on the preparation's properties. Whatever method of sterilization is used, a sterility test is required when a BUD is assigned beyond the limits specified in USP Chapter <797> to ensure safety of the contents. The sterility test must be validated to determine if contaminations can be isolated if they are present and to determine the sensitivity of the assay (refer to Chapter 12 and USP Chapter <71> Sterility Test for more detailed information).[8] See **Table 10-1** for a review of the different types of sterilization, their advantages, and their disadvantages.

TABLE 10-1. Sterilization Methods*

Sterilization Method	Specifications	Advantages	Disadvantages
Dry heat	180°C for 30 minutes, 170°C for 1 hours, or 160°C for 3 hours	Good for heat stable, nonaqueous materials (ie, glass, some oil-based injectables, fats)	Heat sensitivity Requires longer time and higher temperature than moist heat
Steam Heat	Pressure: 15 lb/sq inch Temperature: 121°C Time: 20–60 minutes	Uses biological indicator to verify sufficient heat and pressure	Components that are sensitive to heat and moisture
Filtration	0.2 μm Numerous fibers, size, and load specifications	Filter integrity test verifies filter did not rupture	Filter must be certified for volume and filtrate load Some solutions may be incompatible with filters
γ irradiation	~ 25 kGy Requires very high radiation to be effective	Containers and packaging may remain intact Fewer variables to control	Incompatibilities with some finished products
Ethylene oxide, nitrous oxide, hydrogen peroxide vapor	Depending on gas used, different saturation and permeation	Less invasive Good for heat sensitive components	Highly flammable and highly reactive Possibility of forming residual compounds

* Refer to Chapter 12 for more details.

USP Chapter <797> specifies that nonsterile active ingredients for CSPs must come from an FDA-registered facility and include a certificate of analysis.[1,7] All other components that are not active pharmaceutical ingredients (API) must comply with criteria described in USP monographs, if a monograph exists. The ingredients must come with a certificate of analysis obtained from an FDA-registered facility.[7] All APIs and other components used must be evaluated for suitability for use in sterile drug preparation. Components labeled with "not for pharmaceutical use," "not for injectable use," "not for human use," or an equivalent statement must not be used to compound for these purposes.[7] Bulk or unformulated drug substances and added substances or excipients must be stored in tightly closed containers under the specific temperature, humidity, and lighting conditions identified in official monographs or documentation from suppliers. Also, the date of receipt in the compounding facility must be clearly and indelibly marked on each package of ingredient that lacks an expiration date. Upon receipt of each lot of the ingredient, a visual inspection of the lot for evidence of deterioration or other types of unacceptable quality and mislabeling must be performed as described in a written protocol.

Processes Involved in Compounding

There are two types of methods used to process CSPs, aseptic processing and terminal sterilization. Both methods are defined in USP Chapter <797> and *Current Good Manufacturing Practice—Guidance for Human Drug Compounding Outsourcing Facilities Under Section 503B of the FD&C Act.* Regardless of method used, it is critical that the safety, quality, identity, potency, and purity of the CSP is maintained and stated per the label. Aseptic processing is done by maintaining the sterility of sterile components as they are manipulated throughout the compounding process or by compounding from one or more nonsterile components followed by sterilization by filtration. Depending on the CSP components needed, initial components could be sterile or the CSP may need to be sterilized prior to its final presentation.

Terminal sterilization occurs if the prepared CSP in its final container is compatible with a sterilization process. Examples of the types of terminal sterilization can be seen in Table 10-1. Terminal sterilization requires a sterility assurance of 10^{-6}, which means that the chance of a contaminated unit occurring is 1 in 1 million units. Terminal sterilization should not alter the safety, quality, identity, potency, and purity of the final product. Please see Chapter 12 for more in-depth discussion regarding sterility assurance.

WRITTEN PROCEDURES

Personnel who work with CSPs should develop and comply with the following written procedures, which are explained in detail in Chapters 28, 30, and 33:

- There must be a specifically designated and adequate area for the orderly placement of equipment and materials to be used in compounding. CSPs should be prepared in a separate and distinct area from nonsterile compounding.[1]
- Presterilization procedures for components that are nonsterile, such as weighing and mixing of nonsterile powders, must be completed in at least an International Organization for Standardization (ISO) Class 8 environment.[7]
- For the safety of personnel, antineoplastic hazardous drugs and any hazardous API should be stored in an environment that is negative pressure and ventilated to the outside with a minimum of 12 air changes per hour. This is recommended by the National Institute for Occupational Safety and Health and required by USP Chapter <800> Hazardous Drugs—Handling in Healthcare Settings.[8]
- Careful selection of respiratory and personal protective equipment (PPE) is crucial for protecting staff. Additionally, appropriate engineering controls need to be applied and followed (see Chapter 27).
- Liquid preparations are especially hazardous because vapor easily passes through filtration-based transfer systems, rendering them ineffective for exposure control.[10]
- Any hazardous components requiring manipulation should follow USP Chapter <800> and its assessment of risk, primary and secondary engineering controls, and SOPs (see Chapter 27).

Pharmacists must ensure that the sterile components under their supervision meet acceptable criteria of stability and sterility by doing the following[11]:

- Expiration dates must be observed, and the oldest stock must be dispensed first. The BUD of a CSP must not exceed the expiration date of any of the components used in compounding. Not all chemicals used in pharmaceuticals have been assigned an expiration date by the manufacturer.
- Components should be stored under the environmental conditions stated in their individual monographs and labels.
- If a component has undergone a physical change not explained in the labeling, the CSP should never be dispensed. Visual checks are of limited value in this setting, as the best observations will detect particles 20 to 50 µm in diameter. Although a microscope enhances the size of the particles, the volume needed for testing is quite large according to USP Chapter <788> Particulate Matter in Injections, which would cause excessive waste.[12] A light obscuration particle sizer is the ideal instrument because it can detect fine precipitates that may occlude small blood vessels (4 to 9 µm in diameter).
- Sterility testing must be conducted using the validated procedures outlined in USP Chapter <71>.[8] Sufficient numbers of test samples are required for adequate strength of the analysis. Sterility testing by membrane filtration is the ideal methodology,

but viscous liquids cannot pass the 0.4 μm filters used. For samples that cannot be filtered, an inoculation test may be used, but it has a much lower capacity to catch microbial contamination.[8] Visual observations are not an effective measure of sterility. If there is evidence that the integrity of a seal of a final CSP has been violated, the CSP must be considered suspect with a potential of microbial contamination.

- It is necessary to practice proper handling and labeling of preparations that are repackaged, diluted, or mixed with other products.
- Dispensing must be done in the proper container with the proper closure.
- Using sterile compounding equipment that is appropriate in design, size, and composition is required so that surfaces contacting components are not reactive or adsorptive. These surfaces should not alter the required safety, identity, strength, quality, and purity of the components.[7] Prescription balances and volume measurement devices should meet USP specifications.[13]
- All formulas, calculations, substances, containers, closures, and in-process materials must be inspected and approved or rejected. There should be a written SOP to follow in the event of nonconformance of bulk chemicals or CSPs.[14]

Pharmacists who compound batches of parenteral preparations must follow a MFR to consistently reproduce CSPs that meet all requirements. For more information on batch compounding, refer to Chapter 28. Additionally, refer to Chapter 12 for sterility assurance, Chapter 17 for labeling compounded preparations, Chapter 18 for finished preparation release checks and tests, Chapter 20 for the stability and incompatibility of drugs, and Chapter 30 for documentation.

COMPONENTS

Components are any ingredients used in compounding, whether they appear in the final preparation or not (ie, intermediate ingredients). Commercially sterile components should be used whenever available. Every effort should be made by the compounder to procure conventionally prepared sterile products from FDA-inspected manufacturers when compounding CSPs. USP Chapter <797> identifies two specific sets of criteria for choosing components when selecting API and other components required for the formulation. As shown in **Table 10-2**, API must be obtained from an FDA registered facility. However, when selecting components that are not API, there is some leeway as long as the appropriate documentation and/or testing is completed to ensure the strength, quality, identity, and purity of the component.[7]

The FDA, in consultation with the Pharmacy Compounding Advisory Committee and USP, determines if a bulk substance should be placed on the 503A bulks list. To be considered, they look at the physical and chemical characteristics of the substance, the safety of the substance, the efficacy of the substance, and its historical use in compounded products. As of this publication, six bulk substances have been approved.[15]

For a 503B, facilities may compound using bulk substances under either of the following circumstances[16]:

- The bulk drug substance appears on a list identifying bulk drug substances for which there is a clinical need (the 503B bulks list).
- The product compounded from bulk drug substance appears on FDA's drug shortage list at the time of compounding, distribution and dispensing.

Vehicles

Vehicles for most liquid sterile preparations should have no therapeutic activity or toxicity. Instead, they serve as solvents or mediums for the administration of therapeutically active ingredients. For parenteral preparations, the most common vehicle is water. Vehicles must meet USP requirements for pyrogen or bacterial endotoxin tests.[17;18]

Sterile Waters for Compounding

Various waters may be used for compounding depending on their intended application. Compounders should not assume that all sterile waters are the same. Pharmacists

TABLE 10-2. CSP Component Selection Considerations

Selecting API for CSP	Selecting Components Other Than API for CSP
• Must comply with criteria in the *USP–NF* monograph (if one exists)	• Must comply with criteria in the *USP–NF* monograph (if one exists)
• Must have a COA that includes the specifications and test results and shows that the API meets the specifications	• Must be accompanied by documentation (eg, COA, labeling) that includes the specifications and test results and shows that the component meets the specifications
• Must be obtained from an FDA-registered facility	• Should be obtained from an FDA-registered facility

API = active pharmaceutical ingredient; COA = certificate of analysis; CSP = compounded sterile preparation; FDA = U.S. Food and Drug Administration; *USP–NF* = *United States Pharmacopeia–National Formulary.*

should familiarize themselves on the types of sterile water available, including their uses and limitations. This section focuses on sterile monographed waters typically seen in compounding, which include sterile water for injection, sterile water for irrigation, sterile water for inhalation, and bacteriostatic water for injection.

Water for Injection is used as a generalized definition, and compounders may sometimes use it interchangeably when speaking of the types of waters available. USP defines *water for Injection* as an excipient (vehicle) in which product endotoxin must be controlled. Water for injection is purified by distillation or other means that depend on the type of water used and its validated method.

Sterile water for injection is not intended for direct injection. Its low tonicity causes hemolysis of the cells and may be fatal. It is packaged in containers ranging in size from 10 mL to 3 L. Sterile water is used for the preparation of bulk substances, reconstitution of lyophilized powders, or cleaning of components where a validated water system is not in place. As such, it is required to meet the specifications outlined in USP Chapter <788> Particulate Matter in Injections.[12]

Some types of water cannot be used for the preparation or administration of an injectable product. Sterile water for irrigation does not comply with USP Chapter <788>, so it is not allowed to be used. Sterile water for inhalation is sterilized and packaged in single-dose containers that are labeled with their full name. It may be used in conjunction with inhalers and nebulizers or used as a diluent with another component. However, sterile water for inhalation does not need to comply with USP Chapter <788>, therefore it is not suitable for use in injectable applications.[12]

Bacteriostatic water for injection is sterilized and contains one or more bacteriostatic agents to inhibit microbial growth. It can be used in the preparation of injectable medications similar to what is seen with sterile water for injection. It is typically seen in the preparation of multidose vials. However, if benzyl alcohol is used as a bacteriostatic agent, it is contraindicated in the preparation of parenteral medications for use in newborns or as a component in the preparation of CSPs intended for use in spinal or epidural use.[19]

Aqueous Isotonic Vehicles

Aqueous isotonic vehicles are often used in sterile preparations. A common example is an injectable solution of 0.9% sodium chloride (ie, normal saline solution) that is sterilized and packaged in single-dose containers no larger than 2,000 mL. Bacteriostatic sodium chloride injection is a 0.9% sodium chloride injection that contains one or more bacteriostatic agents in a container no larger than 30 mL. Solutions of 0.9% sodium chloride for irrigation are also available in multiple sizes. However, these alternatives to sodium chloride for injection have the same limitations as water for irrigation or bacteriostatic water.

Other isotonic vehicles include Ringer's injection, 5% dextrose injection, and lactated Ringer's injection. None of these components are available in containers larger than 1,000 mL. There are other concentrations of dextrose and saline available. Care should be taken to ensure their osmolality and tonicity are compatible with the preparation and intended patient.[20]

Water-Miscible Solvents

Several water-miscible solvents are used as a portion of the excipient in sterile preparations (ie, as cosolvents). These solvents (eg, ethanol, glycerin, liquid polyethylene glycol, propylene glycol) dissolve drugs with low water solubility. Preparations compounded with these components are usually administered intramuscularly or require significant dilution for intravenous (IV) administration.[21] Examples of drugs in cosolvent formulations include some vitamins, antihistamines, and cardiac glycosides. When the solvent has toxic properties or produces toxic decomposition products (eg, Cremophor), the formulation requires extra caution (eg, limiting the final cosolvent concentrations). Administration of these viscous liquids as an undiluted IV injection has resulted in complications.[22]

Nonaqueous Vehicles

Nonaqueous vehicles, such as fixed oils, can be used to formulate parenteral preparations. USP specifies that fixed oils must be vegetable (ie, metabolizable) in origin, odorless (or nearly so), and have no rancid odor or taste.[23] Examples include peanut, cottonseed, corn, and sesame oils. Some vitamins and hormones can only be solubilized in these oils. Oil-based parenteral drugs can only be given intramuscularly. However, emulsified oils (eg, soybean and safflower) prepared as liposomes mimic the natural chylomicrons that circulate in the bloodstream. Liposomes may be used as vehicles for lipid-based drugs, such as propofol and amphotericin B, or as a source of essential fatty acids in nutrition support.

Sterile compounding of total parenteral nutrition (TPN) may include lipids along with the amino acids and dextrose. These combined products are called 3-in-1 or total nutrient admixtures. Special handling is necessary for these formulations as they are easily contaminated (see Chapter 22 for details). Special limitations for compatibility are required because the destabilized emulsions can lead to pulmonary and immunologic consequences. Review USP Chapter <729> Globule Size in Lipid Emulsions for a detailed method to evaluate stability of IV lipid emulsions.[24]

Solutes

Solute chemicals dissolved in vehicles should be USP grade or better because their contaminants, especially metals (eg, aluminum), can alter solubility and compatibility of other solutes, cause catalytic chemical reactions, or cause toxicity to patients. Added substances can increase stability or usefulness. Some additives have limited effectiveness or a narrow range of usefulness before producing complications. A pharmacist must consider the total formulation of active ingredients and added substances when compounding. No coloring agent should be added to a sterile preparation solely to color it.

Antimicrobial Preservatives

Antimicrobial preservatives may be added up to a concentration that is considered bacteriostatic or fungistatic. Some preservatives, however, have innate toxicity within these concentrations (eg, phenylmercuric nitrate 0.01%, benzalkonium chloride 0.01%, and phenol 0.5%). Because of their toxicity, these preservatives are mostly used in ophthalmics and with multidose injectables intended for intramuscular or subcutaneous injections.

Benzyl alcohol (usually 0.9%) and parabens (eg, methyl 0.18% combined with propyl 0.02%) are commonly used in injectables. In oleaginous preparations, no antimicrobial is highly effective. However, hexylresorcinol 0.5% and phenylmercuric benzoate 0.1% are reported to be moderately bacteriocidal.[25] An antimicrobial agent may be effective in one formula of ingredients but not in another. For example, large molecule components (eg, polysorbate 80, polyvinylpyrrolidone, and polyethylene glycol) form complexes that inactivate the parabens. To select a preservative, an appropriate reference should be consulted, and its effectiveness should be verified.[26] USP provides a test for the efficacy of antimicrobial preservatives.[27] USP Chapter <797> limits antimicrobial effectiveness in multidose vials to 28 day or as described by the manufacturer.[7]

Note that simply adding a preservative to a CSP does not automatically extend the BUD unless the compounder has a verifiable sterility testing program in place.

Preservatives should be avoided with preparations for neonates and premature infants. Surfactant-based preservatives are toxic to neurologic tissue and must be avoided in injectables for intrathecal administration.

pH Buffers

Buffering agents stabilize an aqueous solution of a chemical, which prevents degradation. Buffer systems are formulated at the lowest concentration needed for stability so that the body's physiologic pH is not disturbed. Acid salts, such as citrates, acetates, and phosphates are commonly used as buffers. The use of sodium bicarbonate should be limited when neutralizing acids in an injection, as it can form gasses as a reactant and precipitate salts.

Cysteine is added in pediatric and neonatal parenteral nutrition compounding solutions. It reduces pH and enhances the solubility of calcium and phosphate, which normally forms a precipitate. Tables are available to predict the limits of calcium and phosphate in solutions of varying amino acid concentrations. It must be noted that these are probability tables that do not consider other additives that may contribute to precipitate formation. The consequences of a lack of understanding of this phenomenon have resulted in patient complications.[28] Despite the use of solubilization enhancers, a filter should always be used with parenteral nutrition solutions because while the potential for precipitation can be significantly reduced, it cannot be eliminated.

Antioxidants

Antioxidants help prevent oxidation of an active drug. The most common antioxidants are sodium and potassium salts of metabisulfite and sulfite ions.[21] However, the choice of salt depends on the pH of the system to be stabilized. Metabisulfite is used for low pH values, bisulfite for intermediate pH values, and sulfite for high pH ranges. The administration of large amounts (500 mg/L) of sodium bisulfite in peritoneal dialysis fluids causes toxicity when large volumes (10–40 L/day) are used. Allergic reactions have been noted due to this preservative. Other antioxidants include acetone metabisulfite, ascorbic acid, and cysteine hydrochloride.

Chelating Agents

Chelating agents enhance the effectiveness of antioxidants. They form complexes with trace amounts of heavy metals, thereby eliminating the catalytic activity of metals during oxidation. The most commonly used chelating agent is edetate disodium.[21]

Tonicity Agents

Some injectable preparation monographs require osmolar concentrations be included on the preparation's label. Ideally, parenteral preparations are formulated to be isotonic by use of an isotonic vehicle (eg, normal saline). In peripheral parenteral nutrition (PPN), the solution is administered through one of the smaller veins. PPN requires the overall osmolarity of the combined ingredients to be below 900 mOsm/L to maintain the integrity of the vein.

Solubilizers

Pharmacists must know the solubility characteristics of new drug substances (especially in aqueous systems) because they must possess some aqueous solubility to elicit a therapeutic response. To maintain some drugs in solution, pharmacists may have to include either a miscible cosolvent or a chemical solubilizer (see **Table 10-3**). Polyethylene glycols 300 and 400, propylene glycol, glycerin, and ethyl alcohol are frequently used. However, toxic levels of these solvents and amounts that make the preparation too viscous for parenteral use must be avoided.

Emulsifiers

Some drugs are minimally soluble in water. Emulsifiers are used to suspend tiny oil globules in water. They help create an emulsion that contains a uniform concentration of the active drug throughout the volume of the liquid. Emulsions may serve as a caloric source in parenteral nutrition. One example is soybean oil and water emulsion that is manufactured with egg yolk phospholipids 1.2% and glycerol 1.7% as emulsifiers. An example of an active drug is propofol that is dissolved in soybean oil, which is emulsified at a concentration of 10 mg/mL in water using glycerol (22.5 mg/mL) and egg lecithin (12 mg/mL) as emulsifiers. Lipids are also used to encapsulate the active pharmaceutical ingredient.

TABLE 10-3. Modalities to Improve Solubility of Parenteral Formulations

Intervention	Issues	Advantages
Lyophilization	Requires a sugar to structure crystal formation	Has stability against hydrolysis Enhances speed of dissolution of reconstituted powders
Cyclodextrin	B-cyclodextrins are associated with nephrotoxicity	α, β, and γ types contain 6, 7, and 8 glucopyranose units
Surfactants	Castor-oil-based has higher incidence of side effects	Allows lipophilic drugs to have aqueous solubility
Liposomal (emulsions)	Limits on droplet size based on USP Chapter <729> standards PFAT5	Can target droplets for immune clearance (amphotericin) Or can be designed for stealth mode and avoid immune clearance (doxorubicin)

PFAT5 = percentage of fat residing in globules larger than 5 μm.

Containers

Containers are defined as "that which holds the article and is or may be in direct contact with the article. The closure is part of the container."[29] All containers for sterile preparations must be sterile and free of particulate matter and pyrogens. These containers should not interact physically or chemically with formulations in a way that alters their required strength, identity, quality, or purity. Containers must also permit inspection of their contents.[30]

Container volumes are specified by USP standards. Each container of an injection is filled with liquid that is slightly in excess of the labeled size or volume that is to be withdrawn. USP provides a guide showing recommended excess volumes for both mobile and viscous liquids.[23]

Container Incompatibilities

Pharmacists must be cognizant of any incompatibilities between the compounded solution and the container and container closures. Examples of incompatibilities are adsorption and leeching. *Adsorption* is when a drug that is in solution adheres to the sides of the container. One example of this is insulin and its adsorptive properties with polyvinyl chloride (PVC) bags and tubing. Adsorption can lower the concentration of insulin available to the patient. *Leaching* is when a reaction occurs between the final container or container closure and the solution. This reaction causes components of the final container or container closure to break down into the drug solution.[31] An example of this is a cyclosporine injection placed in a PVC container, which causes it to leach the plasticizer Di(2-ethylhexyl)phthalate (DEHP). DEHP has been identified in patient bloodstreams. At this time, it is not known what toxicological effects, if any, it may have on a patient.[30]

Rice and Markel reviewed parenteral medications that require selected containers due to the adsorption or leaching of plasticizers from PVC plastic bags.[30] Lipophilic drugs can leach the plasticizer from the container into the patient. Avoid lipids and lipophilic drugs when using PVC containers. PVC containers also allow for evaporation of fluid over time and should not be stored outside protective overwrap for extended periods.

Single or Multidose

Sterile single-dose containers are intended for parenteral, inhalation, irrigation, otic, and ophthalmic administration. Examples include prefilled syringes, cartridges, ampuls, and vials (when labeled as single-use). Multidose containers permit withdrawal of successive portions of their contents without changing the strength, quality, or purity of the remaining portion. Sterile multidose containers are available for preserved parenterals, ophthalmics, and otics.[31]

Glass

Glass is a common material used for sterile preparation containers. USP classifies glass as Type I (borosilicate glass), Type II (soda-lime-treated glass), Type III (soda-lime glass), or Type IV (soda-lime glass unsuitable for parenteral containers [NP]). Because most pharmacists do not have the time or infrastructure to perform glass chemical interaction studies, they should only use Type I glass to minimize sterile preparation incompatibilities.[32]

Syringes

Syringes are used in plastic and glass presentations. Polypropylene syringes are not considered an approved, long-term storage container for compounded medications.[33] Although packaging some medications in a syringe enhances the ready-to-use concept to improve patient care, packaging in a syringe is only for short-term use.

There are typically two methods of filling syringes. When using plastic, it is filled from the tip. Glass syringes can be filled from the tip or, more commonly, from behind. The second method is referred to as the nesting method, in which solution is filled into the barrel from the rear of the syringe and the stoppers and plungers are inserted after.

Plastic

Plastic polymers can be used as sterile preparation containers (as vials and syringes), but they present three problems:

- Permeation of vapors and other molecules in either direction through the container

- Leaching of constituents from the plastic into the preparation
- Adsorption of drug molecules onto the plastic

Plastics must meet USP specifications for biological reactivity and physicochemicals.[23] It is difficult to inspect the contents of plastic containers because they are not clear.

Closures

Rubber closures must be rendered sterile and free of pyrogens and surface particles. To meet these specifications, they must be washed and autoclaved multiple times. Closures are made of natural, neoprene, or butyl rubber. Rubber also contains the following substances[34]:

- Sulfur as a vulcanizing agent
- Guanidines or sulfide compounds as accelerators
- Zinc oxide or stearic acid as an activator
- Carbon, kaolin, or barium sulfate as a filler
- Dibutyl phthalate or stearic acid as a plasticizer
- Aromatic amines as antioxidants

Latex closures have been implicated as a risk factor for patients with latex allergies (see Chapter 29 for more details). Removal of the stopper does not alter the latex exposure. Despite the prevalence of latex allergies, there has not been a single documented case of anaphylaxis due to exposure of a latex sensitive patient to a drug prepared from a container with a latex stopper.

The rubber sealing of a vial or the plug in a syringe is a complex material that can interact with the ingredients of a formula. Rubber closures are also subject to coring. Therefore, pharmacists should consult compendial or literature standards when selecting a rubber closure for sterile preparations.

Parenteral Preparations

Parenteral preparations are classified into six general categories according to USP Chapter <1>[23]:

- Solutions
- Sterile Powders for Solutions
- Suspensions
- Sterile Powders for Suspensions
- Liposomes
- Emulsions

Most CSPs are aqueous solutions. Other categories usually require the equipment and expertise of a licensed pharmaceutical manufacturer. In addition to using the appropriate vehicle, solvent, and container, the pharmacist must ensure that the final CSP maintains the appropriate physiologic and physical norms.

Physiologic Norms

When injectable solutions are formulated, every effort should be made to mimic the body's normal serum values for pH and tonicity and to create a pyrogen-free preparation.

pH

Normal human serum pH (ie, a logarithmic measure of the hydronium ion concentration in solution) is 7.4. Drugs that are acids, bases, or their salts must sometimes be buffered to a pH near normal (eg, 3–8) to prevent pain or tissue damage. pH is also considered a critical component in drug stability. CSPs may require buffering with acids or bases to prevent rapid degradation.[35]

Tonicity

Any chemical dissolved in water exerts a certain osmotic pressure (ie, a solute concentration related to the number of dissolved particles [unionized molecules, ions, macromolecules, and aggregates] per unit volume).[36] Blood has an osmotic pressure corresponding to 0.9% sodium chloride. Thus, its common name is normal saline. Normal saline is said to be iso-osmotic with blood and other physiologic fluids.

In the medical setting, the term isotonic is used synonymously with iso-osmotic. A solution is isotonic with a living cell if no net gain or loss of water is experienced by the cell and no other change is present when the cell contacts that solution. Very hypotonic IV preparations can cause hemolysis of red blood cells (eg, sterile water for injection on its own). Very hypertonic injections can damage tissue and cause pain on injection or crenation of red blood cells. Parenteral solutions usually exert an osmotic pressure of 150 to 900 mOsm/kg. Blood has a physiologic norm of 275 to 300 mOsm/kg.[37] The greater the volume of solution to be injected, the closer the parenteral preparation should be to isotonicity.

Pyrogenicity

Pyrogens are fever-producing endotoxins from bacterial metabolism. They are contaminants that are unacceptable in final CSPs. They are large proteins that cannot be removed by normal sterilization procedures. Pyrogens can exist for years in aqueous solution or dried form.

The following are sources of pyrogens in sterile preparations:

- Aqueous vehicles
- Equipment
- Containers and closures
- Chemicals used as solutes
- Human touch

If sterile water for injection is the vehicle, the risk of pyrogens in water is eliminated. Equipment, containers, and closures can be decontaminated by dry heat or by washing or soaking with acids or bases. Dry heat depyrogenation must be used to render glassware or containers, such as vials, free of pyrogens and viable microbes. USP Chapter <797> requires the description of the dry heat depyrogenation cycle and duration for specific load items to be included in written documentation in the compounding facility.[7] The effectiveness of the dry heat depyrogenation cycle must be verified using endotoxin challenge vials (ECVs).[17;18] Performing bacterial endotoxin tests with ECVs ensures that the cycle is capable of achieving a 3-log reduction in endotoxin.

Bulk supplies of chemicals may be specified as pyrogen free, although they usually are not. Therefore, sterile preparations made from bulk chemicals must undergo a USP-approved pyrogen test.[17] The maximum limit of endotoxin in preparations labeled for intrathecal use is set at 0.2 USP endotoxin units/kg/hr.

Physical Norms

Particulates

Parenteral solutions must be free of particulate matter (ie, mobile, undissolved solids not intended for sterile preparations). Examples include lint, cellulose and cotton fibers, glass, rubber, metals, plastics, undissolved chemicals, rust, diatoms, and dandruff. To determine levels of particulates, USP sets limits and provides required tests.[12]

A careful choice of components, containers, and closures can minimize particulate contamination. Filtration can remove particles and bacteria from sterile preparations.[38] USP Chapter <788> states that visual checks for particles are an unreliable method of evaluation because it is only capable of reliably noting particles 150 µm in diameter and larger. It is possible to visually detect smaller particles with enhanced techniques, but nothing smaller than 20 µm is visible. USP sets limits on the number of allowable particles (10 to 25µm) that can be detected using a microscope or a light obscuration device. The automated device has higher reliability.[12]

Stability

Stability of parenteral preparations must be ensured so that patients receive the intended dose. Hydrolytic and oxidative drug degradations are the most common forms of instability, but they rarely show as cloudiness, precipitates, or color changes. The rate of hydrolysis may be affected by storage temperature or pH of the solution. Oxidation is affected by temperature, pH, exposure to light, oxygen concentration of the solution, impurities (eg, heavy metals), and the concentration of the oxidizable drug. Other types of degradation (eg, racemization, polymerization, isomerization, and deamination) can also occur in solution.

The method chosen for stabilization should be indicated and validated. Because many factors affect the stability of drug molecules, pharmacists who compound parenterals from bulk substances should use a conservative BUD or have knowledge based on literature that longer stability exists. Antioxidant and chelation additive systems should be reserved for formulas that are verified in literature as stable for a given period. The choice of packaging is also important for parenteral drug stability. The American Society of Health-System Pharmacists (ASHP) published *Extended Stability for Parenteral Drugs* and *Injectable Drug Information* as guides that contain information about sterile preparation stability and compatibility.

Impurities

The FDA requires large volume parenterals used in TPN to limit the aluminum content to 25 mcg/L.[39] Aluminum may reach toxic levels with prolonged parenteral administration if kidney function is impaired. Premature neonates are particularly at risk because their kidneys are immature, and they require large amounts of calcium and phosphate solutions that contain aluminum.[40] The FDA requires small volume parenterals used to compound TPN display the maximum concentration of aluminum at expiry or state that the product contains no more than 25 mcg/L of aluminum on the containers. Renally-impaired patients who receive more than 5 mcg/kg/day of aluminum may accumulate the aluminum at levels associated with central nervous system and bone toxicity.[40] When formulating TPN, pharmacists should measure and calculate the soluble aluminum load that a patient will receive and notify the patient's physician if the FDA limit will be exceeded.[39] The physician is responsible for making a clinical decision about patient risk for aluminum exposure versus the risk of a reduced or different treatment.

Heavy metals (eg, lead and mercury) must also be minimized in sterile preparations. Heavy metals can be toxic, and they can catalyze the degradation of active ingredients and preservatives. Introduction of these impurities most likely occurs when nonsterile raw materials are used in compounding. This is why the pedigree of a chemical source must meet USP standards or have a written manufacturer certification of analysis and purity.

Concentrations of calcium salts and phosphate salts are of particular concern for formulators of TPN. If either is too high, an insoluble calcium phosphate precipitate results, which has led to patient deaths.[41] Although some pharmacists rely on a magic sum of calcium and phosphorus to prevent calcium phosphate precipitates, this practice is unsafe because many variables affect the likelihood of precipitation, such as the type of calcium salt (chloride or gluconate) or amount of proteins (as amino acids) in a parenteral nutrition solution. A widely used guide, *Trissel's Calcium and Phosphate Compatibility in Parenteral Nutrition*, is available for resolving the calcium phosphate problem.[42]

PARENTERAL FORMULA CATEGORIES

USP Chapter <797> describes additional parenteral formula categories that must be sterile. The categories that must be sterile are inhalation, bath soaks, irrigations for internal body cavities, implants, and ophthalmics. Inhalation formulations that are required to be sterile are those that will be inhaled into the pulmonary tract, such as nebulized solutions.[7]

The American Pharmacists Association (APhA) has published a collection of 168 formulas, some of which are parenteral, organized by therapeutic category, including analgesics, antiemetics, anti-infective agents, and anti-inflammatory agents.[43] The *International Journal of Pharmaceutical Compounding* (*IJPC*) maintains a website (www.ijpc.com) that lists formulas for many parenteral medications, including some products that have been discontinued by pharmaceutical manufacturers.[44] The *IJPC* website lists files for purchase that contain articles and formulations from back issues of the journal, including sterile medication compounding, stability, and compatibility studies.

Ophthalmic Formulations

Ophthalmic preparations share many of the same properties as IV preparations but present additional concerns. For example, ophthalmic formulations may use different added substances (eg, buffers, antimicrobial preservatives, tonicity-adjusting chemicals, and thickening agents). Ophthalmic preparations include solutions (eye drops or washes), suspensions, and ointments. Because pharmacists rarely compound sterile suspensions or ointments, the following discussion is limited to solutions.

Physiologic Norms

Buffers and pH

Lacrimal fluid has a pH of approximately 7.4 and limited buffering capacity. Therapeutic efficacy depends on the bioavailability of the alkaloid base. Ophthalmic solutions of weak bases (eg, alkaloids) are buffered to an acidity that is as near to a pH of 7.4 as possible while keeping the alkaloid in solution after instillation.[45] The buffer system (eg, phosphate or acetate) should maintain pH within the drug's solubility range for the duration of expiration or BUD.[35] A moderately acidic solution does not cause discomfort upon instillation unless the buffer system overcomes the buffer capacity of lacrimal fluid. Nonisotonic ophthalmic solutions below a pH of 6.6 or above a pH of 9 have been associated with irritation, reflex tears, and blinking.[46]

Tonicity

Lacrimal fluid has an osmotic pressure (ie, tonicity) similar to an aqueous 0.9% sodium chloride solution. Eye tissue can tolerate tonicities of 0.5% to 1.8% sodium chloride without much discomfort.[45] However, the tonicity of eyewashes is more important than drops because a larger volume of solution contacts the eye. The tonicity of intraocular solutions should also be as close as possible to the physiologic norm. When formulating ophthalmic solutions, pharmacists can adjust the tonicity to approximate lacrimal fluid by adding another substance, such as sodium chloride. Several methods can be used to calculate the amount of sodium chloride needed.[46]

Viscosity

Viscosity is important in ophthalmic preparations. Viscosity is sometimes increased to extend contact between the solution and eye. Water-dispersible polymers (eg, methylcellulose, hydroxyethyl cellulose, hydroxypropyl methylcellulose, and polyvinyl alcohol) are used as thickening agents. A good review of viscosity agents, including their maximum concentrations, can be found in *IJPC*.[46]

When a heat-labile drug is formulated with a cellulose derivative, all components must be sterilized separately, and then recombined aseptically. The drug in solution is sterilized by filtration, and the cellulose derivative is sterilized by autoclaving.[47] A viscosity of 25 to 50 centipoises improves contact time with the eye, whereas higher viscosity offers no contact advantage and usually leaves a residue on eyelid margins.[46]

Sterility

To ensure sterility of ophthalmic solutions, pharmacists must prepare them in a sterile environment in single-dose containers or use antimicrobial preservatives in multidose containers. The microbe that causes great concern is *Pseudomonas aeruginosa*. Unfortunately, no preservative is 100% effective against all strains of it.[47] It should be noted that preservatives are only used for topical ophthalmic medication and not for injectables because injectables must be preservative free.

The most common preservative is benzalkonium chloride (0.004%–0.02%). High concentrations of it irritate the eye. This preservative is incompatible with large anions (eg, soaps) as well as with nitrates and salicylates. Other preservatives include phenylmercuric acetate and nitrate (0.001%–0.01%) and chlorobutanol (0.5%). Because chlorobutanol is only stable between a pH of 5 and 6, it is only used with solutions within this pH range.

Physical Norms

Required physical characteristics of ophthalmic drugs include clarity, stability, and compatibility. Ophthalmic drugs are made clear or particle free by filtration. To achieve this, nonshedding filters, containers, and closures must be used. Compounded topical eye drops and compounded injectable preparations must be filtered using at least a 5 micron filter if the starting ingredient(s) include a powder.[48]

Stability depends on the chemical nature of the drug, preparation pH, preparation method (especially temperature), solution additives, and packaging. If oxidation is a problem, sodium bisulfite (up to 0.3%), ascorbic acid, or acetylcysteine can be added. Surfactants are used in low concentrations to achieve solution or suspension of active ingredients.[46]

SUMMARY

When there is lack of availability of a conventionally manufactured sterile product to fulfill a prescription or order due to shortages or other issues, pharmacists may be called upon to compound sterile preparations. In many cases, no commercial product is available for a final sterile preparation. It is imperative that compounders ensure the products intended to be administered are sterile. An overview of the components necessary to prepare a sterile compound has been provided in this chapter. It is the compounder's responsibility to ensure all components meet appropriate compendial requirements.

REFERENCES

1. U.S. Food and Drug Administration (FDA). Compounding Quality Act. 2013. **https://www.fda.gov/drugs/human-drug-compounding/text-compounding-quality-act**. Accessed April 16, 2023.
2. U.S. Food and Drug Administration (FDA). *CPG sec. 460.100 hospital pharmacies—status as drug manufacturer*. Washington, DC: U.S. Food and Drug Administration; October 1980.**https://www.fda.gov/regulatory-information/search-fda-guidance-documents/cpg-sec-460100-hospital-pharmacies-status-drug-manufacturer**. Accessed April 16, 2023.
3. U.S. Food and Drug Administration (FDA). *Hospital and Health System Compounding Under the Federal Food, Drug, and Cosmetic Act; Draft Guidance for Industry; Availability*. Washington, DC: U.S. Food and Drug Administration; April 18, 2016.
4. U.S. Food and Drug Administration (FDA), Center for Drug Evaluation and Research. *Guidance for Industry: CGMP for Phase I Investigational Drugs*. Washington, DC: U.S. Food and Drug Administration; July 2008.
5. U.S. Food and Drug Administration (FDA), Center for Drug Evaluation and Research. *Current Good Manufacturing Practice—Guidance for Human Drug Compounding Outsourcing Facilities Under Section 503B of the FD&C Act Guidance for Industry*. Washington, DC: U.S. Food and Drug Administration; January 2020.
6. USP <797> Pharmaceutical compounding—sterile preparations. In: *2020: USP Compounding Compendium.* Rockville, MD: United States Pharmacopeial Convention; May 1, 2020. **https://doi.org/10.31003/USPNF_M99925_06_017**.
7. USP <797> Pharmaceutical compounding—sterile preparations. In: *2023: USP Compounding Compendium.* Rockville, MD: United States Pharmacopeial Convention; 2023; Issue 1. **https://doi.org/10.31003/USPNF_M99925_07_018**.
8. USP <71> Sterility tests. In: *USP Compounding Compendium.* Rockville, MD: United States Pharmacopeial Convention; Official prior to 2013. **https://doi.org/10.31003/USPNF_M98810_01_01**.
9. USP <800> Hazardous drugs—handling in healthcare settings. In: *2020: USP Compounding Compendium.* Rockville, MD: United States Pharmacopeial Convention; July 1, 2020. **https://doi.org/10.31003/USPNF_M7808_07_01**.
10. Centers for Disease Control and Prevention (CDC). *NIOSH A vapor containment performance protocol for closed system transfer devices used during pharmacy compounding and administration of hazardous drugs (NIOSH docket number 288)*. Atlanta, GA: CDC; 2015:CDC-2015–CDC-0075.
11. USP <1119>Stability considerations in dispensing practice. In: *2018: USP Compounding Compendium.* Rockville, MD: United States Pharmacopeial Convention; May 1, 2018. **https://doi.org/10.31003/USPNF_M99910_03_01**.
12. USP <788> Particulate matter in injections. In: *USP Compounding Compendium.* Rockville, MD: United States Pharmacopeial Convention; May 1, 2013. **https://doi.org/10.31003/USPNF_M99586_02_01**.
13. USP <1176> Prescription balances and volumetric apparatus used in compounding. In: *2019: USP Compounding Compendium.* Rockville, MD: United States Pharmacopeial Convention; May 1, 2019. **https://doi.org/10.31003/USPNF_M99890_02_01**.
14. USP <1163> Quality assurance in pharmaceutical compounding. In: *2020: USP Compounding Compendium.* Rockville, MD: United States Pharmacopeial Convention; December 1, 2020. **https://doi.org/10.31003/USPNF_M1373_05_01**.
15. U.S. Food and Drug Administration (FDA). *Section 503A Bulks List Final Rule Questions and Answers; Small Entity Compliance Guide; Guidance for Industry*. Washington, DC: U.S. Food and Drug Administration; May 2019. **https://www.fda.gov/regulatory-information/search-fda-guidance-documents/section-503a-bulks-list-final-rule-questions-and-answers-small-entity-compliance-guide**. Accessed April 2, 2023.
16. U.S. Food and Drug Administration. *Bulk Drug Substances Used in Compounding Under Section 503B of the FD&C Act*. Washington, DC: U.S. Food and Drug Administration. **www.fda.gov/drugs/human-drug-compounding/bulk-drug-substances-used-compounding-under-section-503b-fdc-act**. Accessed April 16, 2023.
17. USP <151> Pyrogen test. In: *2017: USP Compounding Compendium.* Rockville, MD: United States Pharmacopeial Convention; May 1, 2017. **https://doi.org/10.31003/USPNF_M98900_01_01**.

18. USP <85> Bacterial endotoxins test. In: *2018: USP Compounding Compendium.* Rockville, MD: United States Pharmacopeial Convention; May 1, 2018. **https://doi.org/10.31003/USPNF_M98830_02_01**.

19. USP <1231> Water for pharmaceutical purposes. In: *2021: USP Compounding Compendium.* Rockville, MD: United States Pharmacopeial Convention; December 1, 2021. **https://doi.org/10.31003/USPNF_M99956_07_01**.

20. Allen LV Jr. Basics of sterile compounding: vehicles used in sterile compounding. *Int J Pharm Compd.* 2019;23(3):221–228. **https://pubmed.ncbi.nlm.nih.gov/31085791/**.

21. Akers MJ. Basics of sterile compounding: excipients used in injections. *Int J Pharm Compd.* 2017;21(4):301–308. **https://pubmed.ncbi.nlm.nih.gov/28719373/**.

22. Lim TY, Poole RL, Pageler NM. Propylene glycol toxicity in children. *J Pediatr Pharmacol Ther.* 2014;19(4):277–282. doi:10.5863/1551-6776-19.4.277.

23. USP <1> Injections and implanted drug products (parenterals)—product quality tests. In: *2020: USP Compounding Compendium.* Rockville, MD: United States Pharmacopeial Convention; December 1, 2020. **https://doi.org/10.31003/USPNF_M98730_03_01**.

24. USP. Globule size distribution in lipid injectable emulsions *<729>*. Rockville, MD: USP; August 1, 2019. **https://doi.org/10.31003/USPNF_M99505_02_01**.

25. Akers MJ. Considerations in selecting antimicrobial preservative agents for parenteral product development. *Pharm Technol.* 1984;8:36.

26. Ando HY, Radebaugh GW. Property-based drug design and preformulation. Troy DB, ed. In: *Remington: the science and practice of pharmacy.* 21st ed. Baltimore: Lippincott Williams & Wilkins; 2005:720–744.

27. USP <51> Antimicrobial effectiveness testing. In: *2018: USP Compounding Compendium.* Rockville, MD: United States Pharmacopeial Convention; May 1, 2018. **https://doi.org/10.31003/USPNF_M98790_03_01**.

28. Knowles JB, Cusson G, Smith M, et al. Pulmonary deposition of calcium phosphate crystals as a complication of home total parenteral nutrition. *JPEN.* 1989;13(2):209–213. doi:10.1177/01486071890 13002209.

29. U.S. Pharmacopeial Convention. General notices and requirements. In: *United States Pharmacopeia, 43rd Revision–National Formulary.* 38th ed. Rockville, MD: United States Pharmacopeial Convention; 2021.

30. Rice SP, Markel JA. A review of parenteral admixtures requiring select containers and administration sets. *Int J Pharm Compd.* 2002;6(2):120–122. **https://pubmed.ncbi.nlm.nih.gov/23982133/**.

31. Turco SJ. Characteristics. Turco SJ, ed. *Sterile dosage forms, their preparation, and clinical application.* 4th ed. Philadelphia, PA: Lea & Febiger; 1994:28–38.

32. USP <660> Containers-glass. In: *2015: USP Compounding Compendium.* Rockville, MD: United States Pharmacopeial Convention; May 1, 2015. **https://doi.org/10.31003/USPNF_M1757_01_01**.

33. Thompson CA. No syringe is approved as a standalone storage container, FDA says. *Am J Health Syst Pharm.* 2015;72(21):1831–1832. doi:10.2146/news150068.

34. Turco SJ. Large-scale preparation. Turco SJ, ed. *Sterile dosage forms, their preparation, and clinical application.* 4th ed. Philadelphia, PA: Lea & Febiger; 1994:39–56.

35. Allen LV Jr. Sterile Basics: Intravenous Admixture Preparation Considerations, Part 5: pH Considerations. *Int J Pharm Compd.* 2020;24(4):305–309. **https://pubmed.ncbi.nlm.nih.gov/32649304/**.

36. USP <785> Osmolality and osmolarity. In: *2020: USP Compounding Compendium.* Rockville, MD: United States Pharmacopeial Convention; December 1, 2020. **https://doi.org/10.31003/USPNF_M99580_03_01**.

37. Najem O, Shah MM, De Jesus O. Serum Osmolality. In: *StatPearls* [e-book]. Treasure Island, FL: StatPearls Publishing; January 2023. Available from **https://www.ncbi.nlm.nih.gov/books/NBK567764/**. Accessed April 3, 2023.

38. McKinnon BT, Avis KE. Membrane filtration of pharmaceutical solutions. *Am J Hosp Pharm.* 1993;50(9):1921–1936. **https://pubmed.ncbi.nlm.nih.gov/8135243/**.

39. U.S. Food and Drug Administration (FDA). Aluminum in large and small volume parenterals used in total parenteral nutrition: delay of effective date. *Fed Regist.* 2003;68:32979–32981.

40. Smith BS, Kothari H, Hayes BD, et al. Effect of additive selection on calculated aluminum content of parenteral nutrient solutions. *Am J Health Syst Pharm.* 2007;64(7):730–739. doi:10.2146/ajhp060163.

41. Lumpkin MM. Safety alert: hazards of precipitation associated with parenteral nutrition. *Am J Hosp Pharm.* 1994;51(11):1427–1428. doi:**https://pubmed.ncbi.nlm.nih.gov/7942876/**.

42. Trissel LA. *Trissel's calcium and phosphate compatibility in parenteral nutrition*. Bethesda, MD: American Society of Health-System Pharmacists; 2001.

43. Allen LV. *Allen's compounded formulations: complete collection*. Washington, DC: American Pharmacists Association; 2003.

44. International Journal of Pharmaceutical Compounding. International Journal of Pharmaceutical Compounding Website. **www.ijpc.com**. Accessed September 7, 2023.

45. Chowhan M, Lang JC, Missel P. Ophthalmic preparations. Allen LV, ed. In: *Remington: the science and practice of pharmacy*. 22nd ed. London, Philadelphia: Pharmaceutical Press; 2013:907–929.

46. Allen LV Jr. Basics of Sterile Compounding: Ophthalmic Preparations, Part 1: Ophthalmic Solutions. *Int J Pharm Compd*. 2016;20(5):399–404. **https://pubmed.ncbi.nlm.nih.gov/28339375/**.

47. Allen LV Jr. Preservation, sterilization, and sterility testing of ophthalmic preparations. *Int J Pharm Compd*. 1998;2(3):192–195. **https://pubmed.ncbi.nlm.nih.gov/23989541/**.

48. American Society of Hospital Pharmacists. ASHP technical assistance bulletin on pharmacy-prepared ophthalmic products. *Am J Hosp Pharm*. 1993;50:1462–3.

MICROBIOLOGICAL ISSUES IN COMPOUNDING STERILE PREPARATIONS

11

Abby Roth

INTRODUCTION

Microbiology affects every aspect of sterile compounding, such as facility design and functionality, competencies, and the sterility of a final compounded sterile preparation (CSP). Although the goal is to make a sterile preparation, it is important to understand that microorganisms are everywhere, and the environments where CSPs are prepared are not sterile even though they are well controlled. Sterility assurance comes from more than just passing a sterility test or wearing proper garb. It comes from a variety of processes and procedures that are designed to control microbial contamination, such as good aseptic technique, proper behavior, collecting meaningful viable air and surface samples, and reacting to exceeded levels.

In addition to environmental microbiological control, there are a variety of microbiological tests that are relevant to CSPs depending on organizational operations. Antimicrobial effectiveness testing, bioburden testing, sterility testing, and endotoxin testing may be necessary based on the CSPs prepared and beyond-use dates (BUDs) assigned. Although most organizations will outsource these tests to a contract microbiology laboratory, it is critical that those responsible for compounding operations understand the purpose and general procedures of these tests.

This chapter provides an overview of the microbiological aspects related to sterile compounding. These aspects affect every sterile compounding organization and, depending on operations, more detailed information may be beneficial in making operational decisions.

Maintaining a State of Control

This section addresses the microbiological aspects associated with maintaining facility control and aseptic technique. These are the foundation of every sterile compounding operation.

ASEPTIC TECHNIQUE

United States Pharmacopeia (USP) Chapter <797> defines aseptic technique as a "set of methods used to keep objects and areas free of microorganisms and thereby minimize infection risk to the patient. It is accomplished through practices that maintain the microbe count at an irreducible minimum."[1] This is the first time USP defined aseptic technique. Looking at aseptic technique as a set of specific work practices is essential because it's more than sanitizing gloves with sterile isopropyl alcohol (IPA) and wiping materials. Aseptic technique encompasses all processes and work practices that prevent the microbial contamination of CSPs. These processes and work practices must be established within the organization through standard operating procedures (SOPs), and they must be followed consistently by all compounding personnel. Consistency and a dedication to sterile practices ensures an expected reproducible outcome, a sterile CSP. See Chapter 15 for a discussion of aseptic technique in greater depth.

MICROBIOLOGICAL CONTAMINATION CONTROL

Microbiological contamination control is essential when preparing CSPs, but USP Chapter <797> does not specifically discuss this concept. Three elements make up contamination control: hand hygiene and garbing, material handling, and operator conduct in the compounding environment.[2] By controlling these aspects of the compounding process through SOPs, training, and staff vigilance, microbial contamination does not enter the compounding environment. If it does not enter the compounding environment, it cannot pose a risk to the final CSP. Cleaning and disinfecting (see Chapter 14 for details) is an essential element of sterile compounding operations because it is used

DOI 10.37573/9781585286492.011

to address mistakes in contamination control. Sterile compounding organizations should evaluate their contamination control principles and focus on improving areas that are inad equate.

Microbiological Media and Incubation

The most used forms of media are solid and liquid. Both contain water and nutrients that are necessary for microorganisms to grow in order to be visible. However, solid media (agar) also contains a solidifying agent. There are different categories of media depending on the types of organisms that are to be grown. For the purposes of meeting the requirements of USP Chapter <797>, sterile compounding organizations use a general growth medium that supports the growth of bacteria, yeast, and mold. Trypticase soy agar (TSA) is used for solid agar and trypticase soy broth (TSB), also known as soybean-casein digest medium, is used for liquid broth. Organizations may also choose to use a fungal media, such at malt extract agar (MEA) or sabouraud dextrose agar (SDA) for viable air and surface sampling.[1]

Media is best purchased ready made from a media manufacturer with an ISO accreditation, ensuring a robust quality system. The only time that media needs to be prepared by the pharmacy is as part of a media fill test where nonsterile to sterile compounding techniques are being assessed.

TSA is used for gloved fingertip, viable air, and viable surface sampling. When used for surface and gloved fingertip sampling, the TSA must contain neutralizers, such as lecithin and polysorbate 80. These agents neutralize any cleaning residues that may be on the surface or the compounder's gloves.[3] Media used for air sampling may contain neutralizers, but it is not required and provides no additional sampling benefit.

Viable air sampling media may be in the form of a plate (approximately 100 mm petri dish or approximately 55 mm contact plate) or strip depending on the type of air sampler used. Surface sampling media devices must have a raised, convex surface. They are typically contact plates, but they may also be in the form of paddles or slides. The use of swabs for surface sampling complicates sample collection and processing. If swabs are used, they must be processed in a manner to get a total microbial plate count and not just rubbed on an agar surface. Rubbing on the surface does not provide an accurate count if the result is to be compared with an established action level. In addition, the collection buffer or the plating medium must include neutralizers.

Media must be stored according to the manufacturer's instructions. Agar is typically stored between 2°C and 8°C. However, some manufacturers have agar that can be stored up to 25°C. Agar known to be stored at or below 0°C must not be used, as freezing can damage the gel structure. Agar plates should also come packaged in a sealed container that slows moisture loss of agar.[4] Loss of water content can render the media unable to support microbiological growth and lead to false negative results. Broth is typically stored between 2°C and 25°C.

TSA used for sampling should be sterile and at least double wrapped.[3] It comes from the manufacturer in two ways, aseptically filled or irradiated. Aseptically filled media is cheaper but does not guarantee the media is sterile, while media that is terminally sterilized through irradiation is sterile. If aseptically filled media is used, it should be preincubated before use so that any contamination can grow out and the contaminated plates are not used for sampling.[3] Double or triple wrapped sterile media facilitates the material transfer process and allows for the outer layer to be removed (the inner layer is sterile) as the pack of TSA is transferred into the compounding area.

TSB for sterile-to-sterile process media fills must be sterile. It can be purchased in a variety of containers and volumes. TSB for nonsterile to sterile process media fills is purchased as a nonsterile dehydrated powder. Water is added based on the manufacturer's instructions, and the media is sterilized as part of the media fill procedure.

Certificate of Analysis

USP Chapter <797> discusses the need for having a certificate of analysis for the media used in the media fill test and viable air and surface sampling. However, best practice is to have a certificate of analysis for all microbiological media used by the pharmacy.[3] This document provides assurance from the media manufacturer that the media meets certain established criteria, specifically growth promotion capabilities, appropriate pH, and evidence of sterility (if needed for the media utilized). The certificate of analysis should be readily retrievable.

General Incubation Considerations

Some sterile compounding organizations opt to outsource all incubation and analysis to a contract microbiology laboratory. Others choose to purchase and maintain their own incubators. Either is acceptable, but the pharmacy is ultimately responsible for the proper use of incubators and incubation of samples. If incubation is kept internally, incubators cannot be kept in the perimeter of the segregated compounding area (SCA) or in the cleanroom suite.[1;5] Incubators should be validated to ensure proper installation, operation, and performance, and be part of a cleaning and preventive maintenance program.[5]

USP Chapter <797> specifies that media fill tests and viable air, surface, and gloved fingertip samples must be incubated in incubators. The incubator temperature must be monitored during the incubation period either manually or by a continuous monitoring system. It is essential that these results be reviewed to ensure that samples are incubated at the appropriate temperature.[1] However, it does not mention that the incubators should be calibrated.[1] This should also be considered to ensure proper function of the incubator.

Sample Incubation

Viable air, viable surface, and gloved fingertip samples are incubated inverted using a two-stage incubation. Inverting the samples during incubation prevents potential condensation from dropping onto colonies and causing them to spread over the plate, which could result in a falsely high count or an uncountable plate.[1] Incubation at two temperatures provides the necessary time and temperatures for many of the mesophilic microorganisms typically present in the compounding environment to be recovered.[4]

TSA is incubated between 30°C and 35°C for at least 48 hours, and it is then transferred to 20°C to 25°C for at least 5 days.[1] USP Chapter <797> does not cap the length of incubation, however, leaving the samples in the incubator too long results in desiccation and media that may not support microbial growth. Best practice incubation is 30°C to 35°C for at least 48 hours or up to 4 days, and then incubation between 20°C and 25°C for 5 to 7 days. Incubation times less than three days should be expressed in hours to ensure that the samples have sufficient incubation time for growth.[4] Additionally, the range provides the organization flexibility to read the samples over a period of time and not at a specific hour or day. This is especially helpful if the organization does not operate daily.

Alternatively, two sampling devices can be collected for each sampling location and incubated concurrently in separate incubators. If this strategy is used, both sampling devices could be TSA, or the second device could contain a fungal media (MEA or SDA). One TSA sample is incubated at 30°C to 35°C for at least 48 hours and the other TSA or the fungal media sample is incubated at 20°C to 25°C for least 5 days.[1] Consideration should be given to capping the length of incubation. If both TSA and fungal media devices are used, it is recommended to incubate the TSA at both temperatures to ensure the recovery of bacteria that only grow at 20°C to 25°C.

An incubation of media fill tests also uses a two-stage incubation. TSB is incubated at 20°C to 25°C for 7 days and then at 30°C to 35°C for another 7 days. The order of incubation must be specified in facility SOPs.[1,6] This 14-day incubation period provides the time needed for slower growing organisms to grow.

Personnel Evaluation

USP Chapter <797> requires compounding personnel to demonstrate competency in hand hygiene, garbing, and aseptic manipulation. Competency testing occurs before personnel begin to prepare CSPs independently, and it is then tested every 6 months for those preparing Category 1 and 2 CSPs and quarterly for those preparing Category 3 CSPs.[1] Those that oversee compounding but do not actually compound are required to complete these competencies at least every 12 months.[1] The microbiological testing that accompanies these competencies are gloved fingertip testing, media fill testing, and surface sampling.

Gloved Fingertip Testing

There are two types of gloved fingertip testing. One accompanies the hand hygiene and garbing competency, while the other is part of aseptic manipulation competency. Gloved fingertip testing that is part of hand hygiene and garbing competency is when personnel are required to complete the entire hand hygiene and garbing process as determined by their organization, and then they have their sterile gloved fingertips tested. This testing provides evidence that personnel can properly don sterile gloves without contaminating them. It occurs initially and at designated intervals thereafter based on the CSP Category prepared. Gloved fingertip testing that occurs along with media fill testing is performed before personnel can compound independently, and then repeated at least every three or 6 months thereafter based on the CSP category compounded. This sampling provides data about the cleanliness of the compounder's gloves during aseptic manipulations. In either sampling, sterile IPA cannot be applied to the gloves immediately before sampling because it defeats the purpose of the testing. After testing, the sampled gloves are immediately discarded, and proper hand hygiene is performed.

Gloved fingertip tests are collected using sampling devices filled with TSA containing lecithin and polysorbate 80. Using one device for each hand, gloves are sampled by rolling fingers and thumbs over the surface of the device. Since USP Chapter <797> requires a rolling motion, like collecting fingerprints, there must be sufficient space on the device to collect each finger and thumb, ideally without overlapping. Using larger petri dishes (approximately 100 mm) allows for this rolling motion and the ability to make distinct marks on the plate. The benefit to this, especially with initial gloved fingertip sampling, is that it is possible to identify which finger or thumb was contaminated so the trainer can focus on how those specific fingers become contaminated while donning gloves. However, contact plates are also an acceptable option.

When collecting the sample, there must be enough pressure for microorganisms to be transferred to the agar surface but not so much pressure that the agar breaks.[3] A broken agar surface can result in collected colony forming units (CFUs) growing in a way where one colony may look like multiple colonies, which would yield an inaccurate count. If this occurs during gloved fingertip testing that is part of the hand hygiene and garbing competency, new gloves must be donned and the sampling repeated. Resampling is not possible if the agar surface is broken during the gloved fingertip testing that occurs post media fill testing, as any contamination on the gloves from the media fill test would have been transferred to the first media device.

Gloved fingertip testing that is part of hand hygiene and garbing competency occurs when gloves are donned. This could be in the anteroom, buffer room, perimeter of the SCA, or inside the restricted access barrier system (RABS), such as compounding aseptic isolators (CAIs) and compounding aseptic containment isolators (CACIs). Gloves should not be donned in the laminar airflow workstation (LAFW) or biological safety cabinet (BSC). RABS are the exception, as sterile gloves are donned over the RABS gloves.[1] If the testing occurs in the buffer room, anteroom, or SCA, the person administering the test should hold the plates vertically so they can feel the pressure applied to the plate and provide direction for adjustment. As part of the initial hand hygiene and garbing competency, staff must pass three consecutive gloved fingertip tests.

Gloved fingertip testing that is part of aseptic manipulation competency is performed in a primary engineering control (PEC) after completing the media fill test.[1] Sterile IPA can be used throughout the media fill test, but it cannot be applied to gloves immediately before the gloved fingertip samples are collected. The person administering the test opens plates that are staged in the PEC, leaves them on the work surface of the PEC, and then has the compounder roll their fingers over the surface. They can be left on the work surface because the compounder should know the proper pressure to apply to the plate by this point, as they have already done at least three replicates of gloved fingertip testing during hand hygiene and garbing competency testing. Consideration should be given to administering gloved fingertip testing randomly after compounding to ensure staff vigilance in glove sanitization and good aseptic technique.

The action level for gloved fingertip testing after garbing is greater than 0 CFUs per both hands, and the action level for gloved fingertip testing after media fill testing is greater than 3 CFU per both hands.[1] Exceeding the established action level requires additional action to be taken. This could include additional practice with a master performer, a review of the organization's garbing procedures, and any other identified training.

Table 11-1 summarizes the differences between gloved fingertip testing that occurs with hand hygiene and garbing competency and aseptic manipulation competency.

Media Fill Testing

Media fill testing is performed initially and at least every 6 months from then on for those who compound Category 1 and 2 CSPs and at least every 3 months for those who compound Category 3 CSPs. Those who oversee compounding but do not actually compound are required to complete the media fill test at least every 12 months. Consideration should be given to using the media fill test more frequently as additional verification that compounding personnel utilize appropriate aseptic technique.

A media fill test is designed to "simulate the most difficult and challenging compounding procedures encountered by the person."[1] To ensure the media fill test meets this requirement, organizations must consider developing more than one type of media fill test. For example, if an organization has some technicians who only compound hazardous drugs using a closed system drug transfer device (CSTD) and some who only compound nonhazardous drugs, different media fills must be designed for each. Other variations should be considered, such as using an automated compounding device (eg, a total parental nutrition compounder) and performing nonsterile to sterile compounding.

The media fill test may be read daily so, in the event there is a failure, retraining and retesting can be started in a timely manner. *Failure* is defined as microbial growth in one or more media fill containers.[1] Microbial growth can manifest in different ways and not just render the media uniformly turbid, such as settling to the bottom of the container or clumping. It is important look for turbidity and any other indication of growth.

Media fill test failures must be evaluated and documented, including any corrective actions that are implemented. USP Chapter <797> does not indicate that personnel who fail a media fill test must be removed from compounding. Sterile compounding organizations must evaluate the situation and determine what is best for the compounding operation. For example, removing a new technician who fails their first ongoing media fill is justified, while removing a tenured technician who never before failed a media fill-test may be an overreaction. Regardless of the decision, thorough documentation is required.

TABLE 11-1. Comparison of Gloved Fingertip Testing

	Hand Hygiene and Garbing Competency Test	Aseptic Manipulation Competency Test
Who	All personnel who compound or oversee compounding	All personnel who compound or oversee compounding
Frequency	Initially: 3 times during testing Category 1 and 2: every 6 months Category 3: every 3 months	At the end of testing Category 1 and 2: every 6 months Category 3: every 3 months
Where	Where gloves are donned	In the PEC
Action Levels	> 0 CFU per both hands	> 3 CFU per both hands

CFU = colony forming unit; PEC = primary engineering control.

Source: Adapted with permission of the United States Pharmacopeial Convention. General chapter <797> pharmaceutical compounding—sterile preparations. In: *2023: USP Compounding Compendium.* Rockville, MD: The United States Pharmacopeial Convention; 2023. https://doi.org/10.31003/USPNF_M99925_07_01

Surface Sampling

USP Chapter <797> requires a surface sample be collected as part of aseptic competency testing. A surface sample is collected on the work surface in the direct compounding area (DCA) immediately after the media fill test is complete and before the area is cleaned.[1] Surface sampling post media fill testing is performed initially and at least every 6 months thereafter for those who compound Category 1 and 2 CSPs and at least every 3 months for those who compound Category 3 CSPs.[1]

Viable Air and Surface Monitoring

Viable air and surface monitoring is used to identify microbial contamination (eg, bacteria, yeast, and mold) in the compounding environment. This monitoring is more than checking a box to be compliant with USP Chapter <797>. A robust monitoring program is the key to understanding the microbiological bioburden present in PECs, cleanroom suites, and segregated compounding areas. Viable air and surface monitoring should be a tool for process improvement. By detecting microbiological contamination through sampling, remediation efforts can be implemented to mitigate the contamination from recurring.

Contamination is present in the compounding environment. Even with the best contamination control program, the presence of compounding personnel will result in microbial contamination at some level.[4] This concept is crucial in understanding the purpose of viable air and surface monitoring. The goal is not zero contamination, as this is not possible and unrealistic.[4] The goal is to identify when an established state of microbial control is lost and react with the intention of remediating the issue and improving processes.

There are limitations to viable sampling. Viable air and surface sampling "cannot and need not identify and quantify all microbial contaminates" in the compounding environment.[4] Sampling is also semiquantitative, as the entire surface area and the total volume of air in the compounding environment cannot be sampled, meaning that it cannot provide quantitative data to support the sterility assurance of the final CSP.[4] For example, a sampling session could result in no recovery of any microorganisms. This does not mean that microorganisms are not present in the environment, just that they were not recovered during that sampling session. Sampling is a snapshot in time. It is only capable of collecting the microorganisms present in the air or on the surface when the sample was collected, and only those supported by the media used to sample and the incubation temperatures used will grow. These limitations further support the idea that viable air and surface sampling should be used as a tool to understand the compounding environment and not as a release test for CSPs.

Monitoring Program

USP Chapter <797> indicates that "sterile compounding facilities must develop and implement written procedures for microbiological air and surface monitoring."[1] This is a significant change from the 2008 version of <797>. Previously, only a sampling plan was required, which only had to include the "sample location, method of collection, frequency of sampling, volume of air sampled, and time of day as related to activity in the compounding area and action levels."[7] The 2008 version of USP Chapter <797> indicated that viable sampling occurs as part of the certification and recertification of facilities, but it only required a simplistic version of viable air and surface monitoring.[7] This basic form of a viable air and surface monitoring program resulted in certification professionals assuming the responsibility of developing the organization's sampling plan. The responsibility now returns to the sterile compounding organization.

The monitoring program encompasses all aspects of viable air and surface sampling. The program may require multiple SOPs that cover the development and review of the sampling plan, which is the map with the sampling locations; methods of collection, including the use of sampling equipment and devices; requirements of the sampling session, such as volume of air sampled and the activity occurring in the area; review and trending of data; and investigation and remediation of exceeded action levels. The sterile compounding organization must take responsibility for all these aspects.

In developing the program, the sterile compounding organization must decide who will perform its sampling. If monitoring is performed by compounding personnel, those performing the monitoring must be trained and be able to demonstrate competency every 12 months.[1] Contracted vendors, such as certification providers or a company that specializes in viable air and surface monitoring, can also perform the sampling. However, they are expected to follow the sterile compounding organizations SOPs, including the sampling plan.

Developing the Sampling Plan

When developing a sampling plan, the sample locations should be based on contamination risk to the final CSP.[1] A risk assessment is a valuable tool in determining viable sample site locations. Since the sample locations should be based on risk, the number of locations sampled increases in areas where there is greater potential for contamination to the CSP and where there is significantly more activity. For example, there may be more locations in the buffer room than in the anteroom of a cleanroom suite. To choose locations, observe the workflow of the facility and perform a risk assessment. Although the risk assessment and sampling plan is the responsibility of the sterile compounding organization, collaborating with vendors or those who perform the sampling may be beneficial in determining suitable sampling locations.

USP Chapter <797> does specify some sampling location requirements. Viable air and surface samples are required in all ISO classified areas, including PECs. Surface samples must be collected in the interior of PECs and pass-throughs connecting to classified areas. Additional surface samples should be collected on the following locations:

- Any equipment located within the PEC
- Staging or work areas near the PEC, such as a cart
- Frequently touched surfaces

The identification of frequently touched surfaces could be very subjective. These locations should be identified through the risk assessment and be documented so the rationale used to identify these locations can be shared.

The viable air sample in the PEC must be collected in the DCA. Sampling to the left and right of the DCA does not provide valuable data. If the PEC is a RABS, a viable air sample must also be collected in the transfer chamber if it is ISO classified.[3] The viable surface sample collected in the PEC must be in the DCA. The additional surface samples collected on the equipment in the PEC should be on high touch areas, like touchscreens.

When choosing the locations throughout the cleanroom suite, focus must be on areas that pose the greatest risk of contamination to CSPs. Possible locations for viable air samples in the cleanroom suite include the following:

- In front of the PEC where the operator is working
- Material staging tables or carts

- High traffic routes
- Near refrigerators
- Approximately three feet in front of pass-throughs
- Areas of stagnant air, as identified by the certifier

Possible locations for viable surface samples in the cleanroom suite include the following:

- Staging locations for items placed into the PEC
- Frequently touched surfaces, such as touchscreens, tables, and phones
- Any areas used during the compounding process that may pose a contamination risk

USP Chapter <797> no longer requires viable air sampling in the SCA.[1] However, consideration should be given to include viable air and surface sampling as part of the sampling plan in the SCA. These samples can be used to identify potential contamination that may affect the PEC and to aid in investigating exceeded action levels within the PEC. Since the SCA is unclassified, there are no action levels for these samples. They are for information only. Viable air samples should be conducted at the face of the PEC where the operator is located. Surface sample should done on a staging cart or table for items that are transferred into the PEC.

Sampling Conditions

Viable air and surface sampling must occur during dynamic operating conditions.[1] Sampling during activity provides data to show that the facility and compounding processes are adequate and appropriate to maintain a microbial state of control. Therefore, routine monitoring performed to meet USP Chapter <797> requirements must occur while compounding personnel are present in the compounding area and compounding or simulated compounding is occurring in the PEC. However, there are times when sampling under static conditions is valuable. Collecting static samples can provide insight into the functionality of the engineering controls and the robustness of the cleaning program, especially if there have been exceeded action levels. Sampling under static conditions eliminates variables and helps to narrow the potential root cause of microbial excursions.

Frequency

Viable air sampling must be performed at least every 6 months, and viable surface sampling must be performed at least monthly for locations that compound Category 1 and 2 CSPs. Those who compound Category 3 CSPs, regardless of the frequency, must collect samples more often. Viable air samples are collected at least monthly. Surface samples are collected at least weekly, in the PEC at the end of each batch, and before cleaning.[1] Increased frequency in viable surface sampling is beneficial in identifying microbial trends and improving compounding processes to mitigate contamination. Consideration should be given to more frequent viable air sampling, as this gives a complete picture of the microbial recovery in the controlled environments.

USP Chapter <797> specifies that viable air and surface sampling must be performed when new facilities and equipment are implemented and after the servicing of facilities or equipment.[1] The purpose of this monitoring is to ensure the facility is properly functioning and cleaning was adequate. This sampling is done during dynamic operating conditions. Performing static sampling first can provide evidence that the new build or servicing and cleaning was done appropriately, and then sampling under dynamic conditions proves that the engineering controls and compounding processes are appropriate to maintain the expected microbial state of control. Sampling is also to be performed in response to problems, negative trends, or changes that could impact the compounding environment where the data are used as a tool to better understand the compounding environment and how it may be affecting the CSP.[1]

Viable Air Monitoring

An impaction air sampler is used to collect viable air samples.[1] The type of air sampler dictates the form of the media device (eg, strip, petri dish, or contact plate). Air samplers are used and maintained according to the manufacturer's instructions. The sample volume for each viable air sample is 1000 L of air, which is equivalent to one cubic meter of air. The time it takes to sample is dependent on the type of air sampler and number of liters per minute it can collect. USP Chapter <1116> provides information for selecting viable air samplers.[4]

Surface Monitoring

The media device chosen (eg, contact plate, paddle, or slide) must be rolled over the surface. After sampling, the surface is cleaned and disinfected to remove any media residue left on the surface.

Reporting Results of Viable Air and Surface Sampling

All recovered colony forming units on the sample are counted and recorded regardless of whether two samples were collected at a single location. Viable air sample results are reported as colony forming units per cubic meter of air (CFU/m^3).[1] Surface sample results are reported as colony forming units per sampling device (eg, CFU/plate, CFU/swab, CFU/paddle).

Table 11-2 defines the USP Chapter <797> action levels for both air and surface sampling. Since USP Chapter <797> requires review of SOPs annually, part of this annual review should include an evaluation of action levels, and any changes should be based on trends.[1] The levels may be different than those provided by USP but may not be less stringent.[3]

When the number of CFUs recovered on a sample exceeds the action level, an attempt must be made to identify the recovered microorganisms to the genus level with the assistance of a microbiologist.[1] A genus level identification means the genus name of the microorganism is provided, such as *Staphylococcus* or *Micrococcus*. A Gram stain result or colony description, such as gram-positive cocci or nonsporulating hyphae, is not acceptable unless the laboratory attempted to identify the colony and was unsuccessful.

TABLE 11-2. USP Chapter <797> Viable Air and Surface Action Levels

ISO Classification	Viable Air (CFU/m^3)	Viable Surface (CFU/media device)
ISO Class 5	>1	>3
ISO Class 7	>10	>5
ISO Class 8	>100	>50

ISO = International Organization for Standardization; USP = *United States Pharmacopeia.*

Source: Reprinted with permission of United States Pharmacopeial Convention. General chapter <797> pharmaceutical compounding—sterile preparations. In: *2023: USP Compounding Compendium.* Rockville, MD: The United States Pharmacopeial Convention; 2023. https://doi.org/10.31003/USPNF_M99925_07_01

There are instances where microorganisms are no longer viable after incubation. If this is the case, the laboratory should provide documentation regarding its inability to identify the microorganism.

Although not required, some sterile compounding organizations may decide to identify all recovered growth regardless of whether an action level was exceeded. Others may choose to only identify growth recovered in the PEC or the PEC and the buffer room. This decision should be based on the risk and consideration for the category of CSPs compounded and BUDs. However the organization chooses to handle identifications, it must be clearly documented in SOPs, and it is suggested that rationale for the decision be provided.

Investigation and Remediation of Exceeded Action Levels

Handling exceeded action levels is one of pharmacy's greatest challenges. USP Chapter <797> provides guidance on what needs to be documented, but it leaves the corrective actions to the sterile compounding organization's discretion.[1] This is a benefit, as the corrective actions can be based on specific results from the sampling session and not general chapter requirements. There is no one size fits all answer to handling exceeded levels. Each excursion is unique and must be handled appropriately for the operation, facility design, and number and types of organisms recovered.

USP Chapter <797> states that "the corrective action plan must be dependent on the CFU count and the microorganism recovered," and "the extent of the investigation should be consistent with the deviation and should include an evaluation of trends."[1] This gives the sterile compounding operation the opportunity to make a decision based on the data. For example, if an ISO Class 7 buffer room air sample has 11 CFU of human skin flora, such as *Staphylococcus epidermidis*, the investigation will be minimal compared with an ISO Class 7 buffer room air sample that recovered 11 CFU of mold.

A plan for investigation is not defined by USP. The sterile compounding organization should develop an SOP and form to capture all aspects of the investigation. This ensures consistency in all investigations. The investigation should include the following[8]:

- Microbial control provisions that have occurred since the sampling occurred (eg, cleaning or change in procedure)
- Confirmation that certification testing was performed properly
- Staff interviews and review of work practice logs
- Cleaning the area based on the identification of the microorganisms recovered
- Determining of whether or not the area needs to be removed from service
- Engineering control evaluation and repair if necessary
- Evaluation of BUDs
- Review of past data and resampling to compare with new results
- Personnel retraining
- Documentation of changes to work practices, SOPs, and forms based on the outcome of the investigation

USP also does not address reducing BUDs when an action level is exceeded. The sterile compounding organization is allowed to use their professional judgment. Ideally, this decision is made with guidance from a microbiologist or infection prevention professional. Not all exceeded action levels are the same. A first-time exceeded level in a PEC is more concerning than a first-time exceeded level in the buffer room or anteroom. Therefore, it would be logical to reduce the BUD for compounds made in the PEC until the investigation and resampling is complete. Shutting down the PEC is not always the answer or an option. Patient safety is the number one priority, but there is also the need for patient care, especially for critical access hospitals that may only have one PEC.[9] Finding the balance is key. Compounding in a PEC that only has one data point indicating a possible problem is better than compounding on the counter with no environmental controls for immediate use.

Compendial Testing

This section addresses the compendial tests that may be required depending on the CSPs prepared by a sterile compounding organization. These tests should be outsourced to a contract pharmaceutical microbiology laboratory that has knowledge and experience performing these tasks. There are two general aspects that relate to compendial testing, growth promotion of media and method suitability.

Growth Promotion of Media

Most compendial microbiology tests are growth-based tests. Culture media are the basis for compendial microbiological tests.[5] Therefore, quality control tests should be performed on all prepared media. Tests routinely performed should include pH, growth promotion, inhibition, indicative properties (as appropriate), and periodic stability checks to confirm the expiration dating. Additionally, any reagents used in testing should be verified for appropriateness and function.

Method Suitability

A prerequisite to all growth-based microbiology tests is the ability to recover viable microorganisms in the presence of potentially antimicrobial products or raw materials. Carryover of residual antimicrobial effect from the test article could inhibit growth in the recovery medium, leading to poor microbial recovery.[12] This potential residual activity must be neutralized, and it is necessary to demonstrate the adequacy of neutralization for these tests. This demonstration of neutralization in compendial microbiological tests is known as the demonstration of method suitability. Method suitability testing is also done for bacterial endotoxin testing, which verifies the ability to recover bacterial endotoxin as opposed to the recovery of viable microorganisms.

Antimicrobial Effectiveness Test

To understand antimicrobial effectiveness testing, one must be familiar with antimicrobial preservatives and their purpose. In the case of commercially manufactured, sterile, aqueous-based articles packaged in multidose containers, suitable antimicrobial preservatives are added to inhibit the growth of bacteria, yeast, and mold that may be inadvertently introduced during or after the compounding process. This introduction would be from repeatedly withdrawing individual doses.[10] USP Chapter <797> also discusses the preparation of compounded, multidose containers and how these CSPs may contain antimicrobial preservatives.

One or more antimicrobial preservatives are expected in sterile multidose containers. However, antimicrobial preservatives should not be used as a substitute for good compounding practices to reduce the viable microbial population of a nonsterile and contaminated sterile product. It should also not be used to control the presterilization bioburden of a multidose formulation during preparation. All useful antimicrobial agents are toxic substances. For maximum protection of patients, the concentration of the preservative shown to be effective in the final preparation should be below a level that may be toxic to human beings based on the recommended dosage of the medicinal product. The concentration of an added antimicrobial preservative can be kept to a minimum if the active ingredients of the formulation possess intrinsic antimicrobial activity.

Antimicrobial effectiveness, whether inherent in the preparation or produced because of the addition of an antimicrobial preservative, must be demonstrated through an antimicrobial effectiveness test (AET). This test is required for all aqueous-based injections packaged in multidose containers.[1] For the purpose of the test, *aqueous* is defined as a water activity of more than 0.6.[11] Potential for microbial proliferation in the preparation is one of the factors that must be considered when assigning a *BUD*, which is the date or time after which a compounded preparation must not be used. The BUD for compounded multidose containers after initially entering or opening (eg, needle puncturing) is 28 days if supported by the AET or as designated by the sterile compounding organization.[1]

USP Chapter <51> Antimicrobial Effectiveness Testing is intended to evaluate the performance of antimicrobial preservatives added to inhibit the growth of microorganisms that might be introduced during or after the compounding process.[10] The AET is a suspension test for microbial kill. A controlled inoculum of the challenge organisms is placed in suspension with the sample to be tested, and then the number of survivors is determined by plating at different time points (0, 7, 14, and 28 days) after neutralization of residual preservatives.

Bioburden

Presterilization bioburden is a potential risk to the patient not only because the sterilization process might not be completely effective if the initial bioburden is too high, but also due to the possible presence of residual materials, such as allergens, endotoxins, and exotoxins. It may also have an adverse impact on product quality and stability. Therefore, although bioburden may be confidently killed by destructive sterilization processes or removed by retentive processes (filtration), its proliferation before sterilization should be avoided because the level of bioburden for which the sterilization process was validated may be exceeded.

Bioburden testing should be designed for the recovery of a broad range of microorganisms that are likely to be present in the material being processed. Sterilization processes are implemented to eliminate bioburden in materials and sterile preparations, ensuring both adequate process control and end user safety. Process controls and cleaning programs provide methods for controlling bioburden and support the sampling, enumeration, and characterization of bioburden necessary to ensure that sterilization processes are effective.

Bioburden testing should focus on microorganisms that represent a greater concern in the sterilization process. Total microbial count methods should consider the properties of both the component or CSP under evaluation and the characteristics of the process that may affect recovery. Cultivation methods, diluents, and media selection must be based on experience with the compounding process and test material. The methods listed in USP Chapter <61> Microbiological Examination of Nonsterile Products—Microbial Enumeration Tests may be appropriate for bioburden evaluation, although it may require modification of the methods to meet the requirements of specific test materials.[13]

Sterility Testing

Category 1 CSPs do not require sterility testing. For Category 2 CSPs, sterility testing must be performed if the CSP is assigned a BUD that requires sterility testing. All Category 3 CSPs require sterility testing. As valuable a test as sterility testing is, it comes with limitations. The most concerning is that a passing sterility test does not ensure all CSPs in a batch are sterile. This is because all CSPs cannot be tested. Another limitation is that the sterility test only supports microorganisms able to grow under the conditions of the test. Additionally, the prescribed sample size is so restricted that it provides only a gross estimate of the batch's sterility. Because of these limitations, process and contamination control are the true safeguards of the CSP's sterility. Sterility assurance is gained by robust compounding processes and validated sterilization processes, such as terminal sterilization and sterilization by filtration.

The test for sterility is carried out under aseptic conditions. The precautions taken to avoid contamination must not affect the recovery of any microorganisms in the test. Outsourcing sterility testing to a contract laboratory ensures that the areas in which the tests are performed are monitored regularly and properly maintained.

USP Chapter <797> requires that sterility testing be performed according to USP Chapter <71> Sterility Tests or a validated alternate method, such as a rapid sterility test, that is not inferior to <71> testing.[1] As indicated, the alternate method must be validated, and this is accomplished through the guidance in USP Chapter <1223> Validation of Alterative Microbiological Methods.[14] It is important to note that the validation of an alternate method takes significant time and resources. This must be accomplished by the contract testing laboratory before the method can be used.

USP Chapter <71> Sterility Testing

USP Chapter <71> describes two separate types of tests, membrane filtration and direct inoculation.[15] The membrane filtration method is preferred, but the direct inoculation method can be used when membrane filtration is not suitable.[1] Both methods use the same number of containers and volume of CSP for testing and two different broth media to recover microorganisms that may be in the CSP. Fluid thioglycolate medium (FTM) is used to recover aerobic and anaerobic bacteria and is incubated at 30°C to 35°C. TSB is used to recover aerobic bacteria and fungi and is incubated at 20°C to 25°C. A 14-day incubation period is employed for both media.[15]

To properly perform a sterility test, USP Chapter <71> requires a number of final containers and certain volumes from those containers be tested. USP Chapter <797> indicates that USP Chapter <71> must be followed unless the number of CSPs in a single batch is less than 40 units. In the event that the batch is less than 40 units, sterility testing is done on 10% of the batch and rounded up to the next whole number.[1] This exception is beneficial for reducing drug waste and minimizing expense, but it should be carefully evaluated based on patient risk. It must also be noted that the maximum batch size for all CSPs requiring sterility testing is limited to 250 final yield units.[1]

USP Chapter <71> states that method suitability testing be performed to have a compliant test. Method suitability is critical. It ensures that microorganisms present in a CSP can be recovered using the chosen test method. This is important because carryover of antimicrobial residue from the CSP could inhibit growth in the recovery medium, leading to poor microbial recovery or false negatives. This potential residual activity must be neutralized, and it is necessary to demonstrate the adequacy of neutralization through method suitability testing.

Each specific CSP (defined by concentration of active ingredients, excipients, preservatives, and method of preparation) must be qualified by a method suitability test. This is accomplished by using different challenge microorganisms to demonstrate that the dilution and recovery scheme used is effective at neutralizing any residual antimicrobial properties of the CSP. The method suitability test also defines the methodology of a given sterility test.

Alternative Sterility Test Methods

A method not described in *USP* may be used if the validation results demonstrate that the alternative is at least as effective and reliable as membrane filtration or direct inoculation. There are a variety of rapid sterility test methods available that are considered alternative sterility test methods. The benefit of rapid testing is that test results are available in less than 14 days. However, it is the responsibility of the sterile compounding facility to verify that the rapid sterility test method has been properly validated by the lab and that method suitability is performed for each formulation sent for testing.

Bacterial Endotoxin Testing

Parenteral products need to be sterile and free from harmful levels of bacterial endotoxin (see USP Chapter <85> Bacterial Endotoxin Tests for further details).[16] Bacterial endotoxin is a component of the outer cell membrane of gram-negative bacteria. Purified endotoxin is chemically defined as a lipopolysaccharide (LPS).

Bacterial endotoxin is a concern because it is not destroyed through commonly used sterilization procedures, like steam sterilization, using an autoclave. For example, if a container from a batch is contaminated with a gram-negative microorganism and the batch sits for an extended period before autoclaving, the microorganism could exponentially replicate. Even though the steam sterilization killed the gram-negative microorganism, endotoxin is left behind, putting the patient at risk.

Bacterial endotoxin testing only applies to injectable CSPs. Category 1 injectable CSPs do not require bacterial endotoxin testing. Category 2 injectable CSPs compounded from nonsterile components and assigned a BUD that requires sterility testing and Category 3 injectable CSPs compounded from nonsterile components must be tested.[1] However, the chapter does specify that bacterial endotoxin testing should be performed on Category 2 injectable CSPs compounded from nonsterile components even if they are assigned a BUD that does not require sterility testing. This USP Chapter <797> recommendation is intended to safeguard patients.

The primary procedure used for the measurement of bacterial endotoxin is the bacterial endotoxins test.[16] There are three testing methods mentioned in USP Chapter <85> Bacterial Endotoxins, all of which rely on the reaction between the reagent, limulus amebocyte lysate (LAL), and bacterial endotoxin. The gel clot method looks for the formation of a clot, indicting the presence of bacterial endotoxin. The turbidimetric method utilizes equipment that looks for turbidity in the test sample. The chromogenic method utilizes equipment that looks for a color change if bacterial endotoxin is present. Although the turbidimetric and chromogenic methods are compendial methods, the gel clot method is the reference method in the event testing is questioned.[16]

In the absence of a bacterial endotoxins limit in an official monograph or other CSP formula source, the CSP must not exceed the endotoxins limit calculated as described in USP Chapter <85> for the appropriate route of administration. Epidurally administered CSPs should have the same endotoxin limit as intrathecally administered CSPs.[1] It is critical that personnel responsible for the release of CSPs are familiar with assessing and calculating endotoxin limits.

SUMMARY

Microorganisms continually challenge facility control and CSP sterility. USP Chapter <797> provides minimum requirements for ensuring a microbial state of control and patient safety. Sterile compounding organizations have the responsibility to evaluate their unique facilities and compounding processes to identify contamination control and microbial testing improvements.

REFERENCES

1. General chapter <797> pharmaceutical compounding—sterile preparations. In: *2023: USP Compounding Compendium.* Rockville, MD: The United States Pharmacopeial Convention; 2023. **https://doi.org/10.31003/USPNF_M99925_07_01**.
2. CriticalPoint. *CriticalPoint Pearls of Knowledge—Best Practices for Garbing in Nonhazardous Sterile Compounding Areas.* Totowa, NJ: CriticalPoint, LLC; May 2019.
3. Controlled Environment Testing Association (CETA). *Certification Application Guide Viable Environmental Monitoring for Sterile Compounding Facilities (CAG-009).* Raleigh, NC: CETA; 2020.
4. Chapter <1116> microbiological control and monitoring of aseptic processing environments. In: *USP Compounding Compendium.* Rockville, MD: The United States Pharmacopeial Convention; Prior to 2013. **https://doi.org/10.31003/USPNF_M99835_01_01**.
5. Chapter <1117> microbiological best laboratory practices. In: 2022: *USP Compounding Compendium.* Rockville, MD: The United States Pharmacopeial Convention; Aug. 1, 2022. **https://doi.org/10.31003/USPNF_M613_02_01**.
6. U.S. Food and Drug Administration. Sterile drug products produced by aseptic processing—current good manufacturing practice: guidance for industry. **www.fda.gov/downloads/Drugs/GuidanceComplianceRegulatoryInformation/Guidances/UCM070342.pdf**. Published October 2004. Accessed August 18, 2023.
7. General chapter <797> pharmaceutical compounding – sterile preparations. In: *2022: USP Compounding Compendium.* Rockville, MD: The United States Pharmacopeial Convention; November 1, 2022. **https://doi.org/10.31003/USPNF_M99925_06_01**.
8. CriticalPoint. *CriticalPoint Pearls of Knowledge – Investigation and Remediation of Environmental and Personnel Sampling Excursions.* Totowa, NJ: CriticalPoint, LLC; June 2017.
9. CriticalPoint. *CriticalPoint Pearls of Knowledge – Handling Consecutive and Repeat Viable EM Excursions.* Totowa, NJ: CriticalPoint LLC; April 2019.
10. Chapter <51> antimicrobial effectiveness testing. In: 2018: *USP Compounding Compendium.* Rockville, MD: The United States Pharmacopeial Convention; May 1, 2018. **https://doi.org/10.31003/USPNF_M98790_03_01**.
11. Chapter <1112> application of water activity determination to nonsterile pharmaceutical products. In: *USP Compounding Compendium.* Rockville, MD: The United States Pharmacopeial Convention; Prior to 2013. **https://doi.org/10.31003/USPNF_M402_01_01**.
12. Sutton S. Method suitability control studies for microbial testing: quantitative comparisons. *J. Validation Technology*. 2013;17:2.
13. Chapter <61> microbiological examination of nonsterile products—microbial enumeration tests. In: *USP Compounding Compendium.* Rockville, MD: The United States Pharmacopeial Convention; Prior to 2013. **https://doi.org/10.31003/USPNF_M98800_01_01**.
14. Chapter <1223.1> validation of alternative microbiological methods. In: *USP Compounding Compendium.* Rockville, MD: The United States Pharmacopeial Convention; August 1, 2022. **https://doi.org/10.31003/USPNF_M9153_02_01**.
15. Chapter <71> sterility tests. In: *USP Compounding Compendium.* Rockville, MD: The United States Pharmacopeial Convention; Prior to 2013. **https://doi.org/10.31003/USPNF_M98810_01_01**.
16. Chapter <85> bacterial endotoxins test <85>. In: *USP Compounding Compendium.* Rockville, MD: The United States Pharmacopeial Convention; May 1, 2018. **https://doi.org/10.31003/USPNF_M98830_02_01**.

12

STERILITY ASSURANCE OF COMPOUNDED STERILE PREPARATIONS

Angela W. Yaniv

INTRODUCTION

Sterile products are those that do not contain viable microorganisms. Sterility is an absolute concept. A compounded sterile preparation (CSP) will either be sterile or contaminated with microorganisms.

Many factors contribute to an effective sterility assurance program including[1]:

- Equipment and facilities, including initial qualification, ongoing maintenance, and monitoring programs
- Materials used, including starting ingredients, disposable supplies, and container closure systems
- Personnel training and competence
- Process design and control
- Sterilization and depyrogenation methods

These elements are discussed in detail throughout this text, but this chapter focuses primarily on sterilization and depyrogenation methods.

CSPs Prepared from Sterile Ingredients

In healthcare institutions, the majority of CSPs are prepared by manipulating already sterile ingredients within a closed transfer system, which consists of vials, bags, syringes, needles, and the like. In these compounding scenarios, sterility assurance relies on compounding in the appropriate environment and using the appropriate aseptic techniques to maintain sterility of the components and final preparation.

In traditional patient-specific manual compounding processes that use sterile starting components, contamination rates may be approximated by media fill testing, which has been reported to vary between approximately 5% and 0.005%.[2;3] It is widely accepted and must be assumed that at least 1 in 1,000 CSPs prepared from sterile components will be nonsterile, with the most common cause being touch contamination of critical sites during the compounding process. Contamination rates are affected by the compounding environment and processes and, most importantly, by operator technique and adherence to contamination prevention procedures.[4;5]

CSPs Prepared from Nonsterile Ingredients or Nonsterile Devices

Preparing CSPs from nonsterile ingredients and nonsterile devices presents additional risks in the compounding process, and it requires the product be sterilized effectively before it is administered to a patient.[6] Nonsterile-to-sterile compounding requires a greater degree of expertise and ability to achieve and maintain the sterility of the finished CSP. Compounding personnel undertaking nonsterile-to-sterile compounding must be well versed on the topics of sterility and bacterial endotoxin testing, which must be performed in accordance with USP Chapter <71> and USP Chapter <85>, respectively.[7;8]

STERILIZATION METHODS

Sterilization is a process intended to kill or remove all types of microorganisms. There are two principal sterilization methods:

- Physical (eg, filtration, saturated steam, or dry heat)
- Chemical (eg, ethylene oxide gas or chemical liquids)

Factors determining the method to be used include the chemical and physical properties of the CSP and container closure system.

Filtration is the most common sterilization method used by pharmacists and technicians during extemporaneous compounding of nonsterile-to-sterile CSPs. Regardless

DOI 10.37573/9781585286492.012

of the method, the sterilization cycle must be evaluated to ensure that it was adequate.[6]

Sterility Assurance Level

It is impossible to prove that all microorganisms are destroyed by a sterilization process because the likelihood of survival of an individual organism is never zero. The sterility assurance level (SAL) describes the probability of a single microorganism occurring on an item after a valid sterilization process.[9] In other words, the SAL is the probability that a single item remains nonsterile following a sterilization process (the probability of a nonsterile unit). SAL also describes the killing efficacy of a sterilization process with each log reduction in SAL (10^{-1}) representing a 90% reduction in the microbial population.[10]

Terminally sterilized sterile commercial pharmaceuticals typically have an SAL of 10^{-6} (ie, a probability that one in one million sterilized items will be nonsterile). Pharmacy-prepared CSPs compounded using aseptic methods with no terminal sterilization can only claim an SAL of 10^{-3} (ie, a probability that 1 in 1,000 units will be nonsterile). There are only two possible outcomes of a sterilization process, either the CSP is sterile or not sterile. The sum of the probabilities for both outcomes must equal 100%.[11]

Sterilization by Filtration

Filtration is used to remove viable and nonviable particles from a liquid. It is not considered a terminal sterilization procedure because it does not sterilize the final product. A liquid that has been sterilized by filtration must then be aseptically placed into a container closure system.[1;12]

Filters work by using several mechanisms, including sieving, adsorption, and entrapment.[12;13] A filter considered to be sterilizing must have a nominal pore size of 0.2 or 0.22 µm or smaller. Additionally, the filter must be tested and certified by the manufacturer to retain at least 10^7 microorganisms (specifically *Brevundimonas diminuta*) on each square centimeter of upstream filter surface area. This requirement must be met under conditions similar to those in which the CSP will be sterilized under normal use.[12]

Filter Selection

Filters must be evaluated and selected based on the following criteria:

- Rating for human use
- Pore size
- Compatibility with solution to be filtered
- Characteristics of the solution to be filtered (eg, volume, particulate load, bioburden)

Filter manufacturers publish certificates of quality for their products. These documents typically provide information on the intended use of the filter, the filter's specific bubble point, and prove the filter has been tested for sterility, membrane and housing integrity, microbiological retention, nonpyrogenicity, and extractables.

Pore size

Pore size determines the size of the particles retained within the membrane. For example, a filter with a nominal pore size of 0.2 µm will remove microorganisms, particulates, precipitates, and undissolved powders larger than 0.2 µm in diameter.

Compatibility

The solution to be filtered must be chemically and physically compatible with the membrane material and the filter housing. Most membrane filters are compatible with aqueous solutions, but this cannot be assumed. Consult the manufacturer's technical data sheets to ensure that the drug or solution being filtered is chemically and physically compatible with the filter membrane material and filter housing. They must be compatible at the same pressure and temperature conditions used during the compounding process.

The most common compatibility issues are sorption and leaching. With *sorption*, drugs or another component of the formulation bind to the filter, causing the effluent to be less concentrated than intended. *Leaching* occurs when the solution extracts substances used in the manufacture of the filter, which results in the filtered solution containing unintended components. Substances, such as surfactants, are added to the filter to make it hydrophilic and can leach into filtered solution. These components should not be present in the CSP. However, most membrane filters are designed to be compatible with most pharmaceutical solutions.

Physical compatibility should be considered with large molecular weight drugs, peptides, proteins, or emulsions, which may be adversely affected by filtration. The passage through a small pore size filter may cause shear stress and alter the three-dimensional structure of a drug or solution, potentially rendering them pharmacologically inactive.

Hydrophilic membranes are used to filter aqueous solutions and aqueous solutions containing water miscible solvents. Hydrophobic membranes repel water and are used for filtering solvents (eg, alcohol) and gases (eg, air).[13]

Solution Characteristics

Filtrate Volume

Replacing filters during the filtration process is undesirable because doing so presents an opportunity for inadvertent contamination to occur. Larger filtrate volumes require greater filter membrane surface area to provide a practical flow rate during filtration. In pharmacy compounding applications, the volume of solution might range from a few milliliters to a few liters. Most 25- to 33-mm disk filters used to sterilize solutions have a maximum process volume of 100 mL of solution. When a larger volume is to be filtered, a cartridge filter that has more surface area may be required.[13]

Particulate Load

When pharmaceutical solutions are compounded under controlled environmental conditions, the particulate load of the solution may be quite low. Some preparations may have a large particulate load because the drug being compounded is insoluble or impure. The filter should accommodate the volume and the particulate load without clogging the membrane so that filtration is accomplished without changing filters. When a heavy particulate load is anticipated, a 5- or 1.2-μm prefilter should be placed upstream to decrease the particulate load on the 0.2-μm filter.[12]

Filter Integrity

USP Chapter <797> states that "[f]ilter units used to sterilize CSPs shall also be subjected to manufacturers' recommended integrity test, such as the bubble point test."[6] An integrity test is critical to demonstrate that the filter remained intact during the entire filtration process, which increases the assurance that the filtrate was sterilized. The bubble point test is a simple, nondestructive check of the integrity of the filtration assembly, including the filter membrane.

After the filtration process, liquid is held in the capillary structure of the membrane by surface tension. The minimum pressure required to force the liquid out of the capillary space is a measure of the largest pore in the membrane. This is the *bubble point* of the filter, which is measured in pounds per square inch (psi). Each filter has a manufacturer-specified bubble point. To conduct a bubble point test, the filter is wetted and then challenged with air. A pressure gauge in the system measures the force applied. If air passes through the filter before the manufacturer-specified bubble point is reached, then the filter fails the integrity test.[14] If the filter fails or the test is questionable, the preparation must be resterilized. **Figure 12-1** describes a sample procedure for filter integrity testing of small disk filters.

Although filter integrity testing is required by USP Chapter <797> and is simple to perform, a recent survey of sterile compounding practices found that only 21% of pharmacies are compliant with this practice.[15] Proof of filter integrity when a filter is used to sterilize a solution is critical for sterility assurance and must not be overlooked.

Certain drug preparations may lower the bubble point of the filter, resulting in air passing through it at a lower pressure than expected. Additionally, solutions containing water-miscible alcohols may cause shrinkage of microorganisms to sizes smaller than the filter's nominal pore size.[12] As discussed previously, the chemical and physical compatibility between the solution to be filtered and the filter and housing assembly must be a consideration in filter selection.

General Filter Cautions

- Filters are single-use devices. Do not resterilize or reuse them.
- When filtering using a disc filter, use caution with syringes smaller than 10 mL. The pressure generated by these syringes can exceed the bubble point of the filter (>75 psi). A 20 mL or larger syringe should be used to minimize the pressure generated by the syringe.
- Do not use the same filter to filter solution in both directions.

Sterilization by Steam

Steam sterilization is an advanced compounding procedure. Pharmacists using steam sterilization should consult

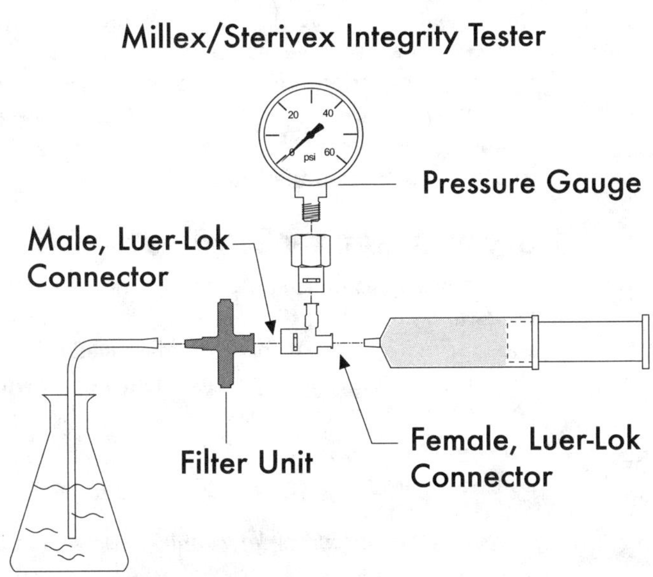

Bubble Point Procedure:

1. Wet the filter with the appropriate fluid, typically water for hydrophilic membranes or an alcohol/water mixture for hydrophobic membranes.
2. Pressurize the system to about 80% of the expected bubble point pressure which is stated in the manufacturer's literature.
3. Slowly increase the pressure until rapid continuous bubbling is observed at the outlet.
4. A bubble point value lower than the specification is an indication of one of the following:
   - fluid with different surface tension than the recommended test fluid
   - integral filter, but wrong pore size
   - high temperature
   - incompletely wetted membrane
   - nonintegral membrane or seal

FIGURE 12-1. Filter integrity testing

Source: Reprinted with permission of Millipore Corporation, Billerica, MA.

with compendial and expert references, such as USP Chapter <1211> Sterility Assurance, USP Chapter <1229.1> Steam Sterilization by Direct Contact, and the Parenteral Drug Association's *Technical Report No. 1*, which was revised in 2007.[1;16;17]

Steam or moist heat sterilization involves the use of an autoclave to expose the articles to moist heat at 121°C under a pressure of 15 psi for a length of time that has been verified to achieve sterility. For most CSPs, the duration of a sterilization cycle is between 20 and 60 minutes.[6] As with filtration, sterilization by steam should be conducted aseptically within a controlled environment by appropriately trained and garbed individuals.

Steam sterilization is a terminal sterilization process, meaning it can be used to sterilize the product and final container. It is the preferred method for sterilizing aqueous solutions and suspensions that have been verified to maintain their chemical and physical stability under the required conditions.

Three values are used to develop the sterilization cycle. The *decimal reduction time* (D-value or D) is the time in minutes at temperature (T) to reduce the microbial population of a specific solution by 90%. This is also called one log cycle. For example, if a population of 100 microorganisms in a solution is reduced by 1 D, the number of microorganisms has been decreased by 90% (ie, 1 decimal place or one log). Ten organisms will have survived the exposure. The *Z-value* (Z) is the number of degrees of temperature required to change the D-value one log unit in time (ie, by a factor of 10). For example, if D at 121°C is 2 minutes and the Z-value is 10°C, then D at 131°C is 0.2 minutes.[18] **Figure 12-2** illustrates the relationship between D and Z.

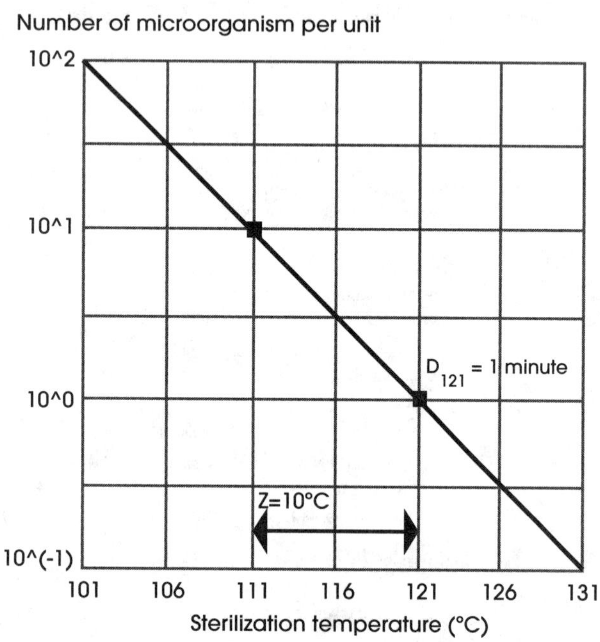

FIGURE 12-2. Relationship of temperature versus log reduction of microorganism

The third value is F_0. F_0 helps us to understand that temperature is not an important factor in sterilization by heat, but lethality is very important. When a material is heat sensitive and cannot be sterilized at 121°C, then exposure time at any temperature that will equal the thermal lethality of 1 minute of exposure at 121°C can be calculated.[19] The time of sterilization can be increased or decreased to ensure lethality at a given temperature.

Sterilization cycles should be validated to ensure that the survival of the most resistant microorganisms is no greater than 10^{-6} under specified operating conditions and parameters (eg, sterilization time and temperature, size and nature of load, and chamber loading configuration). Validation and monitoring of heat sterilization must be documented for each sterilization cycle performed. The specific conditions used, such as temperature, pressure, chamber loading configuration, and number of articles sterilized, must be documented in the compounding record. Monitoring data from each cycle must be recorded to ensure that processes are performed properly and that all critical parameters are within specified limits during the sterilization process.[6]

Steam sterilization has the advantage of rapid penetration of wrapped materials by moist heat, causing the destruction of all viruses and bacteria, including the most resistant spores. The sterilization of some materials is more readily accomplished by steam than with other sterilization processes. However, not all substances and materials are suitable for this method. For example, the interior of a dry sealed container will not be sterilized effectively by steam. A small amount of water must be within the sealed container to sterilize the interior. Oils, waxes, and powders also may not be suitable for sterilization by steam because the exposure to moist heat may adversely affect the material.

The steam autoclave must be maintained in good repair and operated correctly to perform to specifications. Sterilization failure can occur when machines are not regularly serviced. The effectiveness of steam sterilization must be verified using appropriate biological indicators containing *Geobacillus stearothermophilus* (see USP Chapter <1229.5> Biological Indicators for Sterilization) and other confirmation methods, such as temperature-sensing devices.[6;20;21]

Sterilization by Dry Heat

Dry-heat sterilization causes oxidation of cellular constituents and consequently causes cell death. This method is used for materials that might be damaged by moist heat or that are impenetrable by moist heat (eg, powders, petroleum products, and some sharp instruments).

There are two types of dry-heat sterilizers, forced air and static air.

- A *forced-air* or *mechanical convection sterilizer* is equipped with a blower that evenly circulates heated air throughout the chamber. This type of dry-heat sterilizer is discussed in USP Chapter <797>.[6]

- A *static-air sterilizer* is an oven with heating coils in the bottom of the unit. Hot air rises inside the chamber and the chamber is warmed by gravity convection. This type of dry-heat sterilizer is much slower at heating, requires a longer time to reach sterilizing temperature, and is less uniform in temperature control throughout the chamber than is the forced-air type.[22]

The slow rate of heat penetration and microbial killing seen with dry heat makes it a time-consuming method, and the high temperatures are not suitable for most materials. The most common time–temperature relationships for sterilization with dry heat are 170°C (338°F) for 60 minutes, 160°C (320°F) for 120 minutes, and 150°C (302°F) for 150 minutes.

Documentation of the dry-heat sterilization cycle must include duration, temperature, load configuration, and number of articles to be placed in the dry heat oven per cycle. The effectiveness of dry-heat sterilization is verified by temperature sensing devices and use of an appropriate biological indicator containing *Bacillus atrophaeus* spores.[20] *B. atrophaeus* spores are more resistant to dry heat than the *G. stearothermophilus* spores used as biological indicators for steam sterilization.

Sterilization by Gas

Ethylene oxide gas is effective against all types of microorganisms. Its biocidal action is considered to be alkylation of nucleic acids. It is noncorrosive and safe for most plastic and polyethylene materials. Its most common use in pharmacy compounding is for the sterilization of plastic containers, such as dropper bottles. Sterilization by gas is not applicable to liquids or to articles in impervious packaging material.

Ethylene oxide gas is a potential carcinogen and mutagen, therefore it represents a potential occupational health hazard for personnel operating gas sterilizers. Operation of gas sterilizers and aerators should be in strict conformance with manufacturer recommendations and institutional policies. Personnel exposure should be minimized by the use of appropriate ventilation for exhaust gas. A regular monitoring program for personnel should be in place. The use of chemical sterilizers is outside the scope of ordinary pharmacy compounding practice, therefore it must be performed by qualified experts.

Depyrogenation by Dry Heat

Depyrogenation is important for reducing or eliminating endotoxins. A product may be sterile but still pyrogenic because of the presence of bacterial endotoxin.

Endotoxins are lipopolysaccharides that make up part of the gram-negative bacterial cell wall. They are released upon cell lysis and become pyrogenic when released into the bloodstream. It is theorized that humans can tolerate a small amount of endotoxin without adverse events. Endotoxin amounts are expressed as endotoxin units (EU). Acceptable endotoxin limits are defined by dose = K/M, where *K* is the threshold pyrogenic dose of endotoxin per kilogram of body weight and *M* is equal to the maximum recommended bolus dose of product per kilogram of body weight. The endotoxin limit for parenteral drugs is specified in an individual monograph in units such as EU/mL or EU/mg, and so on.[8]

Endotoxins can be difficult to remove from solutions. However, they can be impacted indirectly by controlling bioburden and endotoxin content in starting materials through process controls and direct destruction.[8;23] For this reason, dry-heat depyrogenation continues to be the method of choice for the sterilization and depyrogenation of glassware.

The same devices can be used for depyrogenation and dry-heat sterilization. Depyrogenation uses a higher temperature and shorter duration than dry-heat sterilization (typically 250°C or 482°F) for 30 minutes.[24] Any depyrogenation process must be validated to yield at least a 3-log reduction of reference standard bacterial (*Escherichia coli*) endotoxin.[8;23;24] The resistance of endotoxin to heat is at least an order of magnitude greater than even the most resistant spore. Therefore, a 3-log or more reduction in endotoxin results in a very low probability of nonsterility, far lower in fact than 10^{-6} (SAL $>10^{-6}$).[10]

SUMMARY

Many elements contribute to the sterility assurance of CSPs. When compounding from all sterile ingredients, sterility must be maintained by compounding in the appropriate cleanroom environment and using proper aseptic techniques. Media fills and fingertip sampling provide some information about the ability of compounding personnel to maintain sterility during the sterile-to-sterile compounding process. Compounding with nonsterile ingredients or nonsterile equipment requires a higher level of expertise and understanding. Compounding personnel and supervisors must be familiar with sterilization methods, choose them correctly, and be able to validate that the sterilization process was successful. The CSPs must be able to withstand the sterilization method both physically and chemically. When using filtration to sterilize, the entire process should be evaluated to ensure that risks of postfiltration contamination are minimized. Filters must be tested for integrity after they are used, and results must be recorded. When filter integrity tests reveal that the filter has been compromised, the product must be refiltered. Biological indicators must be used when sterilizing by heat to help ensure that the sterilization cycle was effective.

REFERENCES

1. USP <1211 Sterility assurance. In: *2019: USP Compounding Compendium.* Rockville, MD: United States Pharmacopeial Convention; March 1, 2019. **https://doi.org/10.31003/USPNF_M99930_05_01.**

2. Trissel LA, Gentempo JA, Anderson RW, et al. Using medium-fill simulation to evaluate the microbiological contamination rate for USP medium-risk-level compounding. *Am J Health-Syst Pharm*. 2005;62:285–288.
3. Thomas M, Sanborn MD, Couldry R. IV admixture contamination rates: traditional practice site versus a class 1000 cleanroom. *Am J Health-Syst Pharm*. 2005;62:2386–2392.
4. Trissel LA, Gentempo JA, Saenz LM, et al. Effect of two work practice changes on the microbial contamination rates of pharmacy-compounded sterile preparations. *Am J Health-Syst Pharm*. 2007;64:837–841.
5. Sigward E, Fourgeaud M, Vazquez R, et al. Aseptic simulation test challenged with microorganisms for validation of pharmacy operators. *Am J Health-Syst Pharm*. 2012;69:1218–1224.
6. USP <797> Pharmaceutical compounding—sterile preparations <797>. In: *2023: USP Compounding Compendium*. Rockville, MD: United States Pharmacopeial Convention; 2023. **https://doi.org/10.31003/USPNF_M99925_07_01**.
7. USP <71> Sterility tests. In: *USP Compounding Compendium*. Rockville, MD: USP; Prior to 2013.**https://doi.org/10.31003/USPNF_M98810_01_01**.
8. USP <85> Bacterial endotoxins test. In: *2018: USP Compounding Compendium*. Rockville, MD: United States Pharmacopeial Convention; May 1, 2018. **https://doi.org/10.31003/USPNF_M98830_02_01**.
9. International Organization for Standardization (ISO). ISO 11139:2018: Sterilization of health care products—vocabulary of terms used in sterilization and related equipment and process standards. Geneva, Switzerland: ISO; 2018.
10. Agalloco J, Akers JE, Madsen R. Aseptic processing: a review of current industry practice. *Pharm Technol*. 2004; 28(10):126–150.
11. Mosley GA. Sterility assurance level (SAL): the term and its definition continues to cause confusion in the industry. *PMF Newsletter*. 2008;14(5):2–14. **http://www.microbiologyforum.org/content/file/PMFNews.14.05.0805.pdf**. Accessed April 22, 2023.
12. USP <1229.4> Sterilizing filtration of liquids. In: *2018: USP Compounding Compendium*. Rockville, MD: United States Pharmacopeial Convention; May 1, 2018. **https://doi.org/10.31003/USPNF_M7413_02_01**.
13. McKinnon B, Avis K. Membrane filtration of pharmaceutical solutions. *Am J Hosp Pharm*. 1993;50:1021–1036.
14. EMD Millipore. Integrity testing methods. **https://www.emdmillipore.com/US/en/product/Integrity-Testing-Methods,MM_NF-C537**. Accessed April 22, 2023.
15. Douglass K, Kastango E, Cantor P. What prevents excellence in sterile compounding. *Pharm Purchasing & Products*. 2017;14(10):2. **https://www.pppmag.com/article/2127**. Accessed April 22, 2023.
16. USP <1229.1> Steam sterilization by direct contact. In: *2013: USP Compounding Compendium*. Rockville, MD: United States Pharmaceutical Convention; August 1, 2013. **https://doi.org/10.31003/USPNF_M7409_02_01**.
17. Parenteral Drug Association. Validation of moist heat sterilization processes: cycle design, development, qualification and ongoing control. *PDA J Pharm Sci Technol*. 2007; 61(1 Suppl TR1):2–51.
18. Choudhary A. F0 value, D value, and Z value calculations. Pharmaguideline Website. **www.pharmaguideline.com/2011/03/d-value-z-value-and-f0-value.html**. Accessed April 8, 2023.
19. Choudhary A. Importance and determination of F0 value in sterilization. Pharmaguideline Website. **www.pharmaguideline.com/2014/01/importance-and-determination-of-f0-value.html**. Accessed April 8, 2023.
20. USP <1229.5> Biological indicators for sterilization. In: *2022: USP Compounding Compendium*. Rockville, MD: United States Pharmacopeial Convention; August 1, 2022. **https://doi.org/10.31003/USPNF_M7414_02_01**.
21. USP <1229.9> Physiochemical integrators and indicators for sterilization. In: *2016: USP Compounding Compendium*. Rockville, MD: United States Pharmacopeial Convention; August 1, 2016. **https://doi.org/10.31003/USPNF_M7418_01_01**.
22. Sehulster L, Chinn RYW. Guidelines for environmental infection control in healthcare facilities: recommendations of CDC and the Healthcare Infection Control Practices Advisory Committee (HIPAC). *MMWR*. 2003;52(RR-10):1–44.
23. USP <1228> Depyrogenation. In: *2018: USP Compounding Compendium*. Rockville, MD: United States Pharmacopeial Convention; May 1, 2018. **https://doi.org/10.31003/USPNF_M8097_03_01**.
24. USP <1228.1> Dry heat depyrogenation. In: *2016: USP Compounding Compendium*. Rockville, MD: United States Pharmacopeial Convention; Aug 1, 2016. **https://doi.org/10.31003/USPNF_M8098_01_01**.

13

PERSONNEL CLEANSING AND GARBING

Patricia A. Roberts

INTRODUCTION

Observance of aseptic technique is not the only mechanism to prevent microbial contamination during the compounding of sterile preparations. The careful cleansing of hands and arms, behavior, and donning of personal protective equipment (PPE) by compounding personnel constitute major steps in preventing microbial contamination of compounded sterile preparations (CSPs).[1] USP Chapter <797> delineates garbing and cleansing standards for personnel preparing CSPs (see **Table 13-1** for a summary of the standards). These concepts and additional data will be reviewed further in this chapter. This chapter does not review the use of PPE or garb for handling hazardous drugs (see Chapter 27) or personnel assessment for garbing and aseptic technique (see Chapter 5).

PERSONNEL PREPARATION

Proper personnel preparation prior to compounding is necessary to reduce microbial burden of the compounding environment. The human body can shed squamous cells at a rate of 106 or more per hour, and those particles are laden with microorganisms.[1]

A particle generation study by Whyte demonstrated that 55 humans wearing street or indoor clothing while marching in place dispersed an average of 2,130,000 particles per minute (≥ 0.5 μm) with an average of 2,400 microbe containing particles per minute.[2] When compared with the International Organization for Standardization (ISO) classification of particulate matter in room air (see **Table 13-2**), which is necessary in sterile compounding environments, it is clear that human activity can result in excessive particle generation. In the same study by Whyte, when the 55 participants donned cleanroom garments (polyester coveralls, hoods, disposable gloves, mask, and cleanroom boots), the average number of particles greater than or equal to 0.5 μm dispersed per minute was reduced to 1,020,000 with an average of 177 microbe containing particles per minute.[2] This justifies the importance of appropriate garbing and cleansing to reduce the potential for particle generation and microbial contamination.

Health Status

Particles can be shed at higher rates when individuals are experiencing rashes, sunburn, recent tattoos, weeping sores, conjunctivitis, or active respiratory infections. This increased rate of shedding poses an increased risk of microbial contamination to critical sites of CSPs. Therefore, compounding personnel with these conditions must report the condition to a designated person for evaluation of risk in contaminating a CSP.[1] The designated person should consider the location and size of the skin condition and the symptomatology of the respiratory infection when determining whether the individual will be excluded from working in compounding areas until their conditions are remedied.

Street Clothes and Accessories

Before entering the buffer area or segregated compounding area, compounding personnel must remove personal outer garments (eg, bandanas, coats, hats, jackets, scarves, sweaters, vests); all cosmetics; and all hand, wrist, and other exposed jewelry or piercings (eg, earrings, lip, or eyebrow piercings) that can interfere with the effectiveness of PPE or otherwise increase risk of contamination of the CSP (eg, fit of gloves and cuffs of sleeves).[1] Rings have been found to decrease the efficacy of hand hygiene by increasing the bioload on healthcare workers' hands after hygiene compared with healthcare workers not wearing rings.[3] The wearing of artificial nails, extenders, and polish is prohibited while working in sterile compounding environments.[1] The subungual area of the hands of healthcare workers harbors high concentration of microbes. However, healthcare workers who wear artificial nails have been shown to harbor more gram-negative rods on their fingertips than individuals with natural nails.[4]

Note: The author acknowledges Richard B. Osteen who authored this chapter in the previous edition.

DOI 10.37573/9781585286492.013

TABLE 13-1. Summary of USP Chapter <797> Garbing Standards

Garbing Standard	Category 1 and 2 CSP	Immediate-use CSP	Allergenic Extracts
No skin or respiratory conditions	Yes	No	No
No outer garments	Yes	No	No
No cosmetics or nail products	Yes	No	No
No hand, wrist, or exposed jewelry	Yes	No	No
No ear buds or headphones	Yes	No	No
Low-lint, disposable shoe covers	Yes	No	No
Low-lint, disposable covers for head and facial hair (if applicable)	Yes	No	Yes
Face mask	Yes	No	Yes
Hand cleansing with soap and water	Yes	No	Yes
Low-lint garment	Yes	No	Yes
Alcohol-based hand rub	Yes	No	No
Sterile, powder-free gloves	Yes	No	Yes
Regular application of sterile 70% IPA to gloves throughout compounding	Yes	No	Yes

CSP = compounded sterile preparation; IPA = isopropyl alcohol; USP = *United States Pharmacopeia.*

Source: Reprinted with permission of USP <797> Pharmaceutical compounding – sterile preparations. In: *USP Compounding Compendium.* Rockville, MD: The United States Pharmacopeial Convention; November 1, 2022. DOI: https://doi.org/10.31003/USPNF_M99925_06_01

Natural nails must be kept neat and trimmed. However, USP Chapter <797> does not specify a maximum length of nail to avoid being too prescriptive. Instead, the chapter suggests that facilities adopt other related guidance.[1;5;6] The Centers for Disease Control and Prevention (CDC) recommends keeping nails at a length of less than 1/4 inch.[5]

Garbing and Hand Hygiene Prior to Compounding

Personnel must don the following PPE in an order that reduces the risk of contamination.[1] The order of donning is not specified by USP Chapter <797> because the order of garbing and hand washing depends on the facility's sink placement.[6] However, the general order of garbing can be described as follows:

1. Don shoe covers, head cover, face mask and facial hair cover (if appropriate).
2. Perform hand washing.
    a. Remove debris from underneath fingernails by using a nail cleaner under running warm water.
    b. Wash hands and forearms to the elbows with soap and water for at least 30 seconds. When washing hands, wet hands first with water, then apply an amount of product recommended by the manufacturer to hands. Rub hands together vigorously for at least 15 seconds, covering all surfaces of hands and fingers. Hands should be rinsed with water. If faucet is not automatic, a lint-free towel should be used to turn off the faucet.[5]
    c. Dry hands and forearms completely with low-lint disposable towels or wipers. Hand dryers must not be used.
3. Don a low-lint garment (gown or coverall) that is enclosed at the neck and has sleeves that fit snugly around the wrists.
4. Sanitize hands with alcohol-based hand rub. Apply product to palm of one hand and rub hands together, covering all surfaces of hands and fingers, until hands

TABLE 13-2. ISO Classification of Particulate Matter in Room Air for Key Standards in CSP Environments

ISO Class	Particle Count (> 0.5 μm diameter particles)/m^3
5	3520
7	352,000
8	3,520,000

CSP = compounded sterile preparation; ISO = International Organization of Standardization.

Source: Adapted with permission of USP <797> Pharmaceutical compounding – sterile preparations. In: *USP Compounding Compendium.* Rockville, MD: The United States Pharmacopeial Convention; November 1, 2022. DOI: https://doi.org/10.31003/USPNF_M99925_06_01

are dry. Follow the manufacturer's recommendations regarding the volume of product to use.

5. Don sterile gloves within the classified room or segregated compounding area (SCA).

When compounding personnel leave the compounding area during a work shift, the exterior garment may be removed and retained in a classified area or within the perimeter of SCA if not visibly soiled. It may only be redonned during that same work shift. Shoe covers, hair and facial hair covers, face masks, eye shields, and gloves must be replaced with new ones before re-entering the compounding area, and proper hand hygiene must be performed.[1]

Garbing for Restricted-access Barrier Systems

When restricted-access barrier systems (RABS), such as a compounding aseptic isolator (CAI) or compounding aseptic containment isolator (CACI), are the source of the ISO Class 5 environment, the garbing and gloving requirements for compounding personnel should be as described above with the exception of step five. If using a RABS, disposable gloves (eg, cotton, nonsterile, sterile) should be worn inside the gauntlet gloves and sterile gloves must be worn over gauntlet gloves.[1]

Garbing for Weighing and Measuring of Nonsterile Components for Category 2 Compounded Sterile Preparations

Compounding activities preceding terminal sterilization, such as weighing and mixing of nonsterile ingredients, require compounding personnel to be garbed and gloved the same as when performing sterile compounding in an ISO Class 5 environment.[1]

Garbing for Compounding Category 3 Compounded Sterile Preparations

When Category 3 CSPs are compounded in a cleanroom suite, all compounding personnel entering the cleanroom suite are required to follow additional garbing requirements continuously.[1] The following parameters must be met at all times:

- No skin may be exposed in the buffer room (including face and neck).
- All garb is required to be low-lint and sterile.
- Disposable garbing items cannot be reused.

HAND CLEANSING PEARLS

There are additional factors noted by USP and the CDC related to hand cleansing that must be considered within compounding environments to reduce risk of contamination. These points are outlined as follows:

- A closed system of soap is required for hand hygiene within compounding areas.[1] The CDC also does not recommend adding soap to a partially empty soap container.[5]
- Hot water should be avoided in hand washing due to the increased risk of dermatitis with repeated exposure.[5]
- Use of brushes for hand hygiene is no longer allowed per USP due to the risk of inadvertent irritation or additional shedding.[1;6]
- Use of air hand dryers, including jet air dryers, is not permitted by USP for hand drying due to risk of creating air turbulence and circulating contamination into the compounding area.[6] Low-lint towels or wipers are explicitly identified for hand drying.[1]

ANTIMICROBIAL CLEANSING PRODUCTS

Plain soaps have minimal, if any, antimicrobial activity. Although USP Chapter <797> does not specify a soap with antimicrobial activity be utilized for hand hygiene prior to compounding, the CDC recommends utilizing an antimicrobial soap in all clinical situations, including before donning sterile gloves to insert a central intravascular catheter.[1;5] In 2017, the U.S. Food and Drug Administration issued a final rule determining 24 active ingredients in over-the-counter healthcare antiseptics that are not considered safe or effective due to insufficient data, so they removed them from the market. This rule also resulted in deferral of 6 active ingredients to allow for completion and analysis of ongoing safety and efficacy studies.[7] When an antimicrobial hand washing product is chosen to prepare hands for sterile compounding, efficacy, cost, comfort, dermatitis potential, and the concentration of the active ingredient are important considerations.[5] The infection control committee of a healthcare institution usually specifies the hand cleansing antiseptic agent for use throughout a healthcare institution that can be used for compounding purposes. When selecting cleansers or hand rubs for use, the CDC also suggests consulting the manufacturer of the agent to determine any known interactions with the product, the gloves being used, and other skin care products, such as ingredients in hand lotions or creams.[5]

ALCOHOL-BASED HAND SANITIZERS

USP Chapter <797> requires an alcohol-based hand rub following hand washing and prior to donning sterile gloves. Previous versions of USP Chapter <797> outlined a need for an alcohol-based hand rub with persistent activity, however this is no longer necessary, as USP determined the CDC recommendation to use alcohol-based hand rubs is appropriate for compounding purposes.[6] Most alcohol-based hand antiseptics contain either ethanol, isopropanol, *n*-propanol, or a combination of two. Alcohol solutions containing 60% to 95% alcohol are most effective, with higher concentrations being less effective. This is attributed to alcohol's mechanism of action in denaturing proteins, which is not easily performed in the absence of water. Alcohols are rapidly germicidal when applied to the skin but have no appreciable persistent activity.[5] Alcohol based hand sanitizers are not appropriate to use for visibly dirty hands. It is important that when applying alcohol-based hand rub, individuals follow the manufacturer's guidance for the volume of product necessary to use.

GLOVES

Gloves are available in powdered, nonpowdered, sterile, and nonsterile versions made of different materials. USP Chapter <797> requires the use of sterile, powder-free gloves for use in compounding. The greatest risk of contamination is from touch, so by starting the compounding process with sterile gloves, bioburden can be minimized.[5]

Gloves can be made from latex, neoprene, nitrile, polyethylene, polyurethane, or vinyl. When gloves are used, their selection should be based on the type of compounding to be performed as well as their durability, reliability, comfort, allergenicity, and protection from bacteria or hazardous drug penetration. Although gloves made of different materials have comparable barrier properties when removed from the box, their effectiveness as barriers can be compromised by rigorous hand and finger movements. In one study, latex and nitrile gloves held up better than vinyl gloves.[8] Therefore, it is important to be careful when sanitizing with sterile 70% IPA in the buffer area. **Table 13-3** outlines some known characteristics of certain material gloves.[9;10]

Allergenicity and dermatitis potential should be considered in glove material selection. Latex has the potential to cause three types of skin reactions in individuals, which can impair health and comfort.[11] The first, *irritant contact dermatitis*, results in dry, itchy, irritated areas of skin, which can also be caused by other hand hygiene practices. The second, *allergic contact dermatitis (ACD)*, is an allergic skin reaction that results in a rash with potential for oozing blisters on affected areas of skin. The third is *immediate hypersensitivity to latex*, which can result in skin reactions or more serious reactions, such as runny nose, sneezing, or difficulty breathing. The potential for these types of reactions has led institutions away from utilizing latex gloves. In addition to latex potentially causing ACD, some individuals are found to have a reaction to an accelerant within some synthetic gloves.[12] Individuals may have needs for gloves with alternate chemical composition to ensure health and comfort.

Gloves become contaminated when they contact nonsterile surfaces during compounding activities. Contaminated gloved hands may be disinfected by wiping or rubbing sterile 70% isopropyl alcohol (IPA) to all contact surface areas of the gloves and letting the gloved hands dry thoroughly.[1] Only gloves that have been tested by the manufacturer for compatibility with the hand cleansing and alcohol disinfection agents being used should be worn while compounding. Routine application of sterile 70% IPA must occur throughout the compounding process and whenever nonsterile surfaces (eg, vials, counter tops, chairs, and carts) are touched. Gloves on hands should be routinely inspected for holes, punctures, or tears and replaced immediately if such are detected.[1] Gloves degrade over extended wearing periods. Inferior formulations of glove materials have shown up to 61% of gloves failed a 1000 ml water leak test after 20 minutes of simulated wear.[8]

GARMENTS

When garments are selected, the CSPs to be prepared, type of compounding facility, and cost must be considered. A low-lint garment with sleeves that fit snugly around the wrist is required for compounding per USP Chapter <797>. To be most efficient, garments should be appropriate for the majority of preparations compounded, with only minor exceptions (eg, double gloves for handling hazardous drugs).

TABLE 13-3. Comparison of Glove Materials for Sterile Compounding Gloves

Attribute	Latex	Nitrile	Vinyl
Allergenicity	Allergenic properties	N/A	N/A
Chemical protection	N/A	Strong chemical resistance	N/A
Dexterity	Good dexterity	N/A	N/A
Particulate production	Produces particles	N/A	Low particle production
Durability	N/A	High abrasion and puncture resistance	Low durability
Stretchability	Good stretchability	N/A	Loose fit
Tactile feel	Good tactile feel	N/A	Low touch transfer

The effectiveness of garments in preventing human-borne contamination in the environment depends on garment construction and fabric barrier properties. Garment construction refers to seam containment and closures at the neck, ankles, and wrists. Coverall garments afford the highest surface area coverage and prevention for particle disbursement from individual's street clothes. Individuals require additional space to be seated when donning coveralls. For compounding spaces outside ISO classified environments or with limited space, coat style garments may be preferred. Garment fabrics must provide a barrier for very small particles, must be nonshedding, and must dissipate electrostatic charges (ie, reduce static cling). Garments made of nonwoven fabrics are not particularly durable and are usually limited to a single use, but they provide better protection for workers from the material they are handling.[13] Tyvek by DuPont is a commonly used nonwoven garment material.

Shoe Covers

USP Chapter <797> requires low-lint disposable shoe covers be donned prior to entry into the buffer area and over the line of demarcation. Shoe covers may not be worn outside the anteroom or buffer area. Designated shoes are not an alternative to shoe covers.

Hair Covers

To prevent hair from contaminating the compounding environment, low-lint disposable covers for the head that cover the hair and ears are required. If facial hair is present, a disposable cover for facial hair is also necessary.

Masks

Masks are worn to prevent airborne particles from talking, sneezing, or coughing from spreading. A tightly fitting surgical mask provides some barrier protection against bacteria, but its protective properties are reduced when it becomes wet. Masks with metal nose bridges should be pinched to allow it to follow the contour of the nose. It is never permissible to compound sterile preparations with the mask pulled under the nose. Masks should be changed each time an individual enters the compounding area and whenever their integrity is compromised.

Garment Fit and Integrity

Cleanroom garments must fit properly to prevent billowing and the shedding of particles through openings. Garment cuffs should form a snug seal. To check this seal, a noncontaminating, pencil-sized object can be slid between the wrist and the cuff with the arm hanging straight down. A properly fitting garment will hold the object. If the collar is too large, particles will be emitted. The collar should be snug but not uncomfortable. Garments in enough sizes to fit all sterile compounding personnel must be available. There should also be garbing material on hand for cleaning and maintenance personnel and for visitors (eg, surveyors and inspectors). Sterile garb should be stored in an organized fashion in the anteroom.

SUMMARY

The prevention of contamination in the compounding process of CSPs requires more than proper aseptic technique. Personnel must ensure appropriate grooming, hand washing, and attire. The use of gloves, gowns, hair covers, masks, and shoe covers is critical in preventing microbial contamination of CSPs.

REFERENCES

1. USP <797> Pharmaceutical compounding – sterile preparations. In: *USP Compounding Compendium*. Rockville, MD: The United States Pharmacopeial Convention; November 1, 2022. DOI: **https://doi.org/10.31003/USPNF_M99925_06_01**.
2. Whyte W, Hejab M. Particle and microbial airborne dispersion from people. *Eur J Parenter Pharm Sci*. 2007;12(2):39–46.
3. Salisbury DM, Hutfilz P, Treen LM, et al. The effect of rings on microbial load of health care workers' hands. *Am J Infect Control*. 1997;25(1):24–27.
4. Pottinger J, Burns S, Manske C. Bacterial carriage by artificial versus natural nails. *Am J Infect Control*. 1989;17(6):340–344.
5. Centers for Disease Control and Prevention. Guidelines for hand hygiene in health-care settings. *MMWR Morb Mortal Wkly Rep*. 2002;51:1–45.
6. The United States Pharmacopeial Convention. USP commentary: USP 42-NF 37, second supplement. The United States Pharmacopeia. **https://www.uspnf.com/sites/default/files/usp_pdf/EN/USPNF/usp-nf-commentary/gc-797-commentary-20190628.pdf?_ga=2.232422559.1655015257.1574613191-382423034.1574613191**. Published June 28, 2019. Accessed August 18, 2023.
7. U.S. Food & Drug Administration. Q&A for health care professionals: health care antiseptics. **https://www.fda.gov/drugs/information-drug-class/qa-health-care-professionals-health-care-antiseptics**. Published December 12, 2017. Accessed August 18, 2023.
8. Rego A, Roley L. In-use barrier integrity of gloves: latex and nitrile superior to vinyl. *Am J Infect Control*. 1999;27(5):405–410.
9. Flickinger B. Manufacturers balance cost, comfort and quality to meet changing glove market. *Cleanrooms*. 2006;20:20–25.

10. Mcilvaine R, Tessien B. The importance of gloves. *Cleanrooms*; 2005:14–17.

11. U.S. Department of Health and Human Services. NIOSH alert preventing allergic reactions to natural rubber latex in the workplace. **https://www.cdc.gov/niosh/docs/97-135/default.html**. Published August 1998. Accessed August 10, 2023.

12. Cao LY, Taylor JS, Sood A, et al. Allergic contact dermatitis to synthetic rubber gloves: changing trends in patch test reactions to accelerators. *Arch Dermatol*. 2010;146(9):1001–1007.

13. Whyte W. Cleanroom Clothing. In: *Cleanroom technology: fundamentals of design, testing, and operation*. 1st ed. West Sussex, England: John Wiley & Sons Ltd; 2001:237–262.

14

CLEANING AND DISINFECTING

Erich Brechtelsbauer

INTRODUCTION

In 2011, the Centers for Disease Control and Prevention (CDC) conducted a prevalence survey of hospital acquired infections (HAIs) that generated a national estimate of 687,000 HAIs in U.S. hospitals. About 72,000 hospital patients with HAIs died during their hospitalizations.[1] The costs of HAIs is estimated to be between $28.4 and $33.8 billion dollars annually.[2] Microbial contamination of environmental surfaces can serve as reservoirs of potential pathogens. However, these surfaces generally do not transmit infections directly to staff or patients.[3] Rather, the transfer of microorganisms from environmental surfaces to patients is largely via staff hand contact with surfaces, then hand contact with patients. There are many surfaces within clean rooms that come into contact with compounded sterile products (CSPs), therefore it is imperative that these surfaces are regularly and routinely cleaned and disinfected to prevent transmitting contamination into sterile preparations. Although hand and glove hygiene is more important to minimize the impact of this transfer, an appropriate cleaning and disinfecting program for environmental surfaces is fundamental in reducing a surface's potential contribution to the incidence of HAIs.

Cleaning

Environmental surfaces can be safely decontaminated using less rigorous methods than those used on medical instruments and devices. The following factors influence the cleaning and disinfection procedures for environmental surfaces[3;4]:

- Nature of the surface to be disinfected
- Number of microorganisms present
- Innate resistance of those microorganisms to the inactivating effects of the disinfectant
- Amount of organic soil present on surfaces
- Type and concentration of disinfectant used
- Duration and temperature of disinfectant contact
- Accuracy with which indications and directions for use are followed, if using a proprietary product

Cleaning is the necessary first step in any disinfection process, which is a form of decontamination that prepares the environmental surface for disinfection by removing organic and inorganic matter, salts, and visible soil, all of which interfere with microbial disinfection. The physical action of scrubbing with detergents and surfactants followed by rinsing with water removes large numbers of microorganisms from surfaces. If the surface is not clean before disinfection is started, the success of disinfection is compromised.[3;4]

Many companies sell cleaning supplies designed for use in pharmacy buffer rooms and anterooms (eg, Pharmacy Purchasing & Products).[5;6] Ensuring that buffer rooms and anteroom furnishings are easy to clean is important. Such furnishings include garb dispensers, benches, tables, chairs, carts, shelving and racks, trash receptacles, cabinets, and countertops (Chapter 8).

UNITED STATES PHARMACOPEIA CHAPTER <797>

United States Pharmacopeia (USP) Chapter <797> Pharmaceutical Compounding—Sterile Preparations standards for cleaning and disinfecting apply to primary and secondary engineering controls, immediate use compounding areas, and segregated compounding areas. USP Chapter <797> sets the following requirements for cleaning and disinfecting[7]:

- Responsibility of compounding personnel
  - Trained personnel must write detailed procedures about what cleansers, disinfectants, sporicidal agents, and nonshedding wipe and mop materials can be used and how they are used.

Note: The author acknowledges Ryan A. Forrey who wrote this chapter in the previous edition.

DOI 10.37573/9781585286492.014

    - All personnel responsible for cleaning must be visually observed during the process of performing cleaning and disinfecting procedures during initial personnel training on cleaning procedures, during changes in cleaning staff, and at the completion of any media fill test procedure. After initial observation, compounding personnel must demonstrate competency in cleaning and disinfecting procedures through written or electronic testing every 12 months. Visual documentation must be recorded (eg, sample form for assessing cleaning and disinfection procedures).[8] See **Figure 14-1** for an example.

- Environmental quality and control
    - Carts used to bring supplies from the storeroom cannot be rolled beyond the demarcation line in the anteroom. Carts used in the buffer room cannot be rolled outward beyond the demarcation line unless cleaned and disinfected before being returned.
    - No shipping or other external transport cartons may be taken into the buffer room or segregated compounding area. All supplies in cartons must be decontaminated by removing them from shipping cartons, then wiping or spraying them with a nonresidue-generating sporicidal agent, disinfecting agent, or sterile 70% isopropyl alcohol (IPA) while they are being transferred to a clean and properly disinfected cart or other conveyance for introduction into the buffer room. The agent must be allowed to stay on for the minimum contact time specified by the manufacturer. If 70% IPA is used, it must be allowed to dry.
    - Generally, supplies required for scheduled compounding during a work shift must be wiped down with an appropriate disinfecting agent and brought into the buffer room, preferably on one or more movable carts.
    - Cleaning and disinfecting surfaces in the laminar airflow workbenches (LAFWs), biological safety cabinets (BSCs), compounding aseptic isolators (CAIs), and compounding aseptic containment isolators (CACIs) must be done frequently, including at the beginning of each work shift, before each batch preparation is started, every 30 minutes during continuous compounding periods of individual CSPs, when there are spills, and when surface contamination is known or suspected from procedural breaches.
    - Trained compounding personnel are responsible for developing, implementing, and practicing the procedures for cleaning and disinfecting the direct compounding area (DCA) as described in the standard operating procedures (SOPs).
    - Cleaning and disinfecting must occur before compounding is performed. Items must be removed from all areas to be cleaned, and surfaces must be cleaned by removing loose material and residue from spills (eg, water-soluble solid residues are removed with sterile water for injection or irrigation and low-shedding wipes). This must be followed by wiping with a residue-free disinfecting agent, such as sterile 70% isopropyl alcohol (IPA) that must dry before compounding begins.
    - Work surfaces in ISO Class 7 and 8 areas (ie, buffer rooms and anterooms, respectively) and segregated compounding areas must be cleaned at least daily.
    - Dust and debris must be removed from storage sites for compounding ingredients and supplies. A method that does not degrade the ISO Class 7 or 8 air quality must be used.
    - Floors in ISO Class 7 and 8 areas must be cleaned daily at a time when no compounding operations are in progress.
    - Sterile 70% IPA must remain on surfaces to be disinfected until it is dry before such surfaces are used in the preparation of CSPs.
    - Walls, ceilings, and emptied shelving in buffer rooms and anterooms must be cleaned and disinfected at least monthly.
    - Mopping must be performed by trained personnel using approved agents and procedures described in written SOPs.
    - The schedules of use and methods of application of cleaning and disinfecting agents must be in accordance with written SOPs and followed by janitorial and compounding personnel.
- Equipment and supplies
    - All cleaning materials (eg, wipers, sponges, and mops) must be nonshedding, preferably composed of synthetic microfibers, and dedicated to use in the buffer room, anteroom, and segregated compounding areas. They must not be removed from these areas except for disposal.
    - If cleaning materials are reused (eg, mops), procedures must be developed (based on manufacturer recommendations) that ensure that the effectiveness of the cleaning device is maintained and repeated use does not add to the bioburden of the area being cleaned. Ideally, all cleaning materials are discarded after one use by collection in suitable plastic bags and removed with minimal agitation.
    - Supplies and equipment removed from shipping cartons must be wiped with a suitable disinfecting agent (eg, sterile 70% IPA) delivered

Printed name and position/title of person assessed: ________________________________
Name of facility or location: ____

Cleaning and Disinfection Practices: The qualified evaluator will mark (✔) each space for which the person being assessed has acceptably completed the described activity, prints N/A if the activity is not applicable to the assessment session or N/O if the activity was not observed.

Daily Tasks:

_____Prepares correct concentration of disinfectant solution according to manufacturer's instructions.

_____Uses appropriately labeled container for the type of surface to be cleaned (floor, wall, production bins, etc.).

_____Documents disinfectant solution preparation.

_____Follows garbing procedures when performing any cleaning activities.

_____At the beginning of each shift, cleans all ISO Class 5 devices prior to compounding in the following order: walls, IV bar, automated compounders, and work surface.

_____Uses a lint-free wipe soaked with sterile 70% IPA or other approved disinfectant solution and allows to dry completely.

_____Removes all compounder components and cleans all ISO Class 5 areas as stated above at the end of each shift.

_____Cleans all counters and easily cleanable work surfaces.

_____Mops floors, using the mop labeled "floors," starting at the wall opposite the room entry door; mops floor surface in even strokes toward the operator. Moves carts as needed to clean entire floor surface. Use of a microfiber cleaning system is an acceptable alternative to mops.

_____In the ante-area, cleans sink and all contact surfaces; cleans floor with a disinfectant solution or uses microfiber cleaning system.

Monthly Tasks:

_____Performs monthly cleaning on a designated day. Prepares a disinfectant solution as stated in daily tasks that is appropriate for the surfaces to be cleaned.

_____Cleans buffer area and ante-area ceiling, walls, and storage shelving with a disinfectant solution and a mop or uses a microfiber cleaning system.

_____Once ISO Class 5 area is clean, cleans compounding room ceiling, followed by walls and ending with the floor. Uses appropriate labeled mops or microfiber cleaning system.

_____Cleans all buffer area totes and storage shelves by removing contents and using a germicidal detergent soaked lint free wipe, cleans the inside surfaces of the tote and then the entire exterior surfaces of the tote. Allows totes to dry. Prior to replacing contents into tote, wipes tote with sterile 70% IPA to remove disinfectant residue. Uses new wipe as needed.

_____Cleans all buffer area carts by removing contents and using germicidal detergent soaked lint free wipe, cleans all carts starting with the top shelf and top of post, working down to wheels. Cleans the underside of shelves in a similar manner. Uses a new wipe for each cart. Allows to dry. Wipes carts with sterile 70% IPA wetted lint-free wipe to remove any disinfectant residue. Uses new wipe as needed.

_____Cleans buffer area chairs, the interior and exterior of trash bins, and storage bins using disinfectant solution soaked lint free wipe. Documents all cleaning activities as to who performed such activities with date and time noted.

The person assessed is immediately informed of all unacceptable activities (i.e., spaces lacking a √, N/A, or N/O) and shown and informed of specific corrections.

Signature of Person Assessed	Printed Name	Date
Signature of Qualified Evaluator	Printed Name	Date

(Official June 1, 2008)

FIGURE 14-1. Sample form for assessing cleaning and disinfection procedures

Source: Reprinted with permission of USP <797> Pharmaceutical compounding—sterile preparations. [Revision Bulletin, Appendix V, May 1, 2020]. Rockville, MD: United States Pharmacopeial Convention; 2020. https://www.uspnf.com/sites/default/files/usp_pdf/EN/USPNF/revisions/gc-797-rb-notice-20200424.pdf. Accessed April 8, 2023.

from a spray bottle or other suitable delivery method.

- Before any compounding supplies are introduced into the primary engineering control (PEC), they must be wiped with sterile 70% IPA and allowed to dry before use. When sterile items are received in a sealed container designed to keep the item sterile until use (eg, sterile IV bag within an overwrap, syringes, needles), the item may only be removed from its covering when introduced into the PEC. There is then no need to wipe with sterile 70% IPA.
- Gauze pads wetted with sterile 70% IPA or other particle-generating material must not be used to disinfect the sterile entry points of packages and devices (eg, needle and syringe tips or vial tops).

Surfaces in LAFWs, BSCs, CAIs, and CACIs, which are close to the exposure of critical sites, require disinfecting more frequently than surfaces such as walls and ceilings. **Table 14-1** shows the minimum frequency of cleaning and disinfecting a compounding area required by USP Chapter <797> standards.[8]

USP Chapter <800>

USP Chapter <800> Hazardous Drugs—Handling in Healthcare Settings adds additional requirements for cleaning areas where hazardous drugs (HDs) are handled and compounded. USP Chapter <800> outlines four steps in the process of cleaning equipment used for sterile compounding of HDs, which are deactivation, decontamination, cleaning, and disinfecting.[9]

The first step, *deactivation*, is a process that renders the HD chemically inactive or inert. There is no product that can be used to render all HDs inactive or inert. Thus, it is important that the next step, decontamination, occurs. *Decontamination* is the process of removing the residue from deactivation and any remaining HD residue from the surfaces of the equipment. Because the decontamination process involves transferring the HD residue from the surface of the equipment to the wipes being used to clean, it is important to dispose of the wipes as HD waste. After decontamination, cleaning should be done to remove all contaminants and organic materials (eg, soil, microbial contamination, and HD residue). Cleaning must be followed by *disinfection*, which eliminates all microbial contamination that may be left on the surfaces. **Table 14-2** summarizes the steps for

TABLE 14-1. Minimum Frequency of Cleaning and Disinfecting Surfaces and Applying Sporicidal Disinfectants in Classified Areas and Within the Perimeter of the SCA

Site	Cleaning	Disinfecting	Applying Sporicidal Disinfectant
PECs and equipment inside the PECs	Daily when compounding occurs	Daily for work surface Apply 70% IPA at least every 30 min	Monthly for Category 1 and 2 CSPs Weekly for Category 3 CSPs
Removable work tray of the PEC (when applicable)	Daily when compounding occurs for work surfaces Monthly underneath work surfaces	Daily for work surface Monthly underneath work surface Apply 70% IPA at least every 30 min	Monthly
Pass-throughs	Daily when compounding occurs	Daily when compounding occurs	Monthly for Category 1 and 2 CSPs Weekly for Category 3 CSPs
Work surfaces outside the PEC	Daily when compounding occurs	Daily when compounding occurs	Monthly for Category 1 and 2 CSPs Weekly for Category 3 CSPs
Floors	Daily when compounding occurs	Daily when compounding occurs	Monthly for Category 1 and 2 CSPs Weekly for Category 3 CSPs
Walls, doors, and door frames	Monthly	Monthly	Monthly
Ceilings	Monthly	Monthly	Monthly
Storage shelving and bins	Monthly	Monthly	Monthly
Equipment outside PECs	Monthly	Monthly	Monthly

BSC = biological safety cabinet; CSP= compounded sterile preparation; IPA = isopropyl alcohol; PEC = primary engineering control; SCA = segregated compounding area.

Source: Reprinted with permission of USP <797> Pharmaceutical compounding—sterile preparations. In: *2023: USP Compounding Compendium.* Rockville, MD: United States Pharmacopeial Convention; 2023: Issue 1. https://doi.org/10.31003/USPNF_M99925_07_01.

TABLE 14-2. Cleaning Steps

Cleaning Step	Purpose	Example Agents
Deactivation	Renders compound inert or inactive	As listed in the HD labeling or other agents that may incorporate EPA-registered oxidizers (eg, peroxide formulations, sodium hypochlorite, etc.)
Decontamination	Removes HD residue	Materials that have been validated to be effective for HD decontamination or other materials proven to be effective through testing (eg, alcohol, water, peroxide, or sodium hypochlorite)
Cleaning	Removes organic and inorganic material	Germicidal detergent
Disinfection (for sterile manipulations)	Destroys microorganisms	EPA-registered disinfectant and sterile alcohol as appropriate for use

EPA = Environmental Protection Agency; HD = hazardous drug.

Source: Reprinted with permission of USP <797> Pharmaceutical compounding—sterile preparations. In: *2023: USP Compounding Compendium.* Rockville, MD: United States Pharmacopeial Convention; 2023: Issue 1. https://doi.org/10.31003/USPNF_M99925_07_01.; USP <797> Pharmaceutical compounding—sterile preparations. [Revision Bulletin, Appendix V, May 1, 2020]. Rockville, MD: United States Pharmacopeial Convention; 2020. https://www.uspnf.com/sites/default/files/usp_pdf/EN/USPNF/revisions/gc-797-rb-notice-20200424.pdf. Accessed April 8, 2023.

cleaning HD equipment and areas where HDs are used. A more detailed description of decontamination and deactivation can be found in Chapter 27.

USP Chapter <800> recommends that environmental wipe sampling for HD surface residue should occur at minimum every 6 months. This sampling assists with the identification of contamination and is an indicator of effective decontamination practices. Although, wipe sampling using liquid chromatography mass spectroscopy (LCMS) every 6 months helps identify surface contamination, it does not provide near real-time analysis of effective decontamination. Technologies exist that use lateral flow immunoassay to provide rapid diagnostic insight on surface contamination. This technology can be used more frequently to assess daily, weekly, and monthly practice standards. Surface wipe sampling areas should include interiors of the PEC, pass-through chambers, staging areas within the secondary engineering control (SEC), areas adjacent to the PEC (eg, floors under PEC, supply carts), areas immediately outside of the HD buffer room, and patient medication administration areas. There is no set standard for specific marker drugs, but common markers that can be assayed include methotrexate, doxorubicin, cyclophosphamide, fluorouracil, and platinum containing compounds. If measurable HD residue contamination is detected, it must be documented and contained and everything must be recleaned. Repeat sampling should occur to validate that deactivation and decontamination steps have been effective.[10]

DISINFECTING

Although good cleaning removes many microbes from environmental surfaces, the microbes left behind soon begin to reproduce. Therefore, sterile compounding personnel are required to disinfect at routine intervals throughout a compounding day to kill the bacteria, fungi, and viruses that are present. It is usually not possible to kill all microbes, especially spores, so the purpose of using disinfectants is to significantly reduce the numbers of microbes on surfaces of drug containers and internal surfaces of primary and secondary engineering controls.[11]

USP Chapter <797> on Disinfectants

The USP Compounding Expert Committee (CEC) adopted the use of sterile 70% IPA after considering published data and recommendations from multiple comments.[7] Sterile 70% IPA must be used to disinfect sterile gloves (intermittently), vial stoppers, ampul necks, and injection ports on containers. The CEC felt that because sterile gloves are required to minimize bioburden, the routine and intermittent use of sterile 70% IPA will help enhance the bioburden reduction effort. The CEC discussed the use of sporicidal agents but decided not to recommend them because their drying time (eg, minutes to hours), deposition of residues, chemical reactivity with some compounding materials, and toxicity to personnel were strong disadvantages. The CEC received objective scientific information that argued against the need to rotate disinfectants.[12] However, USP Chapter <1072> Disinfectants and Antiseptics says that it is prudent to augment the daily use of bactericidal disinfectants with weekly or monthly use of a sporicidal agent.[13;14]

Regulatory Framework for Disinfectants

The U.S. Food and Drug Administration (FDA) regulates liquid chemical sterilizers (also called high-level disinfectants by the CDC). Examples of high-level disinfectants are glutaraldehyde, hydrogen peroxide, and peracetic acid. High-level disinfectants are used for cold sterilization of medical equipment, like endoscopes. The Environmental Protection Agency (EPA) regulates and approves product labeling and registration numbers for environmental surface antimicrobial germicides (ie, intermediate- and low-level disinfectants). The labels and product literature for intermediate- and low-level disinfectants specify indications for product use and provide claims for their range of antimicrobial activity. The EPA requires certain preregistration laboratory potency tests for these products to support product label claims. The EPA verifies the manufacturer's claims to inactivate microorganisms through laboratory testing. More than 4,000 antimicrobial products are currently registered with the EPA and sold in the marketplace. Nearly 60% of these antimicrobial products are registered to control infectious microorganisms in hospitals and other healthcare environments.[15]

EPA labeling includes the statement: "It is a violation of federal law to use this product inconsistent with its labeling."[15] This means that janitorial and pharmacy personnel must follow safety precautions and directions for use on the labeling of each EPA-registered product. Not following the specified dilution, contact time, method of application, or any other condition of use is considered misuse of the product. General cleaning agents (eg, detergents and surfactants) do not require EPA registration. But an EPA-registered product is required for cleaning and disinfecting for applications in which germicidal activity is needed.

Disinfectants labeled as "hospital disinfectant" have passed EPA potency tests for activity against three representative microorganisms, *Pseudomonas aeruginosa, Staphylococcus aureus*, and *Salmonella cholerae suis*. Low-level disinfectants are often labeled hospital disinfectant without a tuberculocidal claim because they lack the potency to inactivate mycobacteria.[3] Because mycobacteria have the highest resistance among vegetative bacteria, viruses, and fungi, any disinfectant with a tuberculocidal claim on the label (ie, an intermediate-level disinfectant) is considered capable of inactivating a broad spectrum of pathogens. It is this broad spectrum activity, rather than the product's specific potency against mycobacteria, that is the basis for protocols indicating the appropriateness of using tuberculocidal chemicals for surface disinfection.[16] **Table 14-3** shows examples of microorganisms and their level of resistance to germicidal chemicals.

TABLE 14-3. Descending Order of Resistance to Germicidal Chemicals*

Prions
Bacterial Spores *Bacillus subtilis, Clostridium sporogenes*
Mycobacteria *Mycobacterium tuberculosis var. bovis, nontuberculous mycobacteria*
Nonlipid or Small Viruses Poliovirus, coxsackievirus, rhinovirus
Fungi (spores, vegetative molds, yeast) Trichophyton spp., *Cryptococcus* spp., *Candida* spp.
Vegetative Bacteria *Pseudomonas aeruginosa, Staphylococcus aureus, Salmonella choleraesuis*, enterococci
Lipid-coated or Medium-sized Viruses Herpes simplex virus, cytomegalovirus, respiratory syncytial virus, HBV, HCV, HIV, hantavirus, Ebola virus

HBV = hepatitis b virus; HCV = hepatitis c virus; HIV = human immunodeficiency virus.

*There are exceptions to this list. *Pseudomonas* species are sensitive to high-level disinfectants, but if they grow in water and form biofilms on surfaces, the protected cells can approach the resistance of bacterial spores to the same disinfectant. The same is true for the resistance to glutaraldehyde by some nontuberculous mycobacteria, some fungal ascospores of *Microascus cinereus* and *Chaetomium globosum*, and the pink pigmented *Methylobacterium*. Prions are also resistant to most liquid chemical germicides.

Source: Adapted with permission of Centers for Disease Control and Prevention (CDC), National Institutes of Health (NIH). Appendix B: decontamination and disinfection. In: *Biosafety in Microbiological and Biomedical Laboratories*. 6th ed. Bethesda, MD: Centers for Disease Control and Prevention and National Institutes of Health; June 2020. https://www.cdc.gov/labs/pdf/SF__19_308133-A_BMBL6_00-BOOK-WEB-final-3.pdf. Accessed March 28, 2023.

Choice of Disinfectants

Disinfecting the interior of a PEC (LAFW, BSC, CAI, or CACI) may require intermediate-level disinfection because of the interior surfaces' proximity to critical sites. Chemical germicides with sufficient potency to achieve intermediate-level disinfection include chlorine-containing compounds (eg, sodium hypochlorite or bleach), alcohols (eg, ethanol or isopropanol), some phenolics, and some iodophors.[3] USP Chapter <797> requires sterile 70% IPA and sterile supplies (eg, wipes) to be used when disinfecting the interior of PECs.[7]

SECs, like buffer rooms and anteroom surfaces (eg, floors, walls, ceilings, carts, counters, and shelving), need low-level disinfection, which inactivates vegetative bacteria, fungi, enveloped viruses (eg, human immunodeficiency virus [HIV] and influenza viruses), and some nonenveloped viruses (eg, adenoviruses). Low-level disinfectants include quaternary ammonium compounds, some phenolics, and some iodophors (see **Table 14-4** for more examples).[17] Many disinfectants registered by the EPA are one-step cleaning and disinfecting agents, meaning the disinfectant is formulated to be effective enough to not require a separate cleaning step.

Choice of specific disinfecting agents should be guided by product label claims and instructions from the EPA. Collaborative judgment of infection control officers, janitorial, and pharmacy managers leads to the best selection

TABLE 14-4. Activity Levels of Selected Liquid Disinfectants*

Disinfectant	Aqueous Concentration	Activity Level
Glutaraldehyde†	Variable	High to intermediate
Hydrogen peroxide	3%–6%	High to intermediate
Formaldehyde	1%–8%	High to low
Chlorine compounds‡	500–5,000 mg/L free/available chlorine	Intermediate
Alcohols (ethyl, isopropyl)§	70%	Intermediate
Phenolic compounds	0.5%–3%	Intermediate to low
Iodophor compounds**	30–50 mg/L free iodine up to 10,000 mg/L available iodine	Intermediate to low
Quaternary ammonium compounds	0.1%–0.2%	Low

* These chemical disinfectants are generic formulations. A large number of commercial products based on these generic components can be considered for use. Users should ensure that commercial formulations are registered with the EPA or FDA.

† In general, highly toxic disinfectants, such as glutaraldehyde, are not used on compounding surfaces (eg, floors and countertops).[7]

‡ Generic disinfectants containing chlorine are available in liquid or solid form (eg, sodium or calcium hypochlorite). Although the indicated concentrations are rapid acting and broad-spectrum (tuberculocidal, bactericidal, fungicidal, and virucidal), no proprietary hypochlorite formulations are formally registered with the EPA or cleared by the FDA. Common household bleach is an excellent and inexpensive source of sodium hypochlorite. Concentrations between 500 and 1,000 mg/L chlorine are appropriate for the vast majority of uses requiring an intermediate level of germicidal activity. Higher concentrations are extremely corrosive as well as irritating to personnel, and their use should be limited to situations where there is an excessive amount of organic material or unusually high concentrations of microorganisms (eg, spills of cultured material). USP Chapter <1072> specifies a 0.5% sodium hypochlorite solution.

§ The effectiveness of alcohols as intermediate-level germicides is limited because they evaporate rapidly, resulting in short contact times, and they also lack the ability to penetrate residual organic material. They are rapidly tuberculocidal, bactericidal, and fungicidal but may vary in spectrum of virucidal activity. Items to be disinfected with alcohols should be carefully precleaned, and then totally exposed for an appropriate time (eg, 10 minutes).

** Only iodophors registered with the EPA as hard-surface disinfectants should be used. Manufacturer instructions regarding proper dilution and product stability must be closely followed. Antiseptic iodophors are not suitable for disinfecting devices, environmental surfaces, or medical instruments.

Source: Adapted with permission of Centers for Disease Control and Prevention (CDC), National Institutes of Health (NIH). Appendix B: decontamination and disinfection. In: *Biosafety in Microbiological and Biomedical Laboratories.* 6th ed. Bethesda, MD: Centers for Disease Control and Prevention and National Institutes of Health; June 2020. https://www.cdc.gov/labs/pdf/SF__19_308133-A_BMBL6_00-BOOK-WEB-final-3.pdf. Accessed March 28, 2023.

of cleaning and disinfecting products. A single disinfectant might not satisfy every condition (ie, degree of antimicrobial activity required, nature and composition of environmental surfaces, cost, safety, and ease of use). Select one or two intermediate-level products (eg, sterile 70% IPA and 0.5% sodium hypochlorite solution) to clean the inside of PEC and one low-level disinfectant with antimicrobial and cleaning abilities to clean surfaces in the buffer room and anteroom. McDonnell and Russell provide an excellent review of the mechanisms of action against and mechanisms of resistance to chemicals commonly used in disinfection.[18]

Application of Disinfectants Within Primary Engineering Controls

Simply spraying sterile 70% IPA is not the preferred means of applying this disinfectant to surfaces or pharmaceutical containers. Spraying alone does not physically remove dirt, dust, dried residues, and so on. Rubbing a surface with a lint-free wiper saturated with sterile 70% IPA to remove physical surface contaminants is the best way to disinfect the surface.[19;20]

Wiping surfaces with a wiper is a dual transfer process.[21] Contaminants from the surface are transferred to the wiper and material from the wiper is transferred to the surface. The longer a wiper is used, the more contaminants it will collect and redeposit on the surface. To reduce the redisposition problem, personnel must wipe from the cleanest area toward the dirtiest area within PECs. Pressing a wiper wetted with sterile 70% IPA releases some of the IPA onto the surface. A damp wiper is best for particle removal and prevention of redisposition. IPA also helps dissolve materials like dried salts, greases, or oils. The amount of IPA left behind depends on the degree of saturation of the wiper and the pressure and speed of wiping. A nearly uniform layer of liquid can be left on the surface if desired to lengthen surface contact with a disinfectant.[22] Wipers prewetted with sterile 70% IPA may be more convenient, reasonably priced, and more likely to contain an appropriate amount of IPA.[23] Because there are many types of sterile and nonsterile prewetted wipers, sterile compounding personnel must ensure that only sterile products are used within the PEC. USP Chapter <797> does not recommend saturating cotton gauze pads with IPA for wiping because this increases the particulate load in the environment.[7]

Application of Disinfectants Within Buffer Rooms and Anterooms

To apply disinfectants on buffer room and anteroom surfaces, personnel should apply a mild but effective disinfectant product, using as little of it as possible. A hospital-grade disinfectant (low-level) product for daily hard surface maintenance is suitable unless tougher microbes have been identified through environmental sampling. Some products, primarily those containing quaternary ammonium salts, may be used for cleaning and disinfecting. These products work best on surfaces that are already fairly clean or when they are used twice in a row, once to clean, and then again to disinfect.[11]

Mops can be a serious potential source of contamination.[24] Even when mops are soaked in a phenolic disinfectant overnight, microbes are still present. Therefore, mop heads should ideally be disposable and single use. If a reusable mop head is used, it must be dedicated to the sterile compounding area and laundered and dried before reuse. A bucketless system for applying the disinfectant to the mop head and surfaces is ideal to use in buffer rooms and anterooms because it reduces the effort when cleaning walls and ceilings. If a mop bucket is used, a two- or three-bucket system should be used. One bucket should be disinfectant, one bucket should be water for rinse (with a mop wringer in the two-bucket system), and one empty bucket with a wringer.[25]

Vacuum cleaners might be considered for removing large, visible accumulations of loose material from floors, but exhausting the vacuumed air into the buffer room and anteroom should be avoided to eliminate the risk of bioburden and contamination.[26] Bacterial and fungal contamination of filters in vacuum cleaning equipment is inevitable, and these filters should be cleaned regularly or replaced as per equipment manufacturer instructions.

Pollution Prevention

Because of the potential health risks and impacts on the environment, it makes sense to minimize the amount of disinfectant used.[11] There are four ways to accomplish this:

- Select the right product: Use a product that contains the specific EPA-registered ingredients needed to kill the germs found via environmental sampling. Six ingredients are commonly used as disinfectants in today's janitorial products (see **Table 14-5** for products and their adverse effects). Each of these ingredients can adversely affect janitorial and compounding personnel and the environment in general. Careful storage, mixing, and use of disinfectant products can reduce these impacts.

TABLE 14-5. Adverse Effects of Selected Generic Disinfectant Classes*

	Potential Effects of Each Ingredient			
Ingredient	User	Surfaces	Room Occupants	Environmental Impact
Quaternary ammonium chlorides	Eye and skin burns	Stains floor tile	Usually none	Medium
Phenols	Eye and skin burns	Corrodes plastic surfaces	Usually none	High
Sodium hypochlorite (bleach)	Eye and skin burns, harmful vapors	Corrodes metal surfaces	Affects indoor air quality	Medium to high
Hydrogen peroxide	Eye and skin burns, harmful vapors	Corrodes metal surfaces	Affects indoor air quality	Medium
Alcohols	Absorb thru skin, harmful vapors	Usually none	Affects indoor air quality	Low to medium
Iodine	Eye and skin burns	Stains many surfaces	Usually none	High

* Take care to review each product's safety data sheet for other ingredients that may harm the user. For example, be wary of combined cleaners and disinfectants that contain 2-butoxyethanol or ethanolamine. For information on a specific product, refer to supplier instructions and safety data sheets.

Source: Adapted with permission of Barron T, Berg C, Bookman L, United States Environmental Protection Agency (EPA) Region IX. How to select and use safe janitorial chemicals: Project completion report. Pollution prevention incentives for states. https://citeseerx.ist.psu.edu/document?repid=rep1&type=pdf&doi=539713d7f34066ddc349a818627b3d32430eeb6e. Published December 1999. Accessed August 31, 2023.

- Adhere to schedules: Use the cleaning and disinfecting schedules for buffer room and anteroom surfaces published in USP Chapter <797> (see Table 14-1).[8]
- Control product mixing: Train personnel to dilute concentrated disinfectant products according to EPA-approved labeling.
- Use correct methods: Disinfectants need to be in contact with the germs they are intended to kill. This means the surface must first be cleaned to the point where it is free of dirt, grease, and oil. Then the disinfectant must be thoroughly applied and left in place for the product-specific contact time, often 10 to 15 minutes. It may be necessary to do the work in a sequence to allow for this longer contact time (eg, precleaning the surfaces, then applying the disinfectant, and then emptying the trash while the disinfectant is at work).

Buffer Room and Anteroom Surfaces

The number and types of microorganisms present on buffer room and anteroom surfaces are influenced by the following factors:

- Number of people in the environment
- Amount of activity
- Amount of moisture and air humidity
- Presence of soil and other material capable of supporting microbial growth
- Rate at which organisms suspended in the air are removed
- Type of surface and its orientation (ie, horizontal or vertical surfaces)[27]

Disinfection relates to the saturation and penetration of the cell wall of microbes by the disinfectant agent.[28] Specific contact time (also referred to as dwell time) is sometimes difficult to achieve because the movement of air tends to dry the disinfectant liquid on housekeeping surfaces.

Floors

Strong (ie, intermediate-level) disinfectant cleaning and decontamination of floors in buffer rooms and anterooms is generally unwarranted.[3] Healthcare institutions usually employ a low-level, EPA-registered detergent and disinfectant for cleaning low-touch surfaces, like buffer room and anteroom floors. Wet mopping is the best method for cleaning these nonporous floors.

Part of the cleaning strategy is to minimize contamination of cleaning solutions and cleaning tools. Disposable mop heads are the preferred option. Bucket solutions become contaminated almost immediately during cleaning. Continued use of the solution transfers increasing numbers of microorganisms to each subsequent floor to be cleaned. Cleaning solutions should be replaced frequently. A variety of bucket methods (eg, two-bucket, three-bucket) have been devised to address the frequency with which cleaning solutions are replaced.

Another source of contamination in the cleaning process is the wiper or mop head, especially if left soaking in dirty cleaning solutions. A simplified approach to cleaning involves replacing soiled mop heads with clean mop heads each time a bucket of detergent or disinfectant is emptied and replaced with fresh, clean solution. Floor mats with tacky surfaces act as reservoirs for dust and contaminants, therefore they must not be placed within ISO-classified areas.

Counters and Shelves

High-touch surfaces in sterile compounding areas (eg, doorknobs, counters, sinks, carts, light switches) should be cleaned and disinfected more frequently than surfaces with minimal hand contact. Table 14-1 provides more specific details about cleaning and disinfecting schedules.

Disinfectant Rotation

A few microbes appear to develop resistance to commonly used disinfectants (eg, phenolics and quaternary ammonium compounds).[29;30] USP Chapter <1072> advises that successful cleaning and disinfection methods be included in written procedures on disinfection rotation.[13] If a disinfectant rotation program is required (eg, environmental sampling that shows spores), it should include disinfectants that control a wide variety of microbes and mitigates damage to buffer room and anteroom surfaces. An effective three-part rotation program is described below[31]:

- Routine disinfectants should be used for cleaning and disinfecting buffer room and anteroom surfaces. They should also effectively control vegetative bacteria and remove soil while minimizing damage to surfaces and risks to personnel working in the area.
- Because routine disinfectants are generally not effective against bacterial spores, such as *Bacillus* species, a sporicidal agent should also be applied periodically. Most sporicidal disinfectants are either highly toxic or very corrosive. Thus, they should not be considered for daily use on surfaces in buffer rooms and anterooms. The rotation frequency should be driven by germicidal performance that is verifiable through environmental microbial sampling data. USP Chapter <1072> suggests augmenting the daily use of a low-level hospital disinfectant with weekly or monthly use of a sporicidal agent.[13]
- Because some types of disinfectants leave residues, a residue-removal agent (eg, 70% IPA) should be used as needed.

Janitorial Procedures

Buffer room and anteroom surfaces require regular cleaning and removal of soil and dust. Dry conditions favor the persistence of gram-positive cocci (eg, coagulase-negative *Staphylococcus* spp.) in dust and on surfaces. Moist soiled environments favor the growth and persistence of gram-negative bacilli.[3] Fungi are also present on dust and proliferate in moist, fibrous material.

As previously mentioned, many disinfectants registered by the EPA are one-step disinfectants (ie, formulated to be effective in the presence of light to moderate soiling without a precleaning step).[7] Such commercial disinfectant products often contain a surfactant (synthetic detergent) and an antimicrobial agent (eg, phenol, quaternary ammonium compound). The surfactant allows the product to handle a fairly substantial soil load for surfaces (eg, floors). These agents are designed for frequent use and are relatively safe for personnel and surfaces.[32] Personnel should consult disinfecting product safety data sheets (SDSs) to determine appropriate precautions to prevent hazardous conditions during product application. Personal protective equipment (PPE) used during janitorial procedures should be appropriate to the task.

Safe Disinfectant Storage and Mixing

Avoid application of contaminated cleaning solutions, particularly from small quantity aerosol spray bottles. Making enough fresh cleaning solution for daily cleaning, discarding any remaining solution, and drying out the container will help minimize the degree of bacterial contamination. A premixed, ready-to-use detergent and disinfectant solution may be used if available.

The following information includes recommendations for safe storage of and mixing of disinfectants[33]:

- Incompatible products: Products with incompatible ingredients should be stored separately. For example, keep glass cleaner with ammonia away from products containing sodium hypochlorite (bleach). Away from means in a separate room, in a separate cabinet, or on separate shelves (but not one over the other). SDSs for all the disinfectants used should be available to all personnel who handle the disinfectants.
- Strong ingredients: Store products with acids or other strong ingredients in plastic tubs so that any leaks do not harm the storage rack or janitorial closet.
- Stock rotation: Rotate stock of stored products so that the oldest ones are used first. Some janitorial products (eg, bleach) have a shelf life. Be sure all such products are used before their time expires.
- Spill kits: Keep spill cleanup kits in or near every buffer room and anteroom, and train workers in their use.
- PPE: Janitorial personnel must protect themselves by wearing gloves and goggles when handling harmful disinfectants. Sodium hypochlorite and other products with strong chemicals pose the greatest risks, especially when housekeepers are handling concentrates. To reduce personnel risks during mixing, follow these instructions:
    - Janitorial personnel should be trained in safe work procedures.
    - Have a supervisor do all mixing of concentrated toxic chemicals.
    - Insist that protective gloves and goggles or face shields be worn when the supervisor is handling concentrated products.
    - Safety showers and eye wash stations must be situated in the work areas where disinfectant solutions are prepared.[11] The Occupational Safety and Health Administration regulations require that a 15 minute full-flow eye wash station be provided in any area where workers are exposed to corrosive chemicals.
    - Many accidents and injuries occur when a worker lifts a full mop bucket to pour its contents into a janitorial sink. Teach personnel safe lifting methods.

SETTING UP A BUFFER ROOM AND ANTEROOM CLEANING AND DISINFECTING PROGRAM

Form a team to develop cleaning and disinfection procedures for a buffer room and anteroom.[34] The team should include a sterile compounding manager, a janitorial manager, and an infection control practitioner. Other valuable members of the team might be a pharmacy technician, an operating room manager, a front-line janitorial staff member, and a product purchasing agent.

Responsibilities of this team should include the following tasks:

- Compiling a list of current decontaminating, cleaning, and disinfecting practices for buffer rooms and anterooms. Note that the same level of cleaning and disinfecting practices are required whether buffer rooms or anterooms are large or small (eg, central pharmacy versus pharmacy satellite).
- Assessing and revising each current cleaning and disinfecting practice, adding practices as necessary.
- Develop and apply a training program that emphasizes the following:
    - What cleaning and disinfecting product to use for each purpose
    - How to check the expiration date on each product container
    - How to check for safe use and PPE required for each product

- How to prepare accurate product dilutions
- How to apply each product with the correct exposure time
- How to ensure that product residues are removed or neutralized so as not to contaminate sterile preparations during compounding

Pharmacy and janitorial supervisors should ask their staff members for feedback on the practicality of the procedures and the effectiveness of the training program. Supervisors should decide how trained staff can demonstrate competency (eg, visual observation during the process of performing cleaning and disinfecting procedures).[7;8] See Figure 14-1 for a sample assessment form. In addition, supervisors should monitor and trend environmental sampling data, change practices to correct excursions outside the normal range, and develop written policies and procedures.

A complete disinfection control program should be comprised of six procedural areas[28]:

- Control what contamination enters the buffer room and anteroom.
- Clean the buffer room and anteroom.
- Collect and analyze environmental sampling data.
- Use environmental sampling data to validate the efficacy of cleaning and disinfecting products.
- Validate the mechanical cleaning and disinfection application methods.
- Train and supervise personnel.

Ideal cleaning policies and procedures should address assignment of responsibility; specify daily, weekly, and monthly cleaning schedules; specify cleaning and disinfecting operations; ensure protection and cleanliness of equipment immediately prior to use; and maintain cleaning and disinfecting records.[13] Cleaning materials must be approved as having no negative effect on aseptic technique or CSPs. A continual maintenance program of equipment and supplies (eg, wipers, mops, and buckets) is needed. Equipment in the buffer room and anteroom should be maintained at proper cleanliness levels.[35;36] Managers should review procedures and training programs regularly and update them as necessary. Reviews should include adequacy of the cleaning and disinfecting products in controlling microbes found in the facility, cost of the program, and safety and pollution issues. (**Appendix 33-A** in Chapter 33 shows a model policy and procedure for cleaning and disinfecting a buffer room and anteroom.)

Environmental sampling data should be used to validate the efficacy of cleaning and disinfecting products. A review of isolates from environmental sampling helps determine which cleaners, disinfectants, and sporicides are required.[28] M. Jeffrey laid out a solid program for sterile compounding area cleaning and disinfection.[37] Collecting and analyzing environmental sampling data are covered in Chapter 31.

Routine janitorial processes are often handled by staff after a day's work is done, usually late in the evening or during the night shift. Managers of sterile compounding areas must observe janitorial personnel regularly to ensure that written procedures are being followed. Janitorial personnel must be trained at least annually and more often if environmental sampling shows excursions of samples that require corrective actions. Frequent turnover occurs among hospital janitorial personnel and managers. Thus, it is helpful for the pharmacy department to train its own staff to handle janitorial procedures in buffer room and anterooms.

SUMMARY

Appropriate and routine cleaning and disinfecting of gloves, DCAs, and primary and secondary engineering controls are mandatory. When selecting a disinfectant for sterile pharmaceutical compounding areas, the following points should be considered:

- Number and types of microorganisms present
- Spectrum of commercially available disinfectants
- Reputation of the disinfectant supplier
- Sterilant claims
- Whether disinfectant or sanitizer is supported by EPA registration
- Concentration, application method, and contact time of the disinfectant
- Nature of the surface material being disinfected and its compatibility with the disinfectant
- Amounts of organic compounds on the surface that may inactivate a disinfectant
- Possible need to maintain a residual bactericidal activity of the disinfectant on the surface
- Corrosiveness of the disinfectant to equipment with repeated application
- Safety considerations for operators applying the disinfectant
- Compatibility of the disinfectant with cleaning agents and other disinfectants
- Steps that should be taken to avoid the contamination of compounded preparations by the disinfectant[38]

Compounding and janitorial personnel must carefully apply disinfectants according to written policies and procedures that include the schedule for applications. To prevent breakthrough growth of resistant pathogens in sterile compounding areas, compounding personnel must monitor the effectiveness of the cleaning and disinfecting program by environmental sampling according to written policies and procedures, which include the schedule for sampling, documentation, and data evaluation. Excursions beyond the normal colony forming units and types of microbial flora require personnel to review their cleaning and disinfecting practices in in the following areas:

- Personnel training and work practices
- Choice and application of disinfectants
- Sources of environmental contamination (eg, heating, ventilation, and air conditioning system, including high-efficiency particulate air filter, temperature, and humidity)
- Traffic patterns of personnel, equipment, and supplies
- Hand hygiene and garbing practices

Sources of excess microbial growth must be eliminated, the affected area cleaned, and resampling performed.[3]

REFERENCES

1. Magill SS, O'Leary E, Janelle SJ, et al. Changes in Prevalence of Health Care-Associated Infections in U.S. Hospitals. *N Engl J Med*. 2018;379(18):1732–1744. doi:10.1056/NEJMoa1801550.
2. Scott RD II. The direct medical costs of healthcare-associated infections in U.S. hospitals and the benefits of prevention. Centers for Disease Control and Prevention (CDC). **www.cdc.gov/hai/pdfs/hai/scott_costpaper.pdf**. March 2009. Accessed March 28, 2023.
3. Sehulster L, Chinn RY. Guidelines for environmental infection control in health-care facilities. Recommendations of CDC and the Healthcare Infection Control Practices Advisory Committee (HICPAC). *MMWR Recomm Rep*. 2003;52(RR-10):1–42. **https://pubmed.ncbi.nlm.nih.gov/12836624/**.
4. Rutala WA, Weber DJ. *Guideline for Disinfection and Sterilization in Healthcare Facilities, 2008*. Chapel Hill, NC: Centers for Disease Control and Prevention; May 2019. **https://www.cdc.gov/infectioncontrol/pdf/guidelines/disinfection-guidelines-H.pdf**. Accessed March 28, 2023.
5. Special PP&P buyer's guide: liquid disinfecting cleaners and pre-saturated and dry wipes. *Pharmacy Purchasing & Products*. 2015;(Jan):12–14.
6. Douglass K. Establishing sound practices for cleaning your cleanroom: cleaning products and procedures for USP <797> compliance. *Pharmacy Purchasing & Products*. **www.pppmag.com/documents/V2N5/v2n5pp16_cleancleanroom2.pdf**. Accessed March 28, 2023.
7. USP <797> Pharmaceutical compounding—sterile preparations. In: *2023: USP Compounding Compendium*. Rockville, MD: United States Pharmacopeial Convention; 2023: Issue 1. **https://doi.org/10.31003/USPNF_M99925_07_01**.
8. USP <797> Pharmaceutical compounding—sterile preparations. [Revision Bulletin, Appendix V, May 1, 2020]. Rockville, MD: United States Pharmacopeial Convention; 2020. **https://www.uspnf.com/sites/default/files/usp_pdf/EN/USPNF/revisions/gc-797-rb-notice-20200424.pdf**. Accessed April 8, 2023.
9. USP <800> Hazardous drugs—handling in healthcare settings. In: *USP Compounding Compendium*. Rockville, MD: United States Pharmacopeial Convention; July 1, 2020. **https://doi.org/10.31003/USPNF_M7808_07_01**.
10. Gabay M, Johnson P, Fanikos J, et al. Report on 2020 Safe to Touch Consensus Conference on Hazardous Drug Surface Contamination. *Am J Health Syst Pharm*. 2021;78(17):1568–1575. doi:10.1093/ajhp/zxab134.
11. Barron T, Berg C, Bookman L, United States Environmental Protection Agency (EPA) Region IX. How to select and use safe janitorial chemicals. How to select and use safe janitorial chemicals: Project completion report. Pollution prevention incentives for states. **https://citeseerx.ist.psu.edu/viewdoc/download?doi=10.1.1.387.9389&rep=rep1&type=pdf**. Published December 1999. Accessed August 31, 2023.
12. U.S. Pharmacopeia. *Additional Commentary to USP 31-NF 26 Second Supplement General Chapter <797> Pharmaceutical Compounding—Sterile Preparations*. Rockville, MD: United States Pharmacopeial Convention. **https://www.uspnf.com/sites/default/files/usp_pdf/EN/USPNF/2008-07-18_USP_31_2S_Commentary_Chapter_797.pdf**. Accessed April 8, 2023.
13. USP <1072> Disinfectants and antiseptics. In: *USP 42–NF 37*. Rockville, MD: United States Pharmacopeial Convention; 2019.
14. Sutton SV. Disinfectant rotation—a microbiologist's view. *Controlled Environments*. 2005;(Jul):9–14.
15. U.S. Environmental Protection Agency (EPA). What are antimicrobial pesticides? **www.epa.gov/pesticide-registration/what-are-antimicrobial-pesticides**. Updated March 22, 2023. Accessed March 28, 2023.
16. Occupational Safety and Health Administration (OSHA). Occupational exposure to bloodborne pathogens—OSHA. Final rule. *Fed Regist*. 1991;56:64004–64182. **https://pubmed.ncbi.nlm.nih.gov/10115865/**.

17. Centers for Disease and Control Prevention (CDC), National Institutes of Health (NIH). Appendix B: decontamination and disinfection. In: *Biosafety in Microbiological and Biomedical Laboratories*. 6th ed. Bethesda, MD: Centers for Disease Control and Prevention and National Institutes of Health; June 2020. **https://www.cdc.gov/labs/pdf/SF__19_308133-A_BMBL6_00-BOOK-WEB-final-3.pdf**. Accessed March 28, 2023.

18. McDonnell G, Russell AD. Antiseptics and disinfectants: activity, action, and resistance. *Clin Microbiol Rev*. 1999;12(1):147–179. doi:10.1128/CMR.12.1.147.

19. Cockcroft MG, Hepworth D, Rhodes JC, et al. Validation of liquid disinfection techniques for transfer of components into hospital pharmacy clean rooms. *Hosp Pharm*. 2001;8:226–232.

20. Hiom SJ. Validation of disinfectant techniques in hospital aseptic dispensing units. *Pharm J*. 2000;265:277–278.

21. Cooper DW. Basics of effective wiping. *A2C2*. 2001; May:47.

22. Cooper DW. Applying a uniform layer of disinfectant by wiping. *PDA J Pharm Sci Technol*. 2000;54(1):44–58. **https://pubmed.ncbi.nlm.nih.gov/10778308/**.

23. Siegerman H. Chapter 4: making practical choices in the real world of cleaning. *A2C2*. 2003; Apr:21-3.

24. Murtough SM, Hiom SJ, Palmer M, Russell AD. A survey of disinfectant use in hospital pharmacy aseptic preparation areas. *Pharm J*. 2000;264:446–448.

25. Sandle T. Cleanroom cleaning and disinfection: eight steps for success. **https://www.researchgate.net/publication/307600889_Cleanroom_Cleaning_and_Disinfection_Eight_Steps_for_Success**. Published March 2012. Accessed April 8, 2023.

26. Veillette M, Knibbs LD, Pelletier A, et al. Microbial contents of vacuum cleaner bag dust and emitted bioaerosols and their implications for human exposure indoors. *Appl Environ Microbiol*. 2013;79(20):6331–6336. doi:10.1128/AEM.01583-13.

27. Collins BJ. The hospital environment: how clean should a hospital be? *J Hosp Infect*. 1988;11(suppl A):53–56. doi:10.1016/0195-6701(88)90166-1.

28. McDonnell G, Russell AD. Antiseptics and disinfectants: activity, action, and resistance. *Clin Microbiol Rev*. 1999;12(1):147–179. doi:10.1128/CMR.12.1.147.

29. Bauerfeind A, Burrows RR, Petermuller C. Genetically determined changes in sensitivity to components of disinfectants by *Enterobacteriaceae*. *Hyg Med*. 1981;6:310–313.

30. Chaplin CE. Bacterial resistance to quaternary ammonium disinfectants. *J Bacteriol*. 1952;63(4): 453–458. doi:10.1128/jb.63.4.453-458.1952.

31. Sartain EK. Rotating disinfectants in cleanrooms: avoid going in circles. *A2C2*. 2005; Mar:32-3.

32. Sartain EK. The ABCs of disinfectant validation. *Semiconductor Digest*. 2005. **https://sst.semiconductor-digest.com/2005/03/the-abcs-of-disinfectant-validation/**. Accessed March 28, 2023.

33. Janitorial Chemicals Workshop. Managing your chemicals. **https://p2infohouse.org/ref/14/13715/wbc4.pdf**. Published July 1999. Accessed March 28, 2023.

34. Denny VF, Kopis EM, Marsik FJ. Elements for a successful disinfection program in the pharmaceutical environment. *PDA J Pharm Sci Technol*. 1999;53(3):115–124. **https://pubmed.ncbi.nlm.nih.gov/10754700/**.

35. Zytka D. Designing/building/constructing your cleanroom. *Semiconductor Digest*. 1997. **https://sst.semiconductor-digest.com/1997/01/designing-building-constructing-your-cleanroom/**. Accessed March 28, 2023.

36. Sartain EK. Designing a cleanroom disinfectant program to meet production requirements and regulatory expectations. *A2C2*. 2004; Dec:21-24.

37. Jeffrey M. Is your cleanroom clean? An in-depth look at cleaning and disinfecting agents, procedures, and requirements for the compounding pharmacist. *Int J Pharm Compd*. 2006;10(2):113–119. **https://pubmed.ncbi.nlm.nih.gov/23974185/**.

38. Denny VF, Marsik FJ. Current practices in the use of disinfectants within the pharmaceutical industry. *PDA J Pharm Sci Technol*. 1997;51(6):227–228. **https://pubmed.ncbi.nlm.nih.gov/9448431/**.

15

ASEPTIC TECHNIQUE

Linda F. McElhiney

INTRODUCTION

All compounded sterile preparations (CSPs) must be prepared under strict, sterile environmental conditions by trained personnel using aseptic technique. The *United States Pharmacopeia* (USP) defines *aseptic technique* as "a set of methods used to keep objects and areas free of microorganisms and thereby minimize infection risk to the patient. It is accomplished through practices that maintain the microbe count at an irreducible minimum."[1] The components can either be purchased as sterile or, when starting with nonsterile components, can be separately sterilized via membrane filtration or autoclaving prior to combining. Although various methods for aseptic technique are used in different areas in healthcare, this chapter focuses on the application of aseptic technique in pharmacy practice.

While the importance of sterility was first recognized in the late 1800s, the concept of aseptic technique was not described until years later.[2;3] The need to sterilize solutions and equipment became accepted in the 1920s and 1930s.[4–6] The development of sterile and pyrogen-free products and their applications continues today.

In the late 1960s, improperly manufactured and compounded parenteral solutions caused a rash of complications in patients.[7–12] After these incidents, the National Coordinating Committee on Large Volume Parenterals (NCCLVP) was established. They published recommendations for compounding sterile preparations by pharmacists and other healthcare professionals.[13–19]

In response to the problems with CSPs, the American Society of Health-System Pharmacists (ASHP) published a *Technical Assistance Bulletin* and USP published USP Chapter <1206> to provide guidance on how to properly prepare sterile preparations. However, these guidelines were often not followed by practitioners because they were not legally enforceable.[20;21] In 1938, the U.S. Congress passed the Federal Food, Drug, and Cosmetic Act, which recognized all of the chapters with numbers lower than 1000 in USP as legally enforceable standards and requirements for pharmacy practice.[22] USP revised Chapter <1206> and published USP Chapter <797> on sterile compounding on January 1, 1997, which emphasized the need to maintain high standards for the quality and control of processes, components, environments, and properly trained and verified compounding personnel.[23] The USP Chapter <797> is continuously reviewed and revised by the USP Committee of Experts for Compounding to further improve the quality of CSPs and patient safety.[24;25] USP has since published another revision to Chapter <797> to further improve the quality of CSPs and patient safety.[1]

REQUIREMENTS FOR ASEPTIC TECHNIQUE

The quality of CSPs is only as good as the aseptic technique used. If a person is not properly trained on handwashing and garbing, how to use equipment correctly, working in clean environments, cleaning and disinfecting surfaces, equipment and supplies, sterilization methods, performing quality assurance, and aseptic manipulation skills, the sterility of a CSP may be compromised. Aseptic technique is a specific skill set performed by the compounder to ensure that sterile preparations are compounded without introducing microbial contamination from the compounder. Good aseptic compounding skills do not eliminate the need for proper equipment and environments. Conversely, good equipment and a proper environment does not ensure good quality sterile preparations if the person's aseptic technique is substandard.

The standards in USP Chapter <797> for traditional pharmacies require the following:

> All personnel who compound or have direct oversight of compounding personnel must be initially trained and qualified by demonstrating knowledge and competency in compounding CSPs. . . before being allowed to perform their job functions independently. Designated person(s) are responsible for creating and implementing a

DOI 10.37573/9781585286492.015

> training program for personnel and for ensuring that compounders, personnel who have direct oversight of compounders, and personnel who perform restocking or cleaning and disinfection duties are initially trained and qualified by demonstrating knowledge and competency in maintaining the quality of the sterile compounding environment before being allowed to perform their job functions independently. Training and observation may be performed by the designated person(s) or an assigned trainer. Personnel who compound or have direct oversight of compounding personnel must complete training initially and at least every 12 months in appropriate sterile compounding principles and practices.[1]

Chapter 5 addresses personnel training and competency. This chapter provides information and instruction on the practical skills necessary for aseptic technique.

Equipment and Environment

Sterile compounding is done in a primary engineering control (PEC) that provides an International Organization for Standardization (ISO) Class 5 environment for the exposure of critical sites, the exception being emergent medical situations that may require preparation at the point of care. Proper placement of PECs, such as laminar airflow workbenches (LAFW), is discussed in detail in Chapter 6. For hazardous sterile compounding, a biological safety cabinet (BSC) or a compounding aseptic containment isolator (CACI) is used to provide an ISO Class 5 environment and to protect the compounder from exposure to hazardous substances. These PECs are discussed in detail in Chapter 6 and Chapter 27.

Any component or fluid pathway surface (eg, vial septa, injection ports, opened ampules, needles, or hubs) that is exposed and at risk of direct contact with air, moisture, or touch contamination is called a *critical site*. The key principle in the use of PECs is that nothing should disrupt or block the unidirectional airflow between the high-efficiency particulate air (HEPA) filter and the critical sites where the sterile fluid pathway is created. This aseptic compounding space is called the direct compounding area (DCA). The unidirectional airstream from the HEPA filter is essentially particulate-free and is referred to as *first air*. Items placed in the way of first air can potentially contaminate critical sites with particulates or microorganisms by blowing them onto the injection port, opened ampule, needle, or syringe. Large items placed within the PEC can also disrupt the unidirectional airflow, causing a zone of turbulence that may pull or allow contaminated room air or contamination from the compounder's body into the PEC and potentially contaminate the DCA and critical sites. The risk of contamination increases with the size of the openings and exposure time.

Placement of objects in the PEC is critical in the aseptic technique process. To avoid zones of turbulence, objects should be placed at least six inches from the sides and front open edge of the PEC without blocking air vents or obstructing the airflow. Personnel should keep their hands out of the first air space to avoid blocking the airflow. When

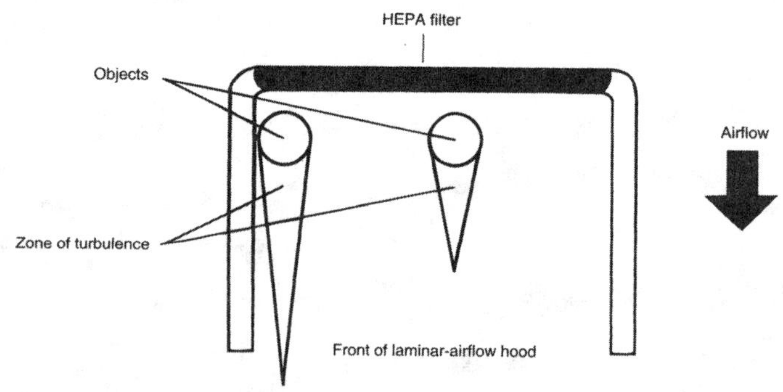

FIGURE 15-1. Zone of turbulence

unidirectional airflow is accessible to all sides of the object, the zone of turbulence is approximately three times the diameter of the object. However, when the airflow is not accessible on all sides, the zone of turbulence may be six times the diameter of the object. Ideally, the object should be placed in the middle of the PEC (see **Figure 15-1**).

The following are general principles for the proper use of PECs as part of good aseptic technique:

- A PEC should operate continuously and should not be turned off when not in use. If the PEC needs to be turned off, it should not be used for a specified time recommended by the manufacturer when turned back on. This downtime allows all of the contaminated room air to be purged from the direct compounding area.
- Before use, all interior working surfaces of the PEC must be cleaned with a sterile cleaning agent followed by disinfection with sterile 70% isopropyl alcohol (IPA) using sterile, nonshedding, lint-free wipes. A sterile sporicidal agent must be used at least monthly for entities compounding Category 1 and 2 preparations or weekly for entities compounding Category 3 preparations to eliminate any fungal contamination within the PEC. Cleaning should be performed from the back to the front and top to bottom so that contaminants are moved away from the HEPA filter. In other words, the compounder should clean from the cleanest part of the PEC to the dirtiest part. According to USP Chapter <797>, the PEC should be disinfected frequently on days when compounding occurs, including at the beginning of the work shift, before the start of each batch, every 30 minutes during continuous compounding periods, when there are spills, and when there is known or suspected contamination from a lapse in the aseptic technique process.
- Nothing should touch the HEPA filter. Spray bottles containing the sterile cleaning and disinfecting agents should not be used in the PEC because the chemicals can damage the HEPA filter. Solution from a syringe should not be pushed out toward the filter for the same reason. Ampules should not be

broken directly toward the filter because the shards of glass could also damage the filter.

- Actions, such as talking or coughing, should be directed away from the DCA, and unnecessary motion should be avoided to minimize airflow turbulence.
- Only objects essential for compounding sterile preparations should be placed in the PEC (eg, no paper, pens, labels, or trays). All items that are needed for compounding must be wiped down with sterile 70% IPA before placing them in the PEC.
- PECs must be tested and certified by qualified personnel or contractors every 6 months or as specified by USP Chapter <797> standards or current good manufacturing practices (CGMP). Details of the required testing are discussed in Chapter 6. They should also be tested whenever the PEC is moved and if there is suspected damage to the HEPA filter.[26]

Personnel Cleansing and Gowning

The most common source of contamination of a CSP is by touch. The human body sheds skin cells at a rate of at least 10^6 per hour, and each particle has the potential to transport microorganisms.[25] Although proper gowning and personnel cleansing does not eliminate all particles, it can reduce the particulate burden. Proper personnel cleansing and gowning are among the most critical aspects of aseptic technique.

The following steps are general principles for proper hand hygiene and gowning as part of good aseptic technique. Facilities compounding Category 3 CSPs must meet additional requirements, which are elaborated on in Chapter 13.

1. Don the head cover, shoe covers, facial hair covers, and face mask first in an order defined by the facility's standard operating procedures because these body areas are the dirtiest.
2. The first steps of hand hygiene should be performed in the anteroom and before donning the nonshedding gown. Since the water for handwashing is tap water, the gown should not be put on before handwashing to avoid contamination by water-borne microorganisms splashing onto the gown.
3. Remove any visible debris from underneath the fingernails under warm, running water using a disposable nail pick or cleaner.
4. Wash hands and forearms up to the elbows for at least 30 seconds with soap and water. A closed system of soap (ie, nonrefillable container) must be readily available near the sink.
5. Do not use antimicrobial scrub brushes because they can irritate or damage the skin and can actually increase skin shedding.
6. Completely dry the hands and forearms using lint-free disposable wipes. Electric hand dryers must not be used.
7. After handwashing, don a nonshedding gown with sleeves that fit snugly around the wrists and that is enclosed at the neck.
8. Apply an alcohol-based hand rub and allow hands to dry completely before donning sterile, powder-free gloves.
9. Sterile gloves must be donned as the last step of hand hygiene and garbing. Gloves must be donned in a classified room or inside the line of demarcation in a segregated compounding area before touching anything in the ISO Class 7 buffer room. The gloves are only sterile until the wearer touches something. USP Chapter <797> recommends frequently disinfecting the gloves with 70% sterile IPA during the compounding process, when nonsterile items are touched, and when inspecting gloves for holes, punctures, or tears. Gloves should be replaced as needed. Even though the sterile gloves become quickly contaminated, it has been shown that sterile gloves that were repeatedly disinfected with IPA decreased the contamination rate of pharmacy-compounded preparations from 5.2% to 0.34%.[27] Commercial sterile gloves are also free of endotoxins and particulate contamination.[1]

Syringes

In addition to the proper use of PECs and personnel cleansing and gowning, aseptic technique requires the correct use and handling of sterile equipment and supplies, including syringes, needles, vials, and ampules.

Syringes are made of either glass or plastic. However, plastic is readily available and primarily used in practice settings, such as pharmacies, hospitals, and clinics. Disposable sterile plastic syringes cost less, reduce the risk of transmitting blood-borne pathogens, and are resistant to breaking. Syringes are composed of two main parts, the barrel and the plunger (see **Figure 15-2**). The plunger, which fits inside the barrel, has a flat disk or lip at one end and a rubber or silicone piston at the other. The top collar of the barrel prevents the syringe from slipping during use, and the tip is where the needle attaches. Most syringes have threaded locking mechanism called a Luer-Lok at the tip, which secures the needle.

Syringes are available in many sizes, with volumes ranging from 0.5 to 50 mL. Graduation marks on the syringes represent different increments depending on the size of the syringe. For example, each line on a 1 mL syringe represents 0.01 mL; on a 10 mL syringe, each line represents 0.2 mL; and on a 30 mL syringe, each line represents 1 mL. To maximize measuring accuracy, the smallest syringe that can hold the desired amount of volume should be used.

USP standards require that the stated amount, concentration, or volume of drug must be within a range of 10%.[28] Erstad et al. found that accuracy and reproducibility of delivery of a nominal 0.5 mL fluid volume decreased as syringe size increased from 1 to 5 mL. Error tended toward delivery of excess volume, creating a 16.8% error in measurement when a 5 mL syringe was used to measure a 0.5 mL volume.[29]

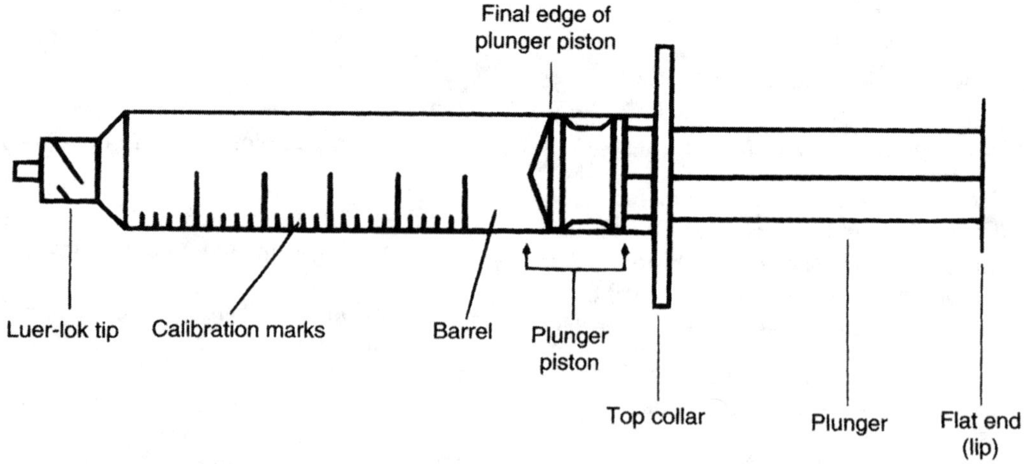

FIGURE 15-2. Parts of a syringe

When measuring fluid in a syringe, the user should line up the final edge of the plunger piston to the desired graduation mark on the barrel (see **Figure 15-3**). To maintain sterility, only the barrel, top collar, and flat end of the syringe may be touched. The tip and the plunger cannot be touched.

Sterile syringes are sent from the manufacturer already assembled and individually packaged in a paper or plastic overwrap or plastic cover. Sterility is guaranteed until the manufacturer's expiration date as long as the outer package remains intact. Inspect the outer package for damage before use and discarded if damaged. The syringe package should be opened in the PEC to maintain sterility. If the sterile syringe is packaged with a protector over the tip, it should not be removed until the needle is ready to be attached.[1;30]

Needles

Needles are available in many sizes, which are described by gauge and length. The gauge of the needle corresponds to the diameter of its bore. The higher the gauge number, the smaller the bore of the needle. Very small needles have a gauge of 30 and the largest have a gauge of 13. The length of a needle shaft usually ranges from 3/8 of an inch to 3 inches. The most common needle sizes used in compounding CSPs range from gauge 18 to 22 and length 1 to 1.5 inches. Some needles also have a 5-µm filter in them to filter out particulate matter.

The components of a simple needle are the shaft and the hub (see **Figure 15-4**). The hub attaches the needle to the syringe and is often color-coded to indicate a specific gauge size. The tip of the needle shaft is slanted to form a point. This slant is called a bevel, and the point is the bevel tip. The opposite end of the slant is the bevel heel.

Like sterile syringes, needles are sent from the manufacturer individually packaged in paper and plastic overwraps with an attached sterile protective cover over the needle shaft (needle cap). They are sterile as long as the packaging

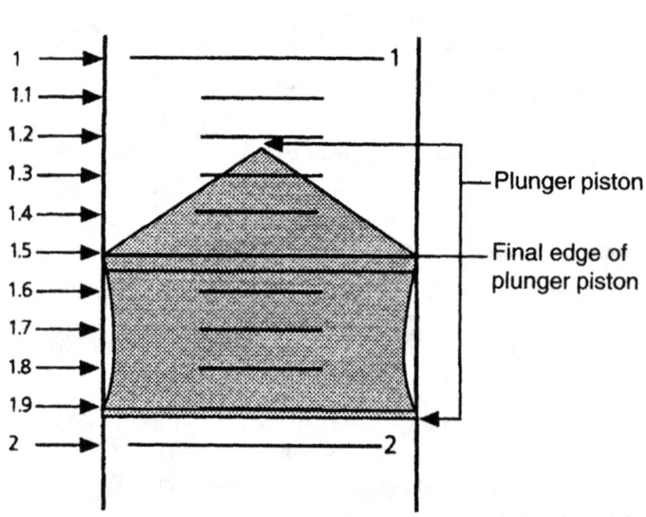

FIGURE 15-3. Syringe markings on a barrel with 1.5 mL withdrawn

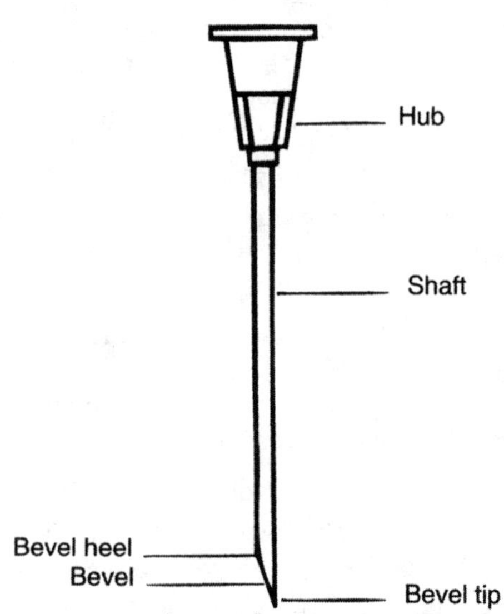

FIGURE 15-4. Parts of a needle

is intact. The hub of the needle should not be touched when removing the overwrap.

A needle shaft is usually metal and lubricated with a sterile silicone coating for smooth, easy penetration through vial closures and injection port septa. Therefore, needles should never be swabbed with alcohol or touched. They should only be handled by the protective cover and the cover should remain in place until the needles or syringes are used. Used needles should not be recapped to prevent an accidental needle stick injury to the user and should be discarded into a sharps container while still attached to the syringe.[1;30]

Vials

Injectable medications are supplied in vials or ampules, each requiring different techniques for withdrawal of the medication. A vial is a plastic or glass container with a rubber or plastic stopper secured to its top with a metal ring. Multidose vials contain preservatives that allow the contents to be used after the stopper has been penetrated. The stopper is usually covered by a plastic flip top or metal cap, but these caps do not assure sterility of the stopper. Once the vial is placed in the PEC and the cap is removed, the stopper must be swabbed with a sterile 70% IPA swab and allowed to dry before needle entry. The correct technique for swabbing the vial is several firm strokes of the swab in the same direction over the rubber stopper. The swabbing is effective in the following ways:

- The alcohol acts as a disinfecting agent.
- The physical act of swabbing removes particles from the stopper.

Although 70% IPA is a chemical disinfectant, there are resistant spores that can thrive in it. Spray or bulk bottles of sterile 70% isopropyl alcohol should not be used to disinfect vial stoppers. Only sterile swabs from a manufacturer must be used.

When vial stoppers are punctured with needles, there is a possibility that cores or fragments from the stopper can be pushed into the sterile liquid in the vial. To prevent this problem, the needle should be inserted in the center of the stopper at the same point with both the tip and heel of the bevel facing up. This noncoring technique is accomplished by first piercing the closure with the bevel tip and then applying lateral pressure (away from the bevel) and downward pressure to insert the needle (see **Figure 15-5**).

Vials are closed-system containers. Air and fluid cannot pass freely in or out of them. Therefore, the volume of fluid to be removed from a vial should be replaced with an equal or near-equal volume of air before withdrawing the fluid to avoid creating a vacuum. This technique should not be used with drugs that produce gas when reconstituted (eg, ceftazidime) or with hazardous drugs. Closed system drug-transfer devices (CSTDs) are commercially available. They allow solutions to be added to or withdrawn from vials while equalizing pressure in a closed system and preventing exposure to hazardous drug droplets. These devices are required

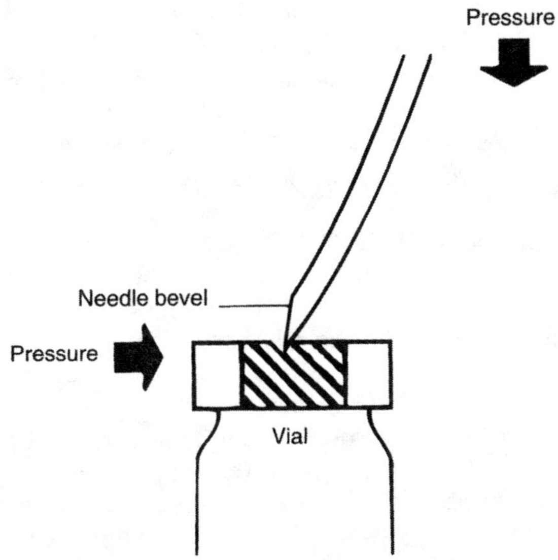

FIGURE 15-5. A noncoring method of piercing a vial with a needle

when working with hazardous drugs. Chapter 27 provides more detailed information on the use of these devices.

If a drug within a vial is in a powdered or lyophilized form, it must be reconstituted first. The desired volume of diluent is injected into the vial. The manufacturer's label should be checked for the recommended volume because the powder may also take up volume. After the diluent is added, an equal or near-equal volume of air must be removed to prevent a positive pressure from developing inside the vial and causing the contents of the vial to spray all over the inside of the PEC. This procedure may be accomplished by allowing air to flow into the same syringe before removing the needle from the vial. Although most drugs dissolve rapidly when a diluent is added and the vial is shaken or swirled, personnel must be sure that the drug is completely dissolved before proceeding. The manufacturer's label should be checked for information about how to mix the diluent with the drug. Some drugs cannot be shaken because the agitation may inactivate them, and they may require gentle swirling, rolling the vial, or simply allowing the vial to sit for several minutes.[1;30]

Ampules

Ampules are primarily made of glass, although there are newer plastic ampules now available. Once an ampule is broken, it becomes an open system, single-use container. Since air or fluid may now pass freely in and out of them, the volume of fluid removed does not have to be replaced with air. Before an ampule is opened, any visible solution in the top portion or head of the ampule should be moved to the bottom or body by one of the following methods:

- Swirling the ampule in an upright position
- Tapping the head with one's finger
- Inverting the ampule and then quickly swinging it into an upright position

To properly open an ampule, its neck should be cleaned with a sterile 70% IPA swab and the swab should be left in place wrapped around the neck. This swab is used to protect the compounder from accidental cuts to the fingers and the spraying of glass particles and aerosolized drug. There are also commercial devices available to prevent these accidents. These devices are not sterile and must be completely disinfected with sterile 70% IPA before use. They slip over the head of the ampule. The head of the ampule should be held between the thumb and index finger of one hand, and the body should be held with the thumb and index finger of the other hand. Pressure should be exerted with both thumbs, pushing away from oneself in a quick motion to snap the ampule open at the neck. Ampules should not be opened toward the HEPA filter of the PEC or toward other items in the direct compounding area. Extreme pressure may result in crushing the head between the thumb and index finger. Most ampules are scored or have a weak point in the neck, so if the ampule does not open easily, it should be rotated so that the pressure on the neck is exerted at a different angle.

To withdraw medication from an ampule, it should be tilted, and the bevel of the needle should be placed in the upper corner space or shoulder near the opening. Glass particles generally settle to the bottom of the ampule, and this technique reduces the risk of aspirating glass into the syringe. Surface tension should keep the solution from spilling out of the tilted ampule. The syringe plunger is then pulled back to withdraw the solution.

The use of a sterile filter needle or straw eliminates glass or paint chips that may have fallen into the solution from being drawn up into the syringe. A filter needle contains a 5-µm filter in the hub. It can be attached to the syringe before the solution is withdrawn from the ampule or after the solution has been withdrawn. If it is added before withdrawing the solution from the ampule, the filter needle must be removed after the solution is withdrawn and replaced with a new sterile needle before adding the drug to another container. If the solution is withdrawn from the ampule with a regular sterile needle, that needle should be replaced with a filter needle before adding the drug to another container. Suspensions should be withdrawn from an ampule using the latter technique. In all cases, the same filter needle should not be used for both withdrawing and injecting because it will nullify the filtering effort. Filter straws may only be used to draw up the solution from the ampule. The straw must then be changed to a regular needle before the medication can be injected into another container.[1;30]

Final Containers

Sterile preparations may be compounded in various final containers, including flexible plastic bags, glass bottles, semirigid plastic containers, syringes, and vials. Flexible plastic bags made of polyvinyl chloride (PVC) or polyolefin are easy to store compared to glass bottles, less likely to break, and do not require venting.

PVC bags are available in several sizes and solution types. These bags are supplied in plastic overwraps, which limit fluid loss, discourage tampering, and help maintain the sterility of the primary bag. After this overwrap is removed, the primary bag of solution should be used according to the manufacturer's recommendations. The injection port or critical site of the bag is covered by a protective tip or septum, and it should be positioned toward the HEPA filter when an intravenous (IV) admixture is prepared so that the first air is not obstructed and air turbulence is minimized in the DCA.[1;30]

COMPOUNDING A STERILE PREPARATION

Before compounding, all materials should be obtained before entering the buffer area. Vials, ampules, parenteral solutions, and all sterile containers should be inspected for cloudiness, particulate matter, cracks or punctures, expiration dates, and any indications of defects.

Before placing items in the PEC, the outer package must be wiped down with sterile 70% IPA to disinfect it and remove excess particulate matter from the packaging. However, USP Chapter <797> states, "When sterile items, are received in sealed containers to keep them sterile until opening, the sterile items may be removed from the covering as the supplies are introduced into the ISO Class 5 PEC without the need to wipe the individual sterile supply items with sterile 70% IPA."[1] To minimize contamination, the discarded packaging should not be laid on any surface within the PEC.

Next, all injection surfaces or critical sites must be disinfected with sterile 70% IPA swabs. Drug fluid should be withdrawn from its container in the amount needed using the appropriate size syringe that will hold the desired volume. To obtain an accurate measurement, any air bubbles should be removed by the following method:

1. Pull back slightly on the plunger to remove any trapped fluid in the needle.
2. Hold the syringe vertically with the needle pointed up and tap the syringe to force the air bubbles to the top.
3. Depress the plunger to push out only the air.

The injection of drug into a bag requires insertion of a needle into the IPA-swabbed injection port and adding the drug by fully depressing the plunger. The injection port has two diaphragms that must be pierced (see **Figure 15-6**):

- Outer septum
- Inner diaphragm about 3/8 inch inside the injection port

To ensure fluid transfer into the IV bag, a needle longer than 3/8 inch must be used.

Adding medication to a glass infusion container begins with the removal of the protective cap from the IV bottle. The stopper is not guaranteed sterile, so it must be disinfected in the same manner as discussed in the vial section of

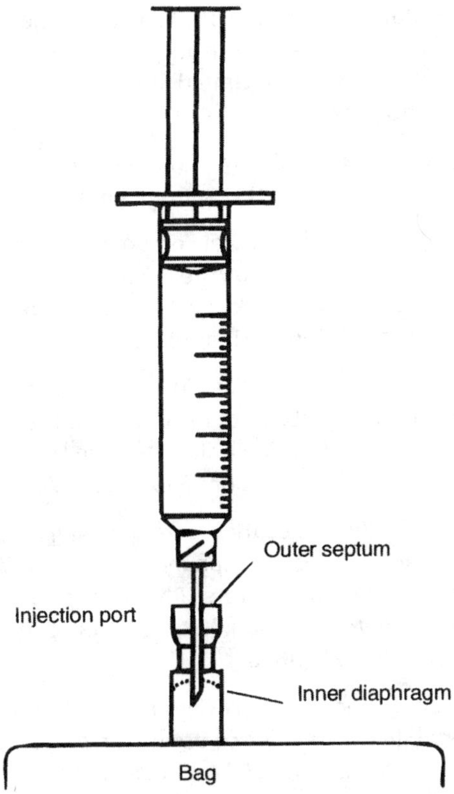

FIGURE 15-6. Injection of drug solution into an IV container

this chapter using a sterile 70% IPA swab. Needles should be inserted through the stopper using the same noncoring technique used for vials. Following admixture, the stopper should be disinfected again and allowed to dry, and a protective seal should be placed over the stopper before it is removed from the PEC. If the glass bottle is evacuated or has an internal negative pressure, no air needs to be removed as the volume of drug is added. If the glass bottle is not evacuated, the bottle may need to be vented while the fluid is being added to the bottle. This can be achieved by inserting a venting needle or device into the alcohol-swabbed stopper before adding the solution or drug, keeping it in the stopper until the solution or drug is added, and then removing it before adding the protective seal.

If the final preparation is in a syringe, the needle used in compounding must be removed and discarded. Before removing the syringe from the PEC, the syringe must be capped with a sterile cap or tip. A small amount of air or overfill may be left in the syringe for priming the needle or tubing before administering the dose. The syringe can be placed in a plastic bag or other container for transport to minimize the potential for plunger depression and or leakage. Commercial, sterile, tamper-evident caps are also available to prevent tampering with the contents of the syringe. Syringes and needles used in the compounding of a sterile preparation should be discarded according to institutional policies and regulatory requirements. Syringes and uncapped needles should be placed in puncture-resistant, sealable containers for proper disposal.

After the sterile preparation is compounded, it should be properly labeled and visually inspected for expected appearance, cores, and absence of particulates. All drug and IV solution containers should be checked by a pharmacist to verify that the compounder added the proper amount of the correct drugs to the correct IV solution and the correct label affixed to the compounded preparation.[1;30]

SUMMARY

Aseptic technique is essential to compounding sterile preparations. It requires that compounding personnel have specialized training and can demonstrate competency. Proper use of PECs, strict aseptic technique, and conscientious work habits are critical in preventing contamination. To assure accuracy and completeness, the label and final preparation must be approved by a registered pharmacist before dispensing and use.

REFERENCES

1. USP <797> Pharmaceutical compounding—sterile preparations. In: *USP Compounding Compendium*. Rockville, MD: United States Pharmacopeial Convention; 2023: Issue 1. **https://doi.usp.org/USPNF/USPNF_M99925_07_01.html**.
2. Griffenhagan GB. The history of parenteral medication. *Bull Parenter Drug Assoc*. 1962;16:129.
3. Howard-Jones N. The origins of hypodermic medication. *Sci Am*. 1971;224(1):96–102.
4. Seibert FB. Fever producing substances found in distilled water. *Am J Physiol*. 1923;67:90–104.
5. Masson AH. The early days of intravenous saline. *Pharm J*. 1976;217:571–580.
6. Dudrick SJ. Rational intravenous therapy. *Am J Hosp Pharm*. 1971;28(2):82–91.
7. Maki DG, Goldmann DA, Rhame FS. Infection control in intravenous therapy. *Ann Intern Med*. 1973;79:867–887.
8. Deeb EN, Natsios GA. Contamination of intravenous fluids by bacteria and fungi during preparation and administration. *Am J Hosp Pharm*. 1971;28(10):764–767.
9. Letcher K. In-use contamination of intravenous solutions in flexible plastic containers. *Am J Hosp Pharm*. 1972;29(8):673–677.
10. Curry CR, Quie PG. Fungal septicemia in patients receiving parenteral hyperalimentation. *N Engl J Med*. 1971;285(22):1221–1225.

11. McGowan JE. Six guidelines for reducing infections associated with IV therapy. *Am Surg*. 1976;42:713–715.

12. Duma RJ, Latta T. What have we done – the hazards of intravenous therapy. *N Engl J Med*. 1976;294:1178–1180.

13. National Coordinating Committee on Large Volume Parenterals. Recommended methods for compounding intravenous admixtures in hospitals. *Am J Hosp Pharm*. 1975;32:261–270.

14. National Coordinating Committee on Large Volume Parenterals. Recommended system for surveillance and reporting of problems with large-volume parenterals in hospitals. *Am J Hosp Pharm*. 1975;32:1251–1253.

15. National Coordinating Committee on Large Volume Parenterals. Recommendations for the labeling of large-volume parenterals. *Am J Hosp Pharm*. 1978;35(1):49–51.

16. National Coordinating Committee on Large Volume Parenterals. Recommended procedures for in-use testing of large-volume parenterals suspected of contamination or of producing a reaction in a patient. *Am J Hosp Pharm*. 1978;35(1):678–682.

17. National Coordinating Committee on Large Volume Parenterals. Recommended guidelines for quality assurance in hospital centralized intravenous admixture services. *Am J Hosp Pharm*. 1980;37(5):645–655.

18. National Coordinating Committee on Large Volume Parenterals. Recommended standards of practice, policies, and procedures for intravenous therapy. *Am J Hosp Pharm*. 1980;37(5):660–663.

19. Barker KN, ed. *Recommendations of the NCCLVP for the Compounding and Administration of Intravenous Solutions*. Bethesda, MD: American Society of Hospital Pharmacists; 1981.

20. American Society of Health-System Pharmacists. ASHP Technical Assistance Bulletin on Quality Assurance for Pharmacy-Prepared Sterile Products. *Am J Hosp Pharm*. 1993;50(11):2386–2398.

21. USP <1206> Sterile drug products for home use. In: *USP 23rd Revision and the National Formulary*. 19th ed. Rockville, MD: The United States Pharmacopeial Convention; 1995.

22. 75th United States Congress. Federal Food, Drug, and Cosmetic Act. 1934. 21 U.S. Code §§ 301–392.

23. USP <797> Pharmaceutical compoundingsterile preparations. In: *USP, 20th Revision, and the National Formulary*. 15th ed. Rockville, MD: The United States Pharmacopeial Convention; 1997.

24. USP <797> Pharmaceutical compoundingsterile preparations. In: USP 27th Revision, and the National Formulary. 22nd ed. Rockville, MD: The United States Pharmacopeial Convention; 2004:2350–70.

25. USP <797> Pharmaceutical compoundingsterile preparations. In: *USP Compounding Compendium*. Rockville, MD: United States Pharmacopeial Convention; May 1, 2020. **https://doi.org/10.31003/USPNF_M99925_06_01**.

26. USP Compounding Expert Committee. Strength and stability testing for compounded preparations. Published January 13, 2014. Revised May 11, 2015. **https://www.usp.org/sites/default/files/usp/document/FAQs/strength-stability-testing-compounded-preparations.pdf**. Accessed August 11, 2023.

27. Trissel LA, Gentempo JA, Saenz LM, et al. Effect of two work practice changes on the microbial contamination rates of pharmacy-compounded sterile preparations. *Am J Health-Syst Pharm*. 2007;64(8):837–841.

28. Douglass K. Best Practices for compounding garbing. *Pharmacy Purchasing & Products*. January 2017. 14(1):6.

29. Erstad AJ, Erstat BL, Nix DE. Accuracy and reproducibility of small-volume injections from various-sized syringes. *Am J Health-Syst Pharm*. 2006;63(8):748–750.

30. Thane E. Understanding primary engineering controls in the lab. *MedicalLab Management*. April 2019;8(4):4-9.

16

ESTABLISHING BEYOND-USE DATES

Kevin N. Hansen

INTRODUCTION

It is the responsibility of the pharmacist or designated person to ensure that all compounded sterile preparations (CSPs) are assigned an appropriate beyond-use date (BUD) that considers both sterility and stability factors from the time the CSP is initiated, through storage, and up to the date and time the CSP is administered. BUDs should be established conservatively to ensure that the CSP maintains required characteristics (eg, stability, sterility) prior to administration. United States Pharmacopeia (USP) General Chapter <797> provides a standard on establishing BUDs for CSPs and provides guidance for compounders on assessing myriad factors that may limit a BUD, in addition to quality assurance testing, sterilization methods, or storage conditions that allows compounders to assign longer BUDs. It is crucial that compounders (eg, pharmacists, technicians) understand the principles for BUD assignment of CSPs and are able to effectively communicate to the administering personnel (eg, nurse)—usually through labeling—the intent of the BUD and what actions are required when the BUD date/time has been reached or surpassed. Establishing an appropriate BUD for a CSP embodies the array of the core purposes of USP Chapter <797>, through minimizing harm or death that could result from (1) microbial contamination, (2) excessive bacterial endotoxins, (3) variability for intended strength of correct ingredients, (4) physical and chemical incompatibilities, (5) chemical and physical contaminants, and (6) use of ingredients of inappropriate quality.[1]

TERMINOLOGY COMPARED

When communicating a BUD, it is essential to differentiate a BUD from an *expiration date*, *infusion-time* or *hang-time*, and *in-use time* (**Table 16-1**). The pharmacist must know how to handle situations when the respective date/time is reached and the appropriate actions to take. For example, a product with a listed expiration date must never be used past the listed dated, however a BUD may be used after the listed date/time if administration has already begun; or else it must be discarded. Misinterpretation or mix-ups between these terms could lead to either administration of a preparation that is outside of acceptable quality, or prematurely discarding a preparation that is acceptable for use leading to avoidable waste.

The term *in-use time* is not used nor defined in USP Chapter <797>, however it is often used in approved labeling of conventionally manufactured products and is used by the FDA. An in-use time is similar to that of a BUD, however the use is generally defined differently, since the product with the assigned in-use time is not intended as the final dosage form for CSP and is often used as a component of a CSP. For example, a conventionally manufactured drug vial may have a listed in-use time of 6 hours once punctured, however this is only referring to the use of the vial, and any remaining drug in the vial, and is not intended to limit the BUD of the final CSP created from the product. The in-use time—like a BUD—is not intended to limit the time during which the CSP is administered. In some cases, a manufacturer's in-use time may also include the administration or infusion time, and thus it is important to evaluate the labeling for specific information in how the in-use time is being defined and used. For example, the package insert for generic docetaxel injection intended for intravenous (IV) infusion over 1 hour states "docetaxel injection final dilution for infusion, if stored between 2°C and 25°C (36°F and 77°F), is stable for 4 hours. Docetaxel injection final dilution for infusion (in either 0.9% Sodium Chloride solution or 5% Dextrose solution) should be used within 4 hours (*including the 1 hour intravenous administration*)."[10] Therefore, assigning a BUD for this preparation of 4 hours is not appropriate, as it would violate the approved labeling for in-use time if administered at the end of the BUD. Thus, an approach should be to assign a BUD of 3 hours, which would be appropriate and include the maximum in-use time of 4 hours if administration begins within the BUD.[10]

DOI 10.37573/9781585286492.016

TABLE 16-1. Beyond-use Date Terminology Comparison

	Expiration	Beyond-Use Date	Infusion-Time or Hang-Time	In-Use Time
Definition	The time during which a product can be expected to meet the requirements of the *USP-NF* monograph, if one exists, or maintain expected quality provided it is kept under the specified storage conditions.[1]	The date, or hour and the date, after which a CSP must not be used, stored, or transported. The date is determined from the date and time the preparation is compounded.[1]	Allowable length of time for an infusion to be used before it must be taken down or exchanged. The time is determined from the date and time the infusion is spiked or accessed with administration set.[2;3]	The maximum amount of time that can be allowed to elapse between penetration of a container-closure system containing a sterile drug product, or after a lyophilized drug product has been reconstituted, and before patient administration.[4]
Applies to	Conventionally manufactured products, APIs, added substances	CSPs	Infusions (ie, CSPs or conventionally manufactured products)	Conventionally manufactured drug products
Based on	Extensive analytical and performance testing using validated methods following CGMP	Conservative risk-based estimates based on available data or limited testing and following USP Chapter <797>	Conservative risk-based estimates based on type of medication being infused, ability to support microbial growth, and following guidance from CDC and INS	Intended use (eg, single-dose, multiple-dose, bulk container) and with appropriate testing (eg, USP Chapter <51> antimicrobial effectiveness testing)
Assigned by	Manufacturer	Pharmacy	Nursing	Manufacturer
Guidance	FDA[5]	USP[1;6], ASHP[7]	CDC[8], INS[9]	FDA[4]

LABELING

The verbiage on the label that describes the assigned BUD can be used to effectively communicate with the administering user (eg, nurse). Establishing label design and verbiage with multidisciplinary involvement can ensure alignment and proper interpretation by individuals who compound, store, handle, or administer CSPs. It is prudent to evaluate the labeling software and design for any limitations to desired terms, which may be limited by character length or space. Listing the BUD on the label following the term "beyond-use date" or "BUD" may be desired, however it is not always clear on how to interpret this without providing education. With this, many organizations use alternative terms to "BUD" on the label with the intent of improving the communication of the listed BUD. Some terms used may be misleading and create additional concerns for inappropriate use, and thus should be avoided, while other terms may provide clarity, intuitiveness, and promote safe practices.[7]

Misleading Terms:

- **Expires:** This term does not communicate the intent of a BUD and may lead to prematurely wasting quality medication in addition to unnecessary aseptic manipulations to patient lines (eg, intravenous set), which may increase opportunities for contamination and patient harm.
- **Use by:** This term may have a similar interpretation as an expiration date and may lead to the same outcomes.
- **Administer by:** This term may imply that the administration must be completed or finished by this time, which is not the intent of a BUD.

Improved Terms:

- **Start administration by:** This term more clearly communicates the intent of the BUD and applies to all CSPs. Shortening "administration" to "admin" may allow for this term to be used based on label software or design.
- **Spike by:** This term is also improved, however it only applies to CSPs that involve an administration set with a spike (eg, IVPB), and does not apply to other CSPs (eg, ophthalmic injections, syringe infusion).

Once the administration of a CSP starts, it will be prudent for the administering user (eg, nurse) to follow organizational policy for allowable infusion- or hang-time of the preparation. In general, this time frame should not exceed 96 hours for most CSPs, which also may align with secondary tubing set change requirements.[2;3] For continuous infusions preparations, this may require that a new date be placed on the label/preparation to identify this allowable "infusion" or "hang-time," similar to how infusion lines are labeled. While the organization may have a blanket policy identifying this maximum allowable time frame, it will be key to identify certain preparations where the period should be much shorter (eg, lipid emulsions, TPN, blood products, etc.) or if indicated by the manufacturer's approved labeling.

STABILITY OVERVIEW

The *stability* of a CSP is an important factor—in combination with sterility factors—that must be determined when establishing a BUD for a CSP. The term "stability" when applied to CSPs refers to "The extent to which a product or preparation retains physical and chemical properties and characteristics within specified limits throughout its expiration or BUD."[1] There are five main generally recognized categories of stability that should be evaluated for a CSP when establishing a BUD, including: 1) chemical, 2) physical, 3) microbiological, 4) therapeutic, and 5) toxicological[11] (**Table 16-2**).

The overall stability of a CSP can be impacted by environmental conditions and dosage form factors (**Table 16-3**). Pharmacists must perform due diligence to ensure proper conditions are maintained throughout the assigned BUD based on available information from a manufacturer, published studies, or through performing a stability-indicating method study. This should include reevaluation of BUD assignment if any alterations of the CSP are made. For certain CSPs, seemingly negligible changes can have profound degradation effects and may show no visual signs that something adverse has occurred.[11]

When beginning to evaluate the stability of a specific CSP, there are several initial starting elements to review, including:

- **Active Ingredient(s)** (eg, cefazolin)
- **Diluent type** (eg, 0.9% sodium chloride, 5% dextrose in water)
- **Final Concentration(s)** (eg, 20 mg/mL)
- **Container closure system** (eg, IV bag)
- **Composition of container closure system** (eg, polypropylene)
- **Intended storage conditions** (eg, refrigerator)
- **Medication specific factors** (eg, protect from light, do not shake)

Evaluation of these basic elements should give the compounder an initial indication on the overall stability of the CSP and to determine if stability factors or sterility factors will be the rate limiting step for determination of a BUD. See the "Evaluating Stability Information" section in this chapter for a more in-depth review of stability factors and evaluation of stability data.

STERILITY OVERVIEW

The *sterility*—or more appropriately referred to in context as *sterility assurance*—of a CSP is an important factor for establishing a BUD and is often the limiting factor. The term "sterility" by its most strict definition includes the *complete* absence of viable microorganisms. This term may be misleading when applied to a CSP as *absolute sterility* cannot be practically demonstrated without the physical destruction of every article produced in addition to limitations in the sterility testing itself.[12;13]

There are two broad categorical approaches to sterilization methods for CSPs, including *aseptic processing* and *terminal sterilization*. Terminal sterilization involves a sterilization process (eg, dry heat, steam, radiation, etc.) of a CSP that produces measurable physical conditions that are lethal to microorganisms. Terminal sterilization processes are measurable and achieve validated performance of not more than 1 nonsterile unit in 1 million units produced, and

TABLE 16-2. Categories of CSP Stability

Type of Stability	Conditions Maintained
Chemical	Each active ingredient retains its chemical integrity and labeled potency, within the specified limits.
Physical	The original physical properties, including appearance, palatability, uniformity, dissolution, and suspendability, are retained.
Microbiological	Sterility or resistance to microbial growth is retained according to the specified requirements. Antimicrobial agents that are present retain effectiveness within the specified limits.
Therapeutic	The therapeutic effect remains unchanged.
Toxicological	No significant increase in toxicity occurs.

TABLE 16-3. Environmental and Dosage Form Factors Impacting Stability

Environmental Factors	Dosage Form Factors
Temperature, light, humidity, oxygen, carbon dioxide	Particle size, pH, solvent system composition, computability of anions and cations, solution ionic strength, primary container, specific chemical additives, molecular binding and diffusion of drugs and excipients

thus terminally sterilized products represent the lowest risk of the two methods. There are specific medications and container closure systems that cannot withstand the physical conditions produced during terminal sterilization cycles, and thus these must be prepared using alternative methods. *Aseptic processing* involves preventing introduction of microorganisms during the preparation process. This can be achieved by using only sterile starting ingredients and products or with the physical removal of any microorganisms—when using any nonsterile ingredients—with the inclusion of sterilization-grade filters. With aseptic processing, the sterility of the CSP and materials used must be protected during the entire process until the final preparation is sealed.[1] While either of these methods can be used singularly to produce a CSP, a process that involves both—postaseptic processing terminal sterilization—is superior than either method used alone, as the initial aseptic processing provides control of presterilization bioburden, and thus making subsequently terminal sterilization processes potentially more effective.[12]

USP Chapter <797> establishes CSP Categories: Category 1, Category 2, and Category 3 CSPs. Each of these categories is primarily based on the environment of which the CSP is prepared, the probability of microbial growth during the time they will be stored, and the time period for use of the CSP. There are myriad factors that may impact the likelihood of microbial growth, and thus USP Chapter <797> outlines specific requirements for each Category that also includes, but not limited to: personnel garbing practices, type and frequency of training & competency, cleaning and disinfecting, application of sporicidal agents, and environmental monitoring.[1]

ESTABLISHING BUDS

When establishing a BUD for a CSP it is prudent to determine the main limiting factor—sterility assurance or stability. If the limiting factor is sterility assurance, the CSP should be applied a BUD that corresponds with the CSP Category it was prepared under (ie, when all conditions for that Category are met) in addition to the CSP storage condition. If the limiting factor is stability, the CSP should be assigned a conservative BUD that may be less than the BUD limits outlined in each corresponding CSP Category BUD table. The BUDs that are outlined in the corresponding CSP Category tables are meant to be maximums (ie, limits), and thus cannot be exceeded. Within each of the CSP categories, there are additional factors that must be assessed for proper BUD assignment, including storage conditions, starting ingredients/components, sterilization method, and whether sterility testing will be performed with subsequent passing result.

Storage Conditions

CSPs can either be stored at controlled room temperature (20–25°C), in the refrigerator (2–8°C), or in the freezer (–25 to –10°C). CSPs that are stored in colder conditions (ie, refrigerator, freezer) can generally be applied longer BUDs compared to those stored at controlled room temperature, as these conditions have been shown to slow the growth of most microorganisms.[1] Certain CSPs cannot be stored in these colder conditions as it may adversely impact their chemical and physical stability (eg, precipitation). Further, certain container closure systems may be damaged by frozen conditions rendering them compromised (eg, cracking). Proper storage of CSPs should be evaluated as part of the BUD evaluation and assignment.

Starting Ingredients/Components

The starting ingredients or components must be assessed prior to assigning a BUD in whether they are sterile or nonsterile. The use of some or all nonsterile starting ingredients or components can be used for either Category 1, Category 2, or Category 3, however they must be subject to a sterilization step to ensure the final CSP is sterile. When using any nonsterile ingredients, components, supplies, or equipment to prepare a CSP, the use of mitigation strategies must be used to ensure the safety of the final CSP. This should include a quality evaluation of each component, ensuring the effectiveness of the sterilization step, and the use of bacterial endotoxin mitigation strategies. When using only sterile starting ingredients, the sterility of each component must be maintained throughout the compounding process.[1]

Sterilization Method

There are two main categories for sterilization methods of CSPs, including aseptic sterilization and terminal sterilization. Aseptic sterilization may be performed by using proper aseptic technique within a primary engineering control and only using sterile starting ingredients, components, supplies, and equipment. An alternative aseptic sterilization method is sterilization by filtration. For this method, a sterile, depyrogenated, pharmaceutical grade sterilization filter with a nominal pore size of 0.22-micron or smaller is used to filter a CSP or ingredient. If a sterilization filter is used, the filter must undergo an integrity test (eg, post-use bubble point test) to verify the filter was intact during filtration and was not damaged or torn. Terminal sterilization refers to a different type of sterilization method which applies a lethal process to an ingredient or CSP to conditions. These conditions can be achieved by steam heat, dry heat, or irradiation. Terminal sterilization has distinct advantages compared to aseptic processing as each process is intended to achieve a probability of a nonsterile unit (PNSU) of less than one nonsterile unit for every one million units produced, and the effectiveness of each terminal sterilization cycle can be determined using appropriate biological indicators. Due to the harsh conditions created by terminal sterilization cycles, it may not be appropriate for certain medications (eg, proteins), or container closure systems (eg, plastic syringe), as it may result in drug degradation or unintended alterations in the container closure system.[1]

Sterility Testing

The use of a sterility test is used to aid in the sterility assurance of a CSP, or batch of CSPs, and thus can generally be assigned a longer BUD compared to a CSP without sterility testing. Due to the destructive nature of sterility testing, a minimum of 2 CSPs must be compounded, of which one will be tested for sterility, while the other is held until the results of the sterility test have been finalized.[1] The traditional USP Chapter <71> sterility test is performed by using membrane filtration or direct inoculation. The samples are incubated for a minimum of 14 days and result as either sterile or not sterile. USP Chapter <71> outlines the specific number of samples that must be sent for testing based on the batch size, type of CSP (eg, parenteral solution, topical ophthalmic, antibiotic solid), and the volume of the CSP (eg, large-volume parenteral).[14] USP Chapter <1> defines large-volume injections where the container is labeled containing more than 100 mL.[15] The use of alternative sterility testing methods can be used, as long as they are validated for their intended purpose and shown to be noninferior to USP Chapter <71> testing methodologies.[1;16]

BUD FOR FINISHED CSP

Category 1 CSPs

Category 1 CSPs are prepared under the least controlled environmental conditions, and thus are assigned BUDs that are more restrictive, compared to Category 2 or Category 3 CSPs. The use of a primary engineering control (PEC) that produces ISO Class 5 unidirectional airflow is required for Category 1 CSPs, and the PEC may be placed in a segregated compounding area (SCA). These types of environments do not provide the same protections as seen in a cleanroom suite, further supporting restricted BUDs[1] (**Table 16-4**).

TABLE 16-4. Category 1 CSP Dating

Category 1 CSPs[1]		
Controlled Room Temperature (20–25°C)	Refrigerator (2–8°C)	Freezer (–25 to –10°C)
Either **sterile** or **nonsterile** starting components		
≤ 12 hr	≤ 24 hr	N/A

Source: Adapted with permission of USP <797> Pharmaceutical compounding—sterile preparations. In: *2023: USP Compounding Compendium*. Rockville, MD: United States Pharmacopeial Convention; 2023.

Category 2 CSPs

Category 2 CSPs are prepared within an ISO Class 5 PEC that is placed within a cleanroom suite, also known as a secondary engineering control (SEC). A SEC has additional protections through the use of controlled air environments through the use of HEPA filters, and additional requirements for environmental monitoring, cleaning and disinfecting, and application of sporicidal agents. Thus, BUD limits are higher than that of Category 1 CSPs. BUDs for CSPs aseptically processed that contain one or more nonsterile starting components have restricted BUDs when sterility testing is not performed. When terminal sterilization processes are used, BUDs are less restricted regardless if starting components are sterile or nonsterile[1] (**Table 16-5**).

If performing and passing a USP Chapter <71> sterility test (or a validated alternative method that is noninferior to USP Chapter <71>), the BUD limits for Category 2 CSPs can be further extended[1;16] (**Table 16-6**). USP Chapter <71> outlines the minimum number of articles that must be sampled based on the number of items in the batch (ie, batch size).[14] For batch sizes less than 40 CSPs, USP Chapter <797> provides guidance when additional CSPs must be prepared for sterility testing.[1] While awaiting the result of the sterility test (not less than 14 days for USP Chapter <71> testing), the remaining CSPs should be held in "quarantine" and not used until the passing results have been reported and performing a visual inspection prior to releasing to ensure the preparation meets appropriate quality characteristics. A bacterial endotoxin test following USP Chapter <85> is required for Category 2 CSPs that undergo sterility testing and have any nonsterile starting components and is recommended if using nonsterile starting components but not performing a sterility test. When performing sterility testing on a CSP batch, it is prudent to note that USP Chapter <797> has a maximum batch size of 250 final yield units.[1]

BUD for Additional CSP Types

In addition to finished, single-dose CSPs, there are a few other types of preparations that USP Chapter <797> outlines that has modified and/or additional requirements for establishing a BUD.

TABLE 16-5. Category 2 CSP Dating

	Category 2 CSPs[1]		
	Controlled Room Temperature (20–25°C)	Refrigerator (2–8°C)	Freezer (–25 to –10°C)
Aseptically processed	*One or more* **nonsterile** starting components		
	1 day	4 days	45 days
	Only **sterile** starting components		
	4 days	10 days	45 days
Terminally sterilized	*Either* **sterile** or **nonsterile** starting components		
	14 days	28 days	45 days

Source: Adapted with permission of USP <797> Pharmaceutical compounding—sterile preparations. In: *2023: USP Compounding Compendium*. Rockville, MD: United States Pharmacopeial Convention; 2023.

TABLE 16-6. Category 2 CSP Dating

	Category 2 CSPs[1]		
	Sterility testing performed and passed		
	Controlled Room Temperature (20°–25°C)	Refrigerator (2°–8°C)	Freezer (–25° to –10°C)
	Either **sterile** or **nonsterile** starting components		
	Perform and pass ***sterility test***		
Aseptically processed	30 days	45 days	60 days
Terminally sterilized	45 days	60 days	90 days

Source: Adapted with permission of USP <797> Pharmaceutical compounding—sterile preparations. In: *2023: USP Compounding Compendium.* Rockville, MD: United States Pharmacopeial Convention; 2023.

Proprietary Bag and Vial Systems

The docking of these types of systems to a vial—within an ISO Class 5 PEC—for *future* activation is considered compounding, according to USP Chapter <797>, however, it does not follow the same requirements for Category 1, Category 2, or Category 3 for establishing a BUD. For these types of systems, establishment of the BUD must be in accordance with the approved labeling or supplemental documentation provided by the manufacturer of the system. Each system has specific vial and/or diluent bag requirements that must be followed (eg, vial top diameter, lyophilized powder, liquid volume). These systems can offer distinct advantages for CSP sterility and stability as the drug in the vial and the diluent solution in the bag are not physically combined (ie, activated) until immediately prior to administration. Once activated, the contents should be promptly administered, otherwise the manufacturer's instructions should be followed to assign a BUD.[1]

Multiple-Dose CSPs

Multiple-dose CSPs require additional protections, usually with preservatives, as the container is entered multiple times, each with an opportunity to introduce contamination into the CSP. For these types of preparations, antimicrobial effectiveness testing following USP Chapter <51> must be conducted and passed (once for each formulation and container closure system).[1]

Stock Solution CSPs

Stock solutions generally do not contain any preservatives, and thus, once the finalized stock solution CSP is entered/punctured—within ISO Class 5 or cleaner air—the BUD of the stock solution should be reduced to 12 hours—or shorter based on CSP stability. Within the 12 hours the entire contents of the stock solution should be used, or it must be discarded. The reduced 12-hour BUD only applies to the stock solution that was accessed and is not intended to limit the BUD of the final CSP that is prepared from the stock solution. If extensive waste results from the reduced BUD, a strategy could be to reduce the volume of the stock solution during preparation into smaller aliquots, which may be particularly useful within pediatric or neonatal pharmacy compounding areas.[1]

Multiple-Dose Topical Ophthalmic CSPs

Certain topical ophthalmic products require dispensing for multiple-doses and to be free from preservatives. While preservatives are generally used to reduce risk of microbial proliferation within a multiple-dose CSP, certain preservatives have been known to be toxic to the ocular surface and thus are frequently prescribed without preservatives.[17] This presents a challenge to the compounder to prepare a multiple-dose CSP without preservatives and uncertainty if the CSP will pass antimicrobial effectiveness testing through USP Chapter <51>. For this scenario, USP Chapter <797> outlines specific requirements where a multiple-dose, nonpreserved, aqueous topical or topical CSP may be labeled as multiple-dose and not requiring USP Chapter <51> testing to be performed if the following requirements are met[1]:

- Prepared as a Category 2 or Category 3 CSP
- Prepared only for a single patient
- Labeled to indicate that once the CSP is opened, the BUD must be reduced to a maximum of 72 hours, if stored under refrigeration, or to a maximum of 24 hours, if stored at controlled room temperature

EXTENDED BEYOND-USE DATES

Under certain circumstances, the BUD limits for Category 2 may not be sufficient to meet patient needs, thus compounders may have a desire to assign a longer (ie, extended) BUD for identified CSPs up to a maximum of 180 days. There are 2 distinct pathways that compounders may assign an extended BUD for certain CSPs *when all required conditions are met.* This includes following the requirements for Category 3 CSPs—outlined in USP Chapter <797>—or through utilizing a published USP compounded monograph. Using extended BUDs may be desirable to prepare CSPs that can be placed in automated dispensing cabinets (ADCs) at controlled room temperature within the operating room or emergency department, where urgent access to ready-to-administer medications are needed for patient care. In many of these care areas, access to refrigeration may not be immediately accessible or is limited in capacity and leveraging Category 2 CSP BUDs may result in extensive waste if CSPs are not readily used. For extended BUDs, the CSPs are held for a longer period of time (ie, BUD) which can increase the risk of patient harm if the CSP was contaminated. Thus, significant increases in quality assurance, quality control, environmental monitoring, personnel training and competency assessment, cleaning and disinfecting, and other requirements must be used. Further, extended BUD CSPs require stability data using a stability-indicating analytical method. The CSP must be made according to the exact CSP that was studied, including the exact formulation, ingredients, and container closure system and materials. For a study to be "stability-indicating" it must be able to distinguish or separate the active ingredient from its degradants/impurities in addition to quantifying the active ingredient. This is often accomplished through the incorporation of a forced degradation study that exposes the CSP to varying amount of temperature, humidity, peroxide, acids/bases, and light.[18] It is important to differentiate a stability-indicating method from that of potency. While both methods may utilize high-performance liquid chromatography (HPLC), only a stability-indicating study can be used to deem the true stability of a preparation, as a potency study is unable to resolve the analyte from that of degradant peaks and may give false conclusions about the stability of a preparation. The difference between the two studies is in the methods. A stability-indicating study begins with method development, method validation, followed by carrying out the stability study.[1;6]

Category 3 CSPs

Category 3 CSPs can be prepared using either aseptic processing or terminal sterilization and utilize either sterile or nonsterile starting components. Sterility testing must be performed on every Category 3 CSP batch and passed prior to releasing for patient administration. The maximum batch size for any Category 3 CSP batch cannot exceed 250 final yield units. The longest BUD that can be applied within Category 3 is 180 days, for a CSP that has been terminally sterilized, performed and passed a sterility test, and stored in the freezer[1] (**Table 16-7**).

There are a multitude of conditions that must be met in order to prepare Category 3 CSPs, including[1]:

- **Training and competency:** garbing competency and aseptic manipulation competency increased to at least every 3 months
- **Garbing requirements:** only sterile garb and no exposed skin or hair (usually requires use of goggles) while in buffer room
- **Environmental monitoring:** more frequent surface sampling (each batch, weekly) and air sampling (monthly)
- **Applying sporicidal agent:** more frequently applied in most areas (weekly)
- **CSP testing (one time):**
    - Stability-indicating method study supporting BUD
    - Particulate matter for injections (USP Chapter <788>) or ophthalmic solutions (USP Chapter <789>)
    - Container closure-integrity test (USP Chapter <1207>)
- **CSP testing (each batch):**
    - Sterility test (USP Chapter <71> or validated alternative method in USP Chapter <1223>)
    - Endotoxin test, if using any nonsterile components (USP Chapter <85>)

As the environment of preparation is an important factor in determining the appropriate CSP category, when assigning Category 3 CSPs, the conditions listed above must be continuously met in the buffer room. Therefore, if wanting to prepare Category 2 CSPs in the same buffer room where Category 3 CSPs are prepared, all staff within the buffer room must meet the more strict, additional requirements of Category 3 CSPs (see above).[1]

USP Compounded Monograph

The *United States Pharmacopeia* (USP) has 3 main areas that it publishes, including General Notices, General Chapters,

TABLE 16-7. Category 3 CSP Dating

	Category 3 CSPs		
	Sterility testing performed and passed		
	Controlled Room Temperature (20–25°C)	Refrigerator (2–8°C)	Freezer (–25 to –10°C)
	Either **sterile** or **nonsterile** starting components		
	Perform and pass **sterility test**		
Aseptically processed	60 days	90 days	120 days
Terminally sterilized	90 days	120 days	180 days

Source: Adapted with permission of USP <797> Pharmaceutical compounding—sterile preparations. In: *2023: USP Compounding Compendium*. Rockville, MD: United States Pharmacopeial Convention; 2023.

and Monographs. The General Notices are the default conditions for applying USP standards and contain basic assumptions and definitions that apply to both General Chapters and Monographs. The General Chapters are outline tests and procedures which are referred to in multiple monographs. Lastly, Monographs contain specific information, definitions, specifications, and requirements related to bulk substances, finished dosage forms, and for compounded preparations. In some cases, the information provided in a monograph may differ than the requirements outlined in either the General Notices or General chapters, and in these instances the Monograph supersedes. A USP compounded monograph may contain the following information[6;19]:

- **Definition:** eg, "fentanyl citrate compounded injection contains NLT 90.0% and NMT 110.0% of the labeled amount of fentanyl..."[20]
- **Ingredients and amounts:** eg, "fentanyl citrate 5,000 mcg, sodium chloride for injection (0.9%), a sufficient quantity to make 100 mL..."[20]
- **Assay**: information on performing the assay with specific acceptance criteria
- **Specific Tests:** tests required to perform for quality assurance (eg, "pH <791>: 4.0 – 7.5, Sterility Test <71>, Bacterial endotoxin test <85>, particulate matter in injections <788>...")[20]
- **Additional requirements:** base information on the packaging, storage, labeling, and beyond use date (eg, "after successful completion of sterility and endotoxin testing, NMT 90 day after the date of which it was compounded when stored at controlled room temperature...")[19]

In the example provided above for fentanyl citrate compounded injection, the resulting BUD when all conditions are met is 90 days stored at controlled room temperature. The preparation instructions for this monograph outlines the use of a 0.22-micron filter, which would be considered aseptic sterilization. When comparing the BUD within the monograph to that within USP Chapter <797> for Category 3, aseptically prepared, controlled room temperature, would result in 60-day BUD. Since the information in the monograph differs than that of USP Chapter <797>, the information in the monograph would supersede the information within the general chapter, and thus applying a BUD of 90 days at controlled room temperature would be acceptable.[20]

EVALUATING STABILITY INFORMATION

While having robust stability-indicating method studies for a specific CSP is ideal, these tests are extremely expensive and cost prohibitive to use widely on every CSP produced. Thus, it is important to know how to evaluate the appropriateness of a CSP formulation and BUD assignment based on available information. This often requires analyzing published stability studies, compatibility information, y-site administration data, and other available information that can help the compounder in establishing an appropriate BUD.

Stability Versus Potency or Strength

A stability study will include the potency or strength of a given medication or ingredient within a CSP; however, not all potency tests can determine stability. The difference between a stability-indicating study and a non-stability indicating potency study is within the methods. Stability-indicating method studies can quantify how much of an active pharmaceutical ingredient (API) is within a given CSP sample, but the study is also validated to separate the API from any containing excipients, degradants, or impurities; whereas a potency study is unable to do this. The difference at face value may appear to have limited advantage, especially given the extreme cost differences between these two methods. However, the resultant difference could be a completely degraded API within a CSP that appears to be perfectly stable when using a non-stability indicating potency over time study, as the degradants are not resolved and the peaks on the chromatogram appear to be that of the API, giving false conclusions to the compounder. The utility of a potency over time study is limited; and may be more valuable to perform an initial potency analysis as close to time point zero as possible to validate the compounding calculations and measurements were performed to a certain degree of accuracy.[21]

Manufacturer Information

Sometimes it is not possible to adhere to the product-approved labeling and guidelines. For example, a higher concentration of drug may be prescribed, a different diluent may be required, or a patient may require a preparation for longer periods such as to the home. Pharmacists should consult the product literature or obtain written information from the manufacturer to establish appropriate beyond-use dating. Deviations from information in the package insert should be communicated when requesting stability information, including the strength, diluent, fill volume, and container type (eg, PVC bag, plastic syringe, and elastomeric infusion device).

Published Stability Information

Published stability information, if carefully applied, can help to determine a theoretical BUD for a given CSP. References on drug stability include the *Handbook on Injectable Drugs, Remington: The Science and Practice of Pharmacy, Extended Stability for Parenteral Drugs,* and published research studies.[22–24] Applying published stability data can introduce inaccuracies if the characteristics of the preparation to be compounded differ greatly from the characteristics of the reported products. The equivalency of data for differing characteristics (eg, composition, concentrations of ingredients, fill volume, and container type and material) should not be assumed. The conditions during in-home use (eg, homes without air conditioning in a hot climate) should also be considered. Informational resources used to establish BUDs should be reliable, referenced, and respected. Word of mouth and historical precedent are never acceptable references. BUDs predicted from published resources should not extend beyond the realistic and practical patient care needs and operational capabilities of the pharmacy. Pharmacists should maintain a record of resources used for establishing BUDs and develop policies and procedures for their appropriate assignment. A referenced table or chart of accepted BUDs for commonly prepared products may be helpful, saving time and resources, and ensuring consistency in the organization.

Preparation-specific Experimental Studies

Preparation-specific experimental studies are the only valid evidence of stability from which beyond-use dating should be predicted. The greater the doubt about the accuracy or applicability of available stability data, the greater the need is to establish beyond-use dating experimentally. For example, failure of one preparation to support bacterial and fungal growth under specific conditions should not be extrapolated to other preparations unless specific and reliable data are available. Experimental studies should always be considered for high-risk sterile preparations compounded from nonsterile ingredients. Semiquantitative procedures, such as thin-layer chromatography, may be acceptable for some preparations. Quantitative stability-indicating assays (eg, high-performance liquid chromatography) are more appropriate for critical preparations. Examples include drugs with the following:

- A narrow therapeutic range
- Minimal supporting evidence of an appropriate beyond-use dating period
- A significant margin of safety that cannot be verified for the proposed theoretical period

Container-specific studies should identify other contaminants or byproducts of container or drug breakdown that are not present in the control preparation.

CSP Incompatibility and Instability

Common incompatibilities or instabilities often are classified as physical or chemical, although all incompatibilities are chemical-based phenomena. In some cases, incompatibilities can result from solubility changes or interactions with the container rather than to molecular changes in the active ingredient.

- **Incompatibility:** Refers to a physical or chemical phenomenon that reduces the concentration of the active ingredient(s). Examples include concentration-dependent precipitation and acid-base reactions. Physical or visual incompatibilities are terms that describe visible changes in the appearance of a preparation, such as precipitation, cloudiness or haziness, color change, viscosity change, cracking, and effervescence.
- **Instability:** Usually refers to the chemical processes that result in a degradation or change in the active ingredients, including hydrolysis, oxidation, reduction, and photodegradation reactions. These changes are generally continuous and irreversible, and can form degradation products, which are therapeutically inactive and may exhibit toxicity. Examples include hydrolysis, oxidative, and other heat-catalyzed reactions.[11,18,21,24] Instability incompatibilities can result from solubility changes or interactions with the container rather than to molecular changes in the active ingredient.

Physical Incompatibilities

Many factors can affect the stability of medications.[11] **Table 16-8** provides examples of the most common factors and their causes.[22,23,26]

Solubility

Drugs can be maintained in aqueous solution as long as their concentrations are below the saturation solubility. Supersaturated solutions are likely to precipitate or form crystals. Drugs with poor water solubility are often formulated with water-miscible cosolvents such as ethanol, propylene glycol, and polyethylene glycol (see Chapter 10). For example, dilution of diazepam from the commercial dosage form may result in precipitation at some concentrations, while further dilution below the saturation solubility point can result in a stable preparation.[27–29]

pH Effect on Solubility

The solubility of drugs that are weak acids or weak bases is related to the pH of the diluent solution. Weak acids or weak bases that are insoluble in aqueous diluents are converted into salts to increase their solubility. Weak acids usually are made into salts of weak acids and strong bases (eg, penicillin G potassium, pantoprazole sodium), while weak bases are made into salts of weak bases and strong acids (eg, morphine sulfate, isoproterenol hydrochloride). As a rule, salts of weak acids and strong bases are physically and chemically incompatible with salts of weak bases and strong acids. Salts of weak acids and strong bases (eg, ampicillin sodium) are generally less stable in acidic IV solutions (eg, dextrose 5%) than in neutral or higher pH solutions (eg, normal saline). Some drug products are available in nonaqueous diluents that increase their solubility and stability (eg, diazepam, digoxin, and phenytoin sodium injection). These drugs may undergo a "change of solvent" or pH effect in aqueous IV solutions, resulting in precipitation or chemical instability.

Solubility of Large Organic Ions

Large organic anions and cations also may form precipitates or insoluble complexes. For example, heparin (a large anionic complex) may precipitate with cationic drugs such as

TABLE 16-8. Factors Impacting CSP Stability

Factor	Incompatibility or Instability	Common Examples
Freezing temperature	Inactivation, denaturation, cracking	Heparin, filgrastim, erythropoietin, lipid-containing TPN
Low temperature (refrigerated)	Crystallization or precipitation	5-fluorouracil, furosemide, acyclovir, metronidazole
Temperature above 8 °C	Accelerated chemical degradation reactions	Ampicillin, others
Light (natural and room)	Accelerated chemical degradation reactions	Dobutamine, furosemide, cisplatin, hydroxyzine, carboplatin
Contact with metal (eg, needles or components of devices)	Chemical reaction	Hydralazine, metronidazole (with aluminum)
Large organic anions and cations	Precipitation or formation of insoluble complex	Heparin with aminoglycosides
Plastic containers, sets, in-line filters	Adsorption of lipophilic agents—especially important at low concentrations	Sufentanil, filgrastim, calcitriol, lorazepam, aldesleukin, insulin
PVC or flexible plastic container permeability	Evaporation, with resultant overconcentration of solution	PVC or flexible plastic containers distributed in overwrap bags, small volume bags are most susceptible
Plasticizer content of PVC containers, sets	Leaching carcinogenic plasticizer DEHP from DEHP-containing PVC	Paclitaxel, lipid emulsion, cyclosporine
Saturation solubility exceeded	Precipitation or crystallization	Morphine sulfate, etoposide

DEHP = di-2-ethylhexylphthalate; PVC = polyvinyl chloride; TPN = total parenteral nutrition.

Source: Adapted with permission of USP <797> Pharmaceutical compounding—sterile preparations. In: *2023: USP Compounding Compendium.* Rockville, MD: United States Pharmacopeial Convention; 2023, ASHP's Interactive Handbook on Injectable Drugs [online database]. Bethesda, MD: American Society of Health-System Pharmacists, and Lima HA. Drug stability and compatibility: special considerations for home care. *Infusion.* 1996;2:11–16.

aminoglycosides. This precipitation depends on whether the solubility product of the heparin salt of the cationic drug is exceeded. As a result, precipitation is more likely to occur at high concentrations (if the drugs are not sufficiently diluted).

Solubility Issues in Parenteral Nutrition Solutions and Total Nutrient Admixtures

The complexity of parenteral nutrition formulations (eg, amino acids, dextrose, fat emulsion, multiple monovalent and divalent electrolyte salts, trace minerals, and vitamins) provides ample opportunity for the formation of insoluble salts. The Food and Drug Administration published a safety alert on the hazards of precipitation associated with parenteral nutrition formulations. Medical personnel and patients or caregivers who administer parenteral nutrition formulations should be trained to visually inspect the preparation for precipitation or other evidence of degradation.[30]

Calcium–Phosphate Solubility Issues

The risk of dibasic calcium phosphate salt formation and precipitation is well documented in the literature.[23;30–34] Although dibasic calcium phosphate is nearly insoluble in water, monobasic calcium phosphate is relatively soluble. The pKa is 7.2 for the equilibrium between dibasic and monobasic phosphate ions. Increases in pH will elevate dibasic phosphate ions, which increases the probability of dibasic calcium phosphate precipitation. Highly reactive salts (eg, sodium bicarbonate and calcium chloride) should be avoided as additives, as they can also contribute to precipitate formation. Calcium phosphate precipitation also may be related to temperature. As temperature rises, particle movement increases the probability of a reaction between free calcium and dibasic phosphate ions. This effect may explain the reported occurrence of calcium phosphate precipitation in the lumen of central venous catheters and the parenteral nutrition solution tubing for infants in incubators. Other factors include high concentrations of calcium and phosphate salts, increases in solution pH, increases in temperature, the addition of calcium before phosphate in the admixture process, lengthy time delays or slow infusion rates that increase exposure of the preparation to room temperature conditions, and use of the chloride salt of calcium. Low amounts of amino acids in the final preparation decrease the buffer capability of the solution, which can also contribute to calcium phosphate insolubility.

These factors can improve solubility and enhance the stability of the preparation and individual components when determining an appropriate BUD for parenteral nutrition solutions:

- Increased amino acid concentrations buffer the preparation.
- A lower pH reduces the dibasic phosphate salt available for precipitation with calcium.
- Lower storage (refrigerated) and administration temperature reduces the risk of precipitation.
- Use the more stable salts of calcium (gluconate or acetate rather than chloride) whenever possible.
- When using an automated compounding device, always follow the manufacturer's protocol for additives.
- Base the calculation of the calcium solubility on the volume of the preparation at the time the calcium is added, not on the final solution volume.
- For 2-in-1 solutions (no lipids added), keep the calcium concentration below 10 mEq/L and the phosphorus (phosphate) concentration below 30 mM/L to decrease the risk of precipitation.

Emulsion Integrity Issues with Total Nutrient Admixtures (TNAs)

The 3-in-1 or TNAs (in which dextrose, amino acids, and fat emulsions/lipids are combined in one container) require additional steps to ensure the stability of the resulting emulsion. The mixing order is critical. Lipids should never be added directly to dextrose before amino acids are added. TNA emulsions are not stable below a final pH of 5, limiting their use in pediatric or neonatal parenteral nutrition solutions containing (highly acidic) cysteine hydrochloride.[33] Concentrations of divalent cations, such as calcium and magnesium, should be limited to avoid destabilizing the emulsion. Because no foolproof method has been found to predict TNA stability, the assigned BUDs should be conservative based on all contributing factors.

Sorption

Occurs when drug is lost (from the solution to be administered) by adsorption to the surface or absorption into the matrix of the container material, administration set, or filter. The longer the contact time with the matrix, the more sorption and less availability of the drug in solution. Drugs that exhibit sorption properties include nitroglycerin, diazepam, vitamin A, dactinomycin, insulin, sufentanil, filgrastim, calcitriol, lorazepam, and aldesleukin. Beyond-use dating for these types of drugs is typically very short.

Adsorption

When drugs are administered in small quantities or at low concentrations, a clinically relevant amount may be adsorbed and removed from solution. In these cases, adsorption plays an important role in determining the beyond-use dating. Drugs administered in larger concentrations or doses lose a smaller percentage of the total dose because of saturation of the binding sites on the container surface.

Absorption

Absorption into the matrix of plastic containers and administration sets, especially ones made of polyvinyl chloride (PVC), is a source of loss for lipid-soluble drugs (eg, vitamin A). Phthalate plasticizers are used in some containers to make the plastic soft and flexible, but lipid-soluble drugs diffuse into them. Plastics that contain little or no phthalate plasticizers (eg, polyethylene, polypropylene, and ethylvinyl acetate [EVA]) do not readily absorb lipid-soluble drugs. Because of this difference in absorption potential, specialized containers or administration sets should be used for some solutions of highly susceptible medications (eg, nitroglycerin, amiodarone). Short and small diameter administration sets can further reduce the surface area exposed for absorption. Some lipid-soluble medications can cause phthalate plasticizers to leach from the container or set into the solution. Concerns have been expressed about the extraction of the plasticizer di-2-ethylhexylphthalate (DEHP) by lipid emulsions.[36] To avoid the formation of toxic hydroperoxides, lipid emulsions should be packaged in glass containers only.[37] Repackaging them in plastic IV bags, which are relatively permeable to oxygen, should be avoided. TNAs can be packaged in plastic because the antioxidant from the amino acid product also protects the lipid emulsion; however, non-DEHP-containing bags are preferred, especially for pediatric or neonatal patients. Non-DEHP bags (which utilize alternative plasticizers), EVA bags, and other non-PVC bags and containers are available. Dual-chamber container systems allow for the mixture of less stable or problematic preparations just before administration to the patient. These types of systems may be particularly helpful for advance preparation of multiple days' supply of TNA for patients in alternate site care.

Other Physical Incompatibilities

Other physical incompatibilities that can occur immediately or over time include the following:

- "Salting out" or precipitation of organic drugs in the presence of strong electrolytes
- Complexation phenomena such as the formation of chelates of tetracycline with aluminum, calcium, iron, and magnesium
- Color changes from chemical degradation to a colored decomposition product
- Gas evolution

Chemical Degradation in CSPs

Drugs may undergo degradation or inactivation by various chemical reactions. Although some reactions can produce visible changes, such as color and gas evolution, many chemical incompatibilities are not visually observable.[11]

Hydrolysis, Oxidation, and Reduction

Hydrolysis reactions involve the attack of labile bonds by water in dissolved drug molecules with resultant molecular changes. Hydrolysis rates increase exponentially with increases in temperature; consider the cumulative non-cold exposure time when evaluating the stability of a temperature-labile CSP.[1] Hydrolysis can be accelerated by high or low pH or the presence of specific chemicals as catalysts.[11] Oxidation and reduction reactions involve exchange of electrons and valence changes which can inactivate drug molecules. To control oxidation reactions in commercial parenteral products, manufacturers evacuate oxygen from glass containers and fill any head space with nitrogen. They may also adjust pH, add buffering agents to stabilize pH, add chelating agents such as EDTA (ethylenediaminetetraacetic acid), add antioxidants such as sodium bisulfate, or package in opaque or light-protecting containers.[11] When medications are diluted, these antioxidant, buffering, or antimicrobial properties may be lost.[1]

Photochemical Decomposition

Photodegradation is the catalysis of degradation reactions by light. Photolysis and photo-oxidation decomposition mechanisms involve energy (light) which causes changes at chemical bonds and resultant changes to the chemical entity.[11] The more intense a light source is and the closer the photolabile drugs are to it, the greater is the rate of photodegradation.[25] Ultraviolet light is more destructive than visible light, and daylight has more damaging effects than fluorescent light on photolabile preparations. To preserve the integrity of photolabile drugs, they must be protected from light. Preparation containers and, when necessary, tubing, can be overwrapped with foil or light blocking amber plastic. Drugs identified as extremely photo labile may require light protection from the initiation of compounding through the conclusion of administration. The overwrap on each preparation and final administration container must be properly labeled to facilitate their identity.

Stability Related to Drug Delivery Systems

When assigning beyond-use dating to a CSP, the potential impact of the container type and material, drug delivery system, and the environmental temperature during distribution, storage, and administration should always be considered. Although some practitioners may choose to extrapolate stability test results from one type of container to another, there are many examples of variation in stability data among container types.[22] For example, one study noted that vitamin C (ascorbic acid) and vitamin B1 exhibited more stability in TNA bags made from a multilayered plastic than in EVA bags.[38]

Large Volume Parenterals

Large volume parenteral admixtures are most often used to administer one or more medications or electrolytes over a longer time period or continuously. Multiple-ingredient preparations (such as parenteral nutrition), which must be infused over extended time periods, have a significantly increased potential for drug stability and compatibility problems because of the long contact time and exposure to ambient temperature and light conditions.

Higher Concentration Delivery Systems

Intermittently administered medications are often prepared at greater concentrations than are typical for large volume infusions. For example, medications in small volume containers, such as 25- to 100-mL bags or single elastomeric containers are more concentrated and generally infused over an appropriately short time period. Medications packaged in syringes are usually even more concentrated and are often administered by IV push or syringe pump. Reservoirs of drugs used for controlled intermittent administration via ambulatory electronic pumps may be extremely concentrated, depending on the drug and patient's IV access. If more than one concentrated drug is combined in a syringe, small volume container, or reservoir, the potential for an incompatibility or other instability is increased due to high concentrations as well as prolonged contact time.

Y-site Administration

For patients with limited venous access, a Y-site technique may be the only available method of administering additional medications. Y-site (and piggyback) drug delivery can reduce the potential for incompatibilities by decreasing the contact time of multiple ingredients and solutions.[39] Relatively few combinations of drugs are so chemically unstable that Y-site administration is precluded.[23] However, a study simulating the Y-site administration of 106 drugs into 9 different TNA formulations revealed that 23 were incompatible with one or more components of the TNA; 6 resulted in precipitates, and 17 caused disruption of the TNA emulsion.[40] Practitioners should ensure that the Y-site route will not affect either the administered drug or the contents of the primary container.

Overwrap Removal

The manufacturers of parenteral solutions packaged in PVC containers have established maximum usage times after removal from the commercial overwrap (Table 20-3 in Chapter 20 summarizes the manufacturer recommendations).[22] The primary consideration is aqueous evaporation through the PVC, resulting in decreased volume of the solutions and alteration of additive concentration. Once additives are placed in these containers, the BUD should be the shorter of the drug stability dating or the solution manufacturer's maximum recommended time for use after removal from the overwrap and storage at room temperature.

COMPOUNDING COMPENDIUM RESOURCE

With each CSP that an organization prepares, timely access to proper stability and sterility information should be readily available to compounding staff. Some CSPs require in-depth study of available information and may result in patient care delays, inappropriate BUD assignment, or omission of key quality steps (eg, filtration, container-closure requirements). To remedy this, every organization should develop an internal resource that provides this information readily and should be reviewed on a periodic basis for accuracy, change in manufacturer's labeling, or availability of new stability study information.

The following are considerations of information to include—but not limited to—in an organization's Compounding Compendium Resource:

- **Drug Vial**
    - What is the drug name (generic, brand)?
    - What is the relative cost of the drug?
    - What vial size is used?
    - Is the vial an SDV or MDV?
    - Does the vial contain preservatives?
    - What is the drug dosage form? (ie, lyophilized powder, in solution, etc.)
    - What type and amount of diluent is required?
    - What is the final concentration after dilution?
    - What is the final withdrawable volume after dilution?
    - What is the BUD of the vial once accessed and/or reconstituted?
- **Preparation**
    - Are there any specialized preparation instructions?
    - What specific materials are required for the preparation?
        - Syringe type and size
        - Needle type, length, and gauge
        - Vented needles
    - Does the drug require to be passed through a filter needle?
- **Admixture**
    - What is the preferred infusion solution/diluent?
    - What alternative diluents are compatible?
    - What are common doses used?
    - Does the admixture require a specific concentration to be made?
    - What is the stability of the drug at each diluent and concentration?
    - How will the admixture be prepared (eg, patient-specific, in batches, etc.)?
    - What environment will the drug be prepared in?
    - What BUD should be assigned to the final CSP?
    - Does the drug require filtration during administration? Is filtration contraindicated?
- **Labeling and Storage**
    - Does the drug require it to be protected from light during storage and/or administration?
    - Will the drug be stored at room temperature or will it be refrigerated or frozen?
    - Can the admixture be sent via the pneumatic tube system (ie, do not tube)?
    - What auxiliary labels are required to be applied to the label?

Each CSP review should include appropriate references documented on the Compounding Compendium Resource, and when the information was last updated. The strategy for how the resource will be shared and updated should be considered. One approach could be to provide the information only in electronic format using a spreadsheet and access link. Careful consideration should be given on who is granted edit access to this document to prevent compounding errors that could lead to patient harm. This approach has advantages in that compounding staff are always looking at the most up-to-date version. There are disadvantages of this approach including access limitations if a computer is not readily available or if experiencing network issues, staff may download the file as a "flat file" and thus reference potentially out-of-date information. Another approach could be to only send out a flat file on a routine cadence (eg, monthly). This approach may allow staff to access the most up-to-date version both electronically and have a printed/laminated copy for quick access within the cleanroom. For printed and flat file copies, version control may be an issue. The use of an "expiration date" on the footer of the resource can ensure that staff know when to throw out the old copies and download the new version that is sent out with the routine cadence. Lastly, as updates are made to the resource—whether in print, or electronically—providing updates via a "change log" can greatly assist staff to know what has been added, removed, or modified. In the absence of providing a change log, staff may result to memory for certain compendium entries, and may not reference the document if the information has changed. Providing a change log will alert staff if a change in practice is required.

SUMMARY

Beyond-use dating has important cost and safety implications. Preparations with longer BUDs may allow more efficient batch compounding in pharmacies, less frequent deliveries for home and off-premises care settings, and recycling of unused preparations in hospitals. Batch compounded preparations may be subjected to greater quality control checks.

BUDs for CSPs must be based on stability and sterility considerations. Both physical and chemical breakdowns are possible. Solubility-related problems may occur from changes in pH, temperature, and drug structure. In addition, drug adsorption to and absorption within preparation containers must be considered. Chemical degradation due to hydrolysis, oxidation, reduction, or photolysis can also quickly deteriorate a preparation. Moreover, the method and environment of drug administration can affect the drug's stability.

Sterility is separate from but as important as stability. Although a CSP may be stable for an extended period, sterility also must be a factor in assigning a BUD. The potential for bacterial growth has been widely studied and verified. With an increased use of TPN, TNA, IG, and other sterile preparations in nonacute care settings requiring extended usage and administration time, this issue is of increasing importance. After considering physical, chemical, and delivery system effects, a pharmacist may still have to limit beyond-use dating. Although manufacturers and published references may provide sufficient information regarding extended stability, the pharmacist may need to conduct or contract for separate stability studies using accepted compendial methods.

APPENDIX 16-A. BUD REFERENCE CHART

Sterility Test (performed and passed)	Sterilization Method (aseptic or terminal)	Starting Components (sterile or nonsterile)	Controlled Room Temperature (20-25°C)	Refrigerator (2-8°C)	Freezer (−25° to −10°C)
Category 1 CSPs					
No	Either Method	Sterile or Nonsterile	12 hr	24 hr	N/A
Category 2 CSPs					
No	Aseptic Processing	Some Nonsterile	1 day	4 days	45 days
No	Aseptic Processing	Only Sterile	4 days	10 days	45 days
No	Terminal Sterilization	Sterile or Nonsterile	14 days	28 days	45 days
Yes	Aseptic Processing	Sterile or Nonsterile	30 days	45 days	60 days
Yes	Terminal Sterilization	Sterile or Nonsterile	45 days	60 days	90 days
Category 3 CSPs					
Yes	Aseptic Processing	Sterile or Nonsterile	60 days	90 days	120 days
Yes	Terminal Sterilization	Sterile or Nonsterile	90 days	120 days	180 days

REFERENCES

1. USP <797> Pharmaceutical compounding—sterile preparations. In: *2023: USP Compounding Compendium*. Rockville, MD: United States Pharmacopeial Convention; 2023.
2. Kienle P. Let's get clinical! Best practices for determining appropriate hang time for IV fluids. Cardinal Health Essential Insights. Published February 2014. **https://www.cardinalhealth.com/en/essential-insights/iv-fluid-hang-time.html**. Accessed May 17, 2023.
3. Centers for Disease Control and Prevention (CDC). Appendix B: summary of recommended frequency replacements for catheters, dressings, administration sets, and fluid. *MMWR Recommendations and Reports*. August 2002;51(RR10):29. **https://www.cdc.gov/mmwr/preview/mmwrhtml/rr5110a3.htm**.
4. U.S. Food and Drug Administration (FDA). Information for health care facilities and providers on "in-use time" | Covid-19. **https://www.fda.gov/drugs/coronavirus-covid-19-drugs/information-health-care-facilities-and-providers-use-time-covid-19#footnote1_4y0fyyg**. Published August 4, 2020.
5. U.S. Food and Drug Administration (FDA). Expiration dates – questions and answers. **https://www.fda.gov/drugs/pharmaceutical-quality-resources/expiration-dates-questions-and-answers**. Published October 24, 2022.

6. United States Pharmacopeia. Updates to USP general chapters <795> and <797>: Stability Study reference document for the 2021 proposed revisions to <795> and <797>. **https://go.usp.org/2022_Revisions_795_797**.

7. Pitt RD, Pilz J, Greubel J, et al. *The Pharmacists Guide to Assigning a Beyond Use Date to a Compounded Sterile or Nonsterile Preparation*. Bethesda, MD: American Society of Health-System Pharmacists; 2021. **https://www.ashp.org/-/media/assets/pharmacy-practice/resource-centers/compounding/docs/The-Pharmacist-Guide-to-Assigning-a-Beyond-Use-Date-_final.pdf**.

8. O'Grady NP, Alexander M, Burns LA, et al. *Guidelines for the Prevention of Intravascular Catheter-Related Infections, 2011*. Washington, DC: Centers for Disease Control and Prevention; 2011. **https://www.cdc.gov/hai/pdfs/bsi-guidelines-2011.pdf**.

9. Infusion Nurses Society (INS). *Infusion Therapy Standards of Practice*. 8th ed. Norwood, MA: Infusion Nurses Society; 2021. **https://www.ins1.org/publications/infusion-therapy-standards-of-practice/**.

10. DOCETAXEL-docetaxel anhydrous injection, solution [package insert]. Morgantown, WV: Mylan Institutional LLC; June 2022. Available at: **https://dailymed.nlm.nih.gov/dailymed/drugInfo.cfm?setid=2992d633-08fa-44f3-b14d-41700f24686b**. Accessed May 17, 2023.

11. USP <1191> Stability considerations in dispensing practice. In: *2023: USP Compounding Compendium*. Rockville, MD: United States Pharmacopeial Convention; 2023.

12. USP <1211> Sterilization and sterility assurance of compendial articles. In: *2023: USP Compounding Compendium*. Rockville, MD: United States Pharmacopeial Convention; 2023.

13. USP <1116> Microbiological control and monitoring of aseptic processing environments. In: *2023: USP Compounding Compendium*. Rockville, MD: United States Pharmacopeial Convention; 2023.

14. USP <71> Sterility tests. In: *2023: USP Compounding Compendium*. Rockville, MD: United States Pharmacopeial Convention; 2023.

15. USP <1> Injections and implanted drug products (parenterals)—product quality tests. In: *2023: USP Compounding Compendium*. Rockville, MD: United States Pharmacopeial Convention; 2023.

16. USP <1223> Validation of alternative microbiological methods. In: *2023: USP Compounding Compendium*. Rockville, MD: United States Pharmacopeial Convention; 2023.

17. Goldstein MH, Silva FQ, Blender N, et al. Ocular benzalkonium chloride exposure: problems and solutions. *Eye*. 2022;36:361–368. **https://doi.org/10.1038/s41433-021-01668-x**.

18. Kupiec T, Skinner, R, Lanier, L. Quality control analytical methods – stability versus potency testing – the madness is in the method. *IJPC*. 2008;12(1):50–53.

19. General notices and requirements: applying to standards, tests, assays, and other specifications of the United States Pharmacopeia. In: *2023: USP Compounding Compendium*. Rockville, MD: United States Pharmacopeial Convention; 2023.

20. Fentanyl citrate compounded injection. In: *2023: USP-NF*. Rockville, MD: United States Pharmacopeial Convention; 2023.

21. Allen LV, Bassani GS, Elder EJ, et al. *Strength and Stability Testing for Compounded Preparations*. Rockville, MD: United States Pharmacopeia (USP); January 2014. **http://www.usp.org/sites/default/files/usp/document/FAQs/strength-stability-testing-compounded-preparations.pdf**.

22. Bing C, Nowobilski-Vasilios A, eds. *Extended Stability for Parenteral Drugs*. 6th ed. Bethesda, MD: American Society of Health-System Pharmacists; 2017.

23. ASHP's Interactive Handbook on Injectable Drugs [online database]. Bethesda, MD: American Society of Health-System Pharmacists. **https://www.ashp.org/products-and-services/injectables?loginreturnUrl=SSOCheckOnly**. Accessed May 17, 2023.

24. Allen LV, ed. *Remington: the Science and Practice of Pharmacy*. 22nd ed. Baltimore, MD: Lippincott Williams & Wilkins; 2012.

25. Newton DW. Physicochemical determinants of incompatibility and instability of drugs for injection and infusion. *Am J Hosp Pharm*. 1978;35:1213–1222.

26. Lima HA. Drug stability and compatibility: special considerations for home care. *Infusion*. 1996;2:11–16.

27. Newton DW, Driscoll DF, Goudreau JL, et al. Solubility characteristics of diazepam in aqueous admixture solutions: theory and practice. *Am J Hosp Pharm*. 1981;38:179–182.

28. Mason NA, Cline S, Hyneck ML, et al. Factors affecting diazepam infusion: solubility, administration-set composition, and flow rate. *Am J Hosp Pharm*. 1981;38:1449–1454.

29. Morris ME. Compatibility and stability of diazepam injection following dilution from intravenous fluids. *Am J Hosp Pharm*. 1978;35:669–672.

30. U.S. Food and Drug Administration (FDA). Safety alert: hazards of precipitation associated with parenteral nutrition. *Am J Hosp Pharm*. 1994;51:427–428.

31. Driscoll DF, Newton DW, Bistrian BR. Precipitation of calcium phosphate from parenteral nutrient fluids. *Am J Hosp Pharm*. 1994;51:2834–2836.

32. Robinson LA, Wright BT. Central venous catheter occlusion caused by body-heat mediated calcium phosphate precipitation. *Am J Hosp Pharm*. 1982;39:120–121.

33. Niemiec PW, Vanderveen TW. Compatibility considerations in parenteral nutrient solutions. *Am J Hosp Pharm*. 1984;41:893–911.

34. Wells P. *A Guide to Total Nutrient Admixtures: What You Should Know About This New Approach to TPN*. Chicago, IL: Precept Press; 1992.

35. Trissel LA. *Calcium and Phosphate Compatibility in Parenteral Nutrition*. Houston, TX: TriPharma Communications; 2001.

36. U.S. Food and Drug Administration (FDA). *Safety Assessment of Di(2-ethylhexyl) phthalate (DEHP) Released from PVC Medical Devices*. Rockville, MD: U.S. Food and Drug Administration. **http://icpe.in/pdf/Safety_assessment_Diphthalate.pdf**. Accessed September 7, 2023.

37. Helback HJ, Moltehnik DA, Ames BN. Toxic hydroperoxides in intravenous lipid emulsions used in preterm infants. *Pediatrics*. 1993;91:83–87.

38. Dupertuis YM, Morch A, Fathi M, et al. Physical characteristics of total parenteral nutrition bags significantly affect the stability of vitamins C and B1: a controlled prospective study. *J Parenter Enteral Nutr*. 2002;26:310–316.

39. Leissing NC, Story KO, Zaske D. Inline fluid dynamics in piggyback and manifold drug delivery systems. *Am J Hosp Pharm*. 1989;46:89–97.

40. Trissel LA, Gilbert DL, Martinez JF, et al. Compatibility of medications with 3-in-1 parenteral nutrition admixtures. *J Parenter Enteral Nutr*. 1999;23:67–74.

17

LABELING STERILE PREPARATIONS

Joshua S. Ilenin

INTRODUCTION

A compounded sterile preparation (CSP) must be labeled accurately and completely to facilitate safe administration to the patient. Ensuring the accuracy and thoroughness of the CSP labeling compared with the original provider order, prescription, and the ingredients used to compound the preparation is an integral part of the pharmacist verification process. Primary and auxiliary labels included on sterile preparations communicate proper handling, storage, administration, and drug information to the person administering the drug. The terminology used should be appropriately descriptive based on the knowledge of the end user. The use of abbreviations should be minimized to avoid confusion. All labels should be legible and affixed to the final container so that the information can be read both before and during sterile preparation and administration. If a container is to be inverted for administration, each label must be positioned so that it is right side up while infusing. Light-resistant bags for photosensitive drugs and other overwraps should not impede visibility of the label.

Small containers may require unique methods of affixing the label. For certain syringes, labels may be affixed using the two ends of the label so that syringe markings are not covered or obstructed. This method of attaching the label is called *flagging*. Flagging is also required for CSPs dispensed in small vials and ophthalmic bottles. Very small syringes can be sealed in a larger bag or overwrap, which is then labeled. If the syringe is removed from the bag some point before administration, a second smaller label on the syringe should give key information (eg, drug name, concentration, beyond-use date [BUD], and route). If a CSP undergoes sterilization (eg, steam), final labeling with all required components will need to occur after sterilization.

The exact information on a label varies depending on the preparation type and the patient location and setting, not the *United States Pharmacopeia*'s (USP) CSP category. In 2004, USP required labeling elements for CSPs regardless of where the patient receives the preparation.[1;2] These labeling elements were also required in the revised USP Chapter <797> Pharmaceutical Compounding—Sterile Preparations standards, which became official June 1, 2008.[3] The label requirements have evolved in the most recent update to USP Chapter <797> standards, and they will be discussed in greater detail throughout this chapter.

The general label content is similar, but slight variations exist in addition to the USP standard for patient-specific labeling in institutional and home care settings and for compounded sterile batch preparations.[3-5] This chapter reviews general labeling guidelines, USP labeling requirements for sterile preparations, batch labeling elements (required and optional patient-specific and perioperative labeling elements as specified by the American Society of Health-System Pharmacists [ASHP] and The Joint Commission [TJC]), and other labeling strategies that can be used to help prevent medication errors and facilitate proper disposal of returned preparations, which ensure compliance with the 2003 Health Insurance Portability and Accountability Act (HIPAA) privacy regulations.[4;6-12]

GENERAL LABELING GUIDELINES

To ensure proper labeling, the following guidelines should be followed:

- Labeling is required unless the CSP meets the USP immediate-use provision (ie, labeling is required if it is not administered immediately and completely by the person who prepared the medication or the preparer does not witness the immediate and complete administration of the drug).[1]
- The label must conform to applicable federal, state, and local laws and regulations. Some states require specific labeling elements to be in a larger bold font than the rest of the label information. The Institute for Safe Medication Practices (ISMP)

DOI 10.37573/9781585286492.017

recommends that patient name, generic drug name, and the patient-specific dose be printed in bold typeface on medication labels in a minimum 11- or 12-point font size that is easy to read. Serif fonts are preferred, as sans serif font types may contain decorative details or flourishes that can lead to misinterpretation of label information.[10] USP Chapter <17> Prescription Container Labeling provides standards for prescription container labeling that are focused on standardized formatting and placement of critical information (eg, drug's generic and brand name, strength, and dosing instructions), which use clear, simple language with the goal of increased understanding and reduced medication errors.[11] USP Chapter <7> Labeling provides general labeling standards, which include the amount of each active ingredient per dosage unit and specified warnings for high-risk drug classes (eg, neuromuscular blocking [paralyzing] agents).[12]

- Medication labels must be typed or electronically printed in a standardized format to ensure accurate and complete labeling. The label is legible, easy to read, and free from erasures and strikeovers. The background color for labels enables clear visualization of text and barcodes.[10] Unlabeled CSPs or those with incomplete labeling should be corrected or immediately and safely discarded. ISMP offers guidelines for formatting electronically generated CSP labels, utilizing sterile compounding technology, and recommends matching the format and units of measure of the prescriber's order.[13]
- The appropriate primary and auxiliary labels must be firmly affixed to the container. Pharmacy preparation labels are not to be used as the final CSP product label because they may have different information.[13]
- Metric units of measure should be used instead of the apothecary system.
- Numbers, letters, coined names, unofficial synonyms, prohibited abbreviations, and trademark symbols should not be used to identify medications with the exception of approved letter or number codes for investigational drugs.[10]
- All medications with illegible or worn labels must be properly and safely discarded.
- A uniform, systematic labeling method must be used. One order or drug preparation batch must be filled and labeled at a time.
- Primary and auxiliary labels should be affixed such that they do not cover any critical information (eg, drug name, concentration, expiration, or route of administration) for any diluent solutions containing additives.
- During the hours the pharmacy is open, sterile product compounding and labeling should be done in a pharmacy. Within the pharmacy, only a pharmacist or authorized pharmacy technician or intern under the direction and supervision of a pharmacist may label and dispense medications, make labeling changes, and transfer medications to different containers.

USP Label Requirements for Compounded Sterile Preparations

Minimum standards for CSP labels for all healthcare settings were first established in the 2004 version of USP Chapter <797>.[2] Subsequent revisions of the guidelines further clarified requirements for CSP labels, including clearly defined criteria for immediate-use CSPs and differentiating required label elements for a single-dose container versus pharmacy bulk package.[1;3] The most recent 2022 version of USP Chapter <797> continues to refine labeling guidance.[1] The guidelines clarify the definitions of label and labeling. *Labeling* refers to any written, printed, or graphic material contained on the immediate container and any outer wrapper or packaging other than the original shipping container. A *label* refers specifically to the information on the immediate container or CSP. When considering the information required on a label, it is best to consult available guidance from any regulatory agencies with oversight of where the CSPs will be dispensed and administered. The label information should always be verified to ensure consistency with the medication order, master formulation record, and compounding record.[1] The following information is the minimum required by USP on the immediate container for Category 1, 2, and 3 CSPs.

Figure 17-1 illustrates a sample label that must be present on the surface of the container. The parts of the label are

Voriconazole(2)	**200 mg**(2)
in 5% Dextrose in Water(2)	100 mL(2)
IVPB For IV Use(4)	
Total Volume	**120 mL**(5)

Infuse intravenously(7) over 2 hours(7) every 12 hours(7)

Lot: C04171601(1)
Keep refrigerated(3)
Use before: 10:00 4/18/23(4)
Single-dose(6) compounded preparation
Prepared by: LI(7)

FIGURE 17-1. Sample label per the USP Chapter <797> compounded sterile preparation label standard

described below. The numbers in parentheses corresponds to numbers on the label.

- Assigned internal identification number (1): Each CSP should have a unique identifier in the form of a barcode, alphanumeric prescription, order, or lot number that is featured on the immediate label.[1]
- Names and amounts or concentrations of active ingredients (2): The name of each drug, preferably the generic name, should be legibly printed on a CSP label. If multiple components are used, the names of all drug products or ingredients, including admixture solutions and their corresponding volumes, should be listed on the label. The trade drug name or commonly known name of the preparation may be included in an effort to reduce the potential for error. The amount of each active ingredient per dosage unit or total volume should be the primary expression of strength on the label.[12] Although the admixture solution (eg, dextrose or sodium chloride) is not considered an active ingredient in a CSP, it may be a consideration in certain clinical settings. The admixture solution can affect CSP stability and the BUD and is helpful to include for completeness on a CSP label. For sterile preparations given by intrathecal or intravitreal routes and to neonatal patients, the label should include preservative-free ingredients, admixture solutions, and diluents used in compounding to ensure appropriateness for administration. In some cases, it may be appropriate to label ophthalmic sterile preparations with the concentration of the active ingredients and preservatives.
- Storage conditions (3): Storage instructions can be located on the primary label or added as an auxiliary label. Preparations must be stored in accordance with the conditions stated on the label to ensure the sterility, stability, and maintain the assigned BUD. This can include but is not limited to whether the preparation should be refrigerated, kept at room temperature, protected from light, or not shaken. If the sterile preparation requires refrigeration, it should be stored in a refrigerator dedicated to medications and not comingled with food or other products that could contaminate a CSP.
- Beyond-use date (4): The BUD is the date or time after which a CSP cannot be used, stored, or transported and must be discarded.[1] The BUD is determined from the date or time the preparation is compounded and should be consistent within a healthcare setting and compounding facility. BUDs are assigned based on direct testing or extrapolated from reliable literature sources that consider stability information, sterility, and other critical factors. The methods used to assign actual preparation-specific BUDs are discussed in Chapter 16.
- Total volume of the preparation (5): Total amount or volume is usually expressed in the metric system. For intravenous (IV) piggybacks and continuous infusions, this measurement allows tracking of the patient's total fluid intake. If the volume of the admixture solution is not significantly different from the total volume, these measurements are used interchangeably (eg, for antibiotic solutions). For larger volume solutions with multiple additives, the actual or calculated total volume should be used (eg, for parenteral nutrition admixtures). For syringes and vials that are overfilled, both the overfill volume and the volume of the prescribed medication dose should be clearly shown on the label.
- Designation of whether the end product CSP is a single-dose container or pharmacy bulk package (6): This information is critical in communicating whether the CSP is for one-time single use or contains multiple doses as well as part of the information needed to determine the appropriate BUD as discussed in Chapter 16. Once a single-dose CSP is used, any remainder should be promptly and properly discarded. If a CSP is a pharmacy bulk package restricted to be used within the pharmacy to prepare many single doses, it must be prominently labeled Pharmacy Bulk Package: Not for Direct Infusion.[1] In addition, the label must include or refer to information on the safe use of the product, proper technique of administration, and an appropriate BUD after the bulk container has been entered if it is used and stored properly.[1]

Additional information to include as part of the CSP labeling is outlined below:

- Appropriate routes of administration (7): Although the dosage form or actual physical entity that contains all the ingredients that deliver a dose of the drug may imply the route of administration (eg, IV bag implies IV administration unless labeled otherwise), the appropriate routes of administration should be placed on the preparation label.[11] When a container is used outside the normal pattern or a dosage form has multiple uses, it is especially important that the route is clearly stated to prevent medication errors. Drugs can often only be administered by a certain route. Sometimes the amount and concentration of a CSP is route specific. Preparations used for irrigation, cardioplegia, intrathecal and epidural injections, inhalation, and peritoneal dialysis should be clearly marked and distinctively labeled by size, shape, and the use of auxiliary labels.
- Other information for safe use (7): Other information, including special handling and applicable warning statements, for the safe use of the preparation can be put on the primary label or added as auxiliary labels. This information should include the identification of the responsible compounding

personnel who prepared or verified the preparation and a second unique identifier (eg, the prescription number, lot number, or control number) that is unique to that specific CSP, which is used by the dispensing pharmacy to reference the original order and detailed compounding record.[4] Both are helpful when questions arise about the preparation.

Syringes should be clearly labeled with the intended route of administration (eg, IV push, pump or gravity, epidural or intrathecal, inhalation, intravitreal, intramuscular, or subcutaneous). In some cases, the ramifications of giving a particular drug or dose by an unintended route can be fatal (eg, IV dose given intrathecally). Patient-controlled analgesia (PCA) containers should also be clearly marked because they may be the same for IV and epidural PCA, but the concentration of drug differs.

Use and special handling instructions should include complete directions for the proper clinical administration of the CSP, including the infusion period and the frequency of the dose prescribed. Device-specific settings and instructions can also be placed on the label to reduce the risk of incorrect administration. Simple and concise cautionary statements for the safe use of the preparation can be put on the primary label or added as auxiliary labels or graphics. For drugs with short BUDs, a simple statement for pharmacy not to compound the dose until the patient is ready for it can be added to the label to ensure timeliness of the medication preparation and prevent waste.

Some drugs may require appropriate precautionary labels to facilitate safe handling, use, and disposal. For facilities that ship preparations to recipients outside their own facility, including patients, disposal instructions for out-of-date or unused units should be included.[1] If no warnings are applicable, the preparation should be void of cautionary statements, "so that that those with cautionary statements are immediately apparent."[14] CSPs can be prominently labeled to identify the preparation as a compounded entity. This can be as simple as adding verbiage to the label (eg, "This is a compounded drug" or a similar statement).[15] Note that the label for multidose vial allergen extract CSPs must list the patient's name in addition to an appropriate BUD and temperature storage range.[1]

USP Immediate-use CSP Labeling Requirements

Labels for immediate-use CSPs are not subject to the same requirements as Category 1, Category 2, or Category 3 CSPs.[1] There are no label requirements for immediate-use CSPs if administered by the preparer or if the preparer is a witness to administration. If the preparer is not available to witness administration, a limited amount of information is required to ensure safe administration.

Figure 17-2 illustrates a sample label required for immediate-use CSPs that must bear a label. The parts of this label are described below, and the numbers in parentheses correspond to the numbers on the label.

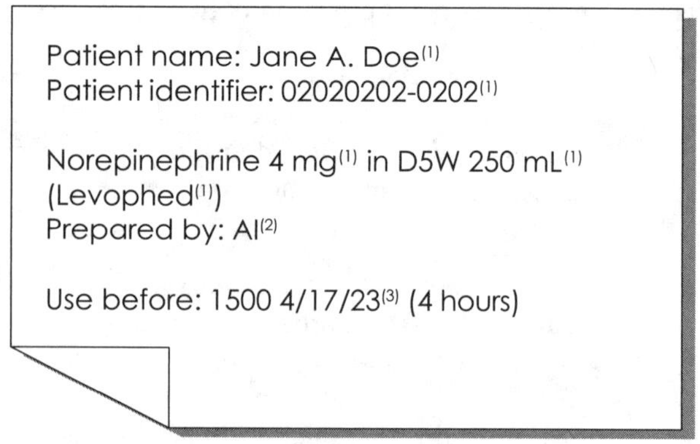

FIGURE 17-2. Sample label per the USP Chapter <797> immediate-use sterile preparation labeling standard

- Names and amounts of all ingredients (1): This section is the same as item 1 on the previous CSP label.
- The name or initials of the person who prepared the IV admixture (2): The identity of the preparer of the sterile preparation should be noted on the label. This information is helpful when questions arise about the preparation.
- The exact 4-hour BUD and time (3): This section is similar to item 3 on the previous CSP label. However, it must note the exact 4-hour BUD and time. A date by itself is not sufficient. The 4-hour BUD is determined from the actual time the preparation is compounded and is generally expressed in military time (eg, 1500 is used to express 3:00 p.m.).

Due to the emergent, critical need of immediate-use CSPs, auxiliary labeling is not required because the process could subject the patient to additional risk due to delays in therapy.

BATCH LABELING

CSPs that are not produced on a patient-specific basis may require slightly different labeling elements beyond the previously described USP labeling items 1 through 7. Batch CSPs are preparations compounded in anticipation of an actual physician's order or prescription. Risk reduction strategies for batch preparation include printing only one batch of labels at a time, printing only the exact number of labels needed for the batch, labeling the batch preparations immediately after compounding, and labeling the batch "separately from other batched products."[16] A copy of the batch label should be included on the required compounding record. Label items 1 through 7 are either exactly the same or slightly different than the ones listed in Figure 17-1. Only

Insulin Adult Standard Drip[2]

Regular Insulin 250 units[2] in 0.9% NaCl 250 mL[2]
Drip concentration = **1 unit/mL**[2] ***INSULIN*** [9]
Total volume: 252.5 mL[4]

FOR IV USE[3]

Lot number: G041706[1]
Prepared on: 4/17/16
Prepared by: LI/SW[8]
Use before: 4/24/23 at 1500[6]
Keep refrigerated[5]
Single-dose container[7]

FIGURE 17-3. Sample label for batch compounded preparations

the differences and additional labeling requirements will be further explained.

Figure 17-3 illustrates a sample label used for batch preparations. The parts of this label are described below, and the numbers in parentheses correspond to numbers on the label.

Required Labeling

- Lot number or control number (1): A lot or control number tracks a preparation back to its batch preparation documentation sheet. These numbers are usually generated internally based on a standard process. They should be readily traceable to documentation of how and by whom the preparation was made and if sterility testing was performed. The date of preparation and either a specifically assigned drug preparation number or daily sterile compounding sequence number is usually included in the numbering logic.
- Name of preparation (2): The commonly known name of a preparation is useful, especially for one with multiple ingredients, because the product can be readily identified. This can be used in addition to but not as a replacement of the required names and amounts or concentrations of active ingredients. The names and amounts of drugs added to a solution must all be listed. Usually for batch preparations, additives, such as preservatives and buffering agents, should be listed. Admixture solutions or diluents, such as 0.9% sodium chloride, 5% dextrose, and sterile water for injection, may affect how a final preparation is used, especially if the preparation contains preservatives.
- Route of administration (3): Route of administration can be specific (eg, for irrigation) or general (eg, for injection) if the preparation can be used safely for more than one route.
- Total amount or volume of the preparation (4): The total amount or volume may be stated as a common metric volume for the final preparation (eg, milliliters) or as a concentration that includes both the amount of drug and the total volume in which it is contained. TJC and ISMP discourage the use of the abbreviations for cubic centimeters (cc) rather than mL for milliliters.[10]
- Storage conditions (5): Storage requirements should reflect preferred conditions before and after the preparation was administered to the patient.
- BUD and time (6): This section is the same as item 3 on the USP label.
- Designation whether the end product CSP is a single-dose container or a pharmacy bulk package (7): This section is the same as item 6 on the USP label.
- Identification of responsible compounding personnel (8): The identity of the preparer and pharmacist who releases the preparation should be noted on the label. This information is helpful when questions arise about the preparation.
- Appropriate auxiliary labeling (9): Although precautionary labeling is covered in the next section, specific high-risk drugs may have graphics or warnings included in their batch labeling.

Although not listed in Figure 17-3, device-specific instructions, when appropriate, should be added to the batch label.[4] This can be in the form of listing the exact pump setting to use when compounding a specific batch CSP or utilizing a specialized drug container (eg, 60-mL blue syringes for inhaled epoprostenol).

Auxiliary and Optional Labeling

Because batched preparations are relabeled with patient-specific information prior to dispensing, auxiliary labels should be minimized to include only relevant essential precautions to take prior to final dispensing to the patient. Any pertinent auxiliary or optional information should be incorporated into the batch label if possible. Use of auxiliary labels may lead to errors if old labels are not removed before dispensing of the relabeled preparation. There may be exceptions when auxiliary labels are pertinent to patient-specific situations and are correctly positioned on the final container in order to be read both before relabeling and at the point of administration to the patient.

LABELS IN INSTITUTIONAL SETTINGS

In addition to the above USP minimum labeling standards, there are other requirements when CSPs are used in institutional settings. Accurate labels not only help staff efficiently prepare and dispense preparations, but also supply needed information to staff or patients and caregivers to safely administer the correct medication to the correct patient.

Patient-specific Labels in Institutional Settings

Figure 17-4 illustrates a patient-specific sample label used in an institutional setting. The parts of this label are described below. Numbers in parentheses correspond to numbers on the label:

Required Labeling

- Patient name and identification number (1): A patient name on a label indicates the dose as ordered and prescribed for that specific patient and to whom it should be administered. Exclusion of a name may indicate that the preparation can be used on other patients, which may lead to errors. The first name, last name, and middle initial of the patient should be used. In addition, a medical record number, account number, or encounter number also identifies each patient in most hospital computer systems and can serve as a second unique patient identifier. This number is critical to drug administration in hospitals that use barcode technology since the barcode is linked to each patient's unique medical record, account number, or encounter number.
- Patient location (2): Location information within a treatment facility helps ensure that the CSP gets to the correct patient in an expedient manner. Transfer or discharge of patients should be tracked so that label information is updated. If the data are not relayed or used, delays in therapy and unnecessary duplicate work can result.
- Name and amount of drugs added and name of admixture solution (3): This section is similar to item 1 on the USP label. However, it includes the names and amounts or concentrations of the drugs added to the CSP in addition to the name of the admixture solution used in compounding. Identification of the admixture solution makes the label more complete and accurate. Diluent information is often not listed on the label when sterile water for injection is required to reconstitute drugs.
- Approximate final total volume of admixture solution (4): This section is the same as item 2 on the USP label. The total volume should be listed for all preparations, including intermittent and continuous IV admixtures, critical care infusions, total parenteral nutrition fluids, irrigations, dialysate fluids, and small volume sterile preparations, such as syringes.
- Time and date of scheduled administration (5): In institutions, the scheduled administration time is generally referred to as the due time and is expressed in military time (eg, 1300 is used to express 1:00 p.m.). This information notifies the nursing staff of the administration schedule maintained in the pharmacy and drives the medication administration record (MAR) contained within an electronic health record. Nurses can make a professional judgment about exactly when to begin administration based on whether the patient is scheduled for a test or procedure out of the patient care area and the number of patients the individual nurse is assigned. Administering a CSP up to one hour before or after the scheduled administration is generally acceptable. However, if both pharmacy and nursing schedules are the same, errors will be minimized. If nurses follow the scheduled administration time and date printed on the label, admixtures will not be used out of sequence. When admixtures are given in incorrect sequence, the oldest ones (with the earliest BUD) expire prior to use and result in unnecessary waste. Institution-specific

Institution's Name
John B. Doe[(1)] E 1010[(2)]
01010101-0101[(1)] Ord #: 24 Bag #: 3

Time due: 4/17/23 17:00[(5)]

Vancomycin[(3)] **1750 mg**[(3)]
NaCl 0.9%[(3)] **250 mL**[(3)]
Total volume **268 mL**[(4)]
IVPB Infuse intravenously[(8)] over 90 minutes[(9)]
every 12 hours[(9)]
Prepared on: 4/17/23[(6)]
Prepared by: LI[(10)]
Checked by: SW[(10)]
Use before: 2000 4/26/23[(7)]
Keep refrigerated[(11)]
Single-dose container[(12)]
This is a compounded drug intended for an adult[(13)]

FIGURE 17-4. Sample label in an institutional setting

standardized administration times also reduce confusion and waste and prevent omitted doses.

- Time and date of compounding (6): The time and date of compounding are needed to determine actual beyond-use times. TJC requires the date prepared for all compounded IV admixtures and parenteral nutrition solutions and a beyond-use time for all preparations with beyond-use periods less than 24 hours.[9] This information may be contained on the label even if it is not stated clearly. For example, the scheduled administration time may indicate when a drug was prepared based on that sterile preparation batch or fill list period. For institutions using an electronic health record (EHR) or other automated system to generate labels, it is important to note how the time and date printed correspond to the actual compounding time. When batching a preparation and dispensing model for patient-specific CSPs is used, a significant number of labels may be printed at once and prepared over a period of time. This could lead to a discrepancy in the time printed on the label and the actual preparation time. Developing a process to capture and correct these discrepancies will help reduce the risk of inadvertently miscommunicating the correct BUD.
- BUD and time (7): This section is similar to item 3 on the USP label. In an institutional setting, the BUD assigned to a preparation is usually the actual time that it is deemed unusable for the patient or a standard time in which it should be returned to the pharmacy. After the preparation is returned, the pharmacist can determine if it should be redispensed or discarded. Methods used to assign actual BUDs are discussed in Chapter 16. For CSPs with beyond-use periods less than 24 hours, a beyond-use time is also required.[9]
- Route of administration (8): This section is the same as item 4 on the USP label.
- Special handling instructions and administration instructions (9): This section is similar to item 7 on the USP label. However, it includes all directions needed for proper administration to a patient in an institutional setting. For intermittent doses, administration instructions should include the duration and sometimes the rate of administration. If the preparation requires activation or some other manipulation prior to patient administration, this information should also be included on the primary label or added as an auxiliary label (eg, break seal and mix prior to administration). For continuous infusions, administration instructions generally include the rate and a stop time. A singular rate should not be included for a continuous infusion that is being titrated because the rate may change without the pharmacy's knowledge and no longer be accurately reflected on the label. This situation could result in a medication error. In these cases, infuse as directed, titrate, or a rate range may be more appropriate to include with a note to refer to the medication administration documentation for further details.
- Identification of the responsible compounding personnel (10): This section has been incorporated into item 7 on the USP label. The identity of the preparer and pharmacist who releases the preparation should be noted on the label or in a dispensing record in the pharmacy. State boards of pharmacy often require the initials of the responsible pharmacist to be on the label. This information is helpful when questions arise about the preparation.
- Storage conditions (11): This section is the same as item 5 on the USP label because storage instructions can be located on the primary label or added as an auxiliary label. This information reminds nurses to refrigerate, protect from light, or not shake a preparation before administration to the patient. Refrigeration of CSPs is often the standard in the institutional setting, so appropriate storage temperature information (eg, refrigerate or do not refrigerate) should be highlighted or otherwise differentiated from other label text for emphasis. Warnings about not shaking the preparation also remind pharmacy personnel that the physical shaking that might occur during pneumatic tube transport can adversely affect the quality of certain CSPs.
- Designation of whether the CSP is a single-dose container (12): This section is the same as item 6 on the USP label. In institutional settings, most end product CSPs are single-dose containers.
- Warning statements if applicable (13): This section is the same as item 7 on the USP label. Cautionary statements are required only if there are any pertinent handling or disposal precautions that should be adhered to regarding patient, family, and caregiver safety (eg, "Warning: Paralyzing Agent" for neuromuscular blocking drugs). This section can also include who the CSP is intended for (eg, for adults and not for children).

Figure 17-5 illustrates a patient-specific sample label used in an institutional setting where the CSP is shipped outside the institution's own facility. All parts of the label are the same as described above with the one exception listed below (numbers in parentheses correspond to numbers on the label):

- Name, address, and contact information of the compounder if the institution ships compounded preparations to recipients outside their own facility (14): This information provides an easy mechanism for another facility or the patient to contact the dispensing pharmacy when questions arise about product preparation, delivery, storage,

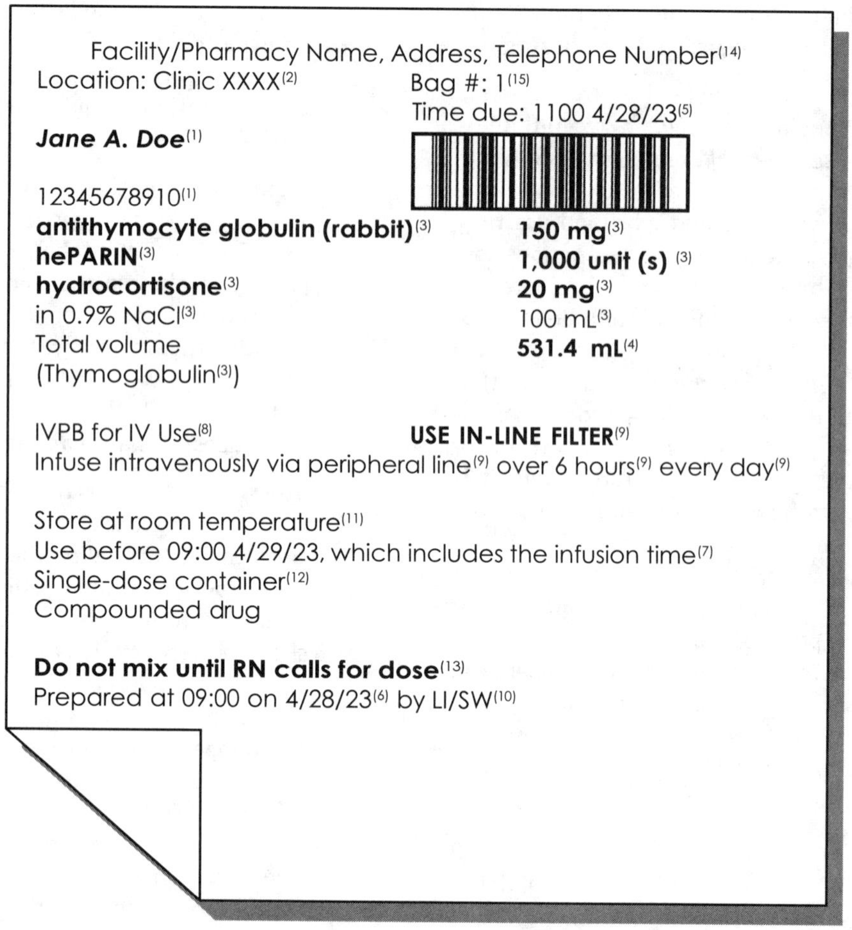

Facility/Pharmacy Name, Address, Telephone Number[14]

Location: Clinic XXXX[2] Bag #: 1[15]

Time due: 1100 4/28/23[5]

Jane A. Doe[1]

12345678910[1]

antithymocyte globulin (rabbit)[3]	**150 mg**[3]
hePARIN[3]	**1,000 unit (s)** [3]
hydrocortisone[3]	**20 mg**[3]
in 0.9% NaCl[3]	100 mL[3]
Total volume	**531.4 mL**[4]
(Thymoglobulin[3])	

IVPB for IV Use[8] **USE IN-LINE FILTER**[9]

Infuse intravenously via peripheral line[9] over 6 hours[9] every day[9]

Store at room temperature[11]

Use before 09:00 4/29/23, which includes the infusion time[7]

Single-dose container[12]

Compounded drug

Do not mix until RN calls for dose[13]

Prepared at 09:00 on 4/28/23[6] by LI/SW[10]

FIGURE 17-5. Sample label in an institutional setting for use outside of the original facility

Note: Facility or pharmacy name, address, and telephone number (14) are only required if the CSP is sent outside the facility that compounded the preparation.

administration, and disposal. Some compounding facilities and pharmacies also supply the recipient with an emergency contact number on the label or as an insert in the package with the compounded medication.

OTHER CONSIDERATIONS

When human drug CSPs are purchased from a Section 503b registered outsourcing facility, the CSP label must meet the U.S. Food and Drug Administration's (FDA) Compounding Quality Act labeling of drugs standard.[15] Unique 503b labeling requirements that differ from USP Chapter <797> standards include the phrase "not for resale," a statement that the CSP is a compounded drug, the National Drug Code number if applicable, and use of the phrase "hospital/office use only" under specific circumstances.[8] The FDA regulates the outsourcing facilities. States may establish additional requirements that should be followed based on the state in which the preparation will be administered. For more information on outsourcing the compounding of sterile preparations, refer to Chapter 34.

AUXILIARY LABELING

Auxiliary labeling provides supplemental instructions and precautions similar to item 7 on the USP label without the space limitations of preformatted or computerized labels. Auxiliary labels should not be used judiciously and should avoid cluttering the CSP with unnecessary information. They should be limited to essential information needed for safe and effective administration. Auxiliary labels have an added advantage of highlighting the information in a different font, color, design, or style than the CSP label. Auxiliary labels also help staff follow the manufacturer recommendations and the pharmacy guidelines for storage prior to distribution. **Figure 17-6** illustrates sample auxiliary labels.

The same auxiliary labels should be used each time a particular sterile preparation is dispensed to prevent confusion and highlight the importance and validity of the

FOR THE EYE

NOT FOR IV USE

PROTECT FROM LIGHT

DO NOT REFRIGERATE

REFRIGERATE

USE IN-LINE FILTER

DO NOT SHAKE

FOR IRRIGATION ONLY

EPIDURAL

FIGURE 17-6. Sample auxiliary labels

information. Auxiliary labels are often used for information about the following:

- Light protection (eg, protect from light)
- Final filters (eg, use in-line filter)
- Rate precautions
- Storage conditions (eg, refrigerate, do not refrigerate, or do not shake)
- Drug concentration
- Handling precautions (eg, chemotherapy or hazardous drug)
- Routes of administration (eg, for the eye, not for IV use, or for irrigation only)
- Other information for safe use (eg, break seal and mix prior to administration, warning: paralyzing agent, or STAT)

All information for the preparation's safe use is now required to be part of the labeling, which can be located either on the primary label or on auxiliary labels.

OPTIONAL LABELING

- Bottle or bag sequence number (15): The sequence number of the container may be important, depending on the type of drug or number of doses ordered. The total number of doses given should be tracked to prevent bags given out of sequence or doses being lost. The sequence number can also help prevent unnecessary waste due to CSP expiration. In the institutional setting, the order number along with the bag number and patient name also provide a unique assigned internal identification number for each CSP. (Refer to Figure 17-5.)

Perioperative and Other Procedural Area Settings

Figure 17-7 illustrates a sample label used in perioperative and other procedural areas for medications both on and off the sterile field that are not immediately administered.[9] Verification of all medication labels should be performed verbally and visually by two qualified healthcare professionals whenever the person preparing the medication is not the one administering it.[9] A culture of no tolerance for unlabeled medications or containers is paramount in improving patient safety.[17] Medications should be labeled as soon as they are prepared unless they are taken directly to the patient and administered without any breaks in the process.[7] Other risk reduction strategies include providing preprinted or blank labels with sterile markers to improve labeling compliance and conducting regular safety observations to assess labeling compliance and promote consistency.[17;18] If any containers are found unlabeled in the procedural environment, they should be immediately discarded. The contents of this label are described below. Numbers in parentheses correspond to numbers on the label.

Required Labeling

- Name and amount of drugs added or final concentration and strength (1): The names and amounts of all active drugs added to a solution should be included. The commonly known name of a preparation is useful, especially for one with multiple ingredients, because it can be readily identified.
- Diluent name and volume if not apparent from the container (2): Admixture solutions or diluents, such as normal saline, 5% dextrose, and sterile water for

EPINEPHrine(1)
Conc. = 16 mcg/mL(1) 10-mL syringe(1)
0.16 mg/10 mL Total Volume(1)
In 0.9% sodium chloride(2)
Use before: 5/05/23 at 2000(3)
Protect from light(4)

FIGURE 17-7. Sample label for perioperative and other procedural settings

injection or irrigation, may affect how a final preparation is used, especially if the preparation contains preservatives.

- BUD and time (3): This section is the same as item 3 on the USP label. If the BUD is less than 24 hours, a BUD time is required. In short procedures, the BUD date and time may not be necessary if such a process is written into the institution's policies and procedures.[9]
- Storage conditions (4): Storage requirements should reflect preferred conditions before and after the preparation is opened or administered to the patient.

LABELS IN HOME CARE SETTINGS

Additional considerations are required when designing labels for use in the home care setting. First, medications administered in the home care setting are considered outpatient prescriptions and are subject to state board of pharmacy labeling requirements. Label components may vary, so it is important to verify the requirements in the state where the medication is to be administered. Second, the label should convey storage, preparation, administration, and disposal requirements in a language easily understood by the patient or a caregiver.[6] Some states may even require a multilingual label. The label should contain few abbreviations or other confusing terminology. If any manipulation of the CSP is required prior to administration, the label should clearly list each step.[6] The label should serve as an adjunct to other written and verbal instructions given to the patient and caregiver regarding the CSP.

Figure 17-8 illustrates a sample label used in the home care setting.[6] The parts of this label are described below. Numbers in parentheses correspond to numbers on the label.

Required Labeling

- Prescription number, date filled, prescribing physician, and authorized refills (1): This information is typically required by state boards of pharmacy, but it is also used by the dispensing pharmacy to reference the original order.

Facility/Pharmacy Name(7) Local Telephone Number(7)
Street Address(7) 800 Telephone Number(7)
City, State, Zip Code(7)

Rx: 1234567(1) Dispense date: 4/11/23(1)
Patient: **Jane A. Doe**(2) Prescriber: J.R. Smith, MD(1)
110 S. Elm St.
Anywhere, MD(2) Bag: # 1 of 7(8)

Nafcillin 12 gm/240 mL SWFI(4) Total volume: **250 mL**(4)
Administer **Nafcillin 12 gm**(4) intravenously over 24 hours via Eclipse at a continuous rate of 10 mL/hr via PICC(3) **Discard after each use.**(3)

Change bag every 24 hours(3)

Storage: Refrigerate until used; remove 2 hours prior to use(3)
Discard after: 1200 4/25/23(5)
Qty disp: 7
Refills left: 95(1)
Entered by: AI(6)
Single-dose container
This is a compounded drug
Checked by: SW(6)
"Caution: Federal and/or State Law prohibits transfer of this drug to any person other than the patient for whom it was prescribed."

FIGURE 17-8. Sample label in a home care setting

- Patient's full name and address (2): The full name of the patient should be printed as part of the prescription label. Although the address is optional, it may simplify delivery procedures and ensure efficient delivery of the correct medication, equipment, device, or supplies to the correct patient or patient's representative. In an effort to maintain patient confidentiality, the outer shipping container should not be labeled with any information regarding the medication. It may be relevant to include appropriate storage information on any outer shipping container to ensure proper handling.[6]
- Directions to the patient for use of the medication (3): This section is similar to item 9 on the institutional label. However, it should be easy for the patient or caregiver to understand. Clear instructions should be included regarding required manipulations of the sterile preparation (eg, measuring, reconstituting, adding other ingredients, and setting up needed tubing or filters for proper drug administration). Directions should include the route of administration, rate of administration, frequency of administration, and any special precautionary handling or storage requirements (eg, refrigerate or do not shake). If the drugs are to be administered with an infusion device, the device settings should also be included on the label.[6]
- Name and amount or strength of drug added and volume of admixture solution (4): This section is similar to items 3 and 4 on the institutional label. However, the admixture may contain more than one dose. In this situation, the label should indicate the amount of drug in one dose, the appropriate volume for that amount, and the total amount of drug or nutrient within the preparation container (eg, bag, bottle, cassette, syringe, or vial). The total volume of the preparation should be clearly indicated on the label. This information may be helpful in the event that a home care patient is transferred to another care facility.[6] A well-designed label format should avoid misinterpretation of dosage information when multiple doses of a drug are aseptically compounded in one container.
- BUD (5): This section is the same as item 3 on the USP label. The BUD used in home care settings is usually the actual BUD established for the preparation so that a multiple-day supply of the preparation can be dispensed and delivered. BUDs are often maximized for practical reasons, such as the distance of the patient from the pharmacy and to reduce the need for multiple deliveries to the patient. As a result, refrigerated storage may be preferred. The label may also include information regarding the room temperature BUD in the event that the CSP is not consistently stored at a refrigerated temperature. BUDs of CSPs used in ambulatory infusion pumps worn close to the body must consider that these drugs are administered at warmer than room temperatures. Methods used to assign actual BUDs are discussed in Chapter 16. These preparations cannot be redispensed (even if returned unused) since they are considered outpatient prescriptions, and it is impossible to confirm storage conditions when stored at home.
- Initials (or name) of the responsible pharmacist (6): State boards of pharmacy often require that the initials or name of the pharmacist verifying the CSP appear on the label. This information is helpful when questions arise about product preparation.
- Name, address, and telephone number of the compounding facility and pharmacy (7): This section is the same as item 14 on the institutional label. It is typically required by state boards of pharmacy to provide an easy mechanism for the patient to contact the dispensing pharmacy if questions arise about product preparation, delivery, storage, administration, and disposal. Some compounding facilities and pharmacies also supply the patient with an emergency contact number on the label or as an insert in the package with the compounded medication.

Auxiliary Labeling

This section is similar to the auxiliary labeling described on the institutional label. However, federal transfer labeling must be included (as with any outpatient prescription) and the user must be able to easily understand it. Individual state laws or regulations may also require other information. Some states require that compounded medications be identified as such. The International Academy of Compounding Pharmacists recommends the following statement be included on either the primary or auxiliary label of compounded medications for human use. "This medicine was specially compounded in our pharmacy for you at the direction of your prescriber."[19] Such a statement is similar to the label verbiage previously discussed indicating that the preparation is compounded.

Optional Labeling

Bottle or bag sequence number (8): As in the institutional setting, the bottle or bag sequence number can help track the specific number of doses ordered and the total number of doses administered (eg, bag 1 of 7). Refer to Figure 17-8 for an example.

ADDITIONAL LABELING STRATEGIES

Label information should be clear, complete, easy to read, and aid in preventing medication errors. Various strategies can be used to make labeling look unique and draw patient or caregiver attention to critical information. It is unclear if any of these strategies have an impact on patient safety.

Color and Graphics

One strategy to reduce errors associated with CSP preparation and administration is the utilization of color and graphics to draw attention to various critical information on the label. In some instances, using color to highlight preparation information and make various label features or components stand out (eg, drug concentration) has demonstrated some success.[20] For example, different colored font or label colors may be used for different concentrations or strengths of the same drug. Color labels have also been employed in workflow design (eg, making STAT preparations print on a different color label to facilitate efficient and timely pharmacy preparation and delivery as well as nursing administration to the patient). In these examples, color itself is not used as a standard code to classify or identify the therapeutic drug class.

In contrast, ISMP warns that color coding should be used with extreme caution because people identify a color with a function.[20] They suggest that color coding by pharmaceutical vendors and individual healthcare facilities may actually contribute to medication errors. Another factor to consider when utilizing color in label design is that color blindness can influence the effectiveness and potentially contribute to unintended medication errors as well. Based on these considerations, it is not a prudent practice to rely solely on a standard color to classify or identify specific drugs or drug categories, even high-risk medication categories.

Another labeling technique to prevent medication errors involves the use of graphics (eg, octagons or triangles) on labels to note high concentrations of a drug or high alert routes of administration (eg, for epidural medications).[21] These graphics are meant to draw the eye toward an important subset of information regarding the product without detracting from the overall label information. Color or graphic warnings on labels should be used sparingly to "avoid practitioners mentally overriding the information" when reading the exact drug name, strength, and dose they are preparing, dispensing, and administering.[21]

Use of Tall Man Letters on Labels

To reduce medication errors, the FDA launched the FDA Name Differentiation Project in 2001. This project sought to identify look-alike generic drug name pairs and collaborate with manufacturers on the voluntary use of tall man letters (eg, DOBUTamine, DOPamine) to differentiate the selected look-alike drug names on the labels.[22] *Tall man lettering* involves the selective use of upper case to differentiate the look-alike and sound-alike portion of a drug name. The most updated FDA list contains 23 name pairs with suggested tall man lettering. Since this is strictly a recommendation from FDA, the adoption of tall man lettering varies by manufacturer. This has led to inconsistency in labeling from vendor to vendor and sometimes from drug to drug, which can create confusion for those involved in the compounding, dispensing, and administration of these drugs. The FDA and ISMP have continued to expand their list of recommended tall man letters to be used to differentiate look-alike and sound-alike drug names, although the two lists are not consistent with one another.[10;23] Pharmacies can also choose to use tall man characters to distinguish between similar sounding or look-alike drug names on CSP labels. Again, without a set standard, facilities should review guidance from FDA and ISMP to standardize the use of tall man letters for the CSPs and affected letters chosen in their own specific institution.[10] To date, the real world effectiveness of the tall man lettering strategy is unknown. However, Grasha found tall man lettering "reduced drug selection errors by 35% in a simulated pharmacy dispensing environment."[24;25] Similar to color coding or graphics, tall man lettering should be used judiciously as a supplementary tool for increasing the effectiveness and safety of information contained on medication labels.

Use of Barcodes on Labels

The National Coordinating Council for Medication Error Reporting and Prevention recommends the use of both machine-readable codes (eg, barcodes) and human readable medication labels.[26] Each healthcare institution and compounding facility must decide what exact information the barcodes they use will contain. If a barcode medication administration (BCMA) system is utilized, the medication identifier, lot number, and BUD for CSPs can be elements of barcoded information placed on a CSP label.[27] Barcodes can be oriented vertically or horizontally in a standardized location on the label (whichever allows the best readability while the dose is being administered).[10] The standard color for all barcodes printed on a medication label is black.[10]

Prior to dispensing, pharmacy personnel must ensure that the barcode, as read by the scanners used at that institution, represents the correct drug. Multiple barcodes on a preparation are confusing and should be avoided.[16] At the point of administration and as part of the five rights (right drug, right dose, right patient, right route, and right time), the nurse should scan the actual medication to be given and the patient identification wristband. This helps ensure the particular drug and dose has been prescribed for that specific patient before administration. System alerts or other critical safety information can also be programmed into the BCMA system for specific high-risk medications. As with other technologies, shortcuts and workarounds can negate the effectiveness of barcoding as a patient safety tool.

Specialty Labels

HIPAA privacy regulations state that patient confidentiality of protected health information must be maintained.[28] Some companies have designed new label formats that ensure patient privacy and confidentiality whereby the portion of the label that contains the patient name and other identifying information can be peeled off or removed before destruction of any sterile preparation. This design allows for the patient information component of the label to follow the confidential waste stream without the risk of violating privacy regulations. If specially designed labels like this are not used, patient confidentiality and privacy need to be ensured using other methods.

SUMMARY

Accurate labeling of compounded sterile products is a USP requirement for all CSPs regardless of the setting in which the patient receives the dose.[1] The information on the label must be legible, accurate, easy to understand, uniform, and appropriately displayed. There are minor differences in the recommended label information for patient-specific, institutional, and home care settings as well as for compounded sterile batch preparations.

Patient-specific labeling information for CSPs should include but not be limited to the following:

- Patient name and a second unique identifier (eg, patient identification number, lot number, control number, or prescription number)
- Patient location
- Names and amounts or concentrations of all active ingredients, including drugs, admixture solutions, and diluents
- Total amount or volume of the CSP
- BUD (and time if applicable)
- Appropriate routes of administration
- Storage conditions
- Single-dose container or pharmacy bulk package designation (if applicable)
- The fact it is a compounded drug preparation
- Special handling instructions, including the following:
    - Specific administration instructions or directions for use
    - Time and date of scheduled administration
- Warning or precautionary statements when appropriate
- Other information for safe use, including the following:
    - Responsible pharmacist's initials
    - Date of preparation
    - Any additional information to ensure the safe use of the CSP

These labeling requirements can be met on either the primary label or on auxiliary labels. Unique labeling techniques and strategies should continually be studied, utilized, and evaluated for effectiveness in preventing potentially significant medication errors and adverse drug events. Labels should also be designed to ensure patient privacy of protected health information. The goal of any strategy for labeling CSPs should be focused on appropriate and safe drug administration to the patient.

REFERENCES

1. USP <797> Pharmaceutical compounding—sterile preparations. In: *2022: USP Compounding Compendium.* Rockville, MD: The United States Pharmacopeial Convention; November 1, 2022. **https://doi.org/10.31003/USPNF_M99925_07_01**.
2. USP <797> Pharmaceutical compounding—sterile preparations. In: *USP 27–NF 22*. Rockville, MD; United States Pharmacopeial Convention; 2004.
3. USP <797> pharmaceutical compounding—sterile preparations. Revision Bulletin, 2008. **www.usp.org/pdf/EN/USPNF/generalChapter797.pdf**. Accessed July 26, 2022.
4. American Society of Health-System Pharmacists (ASHP). ASHP guidelines on compounding sterile preparations. *Am J Health Syst Pharm*. 2014;71(2): 145–166. doi:10.2146/sp140001.
5. Brzozowski DF, Hale KM, Segal R, Mirtallo JM. Pharmacists' opinions about and compliance with recommendations for intravenous admixture practices. *Am J Hosp Pharm*. 1987;44(9):2077–2084. **https://pubmed.ncbi.nlm.nih.gov/3479020/**.
6. Petroff BJ, Filibeck D, Nowobilski-Vasilios A, et al. ASHP guidelines on home infusion pharmacy services. *Am J Health Syst Pharm*. 2014;71(4):325–341. doi:10.2146/sp140004.
7. American Society of Hospital Pharmacists (ASHP). ASHP technical assistance bulletin on pharmacy-prepared ophthalmic products. *Am J Hosp Pharm*. 1993;50(7):1462–1463. **https://pubmed.ncbi.nlm.nih.gov/8362884/**.
8. American Society of Health-System Pharmacists (ASHP). ASHP guidelines on outsourcing sterile compounding services. *Am J Health Syst Pharm*. 2015;72(19):1664–1675. doi:10.2146/sp150024.
9. The Joint Commission. National Patient Safety Goals effective January 2022 for the hospital program. **https://www.jointcommission.org/-/media/tjc/documents/standards/national-patient-safety-goals/2022/npsg_chapter_hap_jan2022.pdf**. Published October 25, 2021. Accessed September 8, 2023.
10. Institute for Safe Medication Practices (ISMP). Guidelines for safe electronic communication of medication information. **https://www.ismp.org/node/1322**. Published January 16, 2019. Accessed September 8, 2023.
11. USP <17> Prescription container labeling. In: *2020: USP Compounding Compendium*. Rockville, MD: United States Pharmacopeial Convention; May 1, 2020. **https://doi.org/10.31003/USPNF_M5531_02_01**.

12. USP <7> Labeling. In: *2023: USP Compounding Compendium.* Rockville, MD: United States Pharmacopeial Compendium; September 1, 2023. **https://doi.org/10.31003/USPNF_M4908_11_01**.

13. Institute for Safe Medication Practices (ISMP). Guidelines for sterile compounding and the safe use of sterile compounding technology. **https://www.ismp.org/resources/guidelines-sterile-compounding-and-safe-use-sterile-compounding-technology**. Published May 4, 2022. Accessed September 8, 2023.

14. U.S. Pharmacopeia (USP). Medication safety & labeling. **www.usp.org/usp-healthcare-professionals/medication-safety-labeling**. Accessed September 8, 2023.

15. Food and Drug Administration (FDA). Human drug compounding. **www.fda.gov/drugs/guidancecomplianceregulatoryinformation/pharmacycompounding**. Updated April 26, 2021. Accessed September 8, 2023.

16. Cohen MR, Smetzer JL. Mislabeling event with batched drugs: unintended consequences of practice change; morse code imprint; multiple barcodes cause confusion. *Hosp Pharm*. 2014;49(5):415–418. doi: 10.1310/hpj4905-415.

17. Institute for Safe Medication Practices. Strengthen your resolve: no unlabeled containers anywhere, ever! *ISMP Med Safety Alert.* 2014;19:1–4.

18. Vlessides M. Pilot study finds preprinted labeling saves time, ups safety. *Pharm Practice News.* December 10, 2014. **www.pharmacypracticenews.com/Operations-Management/Article/12-14/Pilot-Study-Finds-Preprinted-Labeling-Saves-Time-Ups-Safety/29018**. Accessed September 8, 2023.

19. Allen LV Jr. Editorial: kudos to IACP and the new labeling guidelines. *Compound Today*. 2006;3:1–2.

20. Institute for Safe Medication Practices (ISMP). A spectrum of problems with using color. *ISMP Med Safety Alert.* 2003;8:1–2.

21. Young D. Experts examine problems with labels on parenteral infusion products. *Am J Health Syst Pharm*. 2007;64(4):345–346. doi: 10.2146/news070015.

22. Food and Drug Administration (FDA). FDA name differentiation project. **www.fda.gov/drugs/drugsafety/medicationerrors/ucm164587.htm**. Updated April 28, 2020. Accessed September 8, 2023.

23. Institute for Safe Medication Practices (ISMP). List of confused drug names. **www.ismp.org/tools/confuseddrugnames.pdf**. Published February 28, 2019. Accessed September 8, 2023.

24. Institute for Safe Medication Practices (ISMP). Let us know if "tall man" letters have been effective. *ISMP Med Safety Alert*. 2003;8:3.

25. Institute for Safe Medication Practices (ISMP). For every problem a solution; for every solution a problem. *ISMP Med Safety Alert*. 2004;9:2.

26. National Coordinating Council for Medication Error Reporting and Prevention (NCCMERP). Recommendations for bar code labels on pharmaceutical (drug) products to reduce medication errors. **www.nccmerp.org/recommendations-bar-code-labels-pharmaceutical-drug-products-reduce-medication-errors**. Revised June 5, 2007. Accessed September 8, 2023.

27. Venti E. Enhanced medication labeling to improve patient safety. *Cleanrooms & Compounding.* 2007;410:10–13.

28. Giacalone RP, Cacciatore GG. HIPAA and its impact on pharmacy practice. *Am J Health Syst Pharm.* 2003;60(5):433–442, quiz 443–445. **https://pubmed.ncbi.nlm.nih.gov/12635449/**.

18

FINISHED PREPARATION RELEASE CHECKS AND TESTS

Angela W. Yaniv

INTRODUCTION

Compounding processes must be designed to prevent errors. Checking processes must be designed to detect any errors that occurred during compounding. Although these concepts seem self-evident, there is a long history of compounding misadventures that have led to patient harm. Chapter 1 discusses this in more detail, and there are several articles outlining compounding errors in the United States.[1;2]

The American Society of Health-System Pharmacists (ASHP) published a technical assistance bulletin on the topic in 1993 with subsequent revisions in 2000 and 2014.[3-5] In January 2004, the U.S. Pharmacopeial Convention (USP) published USP Chapter <797> Pharmaceutical Compounding—Sterile Preparations, the first national and enforceable requirements for sterile compounding. USP Chapter <797> was revised in 2008 and again in 2022 (to become official on November 1, 2023).[6;7] The goal of USP Chapter <797> is to prevent harm to patients receiving compounded sterile preparations (CSPs) that could result from microbial contamination, bacterial endotoxins, variability in intended strength of correct ingredients, physical and chemical incompatibilities, chemical and physical contaminants, and/or the use of ingredients of inappropriate quality.[7]

Despite enforceable requirements in place as of 2004, catastrophic compounding errors involving variability from intended strength of ingredients and microbial contamination have occurred.[8-14] Such errors could have been avoided if robust preparation release checks and tests had been in place.

MEDICATION ORDER WRITING AND TRANSCRIPTION

Paper medication orders must be transcribed in some fashion to create a compounding label. Preparation of preprinted order forms may help reduce errors in prescribing the appropriate dose or base solution for a CSP. Preprinted orders may also reduce the need for extraneous calculations. Because errors can occur in transcription, it is necessary to compare the compounding label with the original order. In manual transcription systems, it is helpful to implement double-checks of order entry and preparation labels, especially for medications for populations at high risk for harm (eg, chemotherapy orders, neonatal pediatric patients, and high-alert medications).

When orders are electronically generated and verified, the compounding label represents the electronic order. Electronic medication ordering can be used to standardize concentrations, doses, and base solutions. Properly constructed medication files and electronic order sets can reduce or eliminate the need for extraneous dosing calculations and can ensure that sterile products are ordered in compatible fluids at the appropriate concentrations. Pharmacists with a thorough knowledge of drug dosing and preparation should be involved in constructing drug files and order sets. For batch production of sterile preparations, a master formulation record (MFR) must be defined in writing with all compounding processes detailed so that each batch is made in the same way each time.

GOOD DOCUMENTATION PRACTICES

Review of compounding records is a critical final release check. Good documentation ensures that all steps in the compounding process actually occurred and is the proof that written policies and procedures were followed. Before final release of a CSP, the pharmacist must verify documentation in the compounding record to ensure the following:

- Proper components were used (vials, ampuls, and final solution container).
- Proper compounding methods were used and were verified (eg, reconstitution, solution transfer quantities).

DOI 10.37573/9781585286492.018

- Proper quantities of components were used when compared to desired versus actual yield. For a patient-specific product, the amount of drug needed matches the amount used (ie, two 500-mg vials were used to prepare one 1,000-mg dose). For a batch, the amount of drug used yields the expected number of doses (ie, 10 1-g antibiotic syringes were expected, and 10 syringes were prepared using one 10-g source vial of antibiotic with no residual solution in the source container).
- Correct labels were used. The label accurately reflects the ingredients used in compounding and is applied to the product without obstructing information needed in administration, such as syringe graduations. For a patient-specific preparation, the label includes the appropriate patient information and identifiers. For batched products, the label includes an internal lot number to identify that batch. Also, for batched products, the number of labels printed corresponds with the number of items in the batch. Instances of insufficient or extra labels are investigated, as this indicates a potential error in the compounding or labeling of the batch (see Chapters 17, 28, and 30 for details).

Good documentation provides enough information to determine how a preparation or batch was made without relying on the recollection of the compounder or checking pharmacist. It allows retrospective review of a compounding process and provides traceability in the event of an unexpected or untoward outcome. It must be complete, correct, and legible. Elements of good documentation that must be included in the compounding record are as follows[7]:

- Name, strength or activity, and dosage form of the CSP
- Date and time of preparation of the CSP
- Assigned internal identification number (order number, prescription number, lot number, etc.)
- A method to identify the individuals involved in the compounded process and individuals verifying the final CSP
- Name of each component
- Vendor, manufacturer, National Drug Code (NDC), lot number, and expiration date for each component
- Weight or volume of each component
- Strength or activity of each component
- Total quantity compounded
- Final yield (for batches)
- Assigned beyond-use date (BUD) and storage requirements
- Results of quality control procedures (eg, visual inspection, filter integrity testing, pH testing, etc.) as applicable
- Calculations made to determine and verify quantities and/or concentrations of components if applicable
- MFR reference for batches

COMPONENT STANDARDS

The selection of appropriate ingredients to use in CSPs is critical to the quality of resulting CSPs. Commercially available sterile components should only be sourced from U.S. Food and Drug Administration (FDA)-registered manufacturers, which are required to perform release testing to ensure that the product meets USP monograph requirements for purity and strength. Nonsterile active pharmaceutical ingredients (APIs) and other bulk nonsterile chemicals should also be sourced from chemical manufacturers or repackagers registered with the FDA.

Raw chemical components and APIs (eg, nonsterile powders) are supplied in many levels of purity. The highest purity chemicals are designated as American Chemical Society (ACS) grade and meet or exceed the standards of ACS. Chemicals designated as reagents are high purity, and they are used in many laboratory and analytical applications. Chemicals designated as USP meet or exceed the standards of the USP monograph and are suitable for use in pharmaceutical compounding. Laboratory-grade chemicals may be relatively pure, but the exact level of impurities may be unknown. Laboratory-grade chemicals are not suitable for pharmaceutical compounding. Other designations may include purified, pure, practical, or technical. Chemicals with these indications may be of good quality but have not been tested against an official standard and should not be used in pharmaceutical compounding.[15] Food-grade bulk substances are chemicals that can be used in food and related products. Food-grade substances must be certified as meeting USP standards to be used in pharmaceutical compounding.

USP-grade ingredients are the lowest quality that may be used in pharmaceutical compounding.[7] If a component or API has USP at the end of its drug name (eg, morphine sulfate USP), there is a USP monograph in the USP compendium, and that component or API meets the compendial standards. If a USP-grade component is not available, then a higher-grade component may be used.

Accept bulk chemicals and APIs only when accompanied by a certificate of analysis (COA). A COA details the component's purity, and contains critical information about its quality and release checks performed. A COA is specific to a lot of API. A COA must be obtained for every lot purchased. The pharmacist must evaluate the COA and all other available information to determine whether a component is suitable and safe for pharmaceutical compounding.

COMPOUNDING ACCURACY CHECKS

CSPs must be checked for accuracy before being released or dispensed by the responsible pharmacist. Written policies and procedures for the checking process should be in place and must meet applicable Federal and state regulations. Ideally, compounding and checking should be done by two different people. When this is not possible (pharmacist is preparing and checking), it is critical for the pharmacist to develop and consistently observe a self-check process. Accuracy checks include determining that the CSP was prepared with correct ingredients in the correct amounts, all required procedures were followed, documentation was completed accurately, and the CSP was labeled appropriately.

Over the last fifteen years, a number of technologies have entered the market that allow for enhanced documentation of the compounding process and can assist with accuracy checking. Many of these intravenous (IV) workflow management systems incorporate multiple elements to assist in verification of compounding accuracy. The Institute for Safe Medication Practices (ISMP) encourages the adoption of technology as an error-prevention strategy in sterile compounding and indicates that use of an IV workflow management system is a minimum safety standard for preparing CSPs.[16;17]

Syringe Pull-back Method

In the syringe pull-back method of accuracy checking, the compounder documents the amount of ingredients used and then returns the source containers and the syringes used with the plunger pulled back to the gradation representing the volume added to the CSP to the pharmacist. When using the syringe pull-back method, the pharmacist should verify that the appropriate number of containers was used and that residual amounts in the containers correspond with the preparation. Any variation between documentation and pull-back, the presence of unexpected source containers, or unexpected residuals should result in an investigation with the compounder. If questions are not completely resolved, the dose should be discarded.

Syringe pull-back is a representation of the compounding process, and it requires some faith that the compounder documented and pulled back correctly. It has been shown to provide highly variable results when checked against gravimetric measurements.[18] ISMP states that proxy methods, such as syringe pull-back, should not be used to verify complex CSPs, chemotherapy, pediatric and neonatal doses, or high-alert CSPs, and that when used, the source containers must be present during the checking process.[19]

Visual Syringe Checks and Photographic Documentation

As advocated by ISMP, institutions may require visual syringe checks during the compounding process for certain products, such as chemotherapy, intrathecals, and other high-alert drugs. Such checks can be useful but are difficult to document and even more difficult to trace. They also require that a pharmacist be immediately available in the compounding area to complete the checks.[19]

An alternative is photographic documentation of drugs in the syringes captured during the compounding process. Several IV workflow software solutions incorporate photographic documentation. Required images must be specified in standard operating procedures so that each compounder provides the same photographic elements for each CSP prepared. Photographic documentation can be retrieved easily and can provide a clear record of how a product was made.[20]

Barcode Identification of Ingredients

Many IV workflow systems incorporate barcode identification of ingredients. Barcode identification can prevent compounding errors before they occur by alerting the compounder when an incorrect ingredient is selected and scanned. They also allow tracking of the exact NDC used in compounding. Ideally, the system used is capable of identifying barcodes for all components used to prepare a CSP (eg, drugs, fluid, and diluent for reconstitution).

To work effectively, the IV workflow system must expect the ingredients that will actually be used. This requires that electronic drug files be maintained to properly reflect the compounding process. When this is not the case, the workflow system generates alerts that may lead to alert fatigue or the instigation of workarounds. The database of barcodes must also be maintained because products may be obtained from new sources or the manufacturer may change the product barcode. Controls must be in place to ensure that barcode maintenance is done by a qualified individual. Assigning a barcode to an incorrect ingredient can result in errors.

Gravimetric Checks

Gravimetric (weight) verification provides precise information about the amount of an ingredient used in compounding. With gravimetric measurement, the amount of ingredient transferred is weighed using a precision scale. The weight of ingredient can be obtained as the change in weight from empty syringe to filled syringe, change in weight of the drug vial after fluid withdrawal, and/or change in weight of the bag after the ingredient is added. The precise weight is then converted to volume or dose using the specific gravity of the ingredient.

Multichannel pumps used in compounding parenteral nutrition solutions use gravimetric measurement to confirm the accuracy of the pump. Per the American Society for Parenteral and Enteral Nutrition's *Safe Practices for Parenteral Nutrition* and *ASHP Guidelines on the Safe Use of Automated Compounding Devices for the Preparation of Parenteral Nutrition Admixtures*, the use of gravimetric measurement allows the operator the ability to evaluate the accuracy of the automated compounding device.[21;22] Gravimetric measurement is used in robotic compounding devices as well, and it is incorporated in some IV workflow systems.[23;24] Scales used for gravimetric checks must be properly calibrated daily or per the manufacturer specifications and certified at least annually.

Gravimetric checks rely on association of the weight with the ingredient being weighed. The workflow system or automated compounding device must incorporate a mechanism to identify the ingredient, such as barcode identification or photo recognition of the ingredient vial. For multichannel pumps, a manual check of the pump set up is necessary to ensure that the appropriate channel (and therefore specific gravity) is associated with the appropriate ingredient. Checks should also be made each time a source container is changed.[21] Mismatch of ingredient to pumping channel can be difficult to detect and can lead to potentially devastating results.

Point of Preparation Testing

The ability to quantitatively and qualitatively test each patient-specific CSP at the point of preparation is limited. Refractometry was used more widely in the late 1980s and 1990s to monitor for controlled substance tampering or diversion and to evaluate parenteral nutrition solutions.[25-30] Refractometry detects the refractive index of a solution as expressed in Brix units. The Brix scale describes the percentage concentration of soluble solids in a water solution. It can be used to qualitatively evaluate CSPs quickly but without much specificity. It is not a quantitative test of the solution's actual components or their concentration.

Technologies continue to be developed using a variety of photometric and spectroscopic methods, but few are marketed and in active use at the time of this writing. Enhanced photoemission spectroscopy has been reported to be sensitive and specific at detecting an incorrect medication and out of range concentration variances.[31]

PHYSICAL INSPECTION

Although accuracy in compounding and use of correct ingredients are of utmost concern, all CSPs require a physical inspection prior to final release or dispensing. When compounding verification is completed remotely using IV workflow management systems, a process for physical inspection prior to dispensing must be established. Physical inspection provides basic information about the integrity of the CSP and should include evaluation of the following:

- Container and closure integrity: The container is intact and free from leaks. Seals or caps are intact.
- Particulates: The solution is free of visible particulates and extraneous substances other than gas bubbles.
    - A light or dark background comparison can assist in detecting visible particulates.
    - When infused, particulates may cause immune reactions, create a locus for infection, block capillaries (8 to 15 μm in diameter), or cause direct physical damage to blood vessels.[32]
    - The threshold for visibility is around 150 μm. Smaller, subvisible particles may not be detected through physical inspection. Microscopic evaluation may be warranted for some products if a high subvisible particulate load is suspected.[33;34]
- Appearance: Color, volume, and other detectable characteristics are as expected. Emulsions, such as fat containing parenteral nutrition solutions, are uniform with no phase separation (cracking, creaming, or oiling).
- Labeling: The labeling is clear, legible, and correctly represents the product. Appropriate auxiliary labels are attached.

STERILITY TESTING

Sterility testing is required for all Category 3 CSPs and for Category 2 CSPs assigned a BUD that exceeds the limits defined in USP Chapter <797> Table 13.[7] When sterility testing is conducted, it must comply with USP Chapter <71> Sterility Tests.[7;35] It is important to understand that sterility tests are not designed to ensure that a batch of product is sterile or has been sterilized. Assurance of sterility is accomplished primarily by validation of the aseptic procedures used and the sterilization process.[35] These concepts are discussed in Chapter 12.

Sterility testing has several limitations. The tests are always destructive. Sterility testing can only detect viable organisms if they are present in the samples that are tested and able to grow in the media used. The volume and number of units tested may represent a very small fraction of the volume and units prepared in the batch. Some units in a batch may be contaminated but not detected because of the sample size (false negative). Samples may be contaminated during inoculation procedures leading to growth when the batch is not actually contaminated (false positives).

USP Chapter <71> delineates the types of growth media to use, the minimum quantity and number of articles to be tested in each media, and sterility testing methods. Sterility tests must be conducted using two different media, fluid thioglycollate medium (FTM) and soybean-casein digest medium (SCDM). FTM is used primarily to detect anaerobic bacteria, although it will also detect some aerobic species. SCDM is used to detect aerobic bacteria and fungi. Each lot of media used for sterility testing must be shown to support growth of bacterial and fungal species including *Staphylococcus aureus*, *Pseudomonas aeruginosa*, *Clostridium sporogenes* for FTM and *Bacillus subtilis*, *Aspergillus brasiliensis*, and *Candida albicans* for SCDM. Suitable strains and additional procedures for growth promotion tests are listed in USP Chapter <71>.[35] Commercially available growth media must be accompanied by a COA confirming that growth promotion tests have been conducted by the manufacturer.

The minimum volume of each CSP to be tested is dependent on the volume of the final product and is described in USP Chapter <71>.[35] If the product is less than 1 mL, the entire volume must be tested. If the volume is 1 to 40 mL, half the total volume is tested. If the volume is 40 to 100 mL, 20 mL is tested. If the volume is greater than 100 mL, 10% of the volume is tested (at least 20 mL).

USP Chapter <71> describes minimum articles to be tested as follows[35]:

- Batches up to 100 units: 10% of the articles should be tested with a minimum of four articles tested
- Batches between 100 and 500 units: 10 units should be tested
- Batches greater than 500 units: 2% of the units (up to 20 units) should be tested
- Large volume parenteral: 2% of the units (up to 10 units) should be tested

USP Chapter <797> limits the batch size to 250 articles for CSPs requiring sterility testing and also outlines some exceptions to USP Chapter <71> article requirements for batches of 1 to 39 articles.[7] Consequently, for 503A facilities following USP Chapter <797> (as opposed to 503B facilities following CGMP), the following minimums for articles to test would apply[7]:

- Batches of 1 to 39 units: 10% of the batch should be tested and rounded to the nearest whole number, for example
    - If 1 unit is made, a second unit is required for testing
    - If a batch of 25 units is made, 3 units are required for testing
- Batches between 40 and 100 units: 10% of the articles should be tested
- Batches between 101 and 250 units: 10 units should be tested

The number of units specified must be tested in both FTM and SCDM media. When the total volume of the product allows, the same units should be used to inoculate both media.[35]

Two sterility testing methods are described in USP Chapter <71>. Membrane filtration is the preferred method when it is used with filterable aqueous, oily, or alcoholic preparations and preparations miscible with or soluble in aqueous or oily solvents. In *membrane filtration*, the samples to be tested are filtered through a membrane with a nominal pore size no greater than 0.45 µm. The entire volume of each unit can be run through the filter, which maximizes the ability to detect any microorganisms present in the units tested. The membrane is then incubated in the required media for 14 days. Direct inoculation is the other method described. With *direct inoculation*, the required volume from each unit is combined with the appropriate amount of the growth media and incubated for 14 days. For most products, only a portion of the unit is used to inoculate the media, so this method detects the presence of microorganisms only in the tested portion of each unit. With both methods, the FTM samples are incubated at 30 to 35°C and SCDM samples are incubated at 20 to 25°C. Turbidity indicates growth.[7;35]

When sterility tests indicate that microbial growth has occurred, USP Chapter <71> allows for a retest of the batch under certain circumstances when there is evidence that the positive sterility test can be attributed to a fault in the process.[35] Otherwise, the batch must be destroyed.

Batches undergoing sterility testing should remain in quarantine until sterility test results are available. If a batch is released early, there must be a mechanism in place to recall the batch should the sterility test subsequently show growth. In such an instance, immediate investigation must occur, including identification of patients potentially exposed and appropriate reporting of the event.

Alternative sterility testing methods may be used if they are determined to be equivalent or superior to the methods listed in USP Chapter <71>. Validation of alternative methods is described in USP Chapter <1223> Validation of Alternative Microbiological Methods. Several rapid microbiological methods have been described using signals of microbial presence, including carbon dioxide fluorometric or colorimetric detection, microbial adenosine-kinase enhanced adenosine triphosphate bioluminescence, and direct fluorescent labeling.[36-38]

BACTERIAL ENDOTOXIN TESTING

Endotoxins are lipopolysaccharides that make up part of a gram-negative bacterial cell wall. They are released upon cell lysis and become pyrogenic when introduced into the bloodstream. They can be difficult to remove from solutions but can be rendered inactive or destroyed by heat. Endotoxins cause fever, hypotension, organ failure, and even death when present in large enough quantities.

Endotoxin testing is required for Category 2 and 3 CSPs compounded using nonsterile ingredients or nonsterile equipment and CSPs that require sterility testing.[7] Category 2 injectable CSPs compounded from one or more nonsterile components but assigned a BUD that does not require sterility testing should be tested for bacterial endotoxins.[7] When endotoxin testing is conducted, it must comply with USP Chapter <85> Bacterial Endotoxins Test.[39]

Endotoxin levels are measured in terms of biological activity as endotoxin units (EU) in the United States and international units (IU) in Europe. These units are equivalent. USP Chapter <85> contains general information about preventing pyrogens, depyrogenation, calculation of endotoxin limits, and methods for endotoxin testing.[39] USP drug monographs usually contain specific endotoxin limits in EU/mg of drug or EU/mL of CSP mixture.

USP Chapter <85> describes two endotoxin testing techniques, the gel-clot technique and the photometric quantitative technique. Both techniques use *Limulus amebocyte lysate* (LAL), a reagent derived from the white blood cells of the horseshoe crab. The gel-clot technique requires preparing an appropriate dilution of the CSP that is combined with the LAL reagent. Control samples are also prepared, and all samples are incubated for 1 hour in a dry-heat incubator. A positive result is a gel from an endotoxin-induced, enzyme cascade of clottable proteins in LAL. Instrumented photometric techniques are quicker and more efficient than gel-clot tests, but they require more costly equipment and skilled analysts. At least one technology is available using disposable cartridges containing the reagents with the test being read by a handheld device.

POTENCY AND STABILITY TESTING

Potency tests determine the amount of an active drug that is in a sample at a given time. A potency test may be used, particularly when compounding from bulk chemicals, to determine that the compounding recipe yields a product of the expected potency. USP monographs indicate the acceptable potency or concentration range for each drug. In most cases this is plus or minus 10% of the labeled strength or concentration (between 90% and 110% of label claim).[7;40]

Stability tests determine the extent to which a product retains its initial chemical, physical, and therapeutic characteristics over time. Stability testing may include method development and validation if a method is not specified in the USP monograph or previously published. The stability study itself evaluates both the amount of intact drug and any degradation products over time.[7;34;40]

High-performance liquid chromatography can be used to determine potency and stability when a stability-indicating method is used. Ultraviolet-visible spectrophotometry can be used to test for potency, but it is limited to liquids containing a single drug. Titration is another method used to determine potency.[7;40] Potency testing alone cannot be used to establish a BUD because it does not differentiate drug and degradation products.

It is extremely important to understand the methods used for testing when outsourcing to an analytical laboratory. When designing or interpreting a stability study with the purpose of BUD determination, the data must reflect stability of the drug under the same conditions that will be present in the clinical setting (eg, same concentration, diluent, container closure system, and storage conditions).

pH TESTING

pH testing may be required for some products when the solution requires a pH adjustment for product stability or a specific pH range because of the route of administration (eg, ophthalmic products). When a specific pH is required, an electronic pH meter should be used.

SUMMARY

Compounding processes must be designed to prevent compounding errors from occurring. Finished preparation release checks and tests must be designed to identify any errors that occur before a CSP is dispensed to a patient.

USP Chapter <797> requires that CSPs be physically inspected before release for particulates, container and closure integrity, and any other visible defects. Compounding accuracy checks must include identification of correct ingredients, confirmation that correct amounts of ingredients were used, and that compounding procedures were followed.

Additional tests, including sterility and endotoxin testing, may be necessary for CSPs compounded from nonsterile components or assigned a BUD that exceeds the USP Chapter <797> recommendations. Potency testing is useful in validating compounding recipes using bulk ingredients. Potency testing alone cannot be used to determine stability of a CSP over time. A stability indicating method is required.

REFERENCES

1. Myers CE. History of sterile compounding in U.S. hospitals: learning from the tragic lessons of the past. *Am J Health Syst Pharm*. 2013;70(16):1414–1427. doi:10.2146/ajhp130112.
2. Gudeman J, Jozwiakowski M, Chollet J, et al. Potential risks of pharmacy compounding. *Drugs R D*. 2013;13(1):1–8. doi:10.1007/s40268-013-0005-9.
3. American Society of Health-System Pharmacists (ASHP). ASHP technical assistance bulletin on quality assurance for pharmacy-prepared sterile products. *Am J Hosp Pharm*. 1993;50(11):2386–2398. **https://pubmed.ncbi.nlm.nih.gov/8266973/**.
4. American Society of Health System Pharmacists (ASHP). ASHP guidelines on quality assurance for pharmacy-prepared sterile products. *Am J Health Syst Pharm*. 2000;57(12):1150–1169. **https://pubmed.ncbi.nlm.nih.gov/10911516/**
5. American Society of Health System Pharmacists (ASHP). ASHP guidelines on compounding sterile preparations. *Am J Health Syst Pharm*. 2014;71(2): 145–166. doi:10.2146/sp140001.
6. USP <797> Pharmaceutical compounding—sterile preparations. In: *2020: USP Compounding Compendium*. Rockville, MD: United States Pharmacopeial Convention; May 1, 2020. **https://doi.org/10.31003/USPNF_M99925_06_01**.
7. USP <797> Pharmaceutical compounding—sterile preparations. In: *USP Compounding Compendium*. Rockville, MD: United States Pharmacopeial Convention; November 1, 2023: Issue 1. **https://doi.org/10.31003/USPNF_M99925_07_01**.

8. Centers for Disease Control and Prevention (CDC). Deaths from intravenous colchicine resulting from a compounding pharmacy error—Oregon and Washington, 2007. *MMWR*. 2007;56(40):1050–1052. **https://pubmed.ncbi.nlm.nih.gov/17932481/**.

9. Institute for Safe Medication Practices (ISMP). Fatal 1,000-fold overdoses can occur, particularly in neonates, by transposing mcg and mg. **https://www.ismp.org/resources/fatal-1000-fold-overdoses-can-occur-particularly-neonates-transposing-mcg-and-mg**. September 6, 2007. Accessed March 5, 2023.

10. Paul R. Former pharmacist indicted for manslaughter after med error. *Drug Topics.* September 17, 2007. **https://www.drugtopics.com/view/former-pharmacist-indicted-manslaughter-after-med-error**. Accessed March 5, 2023.

11. U.S. Food and Drug Administration (FDA). Multistate outbreak of fungal meningitis and other infections. **https://www.fda.gov/drugs/drug-safety-and-availability/multistate-outbreak-fungal-meningitis-and-other-infections**. Published November 1, 2016. Accessed March 5, 2023.

12. Moehring RW, Lewis SS, Isaacs PJ, et al. Outbreak of bacteremia due to *Burkholderia contaminans* linked to intravenous fentanyl from an institutional compounding pharmacy. *JAMA Intern Med*. 2014;174(4):606–612. doi:10.1001/jamainternmed.2013.13768.

13. Gupta N, Hocevar SN, Moulton-Meissner HA, et al. Outbreak of *Serratia marcescens* bloodstream infections in patients receiving parenteral nutrition prepared by a compounding pharmacy. *Clin Infect Dis*. 2014;59(1):1–8. doi:10.1093/cid/ciu218.

14. Goldberg RA, Flynn HW Jr, Miller D, et al. Streptococcus endophthalmitis outbreak after intravitreal injection of bevacizumab: one-year outcomes and investigative results. *Ophthalmology*. 2013;120(7):1448–1453 10.1016/j.ophtha.2012.12.009. doi:10.1016/j.ophtha.2012.12.009.

15. Science Company. Chemical grade definitions. **www.sciencecompany.com/Learn-Chemical-Grade-Definitions-from-Highest-to-Lowest-Purity-W53.aspx**. Accessed March 5, 2023.

16. Institute for Safe Medication Practices (ISMP). Technology and error-prevention strategies: why are we still overlooking the IV room? **www.ismp.org/newsletters/acutecare/showarticle.aspx?id=98**. January 15, 2015. Accessed March 5, 2023.

17. Institute for Safe Medication Practices (ISMP). *ISMP Guidelines for Sterile Compounding and the Safe Use of Sterile Compounding Technology*. Plymouth Meeting, PA: Institute for Safe Medication Practices; 2022.

18. Poppe LB, Savage SW, Eckel SF. Assessment of final product dosing accuracy when using volumetric technique in the preparation of chemotherapy. *J Oncol Pharm Pract*. 2016;22(1):3–9. doi:10.1177/1078155214549489.

19. Institute for Safe Medication Practices (ISMP). *ISMP Guidelines for Safe Preparations of Compounded Sterile Preparations.* Plymouth Meeting, PA: Institute for Safe Medication Practices; 2016. **https://www.ismp.org/sites/default/files/attachments/2017-11/Guidelines%20for%20Safe%20Preparation%20of%20Compounded%20Sterile%20Preperations_%20revised%202016.pdf**. Accessed April 2, 2023.

20. Moniz TT, Chu S, Tom C, et al. Sterile product compounding using an i.v. compounding workflow management system at a pediatric hospital. *Am J Health Syst Pharm*. 2014;71(15):1311–1317. doi:10.2146/ajhp130649.

21. American Society of Health-System Pharmacists (ASHP). ASHP guidelines on the safe use of automated compounding devices for the preparation of parenteral nutrition admixtures. Developed through the ASHP Council on Professional Affairs and approved by the ASHP Board of Directors on April 27, 2000. *Am J Health Syst Pharm*. 2000;57(14):1343–1348. doi:10.1093/ajhp/57.14.1343.

22. Mirtallo J, Canada T, Johnson D, et al. Safe practices for parenteral nutrition. *JPEN*. 2004;28(6):S39–S70. doi:10.1177/0148607104028006s39.

23. Yaniv AW, Knoer SJ. Implementation of an i.v.-compounding robot in a hospital-based cancer center pharmacy. *Am J Health Syst Pharm*. 2013;70(22):2030–2037. doi:10.2146/ajhp120649.

24. Reece KM, Lozano MA, Roux R, et al. Implementation and evaluation of a gravimetric i.v. workflow software system in an oncology ambulatory care pharmacy. *Am J Health Syst Pharm*. 2016;73(3):165–173. doi:10.2146/ajhp150169.

25. Gill DL Jr, Goodwin SR, Knudsen AK, et al. Refractometer screening of controlled substances in an operating room satellite pharmacy. *Am J Hosp Pharm*. 1990;47(4):817–818. **https://pubmed.ncbi.nlm.nih.gov/2321661/**.

26. Cheung JF, Chong S, Kitrenos JG, et al. Use of refractometers to detect controlled-substance tampering. *Am J Hosp Pharm*. 1991;48(7):1488–1492. **https://pubmed.ncbi.nlm.nih.gov/1882879/**.

27. Frankenfield DL, Johnson RE. Refractometry of controlled substances. *Am J Hosp Pharm*. 1991;48(10):2129–2130. **https://pubmed.ncbi.nlm.nih.gov/1781464/**.

28. Donnelly AJ, Petryna HM, Newman LM, et al. A simple, reliable, inexpensive method to aid in the detection of diversion of controlled substances by operating room personnel. *Anesthesiology*. 1990;73:A1053.

29. Meyer GE, Novielli KA, Smith JE. Use of refractive index measurement for quality assurance of pediatric parenteral nutrient solutions. *Am J Hosp Pharm*. 1987;44(7):1617–1620. **https://pubmed.ncbi.nlm.nih.gov/3115096/**.

30. Donnelly AJ, Newman LM, Petryna HM, et al. Refractometric testing of alfentanil hydrochloride, fentanyl citrate, sufentanil citrate, and midazolam hydrochloride. *Am J Hosp Pharm*. 1993;50(2):298–300. **https://pubmed.ncbi.nlm.nih.gov/8480789/**.

31. Kaakeh Y, Phan H, DeSmet BD, et al. Enhanced photoemission spectroscopy for verification of high-risk i.v. medications. *Am J Health Syst Pharm*. 2008;65(1):49–54. doi:10.2146/ajhp060626.

32. Bukofzer S, Ayres J, Chavez A, et al. Industry perspective on the medical risk of visible particles in injectable drug products. *PDA J Pharm Sci Technol*. 2015;69(1):123–139. doi:10.5731/pdajpst.2015.01037.

33. USP <788> Particulate matter in injections. In: *2023: Compounding Compendium.* Rockville, MD: United States Pharmacopeial Convention; May 1, 2023. **https://doi.org/10.31003/USPNF_M99586_02_01**.

34. McElhiney LF. End-preparation assessments and tests for compounded sterile preparations. *Int J Pharm Compd*. 2013;17(4):307–311. **https://pubmed.ncbi.nlm.nih.gov/24261146/**.

35. USP <71> Sterility tests. In: *USP Compounding Compendium.* Rockville, MD: United States Pharmacopeial Convention; Official prior to 2013. **https://doi.org/10.31003/USPNF_M98810_01_01**.

36. Gressett G, Vanhaecke E, Moldenhauer J. Why and how to implement a rapid sterility test. *PDA J Pharm Sci Technol*. 2008;62(6):429–444. **https://pubmed.ncbi.nlm.nih.gov/19634346/**.

37. Hiom S, Denyer S, Talbot C, et al. A preliminary investigation into the ability of three rapid microbiological methods to detect microorganisms in hospital intravenous pharmaceuticals. *PDA J Pharm Sci Technol*. 2013;67(4):376–386. doi:10.5731/pdajpst.2013.00928.

38. USP <1223.1> Validation of alternative microbiological methods. In: *2022: USP Compounding Compendium.* Rockville, MD: United States Pharmacopeial Convention; August 1, 2022. **https://doi.org/10.31003/USPNF_M9153_02_01**.

39. USP <85> Bacterial endotoxins test. In: *2018: USP Compounding Compendium.* Rockville, MD: United States Pharmacopeial Convention; May 1, 2018. **https://doi.org/10.31003/USPNF_M98830_02_01**.

40. Allen LV Jr. Basics of compounding: potency and stability testing. *Int J Pharm Compd*. 2013;17(3):220–224. **https://pubmed.ncbi.nlm.nih.gov/24046938/**.

RECEIPT, STORAGE, MOVEMENT, AND DISPOSAL OF COMPOUNDED STERILE PREPARATION COMPONENTS AND FINISHED PREPARATIONS IN THE PHARMACY

19

Joshua S. Ilenin

INTRODUCTION

This chapter covers appropriate handling of sterile commercial products and compounded sterile preparations (CSPs) within the pharmacy. This responsibility begins when a pharmacy assumes custody of products and continues through compounding, internal storage, and waste disposal. To ensure preparation quality as well as employee and patient safety, correct storage and handling procedures are essential. A thorough understanding of regulatory requirements and best practices in each of these areas aids in the development of a robust sterile compounding operation.

This chapter does not cover selection and quality control of nonsterile components and raw materials (see Chapter 10), nor does it discuss the compounding and dispensing of hazardous drugs (see Chapter 27). It also does not cover the delivery of compounded preparations within the institution or outside the institution, for example in home care (see Chapter 20).

RECEIPT

Sterile Components

Proper handling of sterile components begins even before initial receipt within the pharmacy. Components are comprised of active and inactive ingredients, intermediate containers (eg, a syringe used to transfer a drug from one container to another), final containers, closures, and seals. When sterile commercial products are received at loading docks or other receiving areas, they should be transferred to an appropriate storage environment as quickly as possible or within a time period that is consistent with the risk and exposure of the product in the receiving area.[1] This is particularly important for temperature-sensitive products that can reach temperature equilibrium within minutes or hours depending on the product, packaging, and ambient conditions. In general, sterile component manufacturers designate appropriate storage conditions in a package insert or other product information. These documents should be used as the primary source of storage information, and any deviations should be reported to the manufacturer for clarification. In the absence of specific storage information from the manufacturer, *United States Pharmacopeia* (USP) standards can be used as a guide.[1]

All components that will be utilized in sterile compounding should be visually examined at the time of receipt to ensure they are free from damage that could impact product sterility or quality. Delivery documents should be reviewed in the receiving area to ensure that the commercial sterile products have not been subjected to any conditions outside of the manufacturer designated storage requirements. Any deviations that are noted upon receipt should be reviewed with the manufacturer to determine significance before transferring the component to its final storage location. For products that require special handling, such as refrigerator temperature storage conditions, suppliers should provide documented evidence to show that the required temperature range has been maintained during transport.[1] Additional information regarding appropriate packaging and storage, as well as other factors impacting product stability can be found in USP Chapter <659>—Packaging and Storage Requirements and USP Chapter <1119>—Stability Considerations.[2;3] This information can provide valuable insight into best practices for ensuring stability and sterility upon receipt.

Material flow through the clean room environment begins when products are received at the institution. Staff involved in receiving drug ingredients and supplies should be trained to complete a physical inspection for product integrity and compare items received against purchase orders. Once products are verified as suitable for compounding, they should be transported to a designated storage location and stored in accordance with labeling recommendations until just prior to compounding. If storage information is not explicitly stated in product labeling, a standard operating procedure (SOP) should specify how sterile commercial

Note: The author acknowledges Ryan A. Forrey who wrote this chapter in the previous edition.

DOI 10.37573/9781585286492.019

products, sterile ready-to-use containers, and devices (eg, syringes and needles) should be received and stored within the institution. All items used for compounding must be free from material defects, within the manufacturer's expiration dating, and suitable for their intended use. Records should be maintained in the pharmacy to explain the reason for deviation from required storage conditions and any resulting action taken.[1] Quality issues related to drugs and devices should be promptly reported via the MedWatch program to the U.S. Food and Drug Administration (FDA).[4]

USP Chapter <800> Hazardous Drugs—Handling in Healthcare Settings specifies conditions for receipt of hazardous drugs (HDs).[5] External shipping containers and internal packaging of HDs may be contaminated upon receipt in the pharmacy. Additional precautions should be taken to ensure that personnel are not inadvertently exposed to HDs during initial handling. Shipping containers for HD sterile products should be marked as such and handled separately from non-HD containers. The unpacking area must be designated for HDs and be negative or neutral pressure relative to the adjoining spaces. All sterile HD components should be shipped in sealed plastic containers, and appropriate personal protective equipment (PPE) should be outlined in an entity-specific SOP and readily available in the receiving area. See Chapter 27 for more requirements for handling HDs. For handling of nonsterile components and raw materials, see Chapter 10.

COMPONENT AND SUPPLY STORAGE

Intravenous solutions, sterile commercial products, and sterile supplies should be stored according to manufacturer labeling or USP product monographs to preserve stability of ingredients.[2] Most sterile commercial products are aqueous solutions for which hydrolysis, oxidation-reduction, and photolysis are the most common chemical degradation reactions. The rate of a chemical reaction generally increases exponentially for each 10°C increase in temperature.[3] Thus, a hydrolysable drug that is exposed to a 20°C increase in storage temperature, such as being stored at room temperature rather than in a refrigerator, would have a shelf-life decrease of one fourth to one twenty-fifth of its shelf life under refrigeration.[3]

USP limits for storage temperatures are listed in **Table 19-1**.[2] Recommended storage conditions are usually listed in the monograph or stated on the product label. They may include a specified temperature range or a designated place (eg, refrigerate) based on stability studies performed by the manufacturer.[2] Supplemental instructions (eg, protect from light or do not shake) should also be followed carefully. If a commercial sterile product must be protected from light and is in a clear or translucent container enclosed in an opaque outer covering, this covering should not be removed until the contents are to be used.

In the absence of specific storage information on the manufacturer packaging or label, a sterile commercial product should be stored at controlled room temperature away from moisture, excessive heat or cold, and light (eg, away from heating pipes, ventilation ducts, and lighting fixtures).[2] Regardless of labeled storage conditions, pharmacy personnel are responsible for ensuring that sterile commercial products under their control meet acceptable criteria of stability by (1) storing products under the environmental conditions stated in USP product monographs and FDA-approved labeling, (2) using oldest stock first, (3) observing labeled expiration dates, (4) inspecting sterile commercial products for evidence of instability or package defects, (5) dispensing in a proper container closure system, and (6) properly treating and labeling any mixed or repackaged products.[3]

TABLE 19-1. USP Storage Conditions

Condition	Centigrade Temperature Range	Fahrenheit Temperature Range
Freezer	−25 to −10 °C	−13 to 14 °F
Cold	Not exceeding 8 °C	Not exceeding 46 °F
Refrigerator	2–8 °C	36–46 °F
Cool	8–15 °C	49–59 °F
Controlled room temperature	20–25 °C (excursions are allowed between 15–30 °C)	68–77 °F (excursions are allowed between 59 and 86 °F)
Warm	30–40 °C	86–104 °F
Excessive heat	Above 40 °C	Above 104 °F

Source: Reprinted with permission of USP <659> Packaging and storage requirements. In: *USP 40–NF 35*. Rockville, MD: United States Pharmacopeial Convention; 2017.

Controlled Room Temperature

Many starting ingredients or components of compounded sterile products require storage at controlled room temperature. Controlled room temperature has a narrower definition and acceptable range than regular room temperature, and it is critical to understand the implications of these definitions on CSP component stability. Alterations in temperature-related drug stability could potentially compromise the assignment of beyond-use dates (BUDs) to sterile compounded preparations (CSPs). Therefore, USP has further defined *controlled room temperature* as the "temperature maintained thermostatically that encompasses the usual and customary working environment of 20°C to 25°C (68°F–77°F)."[4]

USP further clarifies that storage conditions meet the definition of controlled room temperature provided that the following conditions are met:

- Mean kinetic temperature (MKT) does not exceed 25°C (77°F).
- Excursions between 15°C and 30°C (59°F and 86°F) that are experienced in pharmacies, hospitals, warehouses, and during shipping are allowed.

- Transient temperature spikes of up to 40°C are permitted so long as they last less than 24 hours and the MKT does not exceed 25°C (77°F).

For any temperature excursions above 40°C, the manufacturer should be contacted regarding the resultant impact of product stability. A summary of USP storage conditions and associated ranges is found in Table 19-1.

Hazardous Drug Storage

USP Chapter <800> outlines practice and quality standards related to the storage of hazardous drugs (HDs). The standards state that all hazardous drugs should be stored to limit the risk of breaks or spills. Antineoplastic HDs that require manipulation other than counting or packaging and active pharmaceutical ingredients (APIs) of an HD require additional storage considerations. They must be stored separately from non-HDs in an externally vented, negative pressure room with at least 12 air changes per hour (ACPH).[5] This means refrigerators and freezers that contain antineoplastic HDs must be dedicated to only HDs and must also be in a negative pressure storage room. The storage of refrigerated antineoplastic HDs is often in the buffer room or containment segregated compounding area (C-SCA). If the refrigerator is stored in the buffer room, an exhaust adjacent to the refrigerator's compressor should be considered.[5] The standards do allow for sterile and nonsterile HDs to be kept in a common storage area, but nonsterile HDs should not be kept in a sterile compounding area to minimize the potential for particle introduction. Expired antineoplastic HD products and APIs of HDs must also be kept in a negative pressure room that is segregated from in-date antineoplastic HDs. The storage area must be an externally vented, negative pressure room with at least 12 ACPH to dilute and remove any airborne contaminants.

USP Chapter <800> states that appropriate PPE should be donned whenever HDs are handled, including during receipt, storage, distribution, stocking, and disposal. Appropriate PPE may include chemotherapy-rated gowns; face masks; head, hair and shoe covers; and chemotherapy gloves depending on the activity performed. For receiving and storage within the pharmacy, an SOP should be developed that outlines appropriate PPE. The SOP should take into account the likelihood for exposure and the overall occupational safety plan at the facility.

Monitoring Storage Conditions

To ensure the integrity and potency of a sterile commercial product through its expiration date, pharmacy personnel must monitor conditions in drug storage areas to ensure they remain within manufacturer recommendations. Controlled temperature areas, such as refrigerators, freezers, and incubators, should be monitored at least once daily, and the results should be documented in a temperature log. Continuous monitoring of storage conditions is preferred, as it can provide real-time, updated information and allow for quick identification and resolution of any out of spec fluctuations. Even when continuous monitoring devices are employed, storage conditions should be physically or electronically documented at least once during each working day to comply with regulatory requirements. Compounding personnel must also note the storage temperature when placing a sterile commercial product into or removing a product from the storage unit to monitor any temperature aberrations.

A continuous temperature recording device or a National Institute of Standards and Technology calibrated thermometer with adequate accuracy and sensitivity may be used if properly calibrated and verified for accuracy at least every 12 months or per manufacturer recommendations.[6;7] The temperature-detecting mechanism should be carefully placed so that it accurately reflects the storage condition temperature, humidity, and other conditions. Avoid placing the device near areas with turbulent airflow, such as doors, air returns, air compressors, or heating, ventilation, and air conditioning system vents, as this may arbitrarily raise or lower the temperature tracked by the device, causing inaccurate readings of the storage conditions. Depending on the physical layout of the storage area, it may be necessary to implement multiple monitoring devices to truly understand the storage conditions within the space. Also, remember to consider how these devices will be powered for continual operation. There should be a battery backup or other fail-safe power source to ensure storage conditions are still being monitored in the event of a primary power failure or loss of wireless connectivity.

INVENTORY CONTROL

Sterile commercial drugs and solutions should be inspected periodically to ensure that they are not damaged, soiled, expired, or otherwise unsuitable. Visual product inspection remains one of the most critical aspects of verifying ingredients and supplies before compounding activities commence. Manufacturing, transport, and storage processes present numerous opportunities for product integrity to be compromised, rendering it inappropriate for use in sterile compounding. Staff involved in receiving drug ingredients and supplies and those participating in compounding activities should be trained to review each product for (1) intact packaging, (2) signs of visible damage or leakage, (3) discoloration, (4) visible particulate matter or other changes in solution, and (5) appropriate labeling, including lot number and expiration date.

Pharmacists who supervise sterile compounding must ensure that all ingredients have their correct identity, strength, quality, and purity.[6] There are several ways to verify the identity and strength of ingredients, including visual verification, barcode scanning, intravenous (IV) workflow technology that incorporates photographic documentation, or volumetric and gravimetric systems that verify ingredients. Appropriate SOPs should be maintained to define actions to take in the event of deviation from any required storage conditions. Documentation should be maintained to explain the reason for deviation and whether affected products were dispensed to patients or sent to another healthcare facility.[1]

Before use, each drug, ingredient, and container should be visually inspected for damage, defects, and expiration date.[6] Products that have exceeded their expiration dates or otherwise do not pass a visual inspection should be removed from product storage areas and returned to the manufacturer or disposed. Organizations with computerized perpetual inventory capabilities may generate a regular report to identify and retrieve products about to expire. Although just-in-time ordering has decreased the problem of excessive inventory and expired drugs for some organizations, low-use inventory locations must still be checked carefully.

To permit adequate floor cleaning and avoid water damage, drugs and supplies should be stored on shelves above the floor. The bottom shelf of any storage system must be solid or have a solid plastic liner (if wire) to prevent any backsplash from the floor reaching the drugs and supplies stored on the shelf. This also helps facilitate routine cleaning, disinfection, and sporicidal application in accordance with USP Chapter <797> or entity-specific SOPs.[6] Drugs should be stored no closer than 18 inches from the ceiling so as not to interfere with the fire-control sprinkler system.

Temperature Excursions

With such precise requirements for medication and component storage, it is inevitable that temperature excursions will occur at some point in all facilities. It is essential that a process be in place to identify and address temperature excursions as quickly as possible and evaluate the impact of the excursion on component stability and potency. Various facility design features (eg, larger warehouse style doors, insufficient ventilation or airflow, lack of backup power source) may make temperature excursions more likely and should be remedied whenever possible. If a temperature excursion is identified, a designated person should determine the overall impact on the component.[6] Calculating the MKT based on available temperature data may be helpful in determining the magnitude of a short-term temperature excursion.[1] Component integrity and quality following an excursion can be verified through a review of available literature, contacting the component manufacturer, or analytical testing to confirm the component integrity. Component manufacturers may also retain information regarding the stability outside of labeled storage conditions. If a temperature excursion occurs for refrigerated or frozen components, an alternative BUD may need to be applied. In the event that product integrity cannot be confirmed following a temperature excursion, the product should be quarantined and discarded.[6]

Partially Used Packages

Sterile commercial products used in CSPs may be packaged in single-dose or multidose containers. While single-dose vials are intended for use on a single patient and for preparing a single dose, there are times when a significant portion of the single-dose container contents remains after preparing an individual dose. In such circumstances, the compounder may wish to retain the single-dose container for future use. So long as the container was accessed, remains in an ISO Class 5 or cleaner environment, and maintains any other labeled storage requirements, it may be retained for up to 12 hours after initial puncture. The exception to this is single dose ampules, which must not be retained for any period of time after first access. Multidose containers, which are intended to be penetrated multiple times and may contain a preservative to prevent microbial growth, can be retained for no more than 28 days following first puncture unless otherwise noted in the package insert. Consideration should be given to the route of CSP administration when using a multiple-dose container, as preservative containing components may not be appropriate (eg, intrathecal or neonatal administration). Partial packages of any kind should not be reused if visual inspection detects unauthorized breaks in the container, closure, and seal; the contents do not possess the expected appearance, aroma, and texture; the contents do not pass identification tests specified by the compounding facility; and either the BUD or expiration date has been exceeded.[6]

Product Recall

Each institution should develop and maintain an SOP outlining the appropriate response when a commercial product is recalled. The first step in response to a product recall is to identify whether the affected product is or has been part of the product inventory at the facility.[6] Computerized inventory management systems can help quickly determine whether the pharmacy has the recalled product in stock. Otherwise, a manual review of current inventory and purchase orders must be undertaken to determine the impact of the recall. An entity-specific SOP should outline a process for determining the severity and urgency of the product recall, including how to identify and notify affected patients. Once the extent and impact of the recall has been established, the SOP should address how to recover and dispose of any affected product. A batch record with lot numbers and expiration dates can facilitate a judicious response to a product recall. When a product recall impacts a facility, there needs to be documentation of the recall procedures and associated outcomes. Each institution should also identify the appropriate regulatory agencies to notify in the event of a product recall that impacts the facility.[6]

TRANSPORT INTO CONTROLLED AREAS

The foundation of cleanroom drug and supply storage is limiting the introduction of unnecessary particles or contaminants that can disrupt the ISO classified environment. There are several key strategies to employ that limit particle production in a cleanroom. Access to the classified area should be limited to designated, qualified personnel and air locks, doors, or pass-throughs should be in place to maintain the classified area. Food, drinks, and materials exposed in patient care and treatment areas must not enter ISO classified areas where components and ingredients of CSPs are present.[6] All supplies should be removed from corrugated cardboard or other particle-generating packaging prior to transport into controlled areas. In general, each institution should develop and frequently update or revise product storage and transport policies as they relate to their specific circumstances. One must also consider going beyond creating policies by conducting routine audits of work practices to ensure compliance.

Supplies

Once materials are procured and received, they must be stored appropriately until used in compounding. Compounding personnel must verify that ingredients for CSPs are of the correct identity and appropriate quality based on the following information:

- Vendor labels
- Auxiliary labeling
- Certificates of analysis
- USP monographs
- Safety data sheets
- Direct chemical analysis
- Knowledge of compounding facility storage conditions

Sterile commercial products, sterile ready-to-use containers, and devices are examples of sterile components. An SOP for unit-by-unit physical inspection prior to use must be followed to ensure that these components are sterile, free from defects, and otherwise suitable for their intended use.

Before transferring any supplies to the clean side of an anteroom, into pass-throughs, or into the perimeter of a C-SCA, they should be removed from the outer shipping container or cardboard and visually inspected for any potential contamination. Some manufacturer packaging is acceptable in the cleanroom environment, especially if its purpose is to maintain drug or supply stability or sterility prior to compounding. Any drug ingredients or supplies transported between unclassified storage areas and the clean room suite or between spaces with different ISO classifications should be wiped down with a sporicidal agent, Environmental Protection Agency (EPA)-registered disinfectant, or 70% isopropyl alcohol (IPA) using a low-lint wipe or cloth and gloved hands.[6] If using a sporicidal agent or EPA-registered disinfectant, refer to the product information for specific dwell time required before the item can be transported. If using 70% IPA, it should be allowed to visibly dry before transporting the item. This process helps reduce the risk of contaminants from packaging being inadvertently transported into the buffer room or direct compounding area.

Generally, products should be stored in a manner that limits particle generation. More frequently used items should be stored in the buffer room for easy access during compounding and to limit movement back and forth to the anteroom. Less frequently used items should be stored in the anteroom to limit particle load in the buffer room. All necessary supplies should be gathered before initiating any compounding activities to limit movement in and out of the primary engineering control.

Carts

Carts should be made of nonporous material with casters and wheels that can be easily cleaned. Carts used to bring supplies from unclassified storage areas to classified areas cannot be rolled beyond the demarcation line in the anteroom. Carts used in the buffer room cannot be rolled outside of the classified area unless they are cleaned and disinfected before they are returned.[6] To maintain this segregation, carts can be designated as clean or dirty.

Clean carts can only stay in the buffer room and clean side of the anteroom. Supplies from storage areas are put on dirty carts. At the demarcation line, supplies are decontaminated and transferred to a clean cart. This process minimizes the ingress of particulate and microbial contamination from carts and packaging materials.

HANDLING PRODUCTS IN THE BUFFER ROOM

Products should be stored until just prior to compounding and then gathered for use. Overall, particle burden in the buffer room should be limited, and only the most used essential supplies should be stored routinely in this area. In addition, storing fewer items in this area serves to prevent clutter and confusion from an overcrowded work area. While supplies can be a significant source of particle generation in the cleanroom, the single greatest producer of particles is cleanroom personnel. As a result, limiting movement in and out of the cleanroom is an especially important aspect of determining how medications and supplies should be stored.

Supplies entering the primary engineering control (PEC) should be limited to those needed for the immediate preparation being compounded. They should be arranged in a way that a clear, uninterrupted path of high-efficiency particulate air (HEPA)-filtered first air bathes all critical sites at all times during aseptic compounding.[6] Any supplies coming into contact with CSPs during the compounding process must be sterile or depyrogenated.[6]

Opened or needle-punctured single-dose containers (eg, bags, bottles, syringes, and vials of sterile products and CSPs) must be used within 4 hours if opened in worse than ISO Class 5 air, and any remaining contents must be discarded. Single-dose vials may be used up to 12 hours after initial needle puncture if they are maintained in an ISO Class 5 environment (ie, inside the PEC).[6] Opened single-dose ampules must not be stored for any time period. If single-dose vials are reused on multiple patients or for multiple doses, it is important to verify that institutional billing practice matches compounding practices. Many institutions have chosen to bill for waste with some or all medications. This prevents reuse of single-dose vials in order to maintain compliance with billing practices.

Multidose containers are formulated with antimicrobial preservatives that allow for repeated access over a period of time. Manufacturer packaging for these containers should indicate that they are multidose vials (MDV). The packaging may include guidance on BUDs once the container is accessed. When manufactured MDVs of sterile ingredients are used in CSPs, they should be labeled with the date and time of first access. The BUD after initially entering or opening (eg, needle-punctured) MDVs is 28 days unless otherwise specified by the manufacturer.[2] If an unlabeled MDV is found after initial puncture, it should be treated as expired and disposed of immediately. MDVs do not need to be stored in an ISO Class 5 environment between each use in order to maintain a 28-day BUD. However, the vial stopper should be inspected for physical integrity and disinfected by wiping with a sterile 70% IPA before each use. When contaminants or abnormal properties are suspected or observed in MDVs, the MDVs must be discarded.[6]

After compounding is complete, a closure may be placed on the preparation to enable detection of tampering. A variety of labeling techniques (varying colors, typeface, banners, auxiliary stickers, etc.) may be used to designate HDs, non-HDs, controlled substances, or other high-risk CSPs to facilitate proper handling and disposal by healthcare workers. Used syringes, ampules, vials, and other supplies should be disposed of in a manner that minimizes exit and reentry into the PEC, maintains aseptic technique, and follows applicable waste streams (see Chapter 15 for details).

STORAGE OF COMPOUNDED STERILE PREPARATIONS

Once compounding is complete, CSPs should undergo a visual inspection prior to dispensing or storage to ensure there are no physical abnormalities with the CSP or container closure system.[6] CSPs should also be reviewed to confirm that the finished product and accompanying label match the original medication order. If any defects or issues are noted during the visual inspection of a completed CSP, it should be immediately discarded or physically segregated from acceptable CSPs to prevent inadvertent dispensing. Any defects noted may indicate sterility or stability issues with CSP components or the compounding process and should be thoroughly investigated to determine a possible root cause. When a CSP is not dispensed immediately following preparation, it should be stored according to available product stability information and the BUD assigned on the CSP label. Appropriate controls should be in place to maintain temperature and humidity ranges in the product storage area that are consistent with the assigned BUD. Compounding personnel should routinely verify and document these storage conditions. A subsequent visual inspection should occur just prior to dispensing, and any deviations from appropriate storage conditions should be noted to ensure that the CSP is not damaged or subject to physical or chemical degradation during storage.

One of the most critical components of CSP storage following preparation is determination of the BUD. Sterility and stability of a CSP must be considered when assigning an appropriate BUD because it represents the date and time after which a CSP cannot be used.[6] There are two primary factors that can influence CSP stability and the BUD, which include the physical and chemical stability of all CSP ingredients and the compatibility of these ingredients with the container closure system in which the CSP is stored. With respect to sterility, several factors, including how the CSP is prepared and stored, can impact the BUD. Components of CSP preparation that have an impact on BUD include the following:

- The environment in which the CSP was prepared
- Whether the CSP was prepared aseptically or terminally sterilized during preparation
- Whether the starting components used in the CSP were sterile or nonsterile
- Whether sterility testing was performed
- Storage conditions of the finalized CSP

Varying BUDs are assigned to CSPs based on these factors and the resulting likelihood of microbial contamination or lack of sterility.

The first step in determining the BUD involves identifying the environment in which the CSP is prepared. If a CSP is prepared in an ISO Class 5 environment situated within an otherwise unclassified space (also known as a C-SCA) it is considered a Category 1 CSP. Only Category 1 CSPs can be prepared in a SCA if the PEC meets all requirements outlined in USP Chapter <797>. Given the lack of a classified space surrounding an ISO Class 5 environment, there is a greater risk for microbial contamination or a lack of sterility to occur during the preparation process. The BUD for Category 1 CSPs stored at controlled room temperature (20°C–25°C) is less than or equal to 12 hours and less than or equal to 24 hours for refrigerated storage (2°C–8°C).

If a CSP is prepared in an ISO Class 5 primary engineering control (PEC) situated within a cleanroom suite, it is considered a Category 2 CSP. This layout can include an ISO Class 7 positive pressure buffer room with an ISO Class 8 positive pressure anteroom or an ISO Class 8 positive pressure buffer room if using a pharmaceutical isolator. The physical environment within a cleanroom suite is less likely to contribute to microbial contamination or a lack of sterility, and it allows for longer BUDs to be assigned to Category 2 CSPs. To determine the exact BUD for a Category 2 CSP, further evaluation of the preparation process is required. This evaluation should include a review of the compounding process and any sterility testing performed on the CSP.

If a Category 2 CSP is prepared starting with sterile ingredients or nonsterile starting ingredients that are terminally sterilized, it is considered aseptically processed. Aseptically processed CSPs prepared from only sterile starting ingredients are assigned a BUD of 4 days at controlled room temperature, 10 days under refrigeration, and 45 days if stored in a freezer. If any nonsterile starting ingredients are used, the risk for microbial contamination and a lack of true sterility is higher so shorter BUDs are assigned. These types of CSPs can be stored for 1 day at controlled room temperature, 4 days under refrigeration, and 45 days if stored in a freezer. The BUD of aseptically prepared Category 2 CSPs may be extended if sterility testing is performed in accordance with USP Chapter <71> Sterility Tests or via a test outlined in USP Chapter <1223> Validation of Alternative Microbiological Methods that is noninferior to USP Chapter <71> testing conditions.[8;9] If a batch of aseptically prepared CSPs passes a sterility test, it is assigned an extended BUD of 30 days at controlled room temperature, 45 days under refrigeration, and 60 days if stored in a freezer.

Category 2 CSPs that are terminally sterilized are considered acceptable if the physical and chemical properties of the CSP and container closure system are not compromised. The terminal sterilization process does not include sterilization by filtration. The process used should intend to achieve a probability of a nonsterile unit (PNSU) of 10^{-6}.[6] Examples of acceptable terminal sterilization processes include dry heat, steam, and irradiation. Additional information on terminal sterilization can be found in USP Chapter <1229> Sterilization of Compendial Articles.[10] Terminally sterilized CSPs may also undergo sterility testing to provide an extended BUD. For terminally sterilized CSPs that do not undergo or pass sterility testing, a BUD of 14 days at controlled room temperature, 28 days when stored under refrigeration, and 45 days when frozen is assigned. If sterility testing is performed and passed, terminally sterilized CSPs are assigned a BUD of 45 days at controlled room temperature, 60 days under refrigeration, and 90 days if frozen.

Category 3 CSPs require the same facility engineering controls as Category 2 CSPs, but they must also undergo sterility and bacterial endotoxin testing.[6] There are, however, more stringent requirements for personnel training and competency demonstration, sterile garb, disinfection, and environmental monitoring that are outlined in USP Chapter <797>

TABLE 19-2. USP Chapter <797> BUDs for Category 1 CSPs

Controlled Room Temperature (20–25 °C)	Refrigerator (2–8 °C)
≤ 12 hours	≤ 24 hours

Source: Reprinted with permission of USP <797> Pharmaceutical compounding—sterile preparations. In: *USP-NF*. Rockville, MD: United States Pharmacopeial Convention; 2023.

and described in greater detail in other chapters of this book. As a result, Category 3 CSPs may be assigned a longer BUD than Category 2 CSPs. The exact BUD assigned to a Category 3 CSP is dependent on available stability data for a given CSP and the results of sterility and bacterial endotoxin testing. However, the BUD for a Category 3 CSP cannot exceed what is outlined in USP Chapter <797>. Category 3 CSPs that are aseptically prepared from sterile starting ingredients and pass all applicable sterility and bacterial endotoxin tests are assigned a BUD of 60 days at controlled room temperature, 90 days when stored under refrigeration, and 120 days when frozen. For Category 3 CSPs that utilize one or more nonsterile starting ingredients and undergo terminal sterilization, a BUD of 90 days at controlled room temperature, 120 days when stored under refrigeration, and 180 days when frozen may be assigned.

See **Tables 19-2**, **19-3**, and **19-4** for a summary of USP storage periods before use. Sterility testing may also be performed on aseptically processed CSPs with the same extended beyond-use dates applied.

Redispensed Sterile Preparations

A compounding pharmacist has the sole authority to determine when unopened returned CSPs may be dispensed again.[6] If CSPs are properly stored and transported but go unused, there is potential for them to be returned to the pharmacy and redispensed for another patient. Each institution should develop its own standard operating procedure (SOP) outlining the circumstances in which CSPs can

TABLE 19-3. USP Chapter <797> BUDs for Category 2 CSPs

Preparation			Storage		
Sterilization Method	Sterility Test	Starting Ingredient	Room Temperature	Refrigerator	Freezer
Aseptically prepared CSPs	No	Any nonsterile	1 day	4 days	45 days
		All sterile	4 days	10 days	45 days
	Yes	Sterile/Nonsterile	30 days	45 days	60 days
Terminally sterilized CSPs	No	Sterile/Nonsterile	14 days	28 days	45 days
	Yes	Sterile/Nonsterile	45 days	60 days	90 days

Source: Reprinted with permission of USP <797> Pharmaceutical compounding—sterile preparations. In: *USP–NF*. Rockville, MD: United States Pharmacopeial Convention; 2023.

TABLE 19-4. USP Chapter <797> BUDs for Category 3 CSPs

Preparation	Storage		
Compounding Method	Room Temperature	Refrigerator	Freezer
Aseptically processed, sterility tested, and passing all applicable tests for Category 3 CSPs	60 days	90 days	120 days
Terminally sterilized, sterility tested, and passing all applicable tests for Category 3 CSPs	90 days	120 days	180 days

Source: Reprinted with permission of USP <797> Pharmaceutical compounding—sterile preparations. In: *USP-NF*. Rockville, MD: United States Pharmacopeial Convention; 2023.

be redispensed. CSPs should only be redispensed by compounding personnel who have verified that proper storage was maintained throughout the time that the CSP was outside of the pharmacy. Components of proper storage to consider include sterility, stability, purity, storage temperature, and a lack of physical tampering. Any preparation that is redispensed must use a BUD based on when the CSP was originally dispensed and contain a label with the name and strength of the CSP.

Detecting deviations in storage conditions can be a challenge with sterile liquids, as they often do not result in physically visible changes. Any haze, color change, cloudiness, surface film, particulate or flocculent matter, or gas formation is sufficient reason to suspect possible contamination.[3] CSPs that have left the pharmacy should be disinfected with sterile 70% IPA and returned to a designated storage location for possible redispensing. They should not be returned to the buffer room of an SCA in order to limit potential microbial contamination or particle generation in these areas. CSPs with attached administration sets should be considered opened and not reused unless they were originally attached in a PEC and appear intact.

WASTE MANAGEMENT

Waste Compounding Materials

The CSP preparation process produces drug and nondrug waste. It is important that all waste produced during this process be disposed of in accordance with applicable state and federal guidelines. Drug waste disposal guidance is highly complex and can be very confusing if not fully understood and properly applied during the sterile compounding process. After compounding is complete, used syringes, bottles, vials, and other supplies must be properly discarded based on their waste classification (see **Table 19-5** for details).[11] Needles must be left on syringes and disposed of carefully to prevent possible needle stick injuries. A used needle and syringe should be placed in a puncture-resistant (ie, sharps) container that can be permanently sealed. To further avoid needle sticks, the needle should not be recapped before discarding the needle and syringe. Sharps containers should be sealed and properly discarded when they are no more than three-quarters full. Sharps used in hazardous drug preparation should be disposed of separately from nonhazardous sharps. Red sharps containers used for nonhazardous sharps waste are frequently disinfected by autoclaving or microwaving (not by incineration). These containers pose a risk of exposure to aerosolized hazardous drugs to waste-handling employees. Hazardous sharps should be differentiated from nonhazardous sharps and disposed of in a yellow sharps puncture-resistant container. Properly labeled, leak-proof, and spill-proof containers of nonreactive plastic are required for all areas where hazardous wastes, including sharps, are generated.[8]

Clean paper, plastic packaging, and empty glass and plastic bottles may be discarded in the municipal waste stream. Waste contaminated with blood or other body fluids must not be mixed with hazardous waste. It must be disposed of as regulated medical or biohazardous waste. Under new Environmental Protection Agency (EPA) guidance, empty hazardous waste containers are no longer considered Resource Conservation Recovery Act (RCRA) hazardous waste and can be treated as nonhazardous drug waste.[12]

Hazardous Waste

Healthcare organizations generate hazardous pharmaceutical waste through activities such as sterile compounding, spills and breakage, partially used containers, outdated products, discontinued or unused preparations, and patient personal medications. While each state may have specific guidance on drug waste disposal, federal government oversight is driven by the EPA. For many years, federal guidance on hazardous pharmaceutical waste disposal was based solely on the Resource Conservation Recovery Act (RCRA), which was passed in 1976. The RCRA defined hazardous chemical waste and provided a mechanism for tracking hazardous waste from its generation to disposal.[12] The regulations set forth by RCRA focused primarily on the management of hazardous waste produced on an industrial scale, such as by pharmaceutical manufacturers, rather than those produced by healthcare institutions or reverse distributors. Since the passage of RCRA, there have been numerous advances in drug therapy, and hundreds of drug products

TABLE 19-5. Recommended Pharmaceutical Waste Streams

Pharmaceutical Waste Type	Inactive Drugs	RCRA Ignitable, Hazardous, Toxic, and Other Hazardous Waste	Trace Chemo Sharps	Trace Chemo Soft Waste	Nonhazardous Drugs	Red Sharps	Controlled Drugs	Radiopharmaceuticals
Authority	Local sewer rules	U.S. and state EPAs	OSHA and EPAs	OSHA and EPAs	State Boards of Pharmacy and state EPAs	OSHA	U.S. and state DEAs	Nuclear Regulatory Commission
Waste container*	Sink drain	Black	Yellow	Yellow	White or blue (most common)	Red	Locked storage	Lead protected
Examples of wastes	Inactive contents of returned IVs (eg, D5W, normal saline)	P-, U-, and D-listed drugs, chemo agents (bulk and residue), chemo and hazardous spill cleanup	RCRA empty used vial, syringes and needles from chemo prep and administration	Used gowns, goggles, gloves, sleeves, wipes, tubing, pads IV bags	Endocrine and antivirals (bulk and residue), all nonhazardous waste drugs (including antibiotics and CSPs with active ingredients)	Empty nonchemotherapy ampules, vials, syringes, needles, glass bottles	Unused, returned, outdated controlled drugs	Low-level waste that typically includes RP syringes, needles, and unused liquid held until decayed
Storage prior to disposal	No storage	Central, safe, secure location	Locked storage	Locked storage	Locked storage	Locked storage	Segregated, locked storage	Segregated, protected storage
Ultimate disposition	Publicly owned treatment works	RCRA approved incinerator	Regulated medical waste incinerator	Regulated medical waste incinerator	Regulated medical waste incinerator or waste-to-energy incinerator	Autoclaved, microwaved or regulated medical waste incinerator	DEA registered reverse distributor	Regulated medical waste

CSPs = compounded sterile preparations; DEA = Drug Enforcement Administration; EPA = Environmental Protection Agency; IV = intravenous; OSHA = Occupational Safety and Health Administration; RCRA = Resource Conservation and Recovery Act; RP = recommended practice; P, U, D = acutely hazardous, toxic pharmaceuticals, and hazardous waste.

* Note that colors of waste containers are not standardized nationally. The most commonly seen waste container colors are listed.

Source: Reprinted with permission of Smith CA, Pines E. Managing pharmaceutical waste: a 10-step blueprint for healthcare facilities in the United States. www.hercenter.org/hazmat/tenstepblueprint.pdf. Revised August 2008. Accessed September 8, 2023.

have been brought to market that are considered hazardous by the National Institute for Occupational Safety and Health (NIOSH). The EPA's hazardous drug list has not been routinely updated, and many of these potentially hazardous drugs are not listed as RCRA hazardous waste. For these reasons, healthcare institutions and reverse distributors have struggled for many years to apply RCRA to their practice.

RCRA hazardous waste pharmaceuticals are listed in 40 CFR part 261 subpart D and include P-listed chemicals, U-listed chemicals, and formulations exhibiting characteristics of hazardous waste, which are assigned D codes.[13] Note that these chemicals and drugs overlap with hazardous drugs listed in the NIOSH alert.[14] The NIOSH hazardous drug list is updated much more frequently than the RCRA list, and it is focused primarily on employee protection, whereas the RCRA list is focused on protecting the environment.

- The P list: P-listed drugs are an *acutely hazardous pharmaceutical*, which is defined as an oral lethal dose of less than 50 mg/kg (LD50).[14;15] The current P list includes pharmaceuticals such as arsenic trioxide, epinephrine (excluding epinephrine salts), nicotine, nitroglycerin, physostigmine, physostigmine salicylate, and warfarin above 0.3%.[14;15] For medications on the P list, full, partial, or empty packaging containing the drug is considered hazardous waste.
- The U list: U-listed pharmaceuticals are also considered toxic, however there is no specific LD50 required to designate these agents as hazardous.[14;15] U-listed pharmaceuticals include chemotherapy agents, such as chlorambucil, cyclophosphamide, daunomycin, melphalan, mitomycin C, and streptozocin. There has been significant new drug approval for chemotherapy agents that are structurally similar to these agents, but the RCRA hazardous list only includes those that were approved when the legislation was first promulgated. Other common pharmaceuticals, such as reserpine, selenium sulfide, resorcinol, and chloral hydrate, are also U-listed. Empty containers that once held U-listed hazardous waste can be disposed of as nonhazardous waste via municipal waste streams.[14]
- The D list: The EPA defines four characteristics for hazardous waste: ignitability, toxicity, corrosivity, and reactivity.[14;15] Numerous pharmaceutical products meet the definition of one or more of these criteria and, therefore, should be classified as D-list hazardous waste. The four characteristics are defined as follows:
    - Ignitability: Pharmaceuticals considered ignitable include aqueous solutions containing 24% or more alcohol with a flash point of less than 140°F; nonaqueous solutions having a flash point of less than 140°F; ignitable flammable aerosol propellants; and oxidizers. Several sterile commercial products contain more than 24% alcohol due to its excellent solvent properties.
    - Toxicity: RCRA lists 40 chemicals with specific concentration values above which must be treated as hazardous. Examples of these, which are found in pharmaceuticals as either active ingredients or preservatives, include arsenic, barium, cadmium, chloroform, chromium, *m*-cresol, mercury (including the preservatives thimerosal and phenylmercuric acetate), selenium, and silver. Each of these chemicals have their own regulatory level at which RCRA classifies them as hazardous waste.
    - Corrosivity: Corrosivity applies to strong acids (pH ≤ 2) and strong bases (pH ≥ 12.5). The generation of corrosive hazardous waste is typically limited to chemicals used in pharmaceutical compounding, such as glacial acetic acid and sodium hydroxide.
    - Reactivity: Reactivity applies to highly explosive and water-reactive chemical compounds.

EPA Guidance for Healthcare Facilities

In acknowledgment of the challenges to RCRA implementation and hazardous waste disposal in healthcare settings, the EPA promulgated the "Management Standards for Hazardous Waste Pharmaceuticals and Amendment to the P075 Listing for Nicotine," which was officially published in the National Register in February 2019.[15] This final rule establishes cost-saving, streamlined standards for handling hazardous waste pharmaceuticals that better fit the operations of the healthcare sector while maintaining protection of human health and the environment.[15] The final rule has three main provisions that impact healthcare facilities and reverse distributors.[15-17]

- The ban on sewering of hazardous waste pharmaceuticals.
    - Healthcare facilities and reverse distributors are no longer able to dispose of hazardous waste pharmaceuticals via *sewering* (ie, flushing or pouring down a sink or toilet). This ban is aimed at reducing the amount of hazardous waste pharmaceuticals discharged into the sewer system and publicly owned treatment works (POTW). The ban applies to all RCRA designated hazardous waste, including controlled substances subject to Drug Enforcement Agency (DEA) regulations. The ban is projected to reduce the volume of hazardous waste entering sewer systems by 1,644 to 2,300 tons annually.[16] This ban is more strict than previous EPA regulations and became effective in all U.S. states and territories on August 21, 2019.

- The amendment to the P075 listing for nicotine.
  - Previously, over-the-counter nicotine replacement products, such as gums, patches, or lozenges, were considered P-listed hazardous waste (P075) and subject to RCRA. This new EPA rule exempts these nicotine products from being treated as RCRA hazardous waste, and therefore it allows these products to be disposed of as nonhazardous waste in healthcare facilities and reverse distributors. This exemption does not extend to e-cigarettes, e-liquids, cartridges, or nicotine used in research, which are still considered hazardous waste pharmaceuticals under 266 subpart P.[17]
- Changes to pharmaceutical waste generator categories and requirements.
  - Healthcare facilities were previously required to manage hazardous pharmaceutical waste under 40 CFR part 262, which applies to hazardous waste generators. The new EPA rules dictate that hazardous waste pharmaceuticals from healthcare facilities and reverse distributors be managed under 40 CFR part 266 subpart P. The EPA has created two categories of healthcare facility hazardous pharmaceutical waste, potentially creditable waste and noncreditable waste pharmaceuticals.[17] The major differentiating factor between these two categories of waste is eligibility for manufacturer credit upon disposal. Potentially creditable waste is unused or not administered and less than one year past its manufacturer expiration date. Noncreditable hazardous waste is unlikely to be eligible for credit because it has been removed from the original container, partially administered to or refused by a patient after dispensing, or is greater than one year past its expiration.[17] Each category has different requirements for accumulation, handling, and disposal. Healthcare facilities are responsible for determining whether creditable and noncreditable pharmaceutical waste should be handled as RCRA hazardous waste.[17] Alternatively, a healthcare facility may choose to handle all pharmaceutical waste as RCRA hazardous, eliminating the need for a hazardous determination for both creditable and noncreditable pharmaceutical waste.[17]
- Standards for healthcare facilities that manage noncreditable hazardous waste pharmaceuticals.
  - Healthcare facilities that accumulate solid waste pharmaceuticals must determine whether the waste meets RCRA hazardous criteria and whether the waste is noncreditable. If both of these criteria are met, noncreditable hazardous waste pharmaceuticals must be managed under part 266 subpart P.[17] All noncreditable hazardous waste must be evaluated for potential ignitability or reactivity under RCRA. The waste must be stored separately from all other noncreditable waste or in a container labeled "hazardous waste pharmaceuticals" that is free from damage, spillage, or leakage. Noncreditable hazardous waste pharmaceuticals may be comingled with nonhazardous noncreditable pharmaceuticals so long as they are labeled "hazardous waste pharmaceuticals" and disposed of as hazardous waste. Healthcare facilities can accumulate this type of waste for up to one year without additional permits or status granted by EPA.[17] Records of noncreditable hazardous waste should be maintained in accordance with 40 CFR part 262.20.[17]
- Standards for healthcare facilities that manage creditable hazardous waste pharmaceuticals.
  - Healthcare facilities that accumulate solid waste pharmaceuticals must also determine whether the waste meets RCRA hazardous criteria and is creditable. If both of these criteria are met, waste can be transferred to a reverse distributor for credit and final processing.[17] Healthcare facilities can choose to make a hazardous determination for each potentially creditable waste or comingle all creditable waste and treat it as hazardous under part 266 subpart P.[17] The EPA does not provide any guidance on the type of accumulation containers or the labeling of accumulation areas or containers prior to sending to a reverse distributor. It does provide some recommendations for preventing spills of liquids or aerosol, such as placing the waste in sealed plastic bags or other containers. No time limit on the accumulation of hazardous waste prior to processing by a reverse distributor is noted by the EPA.[17] Healthcare facilities initiating shipments of potentially creditable hazardous waste pharmaceuticals to reverse distributors must retain delivery confirmation for each shipment and shipping papers for a period of three years.[17]

Chemotherapy Waste

See Chapter 27 for a complete discussion of the containment and disposal of HDs, chemotherapy waste, and related materials.

Nonhazardous Drug Waste

In addition to the categories listed above, other applicable rules should be followed regarding controlled drugs, IV bags containing polyvinyl chloride (PVC), investigational new drugs, and radiopharmaceuticals. Drugs that are not on the RCRA P, U, or D list are not considered hazardous waste by the EPA and should be disposed of by incineration.[14] Non-HD waste should be collected in separate containers for incineration at either a regulated medical waste or municipal solid waste incinerator that is permitted to handle nonhazardous pharmaceutical waste.[14] Drugs derived from blood products, including albumin, should be managed as regulated medical waste and ideally incinerated at a regulated medical waste facility. Autoclaving and microwaving are also options. CSPs dispensed in PVC-containing IV bags and tubing should not be incinerated. Incinerating PVC contributes to dioxin formation, which can produce carcinogens or endocrine-disrupting chemicals.[14] Investigational drug waste must be disposed of according to research sponsor protocols. Radiopharmaceutical waste must follow Nuclear Regulatory Commission rules. Pharmacists are advised to check their local and state EPA regulations for guidance in handling all non-HD waste.

Controlled Substance Drug Waste

The EPA's Management Standards for Hazardous Waste Pharmaceuticals and Amendment to the P075 Listing for Nicotine ruling contains a conditional exemption for any hazardous pharmaceutical wastes that are also DEA controlled substances.[15-17] The Controlled Substances Act (CSA) takes precedence in disposal of CSPs containing controlled drugs.[18] Congress passed an amendment to the CSA, the Secure and Responsible Drug Disposal Act, in 2010, authorizing the DEA to promulgate regulations providing options for the safe handling and disposal of controlled substances already dispensed to consumers.[19] In its response to the act, the DEA developed new regulations regarding the disposal of controlled substances by healthcare facilities called Drug Disposal Regulations, which was published on September 9, 2014.[20] These regulations require controlled substances being disposed from the pharmacy's inventory to be incinerated, requiring a transfer between DEA registrants to a reverse distributor. The amount of waste generated after the drug has been dispensed to the patient is now considered to be outside the DEA closed loop. The DEA issued a clarification letter regarding this change in policy.[21] These drugs should be rendered nonretrievable through sewering (if allowed by local and state authorities and not prohibited under EPA's sewering prohibition for hazardous pharmaceutical waste) or through use of a sequestration system that prevents reuse.[16] Due to the ramifications of this major change in policy, the DEA is continuing to issue guidance letters to the industry. It is important to check with local and regional DEA offices and headquarters for additional clarification on specific instances, such as disposal of outdated multidose vials containing controlled substances.

Expired Sterile Commercial Products

All compounding supplies and CSPs should be clearly labeled with an expiration date or BUD to prevent inadvertent use. Some expired products may be returned to the manufacturer for credit. Generally, expired drugs are handled in one of two ways.

- Expired controlled substances (not waste) must be removed from perpetual inventory. In some cases, they may be returned to the manufacturer for credit. Most pharmacies now utilize the services of a DEA-registered reverse distributor for all expired controlled substances, who then issue a Form 222 for controlled substances in Schedule II and provide additional instructions for compliant return of controlled substances in Schedules III through V.
- Unopened expired drugs other than controlled substances should be sent to a reverse distributor for credit evaluation. Some states prohibit drugs that become hazardous waste from being sent through reverse distribution, so it is important to check a specific state's position on this issue.

SUMMARY

Storage and handling of CSPs is of critical importance. Proper procedures for receipt, storage, and control of components must be established and maintained until compounding occurs. After a final CSP has been compounded, it must be appropriately transported within and delivered from the sterile compounding area. Storage and BUD conditions for CSPs differ from those of the original components. Storage conditions should be monitored closely to ensure that stability and sterility of CSPs are always maintained. Finally, management of waste from used supplies and CSPs must be adequately defined in SOPs and comply with local, state, and federal guidance. Strict procedures must be in place to ensure that pharmaceutical waste is handled appropriately to protect both the handler and the environment.

REFERENCES

1. USP <1079> Good storage and distribution practices for drug products. In: *USP 39–NF 34*. Rockville, MD: United States Pharmacopeial Convention; 2016.
2. USP <659> Packaging and storage requirements. In: *USP 40–NF 35*. Rockville, MD: United States Pharmacopeial Convention; 2017.
3. USP <1191> Stability considerations in dispensing practice. In: *USP 39–NF 34*. Rockville, MD: United States Pharmacopeial Convention; 2016.
4. Food and Drug Administration (FDA). The FDA safety information and adverse event reporting system. **www.fda.gov/medwatch**. Accessed September 8, 2023.
5. USP <800> Hazardous drugs—handling in healthcare settings. In: *USP 42–NF 37*. Rockville, MD: United States Pharmacopeial Convention; 2019.

6. USP <797> Pharmaceutical compounding—sterile preparations. In: *USP-NF*. Rockville, MD: United States Pharmacopeial Convention; 2023.

7. USP <1118> Monitoring devices—time, temperature, and humidity. In: *USP 39–NF 34*. Rockville, MD: United States Pharmacopeial Convention; 2016.

8. USP <1223> Validation of alternative microbiological methods. In: *USP 38–NF 33*. Rockville, MD: United States Pharmacopeial Convention; 2015.

9. USP <71> Sterility tests. In: *USP 41–NF 36*. Rockville, MD: United States Pharmacopeial Convention; 2018.

10. USP <1229> Sterilization of compendial articles. In: *USP 36–NF 31*. Rockville, MD: United States Pharmacopeial Convention; 2013.

11. Smith CA, Pines E. Managing pharmaceutical waste: a 10-step blueprint for healthcare facilities in the United States. **www.hercenter.org/hazmat/tenstepblueprint.pdf**. Revised August 2008. Accessed September 8, 2023.

12. U.S. Congress. Resource Conservation and Recovery Act of 1976: Public law 42, U.S. code, chapter 82—solid waste disposal, sections 6901–6992k. 1976. **www.gpo.gov/fdsys/pkg/USCODE-2011-title42/html/USCODE-2011-title42-chap82.htm**. Accessed September 8, 2023.

13. United States Environmental Protection Agency (EPA). Identification and Listing of Hazardous Waste: 40 C.F.R. § 261. 2019. **https://www.ecfr.gov/cgi-bin/retrieveECFR?gp=&SID=c94567294dff611654af7a3944a91d69&mc=true&r=PART&n=pt40.28.261**. Accessed September 8, 2023.

14. Centers for Disease Control and Prevention (CDC). NIOSH list of antineoplastic and other hazardous drugs in healthcare settings, 2016. **https://www.cdc.gov/niosh/docs/2016-161/pdfs/2016-161.pdf**. Published September 2016. Accessed September 8, 2023.

15. United States Environmental Protection Agency (EPA). Management Standards for Hazardous Waste Pharmaceuticals and Amendment to the P075 Listing for Nicotine. Published February 22, 2019. **https://www.govinfo.gov/content/pkg/FR-2019-02-22/pdf/2019-01298.pdf**. Accessed September 8, 2023.

16. United States Environmental Protection Agency (EPA). Frequent questions about the management standards for hazardous waste pharmaceuticals and amendment to the P075 listing for nicotine final rule. **https://www.epa.gov/hwgenerators/frequent-questions-about-management-standards-hazardous-waste-pharmaceuticals-and**. Accessed September 8, 2023.

17. American Society of Health-System Pharmacists. EPA Final Rule: management standards for hazardous waste pharmaceuticals and amendment to the P075 listing for nicotine summary of changes for healthcare facilities. **https://www.ashp.org/-/media/assets/pharmacy-practice/resource-centers/pharmaceutical-waste/summary-epa-final-rule-management-hazardous-pharmaceutical-waste.ashx**. Published 2019. Accessed September 8, 2023.

18. United States Department of Justice, Drug Enforcement Administration. Title 21 CFR, part 1317—disposal. September 9, 2014. **https://www.ecfr.gov/current/title-21/chapter-II/part-1317**. Accessed September 8, 2023.

19. United States Department of Justice, Drug Enforcement Administration. Secure and Responsible Drug Act of 2010. January 5, 2010. **www.deadiversion.usdoj.gov/drug_disposal/non_registrant/s_3397.pdf**. Accessed September 8, 2023.

20. United States Department of Justice, Drug Enforcement Administration. Disposal of Controlled Substances. September 9, 2014. **https://www.govinfo.gov/content/pkg/FR-2014-09-09/pdf/2014-20926.pdf**. Accessed September 8, 2023.

21. Rannazzisi JT. United States Department of Justice, Drug Enforcement Administration letter to practitioners. **https://wasterecycling.org/wp-content/uploads/2022/11/DEA-response-letter-to-AHA-10-17-14.pdf**. October 17, 2014. Accessed September 8, 2023.

MAINTAINING STERILITY, PURITY, AND STABILITY OF DISPENSED AND DISTRIBUTED CSPs

20

Kevin N. Hansen

INTRODUCTION

It is the responsibility of the pharmacist to ensure the stability of dispensed compounded sterile preparations (CSPs) in practice. This can be accomplished by following key principles of dispensing practice, which include the following[1]:

- Dispensing oldest stock first and observing beyond-use dates (ie, first-in, first-out)
- Storing CSPs under appropriate and controlled environmental conditions
- Observing CSPs for evidence of instability
- Treating and labeling CSPs appropriately to ensure conditions are met for CSP quality (eg, protect from light)
- Dispensing CSPs in proper container closure system that maintains quality characteristics
- Promptly and appropriately removing and discarding CSPs of inappropriate quality (eg, temperature excursion, expired)

Pharmacists must recognize environmental conditions and challenges impact CSP quality in various dynamic clinical settings where CSPs are stored in a variety of conditions prior to administration.

STORAGE CONDITIONS

When establishing a beyond-use date (BUD) for a CSP, it is important to consider the storage location before and after dispensing to ensure the preparation maintains its chemical and physical properties through the labeled BUD prior to administration. Colder conditions, such as a refrigerator or freezer, can slow the growth of most microorganisms and should be considered if this storage type is available and doesn't adversely impact the stability of the preparation. Both CSPs stored in a frozen state and their container closure systems must be assessed for stability, as these conditions can cause physical stress to the container and lead to breaking or cracking. *United States Pharmacopeia* (USP) Chapter <797> Pharmaceutical Compounding—Sterile Preparations outlines three storage conditions for CSPs, including controlled room temperature, refrigerator, and freezer. Specific BUD limits are assigned to each storage condition for Category 1, Category 2, and Category 3 CSPs.[2]

Temperature Control and Monitoring

Compounding personnel must be aware of the temperature requirements for CSP storage. The compounding facility and pharmacy temperature-controlled storage areas must be monitored with accurate temperature-sensing equipment and recorded at least daily to ensure that the required drug and CSP storage conditions are met. Areas where CSPs are held must have the temperature monitored every day through manual logging or by a continuous recording device. If a temperature monitoring device is used, the accuracy of the device must be verified at least every 12 months or as required by the manufacturer. **Table 20-1** outlines storage conditions and temperature ranges that correspond with USP standards.[2;3] USP also defines temperatures for cool (8° to 15°C), warm (30° to 40°C), and excessive heat (above 40°C) storage conditions.[3] The storage requirements for CSPs do not fall in these categories.

Temperature Excursions

A *temperature excursion* is defined as an event in which a drug product, preparation, or component is exposed to temperatures outside of the recommended storage range.[4] Temperature excursions may have adverse impacts on the final CSP, including loss of potency or other physical changes (eg, precipitation). Some excursions can be short in duration while others can be prolonged. Excursions may also be slightly outside of the acceptable range or significantly outside of the acceptable range. It may seem easier to determine an excursion from a static temperature change, however, it can be significantly more challenging to notice excursions that happen over a longer duration. Thus, incorporation of time and

DOI 10.37573/9781585286492.020

TABLE 20-1. Storage Conditions and Acceptable Temperature Ranges

Storage Condition	Temperature
Controlled Room Temperature	20°C to 25°C
Refrigerator	2°C to 8°C
Freezer[a]	–25°C to –10°C

[a] If recommended storage is below –20°C, the temperature should be controlled within plus or minus 10°C of the recommended storage condition.

temperature into the equation must be considered, which is accomplished by calculating a mean kinetic temperature (MKT). The *MKT* is a measure of the cumulative thermal stress experienced by a product or preparation over a time. The easiest way to determine the MKT is by using a temperature monitoring device that is equipped with the functionality to automatically calculate it. **Table 20-2** outlines excursion criteria for various storage conditions.[4-7]

For each excursion event, the time, temperature, and MKT should be documented. The designated compounding person must determine whether the CSP is expected to retain its quality or integrity based on the collected information. This assessment may require consulting available literature or additional analytical testing. In the event that detailed information on the excursion event cannot be determined or if multiple temperature excursions have occurred during the CSP's BUD, the CSP should be discarded.[2;3]

Multiple Storage Conditions

While a given CSP may have an intended storage condition after compounding, it is prudent to recognize if additional storage conditions will be used prior to the administration of the CSP. A common example of this is a CSP that is first frozen, then thawed within the refrigerator, and then kept at controlled room temperature prior to administration. The establishment of BUDs for each storage condition for a particular CSP cannot be additive. The storage time for a CSP cannot exceed the original BUD placed on the CSP label for each storage condition. The BUD of the CSP must be reduced to that of the corresponding storage condition and CSP Category as outlined in USP Chapter <797>. CSPs that were once frozen and then thawed should not be placed back into the freezer.[2] See **Figures 20-1** and **20-2** for more details on multiple storage conditions.

USP Chapter <659> states that articles intended for controlled room temperature storage may be alternatively stored or shipped in a cool place or refrigerated unless otherwise specified on the label (eg, do not refrigerate). If this alternative storage is used, this should not be used to determine excursion temperatures outside of controlled room temperature ranges.[3]

TABLE 20-2. Temperature Excursions

Storage Condition	Excursions[a]	MKT
Freezer	If preparation requires storage below –20°C, control within ± 10°C of recommended temperature	
Controlled Cold Temperature	2°C to 15°C *(cannot exceed 24 hours)*	≤ 8°C
Controlled Room Temperature	15°C to 30°C *(cannot exceed 24 hours)* Transient excursion ≤ 40°C	≤ 25°C
Excessive Heat (> 40°C)	Only if manufacturer allows and is supported by stability data	

MKT = mean kinetic temperature.

[a] Excursions are only allowed for brief period of time and they cannot exceed the listed MKT.

PROPRIETARY BAG AND VIAL SYSTEMS

The use of proprietary bag and vial systems may offer benefits and flexibility for dispensing and storing CSPs prior to administration. In general, these systems allow for docking of a particular drug vial intended for intravenous administration to a device that can be activated by personnel immediately prior to administration. This system has several distinct advantages. A ready-to-use drug delivery system can be stored at controlled room temperatures for extended periods of time without adversely affecting the stability of the CSP. This is possible because medication and fluid components are kept physically separate until the device is activated. Additionally, the system may be able to reduce medication errors, needlestick injuries, contamination, preparation time, and drug waste. It also encourages the adoption of medication delivery best practices with the use of a ready-to-use medication.[8]

Each system has specific requirements for the vial that can be docked to the system, such as the diameter of the vial stopper, lyophilized powder vial, or liquid vial with volumetric limitations. These systems may also have specific requirements for the fluid bag, such as the volume, brand, or type of bag, based on the bag and port dimensions. See **Table 20-3** for examples of bag and vial systems.

CSP Storage in Patient Care Areas

Patient care areas designated for CSP and other medication storage should be monitored, and refrigerated storage temperatures should be documented daily or use continuous recording devices.[2] Nursing, pharmacy, and transport personnel must know the institutional policies and requirements for CSP storage, recycling, and reuse. Personnel must always adhere to the BUD of CSPs as labeled. When CSPs are shipped outside the facility, such as to a long-term care

- General CSP Information
    - Category 2 CSP, aseptically processed, sterility test not performed, only sterile starting components
        - Maximum BUD: 45 days frozen
        - Maximum BUD: 10 days refrigerated
        - Maximum BUD: 4 days controlled room temperature
- Example 1: Frozen to Refrigerated
    - Day 0: CSP labeled with 45-day BUD (frozen)
    - Day 15: CSP removed from freezer and placed in refrigerator to thaw, assigned a BUD of 10 days
        - Note: Refrigerated BUD can receive full 10 days because it does not exceed the original BUD time period (15 days + 10 days = 25 days, which is less than 45 days).
- Example 2: Frozen to Refrigerated
    - Day 0: CSP labeled with 45-day BUD (frozen)
    - Day 40: CSP removed from freezer and placed in refrigerator to thaw, assigned BUD of 5 days
        - Note: Refrigerated BUD must receive a reduced BUD of 5 days because it cannot exceed the original BUD time period (40 days + 5 days = 45 days, which is longest the CSP can be stored based on the original assigned BUD).
- Example 3: Frozen to Refrigerated to Controlled Room Temperature
    - Day 0: CSP labeled with 45-day BUD (frozen)
    - Day 20: CSP removed from freezer and placed in refrigerator to thaw, assigned BUD of 10 days
    - Day 25: CSP removed from refrigerator and placed at controlled room temperature, assigned BUD of 4 days
        - Note: The 4-day BUD for controlled room temperature can be used because it does not exceed the previous reduced BUD refrigerated storage condition of 10 days (5 days + 4 days = 9 days, which is less than the original 10 days assigned to refrigerated storage conditions).

BUD = beyond-use date; CSP = compounded sterile preparation.

FIGURE 20-1. Examples of multiple storage conditions

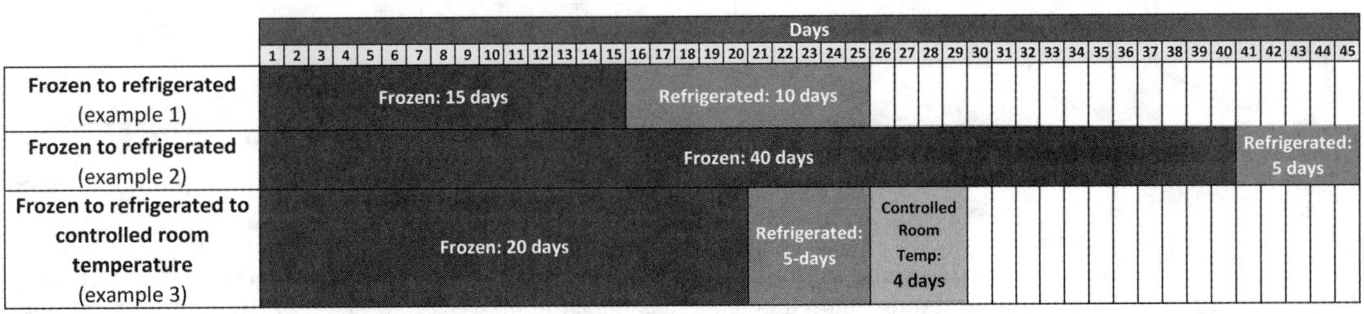

FIGURE 20-2. Calendar representation of examples of multiple storage conditions

facility, offsite ambulatory infusion center, or home infusion patient, compounding personnel need to evaluate the capabilities of the site and educate the patient or facility personnel on appropriate storage of CSPs. Specialized ancillary labeling related to proper storage and use may be necessary for these settings. If a CSP has been exposed to the warmest labeled limit or to excessive heat (ie, exceeds 40°C), the CSP should be discarded. Exceptions to this include pharmacist confirmation of stability either by direct assay or documented stability data.[3]

Clinical Practice

Although most CSPs are generally stored under refrigeration, they are usually warmed to room temperature before administration for patient comfort. Depending on the infusion duration, the preparations can be exposed to ambient temperatures for prolonged periods during administration. Portable infusion devices (eg, ambulatory pumps or elastomeric devices) may expose drugs to near-body temperatures, and some drugs instilled into the reservoirs of implantable pumps remain at body temperature (37°C) for extended periods (eg, 60 days.) The stability of the preparation at its expected delivery temperature and period of use should be considered when establishing the BUD.

Cumulative room temperature storage time also affects the stability of the preparation. For example, sterile preparations may be stored in the pharmacy refrigerator, removed from the refrigerator and warmed to room temperature

TABLE 20-3. Proprietary Bag and Vial Systems

<table>
<tr><th>Device</th><th>Vial Requirements</th><th>Bag Requirements</th><th>Beyond-use Date[a]</th></tr>
<tr><td>Mini-Bag Plus®
(Baxter®)[9]</td><td>20 mm vial stopper diameter (powder and liquid ≤ 10 mL)</td><td>Device pre-attached to Baxter® Mini-Bag Plus® fluid bag (50 mL, 100 mL)</td><td>Once bag is removed from overwrap:
• 50 mL bag = 15 days
• 100 mL bag = 30 days</td></tr>
<tr><td>VIAL-MATE Adaptor®
(Baxter®)[9]</td><td>20 mm vial stopper diameter (powder)</td><td>Baxter® VIAFLEX® fluid bag (50 mL, 100 mL, 250 mL)</td><td>Once device is docked to vial (ie, partial assembly):
• 45 days
Once bag removed from overwrap:
• 50 mL bag = 15 days
• ≥ 100 mL bag = 30 days</td></tr>
<tr><td>addEASE®
(Braun®)[10]</td><td>13 mm, 20 mm vial stopper diameter (powder and liquid)</td><td>Braun® PAB® fluid container (100 mL, 150 mL)
Braun® Excel® fluid container (250 mL)</td><td>Once device is docked to bag:
• Braun® PAB® bag = 70 days
• Braun® Excel® bag = 30 days</td></tr>
<tr><td>ADD-Vantage®
(Pfizer®)[11]</td><td>Specific vials manufactured for use with Add-Vantage® system only (powder and liquid)</td><td rowspan="2">Pfizer® ADD-Vantage® fluid bag (50 mL, 100 mL, 250 mL)</td><td>Once bag is removed from overwrap:
• 30 days</td></tr>
<tr><td>ADDaptor®
(Pfizer®)[11]</td><td>20 mm vial stopper diameter (powder)</td><td>Assembled but not activated:
• 72 hours</td></tr>
<tr><td>Vial2Bag Advanced®
(West Pharmaceutical Services®)[12]</td><td>20 mm vial stopper diameter (powder and liquid)</td><td>All manufacturers' fluid bags (50 mL, 100 mL, 250 mL) that contain an ISO Standard IV port</td><td>Intended only for use immediately prior to administration, not for advanced docking and storage</td></tr>
</table>

IV = intravenous.

[a] This is for storage at controlled room temperature if the system was assembled within an ISO Class 5 primary engineering control but not activated.

before delivery to the patient care unit, and then, if not administered immediately, returned to the refrigerator. In some cases, such as in the hospital setting, unused preparations are returned to the pharmacy and reissued for other patients. The BUD that applies to either the refrigerated or room temperature storage conditions may no longer be valid under these circumstances. When establishing a BUD, the pharmacist must determine the expected stability of the preparation under actual or anticipated storage conditions. When accepting an unused preparation for potential redispensing, credible references should be consulted to determine if the labeled BUD is still valid and if the preparation is suitable for use for another patient.[13-16]

Alternate Site Care Settings

The continued increase of parenteral medications in the home care, ambulatory, and long-term care settings has increased the need for extending beyond-use dating. Longer dating helps minimize costs related to deliveries and can reduce waste. For multidose intermittent infusions via an ambulatory infusion device, the drugs should be stable for a minimum of 24 hours at or above room temperature. When medications have limited room temperature stability, administration using a device that combines the drug with the diluent at administration time is a more common and practical choice.

CSP DELIVERY METHODS

CSPs within the confines of a cleanroom, storage room, and other handling conditions can be mostly controlled. Because CSPs must be transported for use in various patient care settings, handling of these preparations outside the pharmacy or compounding facility must also be considered. Efforts must focus on the acceptability of the sterile preparation for patient use (ie, the sterility, purity, and stability of ingredients) and the reduction of waste and preparation costs. Factors to consider when meeting these requirements include the transfer of the sterile preparation from the sterile compounding area, storage conditions during transport and in the patient care setting, and methods for return, recycling, and disposal.[2;13-20] USP Chapter <1079> Risks and Mitigation

Strategies for the Storage and Transport of Finished Drug Products addresses good storage and distribution practices to implement in order for medications to reach their intended destination (patient or practitioner) with their quality intact.[4] USP Chapter <797> states that compounding personnel are responsible for ensuring that CSPs are stored properly until the BUD is reached or administration to the patient begins.[2] All personnel (including couriers and other nonpharmacy staff) who package, handle, transport, and store CSPs outside the pharmacy must be appropriately trained so that this expectation is met.

Hospital Campuses

CSPs can be delivered by healthcare personnel or by automated means. Many hospitals use a centralized pharmacy to provide CSPs for on-campus ambulatory services and long-term care sites. Procedures and systems to ensure proper training of delivery personnel, product security, and timeliness of delivery remain the responsibility of the compounding facility personnel. With the extensive use of polyvinyl chloride, ethyl vinyl acetate, and other durable, flexible plastic containers for CSPs, rapid turnaround times can be offered by using pneumatic tube systems for delivery. However, some medications and CSPs are not suitable for this method of transport.

In the absence of uniform standards for delivering medications by pneumatic tube systems (and considering the variety of features and capabilities of different brands of these systems), organizations have developed their own guidelines for acceptable use of pneumatic tube systems. Special "Do Not Tube" labels can be affixed to the medication labels to ensure that these medications are handled properly when they are issued and when they are returned to the pharmacy. **Table 20-4** summarizes some representative guidelines for this method of transportation of CSPs.[8;21;22] Syringes may also require special handling to prevent the plunger from depressing and causing leakage into the tube container or system. Padding specifically designed for use in pneumatic tube cartridges can minimize this potential problem.

Home Care and Off-premises Settings

Additional steps to safeguard the integrity of CSPs are required when providing services for home care patients and off-premises care settings, including long-term care facilities, physician offices, and remote site ambulatory clinics. Both the distance from the compounding pharmacy and the drug's stability affect how CSPs are transported for delivery.[16;23]

Temperature control during off-premises delivery of CSPs is very important. The pharmacy must provide appropriate packaging for the preparation that maintains temperatures near the midpoint of the specified acceptable storage range during transit and under expected environmental conditions. Some knowledge of temperature-controlled transport systems is essential. See **Table 20-5** for examples and types of systems employed in the pharmaceutical industry.[24]

The pharmacy should develop and follow written procedures for packaging CSPs for transport. Additional precautions (eg, double-bagging, special labeling) should protect

TABLE 20-4. Suggested Guidelines for CSP and Delivery Using Pneumatic Tube Systems

1. Do not attempt to exceed the weight or size limitations of the tube cartridge that is established by the tube system vendor. This can cause the tube system to fail or result in breakage, damage, or leaking of the contents.
2. If a sterile preparation container is breakable (eg, a glass IV bottle, ampule, vial, or some fragile or brittle plastic bags) or if it could be inadvertently opened or activated by the tube transit process (eg, a syringe), ensure that it is adequately secured and padded in the tube cartridge.
3. Many tube systems have a security feature that facilitates transporting CSPs of controlled substances with a security release code. In these circumstances, appropriate measures should be taken to minimize the risk of diversion. In the absence of this capability, controlled substances should not be sent via pneumatic tubes.
4. When the cost of an ingredient in a sterile preparation is very high, it is difficult to procure and the compounding process is extensive or difficult. It is important to avoid the risk of losing the preparation through an unsecured transport process.
5. Do not transport hazardous, potentially infectious, explosive (eg, freshly prepared CO_2-generating compounds) or flammable materials (eg, medical ethanol for injection) via this method. This includes sterile preparations such as chemotherapy, cytotoxic medications (eg, ganciclovir), caustic agents, radiopharmaceuticals, blood, or blood products.
6. Always avoid the risk of altering the active ingredient or diluent system of CSPs when using a pneumatic tube system. This system can (1) denature or inactivate the ingredients (eg, immune globulins, colony-stimulating factors, monoclonal antibodies, interferons) and crack emulsions (eg, lipids, total nutrient admixtures), and (2) generate foam that will affect the measurement of the dosage, which happens with many protein compounds. If any ingredient in a CSP includes a "Do Not Shake" or similar warnings, the preparation should be transported using another method.

CO_2 = carbon dioxide; CSPs = compounded sterile preparations; IV = intravenous.

Source: Based on Aspden P, Wolcott J, Bootman JL, et al., eds. Medication errors: incidence and cost. In: *Preventing Medication Errors.* Washington, DC: National Academies Press; 2007:105-141, Peak A. Delivering medications via a pneumatic tube system. *Am J Health-Syst Pharm.* 2002;59:1376, Peak A. Delivering medications via a pneumatic tube system. *Hosp Pharm.* 2003; 38:287-90.

TABLE 20-5. Characteristics of Temperature-control Packaging Systems

Ancillary Packaging Components and Systems: These components and systems are the additional means used in combination with the transportation unit (if applicable) to maintain the required temperature during transport. They include active and passive systems.
Active Systems: Systems with active temperature control (eg, air and sea freight containers, refrigerated trucks and cars). In general, active systems are not used by compounding facilities or pharmacies for local or regional deliveries.
Passive Systems: Systems without active temperature control (eg, insulated containers with or without refrigerants or cold packs). These are most commonly used for local or overnight shipments of medications that require storage under refrigerated conditions on arrival at the destination. They may also be used in extreme temperature conditions to prevent temperature excursions that affect the product integrity of noncompounded parenteral medications.

Source: Reprinted with permission of Parenteral Drug Association. Guidance for temperature-controlled medicinal products: maintaining the quality of temperature-sensitive medicinal products through the transportation environment [2007 Revision]. *PDA J Pharma Sci Technol.* 2007;61(2 Suppl TR 39):1-19.

the courier, patient, and caregiver from leakage of any hazardous substances.[20] The courier, patient, and caregiver should be trained to recognize and respond appropriately if there is an accidental spill.[20]

Certain preparations require special packaging for transport to home care and off-campus settings. If the container is fragile or susceptible to jarring (eg, preloaded syringe, glass containers, very full flexible plastic parenteral container), it should be packaged to protect its integrity. Fragile containers may be placed in a hard plastic or cardboard tube, wrapped in bubble packs, or cushioned in clean shipping pellets.

Transport containers and procedures should be evaluated under the most reasonably expected extreme conditions (eg, summer heat, winter cold, significant traffic delays) and documented to ensure that they provide effective temperature control and protection of the contents. These evaluations should be repeated any time the type of container or procedure changes. Postdelivery temperature checks ensure that packaging materials (eg, ice packs, coolers, bubble packs, etc.) maintained adequate control. Temperature sensors can be included inside shipment containers when using common carriers to ensure that the contents are delivered within accepted storage parameters. USP Chapter <1079> calls for the following systems to be applied to the entire life cycle management of drug products[4]:

- Storage management
- Distribution management
- Environmental management
- Risk management

Although a lot of USP Chapter <1079> focuses on large-scale distribution of pharmaceutical products, any compounding facility can develop and validate similar systems and procedures to protect the quality of each CSP throughout its life cycle.

When commercial carriers are used, the pharmacy is responsible for selection and monitoring of these vendors. Before using a carrier, the pharmacy should provide a written statement of shipping requirements, delivery schedules, transit time duration, handling, and external temperature control. Then they should obtain assurance from the carrier that they are capable of fulfilling these requirements. Temperature-sensitive medications should be delivered with the assurance that they are received as intended. Good business and risk management practices include obtaining a signature upon delivery and not leaving medications on the doorstep. Some carriers request special packaging and labeling before they will handle hazardous drugs or biomedical waste. The compounding facility's hazard communication program should specify and standardize the container types, labeling, and other tagging for shipment and handling of CSPs or hazardous drug waste.[20]

Delivery personnel should be aware of the shipping requirements for each package. Ingredient labels generally provide temperature storage parameters. However, because preparations are usually boxed or labels are otherwise concealed, an exterior label should be applied that directs the recipient to open the package immediately and store the preparations as labeled. The recipient should receive instruction to contact the pharmacy if the temperature of the preparations received is not at the expected condition.

CSP STORAGE LOCATIONS

Institutional Setting

After CSPs are delivered to the patient care unit (eg, inpatient, long-term care, or outpatient infusion area), the immediate control over storage conditions shifts from the pharmacy to other healthcare providers. However, the responsibility for ensuring proper storage remains with the compounding personnel.[2] CSPs should be stored in limited quantities and organized in unit refrigerators. Nursing staff should avoid the practice of laying out multiple doses hours before scheduled medication administration times. As part of the patient care unit inspection process, temperatures of medication refrigerators should be monitored and documented daily.[2] If CSPs are removed from the refrigerator long before administration time (eg, at the beginning of a shift), the shorter BUD for room temperature storage conditions apply. This costly and wasteful practice also reduces the ability to recycle unused CSPs in the institution.

Home Care Setting

In the home setting, CSPs are usually stored in the patient's own refrigerator. Patients or caregivers should be instructed to designate a shelf, drawer, or other area segregated from food to avoid contamination of the outside of the container. CSPs should be supplied with an overwrap (eg, resealable plastic bag) to protect the container from other items in the refrigerator and help organize multiple doses. Special care should be taken to ensure that the CSPs do not freeze (ie, do not keep them in the coldest section of the refrigerator).

When the quantity and volume of preparations dispensed are likely to tax the capacity of patient's own refrigerator, a separate refrigerator should be considered. Some home infusion companies may provide a small refrigerator to the patient for storage of bulky parenteral nutrition preparations. Patients should be instructed to store medications (eg, short stability additives) and supplies not requiring refrigeration in a secure, temperature- and humidity-controlled area. Appropriate temperature control in the home is important during administration of these preparations. Labels should specify the storage requirements and the BUD on each dosage unit of a CSP. Patient instruction should include checking preparations for the BUD, verifying refrigerator temperatures daily, and contacting the pharmacy before administration of a medication if a refrigerator malfunctions or they suspect improper storage conditions.

With each patient contact (eg, phone contact, home visit), the pharmacy or nursing personnel should confirm that drug storage is adequate with regard to temperature control, cleanliness, separation of food and drug items, and avoidance of improper preparation use (eg, a single-dose vial used as a multiple-dose container). Improperly stored, soiled, expired, or visibly defective preparations should be removed. During home visits, the pharmacy or nursing personnel should also assess compliance with waste disposal procedures. When the home infusion pharmacy personnel do not directly conduct home visits, the pharmacy staff should provide telephone instruction, reassessment, and reinforcement of medication storage conditions and procedures to the patient or caregiver.

HANDLING RETURNED CSPs

In certain scenarios, a CSP dispensed for a specific patient may not be administered. Thus, it may be available to dispense to another patient if stored appropriately, is within the labeled BUD, and if allowed per state laws. Discontinued or changed orders and extra or duplicate doses are often returned to the pharmacy by normal delivery methods. When these items can be returned to the pharmacy, they should be retrieved as quickly as possible to maximize their recycling potential. If these preparations are left unrefrigerated for pickup until the next scheduled patient care unit delivery, many hours of BUD time can be lost. An active retrieval mechanism for these preparations (eg, pneumatic tube system, special pickup runs) may reduce unnecessary waste in the institutional setting. Any CSP that has been exposed to patient care or treatment areas must not enter anterooms, buffer rooms, or segregated compounding areas unless they have been thoroughly cleaned and disinfected.[2]

Hospitals

Sterile preparations that are returned to the hospital pharmacy may be recycled if the pharmacist knows how they were stored and handled outside the pharmacy. Room temperature BUD parameters apply if the pharmacist is uncertain about the storage and transportation conditions of the preparation. Recycling decisions should be based on the BUD and preparation risk levels. Preparations with very short stability characteristics (less than 24 hours) are usually labeled with an actual BUD and time and are generally not recycled. Other long-stability preparations are labeled with the room temperature standard expiration dates (eg, 24 hours) in the inpatient setting. If the standard expiration date is used, the pharmacist must decide if the returned preparation may be recycled according to its actual BUD (based on stability, infection control guidelines, and storage conditions). Preparations should be used only in time frames that are consistent with published data and the established CSP Category.[2;14;16;25] If a CSP is recycled, this fact should be noted on the label in a manner consistent with facility policies and procedures. If the CSP is returned again, its true preparation time must be identifiable to the pharmacist that determines its suitability for recycling.

Home Care and Long-term Care

CSPs returned from home or long-term care environments are not typically recycled because their storage and handling cannot be verified. Most state boards of pharmacy prohibit return or reuse of any medications once they have left the control of the pharmacy.[26] Reuse of intact items that have not been repackaged (eg, intact vials or commercially prefilled syringes) may be acceptable when allowed by law and regulation only if the packaging is tamper evident, the items are stable at room temperature, and the pharmacist has assurance that controlled temperatures were maintained while the item was in the patient's home or long-term care facility.

WASTING CSPs

Several methods are used to dispose of pharmaceutical waste. Important concerns include prevention of diversion or accidental ingestion and compliance with all local and federal environmental regulations. Heightened awareness of improper drug disposal and the impact on the environment are important issues for pharmacy (see Chapters 19 and Chapter 27 for specifics).[13;20;27-31]

Institutional Setting

Disposal methods vary based on the type of preparation and regulations governing the hospital, outpatient clinic, or long-term care facility. Chemotherapy waste is treated as hazardous and is usually incinerated rather than disposed of in a landfill. The disposal process must meet regulatory requirements specific for destruction of hazardous materials (relative to incineration temperature and duration).[20] For more information, refer to Chapter 27.

Home Care Setting

Patients who administer or receive CSPs in the home setting should be instructed on proper waste disposal for all CSPs and related supplies. When ambulatory or home care patients receive hazardous drugs (eg, continuous chemotherapy), a separate area in the home should be identified for storage of hazardous drug waste in appropriate containers, and all family members should be instructed on the potential dangers of contact with this waste. If needles or other sharps are used in the home setting, the patient should receive a sharps container designated for disposing of used sharps. A schedule for hazardous drug waste or sharps container removal should be developed and agreed on by both the pharmacy and the patient. The schedule must be consistent with local regulations for medical and hazardous waste disposal. Patients should be instructed to contact the pharmacy if waste is not removed according to this schedule.

SUMMARY

The pharmacy retains responsibility for establishing methods to ensure the integrity of CSPs after they leave the compounding facility or pharmacy and up to the point of administration. The pharmacist must ensure that policies, procedures, and resources guarantee proper delivery, storage, return, and recycling of these preparations as well as the appropriate disposal of preparation waste and any hazardous materials.

REFERENCES

1. USP <1191> Stability considerations in dispensing practice. In: *USP Compounding Compendium Revision 43 National Formulary 38*. Rockville, MD: United States Pharmacopeial Convention; November 2019.
2. USP <797> Pharmaceutical compounding—sterile preparations. In: *USP Compounding Compendium Revision 43 – National Formulary 38*. Rockville, MD: United States Pharmacopeial Convention; November 2019.
3. USP <659> Packaging and storage requirements. In: *USP Compounding Compendium Revision 43 – National Formulary 38*. Rockville, MD: United States Pharmacopeia; November 2019.
4. USP <1079> Risks and mitigation strategies for the storage and transportation of finished drug products. In: *USP Compounding Compendium 43 – National Formulary 38*. Rockville, MD: United States Pharmacopeial Convention; November 2019.
5. Seevers RH, Hofer J, Harber P, et al. The use of mean kinetic temperature (MKT) in the handling, storage, and distribution of temperature sensitive pharmaceuticals in pharmaceutical outsourcing. *Pharm Outsourcing*. May–June 2009. 10(3);30–35.
6. Anderson C, Seevers R, Hunt D. The use of mean kinetic temperature to aid evaluation of temperature excursions for controlled cold temperature drugs: proper and improper application. *Pharm Forum*. 2019;45(5).
7. Center for Healthcare Supply Chain Research. *Factbook: The Facts, Figures and Trends in Healthcare (2015–2016)*. 86th ed. Arlington, VA: Center for Healthcare Supply Chain Research; 2016:15.
8. Aspden P, Wolcott J, Bootman JL, et al., eds. Medication errors: incidence and cost. In: *Preventing Medication Errors*. Washington, DC: National Academies Press; 2007:105–141.
9. Baxter – MINI-BAG Plus and VIAL-MATE information from Baxter to PC Kienle on January 25, 2021.
10. BBraun. addEASE Binary Connector with 17 ga. needle. B. Braun Medical Inc. **https://www.bbraunusa.com/en/products/b4/addease-binary-connectorwith17ganeedle.html**. Accessed August 18, 2023.
11. Pfizer – ADD-Vantage information from Pfizer to PC Kienle on January 22, 2021.
12. West – Promotional information sheet #11297 retrieved from **https://www.westpharma.com/products/vial-adapter-systems/vial2bag-advanced-admixture-adapter-drug-transfer-system** on January 22, 2021.
13. American Society of Health-System Pharmacists (ASHP). ASHP guidelines on handling hazardous drugs. *Am J Health-Syst Pharm*. 2018;15;75(24):1996–2031.
14. American Society of Health-System Pharmacists (ASHP). ASHP guidelines on compounding sterile preparations. *Am J Health-Syst Pharm*. 2014;71:145–166.
15. Birdwell SW, Meyer GE, Scheckelhoff DJ, et al. Survey of wastage from intravenous admixture in U.S. hospitals. *Pharmacoeconomics*. 1993;4:271–277.
16. Bing CD, Ross KL. Applying stability data in patient care. In: Bing CD, Nowobilski-Vasilios A, eds. *Extended Stability for Parenteral Drugs*. 6th ed. Bethesda, MD: American Society of Health-System Pharmacists; 2017.

17. Billeter M, Nowak MM, Rapp RP, et al. Waste of IV admixtures in the ADD-vantage system and a traditional minibag system. *Am J Hosp Pharm*. 1990; 47:1598–1600.

18. Mitchell SR. Monitoring waste in an intravenous admixture program. *Am J Hosp Pharm*. 1987;44: 106–111.

19. Salberg DJ, Newton RW, Leduc DT. Cost of wastage in a hospital intravenous admixture program. *Hosp Form*. 1984;19:375–378.

20. USP <800> Hazardous drugs—handling in healthcare settings. In: *USP Compounding Compendium Revision 43 – National Formulary 38*. Rockville, MD: United States Pharmacopeia; November 2019.

21. Peak A. Delivering medications via a pneumatic tube system. *Am J Health-Syst Pharm*. 2002;59:1376.

22. Phyllis Wang, BS, Lynda Nguyen, Update to delivering medications via a pneumatic tube system. *Am J Health-Syst Pharm*. 1 October 2017;74(19):1521–1522. **https://doi.org/10.2146/ajhp150107**.

23. American Society of Health-System Pharmacists (ASHP). ASHP guidelines on home infusion pharmacy services. *Am J Health-Syst Pharm*. 2014;71:325–41.

24. Parenteral Drug Association. Guidance for temperature-controlled medicinal products: maintaining the quality of temperature-sensitive medicinal products through the transportation environment [2007 Revision]. *PDA J Pharma Sci Technol*. 2007;61(2 Suppl TR 39):1–19.

25. ASHP's Interactive Handbook on Injectable Drugs [online database]. **https://www.ashp.org/products-and-services/injectables?loginreturnUrl=SSOCheckOnly**. Accessed March 2023.

26. National Association of Boards of Pharmacy (NABP). *2023 Survey of Pharmacy Law*. Mount Prospect, IL: National Association of Boards of Pharmacy; 2023.

27. Smith CA. Managing pharmaceutical waste—what pharmacists should know. *J Pharm Society Wisc*. November/December 2002:17–22.

28. Young D. News: improper discard of toxic drugs hurts environment, leads to fines. *Am J Health-Syst Pharm*. 2001;58:1576–1578.

29. Saljoughian M. Disposal of hazardous pharmaceutical waste. *U.S. Pharmacist*. 2004;29:HS224.

30. Lavine G. News: EPA inspections of drug disposal practices can be a learning moment. *Am J Health-Syst Pharm*. 2008;65:498, 500.

31. Sherer JT. Commentaries: pharmaceuticals in the environment. *Am J Health-Syst Pharm*. 2006;63:174–178.

SECTION 5: Considerations for Specialized Products and Populations

DOI 10.37573/9781585286492

POINT OF CARE COMPOUNDING AND PREPARATION FOR ADMINISTRATION

21

Ashley Duty

INTRODUCTION

Until approximately 2005 in the United States, sterile compounding was widely performed at the bedside by personnel other than pharmacy staff. Although the extent of compounding was widespread throughout the hospital setting, it was especially prevalent in intensive care units where the presumption was that in this fast-changing, highly intense environment, it was difficult to anticipate the needs of a critically ill patient. However, compounding in nursing units by nurses has continued to decline in practice. Several reasons account for this change. The Joint Commission (TJC) Medication Management Standard MM.05.01.07 states, "a pharmacist, or pharmacy staff under the supervision of a pharmacist, compounds or admixes all compounded sterile preparations (CSPs) except in urgent situations in which a delay could harm the patient or when the product's stability is short."[1] Routine bedside preparation of sterile admixtures does not meet TJC expectations. Additionally, the availability of premixed medication admixtures from pharmaceutical manufacturers has improved over time. The Centers for Medicare & Medicaid Services (CMS) address medication compounding in Pharmaceutical Services (§482.25) and Nursing Services (§482.23) depending on where preparation occurs.[2;3] CMS expects medication preparation to be performed in accordance with state and federal laws and regulations as well as according to accepted standards of practice. In addition, professional organizations, such as the American Society of Health-System Pharmacists (ASHP) and the Institute for Safe Medication Practices (ISMP), advocate that parenteral medication be provided in a ready-to-administer form, such as commercially available premixes or pharmacy-prepared doses.[4;5]

DEFINING IMMEDIATE USE

In 2015, CMS issued updated interpretive guidelines specifying that USP Chapter <797> Pharmaceutical Compounding—Sterile Preparations would be used as the best practice resource for compounding.[3] In 2022, USP Chapter <797> was updated to provide a new definition for immediate use CSPs.

> When all of the following conditions are met, compounding of CSPs for direct and immediate administration is not subject to the requirements for Category 1, Category 2, or Category 3 CSPs:
>
> 1. Aseptic techniques, processes, and procedures are followed, and written standard operating procedures (SOPs) are in place to minimize the potential for contact with nonsterile surfaces, introduction of particulate matter or biological fluids, and mix-ups with other conventionally manufactured products or CSPs.
> 2. Personnel are trained and demonstrate competency in aseptic processes as they relate to assigned tasks and the facility's SOPs.
> 3. The preparation is performed in accordance with evidence-based information for physical and chemical compatibility of the drugs (eg, approved labeling, stability, and compatibility studies).
> 4. The preparation involves not more than 3 different sterile products.
>   a. Batching compounded sterile preparations is permitted for multiple patients. A compounding record is required when preparing compounded sterile preparations for more than one patient.
> 5. Any unused starting component from a single-dose container must be discarded after preparation is complete. Single-dose containers must not be used for more than one patient.
> 6. Administration begins within 4 h following the start of preparation. If administration has not begun within 4 h following the start of preparation, it must be promptly, appropriately, and safely discarded.

DOI 10.37573/9781585286492.021

7. Unless directly administered by the person who prepared it or administration is witnessed by the preparer, the CSP must be labeled with the names and amounts of all active ingredients, the name or initials of the person who prepared the preparation, and the 4 h time period within which administration must begin. [6]

This applies to injections as well as infusions, and it is applicable to immediate-use products that are compounded in the operating room, procedural areas, and other clinical settings, including nursing units. As noted in the definition, administration of immediate use preparations must begin within 4 hours, but there is no requirement for when administration must be finished. Previous versions of USP Chapter <797> required that immediate use compounds be prepared only during an emergency, but this requirement has been removed.[6]

Immediate-use CSPs are singly prepared and are exempt from the requirements of USP Chapter <797> for Category 1 and Category 2.[6] TJC has not yet chosen to adopt the term immediate use for compounding in its accreditation standards. However, as part of the standard MM.05.01.07, TJC defines when compounding outside the pharmacy is acceptable ("in urgent situations in which a delay could harm the patient or when the product's stability is short") and when the use of a laminar airflow hood or other ISO Class 5 environment is required (when "preparing intravenous (IV) admixture or any sterile product that will not be used within 24 hours.").[1] TJC defines an *intravenous* (IV) *admixture* as "a pharmaceutical product whose preparation requires the addition of a measured amount of medication to a 50 mL or greater bag or bottle of IV fluid. It does not include the drawing up of medications into a syringe, the addition of a medication to a Buretrol (inline burette) or the assembly or activation of IV system that does not involve the measurement of an additive."[1]

RISKS ASSOCIATED WITH MEDICATION PREPARATION IN CLINICAL CARE AREAS

Compounding of sterile admixtures in the pharmacy is preferred from a medication safety perspective. It is preferred because there is a greater likelihood of achieving sterility of the final product when trained personnel (using proper hand hygiene and wearing proper garb) prepare a product in a regulated cleanroom suite. The National Institute for Occupational Safety and Health does not allow sterile compounding of hazardous drugs without suitable environmental controls.[7]

Microbial Contamination

Although there is little time for pathogenic microbes to multiply in the solution of a contaminated CSP made for immediate use, the administration of those microbes poses hazards for immunocompromised and critically ill patients. In a systematic review of 16 published studies, Larmené-Beld and colleagues sought to establish and compare the contamination rate of parenteral medications prepared in a clinical environment and a pharmacy environment. Articles included in the study were published between 2000 and 2018, and they accounted for potentially changed working environments and infrastructure in hospitals. This was an improvement upon previously published similar studies. The authors showed that there was a significantly higher contamination rate for the preparation of parenteral medication in a clinical environment compared with a pharmacy environment. A meta-analysis within the systematic review showed that about 1 in 13 parenteral products prepared in a clinical environment were contaminated versus about 1 in 1250 prepared in a pharmacy environment.[8]

Medication Errors

There are other benefits to pharmacy sterile compounding. Having one individual prepare the product while a second individual checks the final product creates an opportunity to catch an error in preparation more often compared to one individual controlling the entire process. Pharmacy technology that is widely available and affordable facilitates CSP checking. This technology uses camera-generated photo images and barcode-driven confirmation to ensure that the right ingredients were selected for inclusion in the final CSP. The ISMP 2018–2019 Targeted Medication Safety Best Practices for Hospitals emphasized the need to perform independent verification of ingredients and volumes even when compounding is completed in patient care units. This best practice can prevent compounding errors, especially when sterile compounding technology is used.[9]

Pharmacy applications provide computer-generated labels that display ingredients in a legible, complete, and standardized manner as well as support product labeling at the time of preparation. However, sometimes it is not feasible to prepare the CSP in the pharmacy to meet the patient's needs, such as an urgently needed medication dose that does not allow time for the pharmacy to prepare and transport it. Another example is limited medication stability (eg, ampicillin injection for pediatric patients) that requires preparation immediately before the time of medication administration in the clinical care area.

With more than an estimated 90% of hospitalized patients receiving some form of IV drug therapy, errors in the preparation or administration have a significant impact on many individuals.[10;11] In their analysis of IV medication errors reported on the MEDMARX database, Hicks and Becker found that 3% to 5% of errors associated with IV medications caused harm.[12] From an observational study of 107 nurses preparing and administering 568 intravenous medications, 69.7% had at least one clinical error and 25.5% were considered serious.[13] The four error types of wrong rate, wrong mixture, wrong volume, and drug incompatibility accounted for over 90% of the errors observed.[13]

In 2012, ISMP published the results of a survey of 540 nurses and their practices with cartridge-type prefilled syringes. The report identified practices wherein nurses would withdraw the medication from the cartridge syringe into another syringe for administration or would reuse the cartridge syringe for subsequent doses for the same patient rather than wasting the medication. Reasons cited for withdrawing the medication from the cartridge syringe into another syringe included a lack of cartridge holders for the cartridge syringes, lack of instruction on how to use this type of syringe, difficulty discerning the markings denoting volume on the cartridge syringe, and a desire to further dilute medication.[14]

An international systematic review and meta-analysis that assessed the overall probability of error in preparing and administering IV medications found the likelihood of making at least one error was 0.73 (95% CI = 0.54–0.9).[15] The error was most likely to happen at the reconstitution step, and removing that step decreased the overall error rate.[15] Errors occurred as a result of slips, lapses, and mistakes, including dose calculation errors, selection of the wrong drug or diluent, omission of a step in the process, poor training, poor labeling of medications, multiple similar medications stored in the same area, insufficient staffing, distractions, and fatigue.[15]

An ISMP survey of over 1,700 practitioners revealed nonstandardized dilution practices as a hazard. Over 83% of nurse respondents reported that they further dilute IV medications even if they have been dispensed by the pharmacy in a concentration that is ready to administer.[16] Another ISMP survey highlighted unsafe practices that were confirmed by observations in U.S. hospitals and outpatient settings.[5] To provide recommendations for safe practices for IV push administration in adult patients, a 2-day summit was held in September 2014 of a cross section of professionals from a variety of healthcare disciplines, regulatory agencies, professional organizations, and product vendors. The summit's objectives for IV push medications included the following[5]:

- Identify the most common risks of administration
- Determine the safest way to administer
- Create and disseminate identified safe practices
- Create standards for knowledge and competency for all healthcare providers

The summit resulted in the publication of a set of recommendations known as the *ISMP Safe Practice Guidelines for Adult IV Push Medications*.[5] Although the focus of this initiative is to address both administration and preparation risks, the recommendations that pertained to preparation of IV push medications were wide in scope and included recommendations to address a lack of standard methodology for preparing doses on nursing units, a lack of recommended solutions for performing dilutions, and the use of containers of normal saline (syringe or infusion bag) when a drug is added but labeling is not updated to reflect the medication and concentration.[5]

Garnerin et al. assessed the influence of human factors associated with manual preparation and arithmetic calculations in the operative setting with anesthesiologists who drew up injections and nurses who drew up oral doses. The human error probability for preparing doses was 3% for nurses and 6.5% for anesthesiologists.[18] In the arithmetic tasks, the human error probability was 23.8% for nurses and 8.9% for anesthesiologists. Error was related to individual nurses to a much greater degree than to individual anesthesiologists, and the results between the two groups were statistically significant.[18] In another study of anesthesiologist accuracy in IV medication preparation, Stucki et al. assessed the contents of 500 unused syringes and found that 29% had drug concentrations outside of the plus 10% of targeted concentration. Of the preparations analyzed, 18% deviated from the labeled dose by over 20%, 8% deviated by over 50%, and 4% exceeded stated concentrations by 100%, suggesting that, in addition to incorrect dilution procedure, other factors were evident, such as selection of the wrong medication vial.[19]

SAFE PREPARATION OF INJECTIONS AND INFUSIONS

Preparing compounded sterile doses in the clinical setting is a decision that must be dictated by patient need and performed to ensure CSP accuracy, sterility, and stability. Compounding of injectable products should be performed only when an equivalent commercial product is not available. The rest of this chapter addresses the safe preparation of injections and infusions, including IV, intrathecal, intradermal, and other sites where administration is made by a needle or catheter. The goal is to provide instruction on preparations conducted by nonpharmacists in areas outside of the pharmacy where laminar flow hoods and cleanroom suites cannot be used. In many cases, the methods for preparing a sterile dose are standardized regardless of the setting or route of administration. However, there may be additional considerations for preparing doses that are administered by less common routes, such as the use of preservative-free ingredients and diluents for medications to be administered via intrathecal, spinal, or epidural routes.

The selection of a workspace for injectable medication preparation is important. The workspace should be a dedicated space, which is clean, uncluttered, and organized so that necessary items to prepare the dose, including the medication, diluents, syringes, needles, transfer sets, disinfectants, and labels, are all readily available. There should be a means to perform hand hygiene close enough to the preparation area so that hands are not contaminated after sanitizing while moving to the preparation area. It is advisable that the medication preparation area is not placed directly next to a sink because microbes reside in drains and can serve as a source of contamination. Ideally, the preparation surface should be nonporous and able to withstand cleaning with appropriate antimicrobial cleaners without affecting the surface material.

Prior to initiating preparation, the prescription or medication order should be reviewed for appropriateness, and a plan for preparing the medication should be developed that includes the following:

- How the medication will be diluted
- Which diluent will be used
- How much diluent will be used
- Final concentration of the diluted medication
- Volume of diluted solution equivalent to the prescribed dose
- Which fluid is appropriate for the final admixture (infusions)
- A second independent double check

Assembly of Materials

All materials should be assembled prior to beginning preparation. The following materials to use include the following:

- Drug vial
- Diluent (if necessary)
- Infusion bag into which diluted injectable medication will be mixed
- Needles
- Syringes
- Sterile alcohol wipes
- Label
- Seals for injection port

The label should be created prior to beginning preparation so that it is ready to be affixed to the medication container immediately after compounding. Labels should include the following minimum information:

- Name of the medicine
- Amount and concentration
- Route of administration
- Diluent and final volume (if an infusion)
- Patient's name and other identifier and location
- Beyond-use date and time (4 hours after preparation)[6]
- Name of the practitioner preparing the medicine

Cleaning the Preparation Surface

The use of a germicidal cleaner is the first step in cleaning the preparation surface. Cleaning agents contain surfactants, and they facilitate the removal of soil, microbes, and other contamination. Cleaning agents include quaternary ammonium compounds, products that contain hydrogen peroxide, peracetic acid plus hydrogen peroxide combination products, or phenolic compounds. Manufacturer instructions should be followed for application of the product and ensuring that proper contact time is maintained for the recommended duration. Staff members that use these products must use personal protective equipment that is recommended by the manufacturer.

Hand Hygiene

Prior to beginning the preparation process, hands must be sanitized. Cousins et al. found that prior to IV drug preparation, nurses did not wash their hands in U.K. hospital patient care areas, only washed hands correctly in 5% of German patient care areas, and washed them properly in 91% of French hospital patient care areas.[20] The option to use either an alcohol-based hand sanitizer or soap and water are supported by the Infusion Nurses Society (INS) and Association for Professionals in Infection Control and Epidemiology (APIC).[21-23] Preparers should follow the instructions for using a waterless, alcohol-based hand sanitizer. If hands are visibly soiled, antibacterial or nonantibacterial soap and water must be used to clean hands rather than an alcohol-based hand sanitizer.

The INS provides evidence-based recommendations for many nursing procedures in the clinical setting in the books *Policies and Procedures for Infusion Therapy* and *Infusion Therapy Standards of Practice*.[21;22] The use of gloves throughout these recommendations is focused on protecting the clinician from exposure to materials or fluids that might cause infectious harm to the nurse. Gloves, per INS, are worn "if there is potential contact with blood, . . . body fluids, mucous membranes, and non-intact skin."[22] Using gloves to prepare injectable medications should be considered a best practice as another method to minimize contamination of the sterile components.

Product Selection and Preparation

Errors in calculating required volumes for drug products and diluents have been documented in literature.[16;24] Enlisting the assistance of a pharmacist to provide instructions for preparing the medication and determining the proper amount of volume that corresponds to the prescribed dose may be beneficial. If this is not an option, enlisting a second professional to provide a double-check for the calculated dose and process is an alternative. The implementation of barcode technology to confirm the correct medication and strength provides safeguards, but it is typically more for medications to be administered in their final dosage form and strength. When immediate-use CSPs are compounded, barcode technology is limited to confirming the proper drug in the vial. Barcode technology will not confirm whether the medication was properly diluted or prepared or whether the correct volume was drawn up.

In the clinical setting, medications are increasingly available through automated dispensing cabinets (ADCs). If the ADC is patient-profiled, it becomes a mechanism to limit access to a medication until a pharmacist has verified the medication order. Even if routine medications appear on patient profiles, ADCs will allow access to other medications through an override function for medications needed urgently. ADC technology allows the use of compartments that stock a single drug product. This feature prevents the selection errors that occur with matrix types of drawers, which provide open access to several drug products. Facilities should ensure that a pharmacist verifies orders prior to preparation. If this is not possible due to urgency, pharmacists should be readily available to help prepare the medication.

To reconstitute a sterile medication in lyophilized form with a sterile diluent, the clinician must use aseptic technique. Manufacturer's instructions (on package inserts) state the proper diluent. After reconstitution, a volume of the sterile medication is drawn into a sterile syringe for administration of the prescribed dose. Some medications may require further dilution in the syringe or in an IV solution to be ready to administer. The prescription order and manufacturer's instructions determine how the medication should be administered.

Clinicians must recognize whether a drug product is in a single-dose vial (SDV) or a multidose vial (MDV). MDVs generally contain preservatives (eg, benzyl alcohol, methyl paraben, and propyl paraben) and are manufactured to be used multiple times within a designated time frame. The Centers for Disease Control and Prevention (CDC) recommends MDVs remain in a separate, clean medication preparation area. If a vial is taken to an immediate patient care area (ie, a setting in which one can touch both the vial and patient), it should be dedicated to a single patient.[25] SDVs do not contain preservatives and are meant for single-use administration. Sometimes SDVs and MDVs do not have clear designations as to how the vials are to be used (ie, "single-dose" or "multiple-dose" are not on the label). If a vial does not explicitly say "multiple-dose," it must be considered single-dose. Misuse of SDVs and MDVs led TJC to publish a Sentinel Event Alert in 2014 entitled Preventing Infection from the Misuse of Vials.[26]

Recommendations for SDVs

- Each SDV should be used for only one dose for one patient.
    - During special circumstances when a single vial is needed multiple times in a short period of time for a single patient (high acuity patient care), an unused needle and unused syringe should be used. Facility policies and procedures should outline appropriate circumstances and locations where an SDV may be used for more than one patient.
- The rubber stopper should be disinfected with sterile 70% isopropyl alcohol before use.
- Opened SDVs should never be returned to an area where it may be accidentally used for another patient.
- Leftover contents from an SDV should never be combined or pooled with other contents.
- If multiple doses of medication are created from an SDV for future use (beyond 4 hours), preparation should occur in an ISO Class 5 environment.

Recommendations for MDVs

- A new needle and new syringe should be used for each entry.
- Needles should not be stored in the rubber stopper of the vial.
- The rubber stopper should be disinfected with sterile 70% isopropyl alcohol before each use.
- Injectable pens are sometimes considered MDVs (see manufacturer labeling for specifics).
- Once punctured, the MDV should be labeled with a beyond-use date (usually 28 days unless specified by the manufacturer).
    - Common exceptions to the 28-day rule are vaccines and injectable pens.

The CDC and the Safe Injection Practices Coalition created the "One and Only Campaign" to create awareness in the healthcare world as to the proper use of needles and syringes.[27] The Injection Safety Checklist, one of many tools created through this campaign, contains important messages on safe injection techniques (see **Figure 21-1**).[28]

Point-of-care Activation Systems

Manufacturers have developed medication vial and infusion bag systems (ie, point-of-care activation systems) that allow for the assembly of the medication vial with the infusion bag, which are kept separated by a physical barrier until it is broken to allow mixing of the medication and solution. Activation is performed just prior to administering the medication to the patient, allowing for a longer dating of the adjoined vial and bag. If assembly is performed in a patient care area "in accordance with the manufacturer's labeling for immediate administration to an individual patient" it is not considered to be compounding as per the latest update to USP Chapter <797>.[6] Staff training on the proper activation process for each proprietary system in use is essential because there have been many examples of Improper activation or failure to activate, which resulted in the delivery of plain infusion solution without the prescribed amount of medication.

Incompatibility with Other Medications

When two medications come in contact with each other in solution, a chemical reaction between the two can change or inactivate one or both ingredients and can cause a physical precipitation of ingredients. This precipitation may or may not be visible. Such reactions or precipitations are termed *incompatibilities*. Drug incompatibilities are different from drug interactions because they take place in the admixture itself rather than within the patient. Besides mixing in the

Injection Safety	Practice Performed?		If answer is No, document for remediation
Injections are prepared using aseptic technique in a clean area free from contamination or contact with blood, body fluids or contaminated equipment.	Yes	No	
Needles and syringes are used for only one patient (this includes manufactured prefilled syringes and cartridge devices such as insulin pens).	Yes	No	
The rubber septum on a medication is disinfected with alcohol prior to piercing vial.	Yes	No	
Medication vials are entered with a new needle and a new syringe, even when obtaining additional doses for the same patient.	Yes	No	
Single dose (single-use) medication vials, ampules, and bags or bottles of intravenous solution are used for only one patient.	Yes	No	
Medication administration tubing and connectors are used for only one patient.	Yes	No	
Multidose vials are dated by HCP when they are first opened and discarded within 28 days unless the manufacturer specifies a different (shorter or longer) date for that opened vial. *Note:* This is different from the expiration date printed on the vial.	Yes	No	
Multidose vials are dedicated to individual patients whenever possible.	Yes	No	
Multidose vials to be used for more than one patient are kept in a centralized medication area and do not enter the immediate patient treatment area (e.g., operating room, patient room/cubicle). *Note:* If multidose vials enter the immediate patient treatment area they should be dedicated for single-patient use and discarded immediately after use.	Yes	No	

FIGURE 21-1. Centers for Disease Control and Prevention injection safety checklist

The checklist items are a subset of items that can be found in the CDC Infection Prevention Checklist for Outpatient Settings: Minimum Expectations for Safe Care. The checklist, which is appropriate for both inpatient and outpatient settings, should be used to systematically assess adherence of healthcare personnel to safe injection practices. Assessment of adherence should be conducted by direct observation of healthcare personnel during the performance of their duties. CDC = Centers for Disease Control and Prevention; HCP = healthcare professional.

Source: Adapted with permission of Centers for Disease Control and Prevention (CDC). Injection safety checklist. https://www.cdc.gov/injectionsafety/pdf/Safe-Injection-Checklist-P.pdf. Accessed Mar 3, 2023., and Centers for Disease Control and Prevention (CDC). Guide to infection prevention for outpatient settings: minimum expectations for safe care. https://www.cdc.gov/HAI/settings/outpatient/outpatient-care-guidelines.html. Reviewed September 4, 2014.

same IV bag, there are other means by which two drugs can come in contact. These include the following:

- Using a Buretrol (inline burette or volumetric chamber) that allows partitioning a volume of IV fluid into which one or more drugs are added.
- Running a medication admixed in a piggyback solution through an infusion line where another medication is infusing.
- Infusing a medication directly through a Y-site into an IV line. The less contact between two medications in the same infusion line the better.

Manufacturer information for each medication that might come in contact with another should be consulted to determine if an incompatibility is likely and how this can be avoided (eg, flushing the line between doses). Alternatively, established IV incompatibility references provide data based on published studies. Not all medications have been studied for compatibility, and pharmacists should carefully consider the risks of combining medications without data.

Medication Labeling

Unlabeled injectables are usually in liquid form and may be indistinguishable from other unlabeled liquids. The ISMP highlighted several incidents where lack of medication labeling resulted in patient harm or death.[29] Examples include the following:

- A 69-year-old woman who died when she was injected with a skin antiseptic instead of contrast media
- A reporter for a local newspaper who died when glutaraldehyde, a preservative, was mistaken for spinal fluid and injected intrathecally
- A physician who applied contrast media with a very basic pH to a male patient's genitalia, believing that it was vinegar, causing the patient to suffer severe burns

Medications prepared in clinical settings are less likely to be labeled. In 2007, the American Nurses Association published the results of a study of over 1,000 nurses on labeling practices. While 97% of nurses who took the survey reported being worried about medication errors and 68% of nurses stated that they believed medication errors could be reduced by more consistent labeling of syringes, only 37% of nurses reported that they always labeled medication syringes. Of note, 28% of nurses who responded stated that they never labeled medication syringes.[30]

With concern for proper labeling, TJC issued specific requirements for labeling medication as part of standard MM.05.01.09 and National Patient Safety Goal NPSG.03.04.01, which set medication (and other solutions) labeling requirements in the operating room and areas where procedures are performed, both on and off the sterile field. Medications are labeled if they are not immediately administered after being placed into an unmarked container.

Preparation of the Infusion for Administration

After an infusion has been compounded, the IV line must be inserted to infuse the medication. In many procedure areas, there may be a practice of prespiking IV infusions, often hours or the day before they are needed. Although there are no definitive data to suggest a specific time limit in advance of administration when an infusion solution may be spiked, the APIC recommends preparing all IV solutions as close to the time of administration as feasible.[23] They recommend doing a risk assessment for any situation that may necessitate an extension of the immediate use definition from USP Chapter <797>.[23] Each institution should create an SOP for proper handling and beyond-use dating of prespiked IV fluid bags. TJC stated that prespiking IV fluid infusions is outside the scope of USP Chapter <797> and facilities will be surveyed to their SOPs.[31]

Another practice issue that can arise is the length of time an IV solution is left in to infuse a patient (otherwise known as *hang time*). There is insufficient data to make overarching recommendations for the hang time of non-lipid-containing parenteral fluids. Per the Healthcare Infection Control Practices Advisory Committee (HICPAC) and the American Society for Parenteral and Enteral Nutrition (ASPEN), lipid-containing solutions (eg, 3-in-1 solutions) are recommended to be completed within 24 hours of hanging the solution and lipid emulsions infused alone are recommended to be completed within 12 hours of hanging the emulsion [32;33]

SUMMARY

Although compounding sterile preparations has transitioned mainly to the pharmacy in most U.S. hospitals, preparation of sterile products does still occur in clinical settings (eg, nursing units, operating rooms, emergency departments, procedure areas, etc.). Those who compound or prepare sterile medication doses in these nonpharmacy settings are nurses, physicians, and other healthcare professionals. Regulatory and accreditation organizations have provided guidelines for when compounding can occur outside the pharmacy and the required environment for this compounding. USP Chapter <797> provides detailed requirements for compounding that occurs in a pharmacy cleanroom setting. However, it does not provide enough details for the specific environmental and process requirements for compounding outside of a cleanroom. Requirements for the preparation of sterile doses outside of a pharmacy were defined in this chapter. The chapter also defined specific types of products and clinical circumstances that might require preparation on an immediate-use basis.

REFERENCES

1. The Joint Commission. Medication management. In: *Comprehensive accreditation manual for hospitals*. Oakbrook Terrace, IL: The Joint Commission; 2022.
2. Department of Health and Human Services (HHS). 42 CFR § 482.23. June 17, 1986. **https://www.ecfr.gov/current/title-42/chapter-IV/subchapter-G/part-482/subpart-C/section-482.23**. Accessed July 10, 2022.
3. Department of Health and Human Services (HHS). 42 CFR § 482.25. June 17, 1986. **https://www.ecfr.gov/current/title-42/chapter-IV/subchapter-G/part-482/subpart-C/section-482.25**. Accessed August 31, 2023.
4. Billstein-Leber M, Carrillo CJD, Cassano AT, et al. ASHP guidelines on preventing medication errors in hospitals. *Am J Health Syst Pharm*. 2018;75(19): 1493–1517. doi:10.2146/ajhp170811.
5. Institute for Safe Medication Practices (ISMP). Safe practice guidelines for adult IV push medications **www.ismp.org/Tools/guidelines/ivsummitpush/ivpushmedguidelines.pdf**. July 23, 2015. Accessed August 31, 2023.
6. USP <797> Pharmaceutical compounding—sterile preparations. In: *2022: USP Compounding Compendium*. Rockville, MD: United States Pharmacopeial Convention; November 1, 2022. **https://doi.org/10.31003/USPNF_M99925_07_01**.
7. Connor TH, MacKenzie BA, DeBord DG, et al. *NIOSH list of antineoplastic and other hazardous drugs in healthcare settings, 2016*. Atlanta, GA: National Institute for Occupational Safety and Health; September 2016.
8. Larmené-Beld KHM, Frijlink HW, Taxis K. A systematic review and meta-analysis of microbial contamination of parenteral medication prepared in a clinical versus pharmacy environment. *Eur J Clin Pharmaco*. 2019;75(5):609–617.
9. Institute for Safe Medication Practices (ISMP). Targeted Medication Safety Best Practices for Hospitals. **https://www.ismp.org/guidelines/best-practices-hospitals**. February 9, 2022. Accessed August 31, 2023.
10. Baranowski L. Presidential address: take ownership. *J Intraven Nurs*. 1995;18(4):162–164. **https://pubmed.ncbi.nlm.nih.gov/7629636/**.
11. Corrigan A. Infusion nursing as a specialty. In: Alexander M, Corrigan A, Gorski L, et al., eds. *Infusion nursing: an evidence-based approach*. 3rd ed. St. Louis: Saunders Elsevier; 2010.
12. Hicks RW, Becker SC. An overview of intravenous-related medication administration errors as reported to MEDMARX, a national medication error-reporting program. *J Infus Nurs*. 2006;29(1):20–27. doi:10.1097/00129804-200601000-00005.
13. Westbrook JI, Rob MI, Woods A, et al. Errors in the administration of intravenous medications in hospital and the role of correct procedures and nurse experience. *BMJ Qual Saf*. 2011;20(12):1027–1034. doi:10.1136/bmjqs-2011-000089.
14. The Institute for Safe Medication Practices (ISMP). ISMP survey reveals user issues with Carpuject prefilled syringes. *ISMP Medication Safety Alert*. 2012;17:1–3.
15. McDowell SE, Mt-Isa S, Ashby D, et al. Where errors occur in the preparation and administration of intravenous medicines: a systematic review and Bayesian analysis. *Qual Saf Health Care*. 2010;19(4):341–345. doi:10.1136/qshc.2008.029785.
16. Institute for Safe Medication Practices (ISMP). Some IV medications are diluted unnecessarily in patient areas, creating undue risk. *ISMP Medication Safety Alert*. 2014;19:1–5.
17. The Joint Commission. *Sentinel event data: contributing factors by error type 2004–2016 (internal communication April 18, 2017)*. Oakbrook Terrace, IL: The Joint Commission; 2017.
18. Garnerin P, Pellet-Meier B, Chopard P, et al. Measuring human-error probabilities in drug preparation: a pilot simulation study. *Eur J Clin Pharmacol*. 2007;63(8):769–776. doi: 10.1007/s00228-007-0319-z.
19. Stucki C, Sautter AM, Wolff A, et al. Accuracy of preparation of i.v. medication syringes for anesthesiology. *Am J Health Syst Pharm*. 2013;70(2):137–142. doi:10.2146/ajhp110654.
20. Cousins DH, Sabatier B, Begue D, et al. Medication errors in intravenous drug preparation and administration: a multicentre audit in the UK, Germany and France. *Qual Saf Health Care*. 2005;14(3):190–195. doi:10.1136/qshc.2003.006676.
21. Infusion Nurses Society (INS). *Infusion therapy standards of practice*. 5th ed. Norwood, MA: Infusion Nurses Society; 2016.
22. Infusion Nurses Society (INS). *Policies and procedures for infusion therapy*. 5th ed. Norwood, MA: Infusion Nurses Society; 2016.
23. Dolan SA, Arias KM, Felizardo G, et al. APIC position paper: Safe injection, infusion, and medication vial practices in health care. *Am J Infect Control*. 2016;44(7):750–757. doi:10.1016/j.ajic.2016.02.033.

24. Parshuram CS, To T, Seto W, et al. Systematic evaluation of errors occurring during the preparation of intravenous medication. *CMAJ*. 2008;178(1):42–48. doi:10.1503/cmaj.061743.

25. The Joint Commission. *Sentinel event 52: preventing infection from the misuse of vials*. Oakbrook Terrace, IL: The Joint Commission; 2014.

26. Centers for Disease Control and Prevention (CDC). Questions about multi-dose vials. **https://www.cdc.gov/injectionsafety/providers/provider_faqs_multivials.html**. Published June 20, 2019. Accessed August 31, 2023.

27. Centers for Disease Control and Prevention (CDC), Safe Injection Practices Coalition (SIPC). One & Only Campaign. **https://www.cdc.gov/injectionsafety/one-and-only.html#:~:text=One%20%26%20Only%20Campaign,-Print&text=Led%20by%20CDC%20and%20the,overall%20safety%20of%20healthcare%20delivery**. Accessed August 31, 2023.

28. Centers for Disease Control and Prevention (CDC). Injection safety checklist. **https://www.cdc.gov/injectionsafety/pdf/Safe-Injection-Checklist-P.pdf**. Accessed March 3, 2023.

Centers for Disease Control and Prevention (CDC). Guide to infection prevention for outpatient settings: minimum expectations for safe care. **https://www.cdc.gov/HAI/settings/outpatient/outpatient-care-guidelines.html**. Reviewed September 4, 2014.

29. Cohen MR, Smetzer JL. Unlabeled containers lead to patient's death. *Jt Comm J Qual Patient Saf*. 2005;31(7):414–417. doi:10.1016/s1553-7250(05)31055-5.

30. Institute for Safe Medication Practices (ISMP). Errors with injectable medications: unlabeled syringes are surprisingly common! **https://www.ismp.org/resources/errors-injectable-medications-unlabeled-syringes-are-surprisingly-common**. Published November 15, 2007. Accessed August 31, 2023.

31. The Joint Commission. Medication Preparation - Spiking Intravenous (IV) Bags in Advance of Administration. **https://www.jointcommission.org/standards/standard-faqs/office-based-surgery/medication-management-mm/000002448/#:~:text=The%20Joint%20**. Updated November 8, 2022. Accessed March 1, 2023.

32. O'Grady NP, Alexander M, Burns LA, et al. Guidelines for the prevention of intravascular catheter-related infections. *Clin Infect Dis*. 2011;52(9):e162–e193. doi:10.1093/cid/cir257.

33. Ayers P, Adams S, Boullata J, et al. A.S.P.E.N. parenteral nutrition safety consensus recommendations. *JPEN*. 2014;38(3):296–333. doi:10.1177/0148607113511992.

22

PARENTERAL NUTRITION COMPOUNDING

Todd W. Canada

INTRODUCTION

Parenteral nutrition (PN) is a potentially life-saving therapeutic intervention for neonates, children, and adults with a dysfunctional gastrointestinal tract (eg, chronic intestinal failure). It is used in a variety of healthcare environments from the intensive care unit (ICU) to the homecare setting. Generally, PN is provided as an intravenous (IV) mixture of crystalline amino acids and dextrose, commonly referred to as a *2-in-1 solution*, while also containing electrolytes, multivitamins, trace elements, or nonnutritive medications. The addition of an IV oil-in-water lipid emulsion (ILE) to PN is commonly referred to as a *total nutrient admixture* (TNA) or *3-in-1 emulsion*, which also contains the same constituents added to a 2-in-1 solution. PN is a complex and high-alert medication that can have stability and compatibility issues depending on the formulation used (ie, 2-in-1 versus 3-in-1). *Stability with PN* refers to the deterioration or degradation of an active drug changing its pharmacologic or pharmaceutical characteristic (eg, oil-in-water ILE coalescence to eventual emulsion cracking). *Compatibility* refers to a disruption in the coexistence of two or more components in the PN formulation (eg, potassium phosphate and calcium gluconate forming the nearly insoluble dibasic calcium phosphate).[1] Pharmacy personnel involved in PN order review and compounding must know the complexity of these stability and compatibility concerns and have knowledge of PN indications, dosing, and monitoring parameters for the individual components. Pharmacist and pharmacy technician involvement in the management and compounding of PN has changed over the past several years, which can be seen in the results from the American Society of Health-System Pharmacists (ASHP) surveys of hospital pharmacy practice over time:

- 2012 results: The 2012 survey showed pharmacists were providing inpatient PN management (eg, initiating, modifying, and monitoring) in 4.7% of hospitals with less than 50 beds and 44% of hospitals with 600 beds or greater (overall mean for all hospitals was 11.1%).[2]
- 2013 results: The 2013 survey showed pharmacists were providing inpatient PN consults (ie, medical record review with oral or written prescriber follow-up) in 45.1% of hospitals with less than 50 beds and 75% of hospitals with 300 to 399 beds (overall mean for all hospitals was 43.2%).[3] It also showed pharmacists were providing inpatient PN management (eg, standing protocol or prescriber delegation) in 32.4% of hospitals with less than 50 beds and 59.7% of hospitals with 400 to 599 beds (overall mean for all hospitals was 55.9%).[3]
- 2014 results: The 2014 survey showed institutions were providing PN as commercially available amino acids/dextrose (2-in-1) in 7.7% of hospitals with 400 to 599 beds and 64.6% of hospitals with 100 to 199 beds (overall mean for all hospitals was 43%). Preparation of PN was outsourced to a compounding facility in 10.6% of hospitals with less than 50 beds and 41.3% of hospitals with 600 beds or greater. The overall mean for all hospitals was 18.6%. Fully 70.1% of hospitals outsourced some compounded sterile preparations (CSPs) with 21.9% of hospitals with 100 to 199 beds and 52.1% of hospitals with 300 to 399 beds partially or completely outsourcing PN. These formulations were compounded with an automated compounding device (ACD) in 1.2% of hospitals with less than 50 beds and 60% of hospitals with 400 to 599 beds (overall mean for all hospitals was 16.8%). PN formulations were compounded by gravity in 16.7% of hospitals with 50 to 99 beds and no hospitals with 600 beds or greater (overall mean for all hospitals was 10.4%). No PN formulations were prepared in 32.5% of hospitals with less than 99 beds because this type of therapy was not used (overall mean for all hospitals was 11.2%). The 2014 survey also showed pharmacy cleanroom compliance with the U.S. Pharmacopeial Convention (USP) Chapter <797> Pharmaceutical Compounding—Sterile Preparations in 43.5% of

DOI 10.37573/9781585286492.022

hospitals with less than 50 beds and 93.5% of hospitals with 600 beds or greater (overall mean for all hospitals was 64.7%).[4]

- 2015 results: The 2015 survey revealed an overall lower percentage (8.7%) of hospitals with a pharmacist assigned to daily nutrition support compared with the 2011 to 2014 (range was 11.6% to 13.6%) surveys. Overall, 2.4% of hospitals with 50 to 99 beds and 56.7% of hospitals with 600 beds or more had a pharmacist assigned to daily nutrition support.[5]
- 2017 results: The 2017 survey reported institutions were providing PN as commercially available amino acids/dextrose (2-in-1) in 24.5% of hospitals with 400 to 599 beds and 71.4% of hospitals with 50 to 99 beds (overall mean for all hospitals was 44.8%). Preparation of PN was outsourced to a compounding facility in 7.5% of hospitals with less than 50 beds and 47.6% of hospitals with 600 beds or greater, with an overall mean for all hospitals of 19.5%. These formulations were compounded with an ACD in 1.3% of hospitals with less than 50 beds and up to 47.6% of hospitals with more than 400 beds (overall mean for all hospitals was 14.3%). PN formulations were compounded by gravity in up to 13.3% of hospitals with less than 199 beds and no hospitals with 600 beds or greater (overall mean for all hospitals was 7.7%). No PN formulations at all were prepared in 33.8% of hospitals with less than 50 beds because this therapy was not used (overall mean for all hospitals was 13.6%). The use of commercially available PN products and outsourcing of PN preparation continued to slowly increase, while gravity compounding of PN continued to decrease.[6]
- 2019 results: The 2019 survey showed pharmacists were routinely responsible for managing medication therapies and PN management occurred in 48.6% of hospitals, which was slightly higher than previous surveys in 2013 (43.2%) and 2016 (46.9%).[7]
- 2020 results: The 2020 survey showed 76.3% of hospitals selectively outsourced PN preparation due to drug shortage management (32.3%), insufficient staff to meet compounding needs (34.7%), and complexity of the PN formulations (31.3%).[8]
- 2021 results: The 2021 survey reported 91.6% of hospitals have a shortage of experienced pharmacy technicians with sterile compounding experience, which is higher than previously reported in 2018 (84.8%).[9]

Clearly, the management and compounding of PN is different based on the size and characteristics of each institution, with most providing between 5 and 15 daily admixtures in combined populations of neonatal, pediatric, and adult patients.[10] The use of standardized, commercial PN is predominantly used in smaller facilities (ie, less than 200 beds), while larger teaching hospitals tend to utilize ACDs more for customized PN. An American Society for Parenteral and Enteral Nutrition (ASPEN) survey revealed that only 60.2% of hospital pharmacies dedicate 0.6 full-time equivalents of a pharmacist position to review, verify, and clarify these complex, high-alert PN orders.[10] Surprisingly, 23.1% of respondents did not allocate any pharmacist time for PN order review and verification. This is especially important because ACDs, which require properly trained personnel, were used in 22.6% to 60% of hospitals with 200 or more beds, and these ACDs rarely (16% to 28%) had an electronic interface with the pharmacy or hospital information system.[4;6;10;11]

The ASPEN survey showed that a pharmacist (54.4%) or a pharmacy technician (27.4%) manually entered the PN order into the ACD.[10] Sacks et al. have previously shown that 39% of PN errors occur during the transcription process (eg, selecting the wrong electrolyte salt or dose, wrong amino acids solution, and drug omission).[12] The extent of the adoption of ACDs has been primarily based on considerations of cost and the risks of manual transcription. Break even analyses have been performed to determine the volume of PN admixtures that need to be compounded each day to justify the costs of an ACD compared to manual compounding, which resulted in 33 to 53 PN formulations per day.[13-15] Besides improvements in efficiency, the value of an ACD offsetting cost has also been reported based on improvements in clinical practice, including implementing a 24-hour PN admixture system, which is recommended by the ASPEN Safe Practices for PN.[16;17] A survey of compliance with pre-USP Chapter <797> standards in hospitals found that more than half of respondents did not validate the accuracy of ACDs, and more than a third of respondents had no plans to change in response to the chapter revision.[18] Errors related to ACDs occurred when actual practices bypassed the safety check system intended to verify the correct sterile product was placed in the right station on the ACD. Manipulating sterile products outside of the laminar flow hood was also a breach in accepted aseptic procedures.[19] The USP, ASHP, and ASPEN have recognized the problems associated with the use of ACDs, and each of these organizations has suggested a standardization of methods used to compound IV admixtures with ACDs and published PN guidelines and standards for safe pharmacy practices.[14;15;17;20-25]

The use of compounding workflow management systems has also emerged to integrate barcode scanning and real-time digital images to standardize the IV process and reduce errors. These management systems have revealed four factors associated with an increased risk of IV compounding errors, including (1) dose preparation during the morning shift, (2) dose preparation on a Sunday or Monday, (3) preparation of doses in ICUs or emergency departments, and (4) technician versus pharmacist compounding.[26] Fortunately, the use of gravity compounding of PN, which does not use any of the above safety features (eg, ACD software, IV management systems), is being utilized less frequently compared with the other methods of preparation across the United States, and it is often only used in smaller hospitals with less than 200 beds.[6]

REPORTED PARENTERAL NUTRITION ERRORS

The importance of pharmacy personnel training cannot be overstated when evaluating the different types of PN errors reported. Wrong dose and wrong drug are the most common PN error observations.[27] Error rates related to PN were the highest of all compounded sterile IV products reported in an observational study of five large hospitals (ie, 400 to 815 beds), in which manual preparation rates were as high as 47.2% and partly automated compounding rates were up to 44.4% at individual hospitals.[19] Some examples of errors that have occurred include the incorrect selection of 5% dextrose for 50% dextrose or 10% dextrose for 70% dextrose parenteral containers due to packaging similarities, substitutions of 70% dextrose for 10% amino acids without barcoding verification on an ACD, incorrect order entry into ACD software with wrong units (eg, mg for mEq), and incorrect use of various electrolytes due to drug shortages (eg, 14.6% and 23.4% sodium chloride, 4 mEq/mL for 2 mEq/mL potassium acetate).[27;28]

Patient deaths reported from PN compounding errors that simulate a pulmonary embolus from precipitated dibasic calcium phosphate and development of unexplained interstitial pneumonitis have also occurred over the last 30 years in the homecare and hospital environments.[29-32] Central venous access loss due to precipitated dibasic calcium phosphate has also been reported, often requiring IV line replacement and patient inconvenience.[33] It should be noted that a pharmacy PN compounding error was not the initial suspicion in any of the above mentioned events, as it was only determined from autopsy or simulation of PN formulations for these unfortunate patients. Drug shortages have also been linked to patient deaths from compounding of nonsterile amino acids solutions with breaches in the mixing, filtration, and sterility testing practices at a compounding pharmacy with administration to patients receiving PN in surrounding hospitals.[34;35] Although hazards of infusing unstable oil-in-water ILE-containing PN have not been reported in humans (ie, unethical to perform such a study), animal models have demonstrated abnormalities in lung histology and lipid deposition in the lungs similar to pulmonary fat embolism syndrome.[36] Patient deaths related to improper use of ACDs have been reported.[17] A fatal zinc overdose occurred in an infant when a pharmacy technician, who had not completed sufficient training for use of the device, compounded the sterile preparation.[37]

A recent international review of published PN patient safety events from 2000 to 2020 found 62% in pediatric (including neonates) and 23% in adult populations (11% of articles included all age groups and 4% did not specify age).[38] The case studies identified PN contamination linked to pharmacy compounding processes or raw materials, extravasation of PN due to incorrectly placed venous access devices, and reports of specific components of PN (eg, trace elements, electrolytes, insulin and dextrose) causing patient harm. Interestingly, they found transcribing, compounding, and dispensing in 43.5% to 63% of all PN errors where the medication processes were described. PN administration was the second most common process for PN incidents, occurring in 29% to 37% of the cases. They noticed from one report that hospital ward nurses were less likely to inform the physician or report the PN errors than ICU nurses. The use of a computerized prescribing tool with the ability to interface with the ACD was successful in three studies by removing the transcribing process as an opportunity for PN errors.[38]

Because PN is considered a USP Category 2 compounded product, pharmacy personnel must pass a written test and validate aseptic manipulative skills using media fill testing initially and every 6 months thereafter or according to state laws governing IV compounding practices.[21] Unfortunately, most facilities are not aware of their microbial contamination rates for Category 2 CSPs (previously classified as medium risk), and rates in published literature range from 0.96% to 5.2%.[39] To further minimize microbial contamination, USP suggests that sterile products with no preservatives used to compound sterile preparations in ISO Class 5 environments should only be used for up to 12 hours after initial needle puncture if labeled storage requirements are maintained during that time period.[21] If labeled storage requirements cannot be maintained, one should consider a shorter in-use time.

SAFETY ASPECTS OF PARENTERAL NUTRITION COMPOUNDING

ASPEN has developed safe practices, consensus recommendations, and clinical guidelines specific to PN as well as a PN safety toolkit (www.nutritioncare.org/pnsafety).[17;22;23] PN safety consensus recommendations also provide a checklist to be completed at each facility for the development of quality improvement initiatives with the PN process.[24] The ASPEN safe practices, consensus recommendations, and clinical guidelines relate to specific pharmacist responsibilities (prescribing PN, reviewing the PN order, compounding and labeling PN, and quality assurance of the PN process).

Prescribing Parenteral Nutrition

The prescribing of PN is a complex process that can have significant impact on patient morbidity and potentially mortality if done inappropriately. Prescribers must know appropriate medical and surgical PN indications, suitable vascular access devices (ie, peripheral versus central IV administration methods), protein and energy requirements, fluid and electrolyte management, micronutrient and vitamin daily allowances, and therapeutic PN goals.[22;23] Physicians are no longer the only prescribers of PN, as physician extenders or midlevel providers (eg, advanced nurse practitioners, physician assistants, residency-trained pharmacists, and certified nutrition support clinician dietitians) are becoming more commonly involved in this role because formal nutrition support teams (eg, physician-led team with nurse, dietitian, and pharmacist) are rarely found in institutions.[40]

The following are consensus recommendations from the ASPEN clinical guidelines:

> Healthcare organizations shall use a standardized process for PN management, and this process shall include clinicians with expertise in the area of nutrition support, preferably from multiple disciplines. PN shall be prescribed using a standardized PN order format and review process applicable to patients of every age and disease state within a healthcare organization. When reordering PN, each PN component should be reordered in its entirety, including full generic names and doses.[22]

Educating healthcare professionals on PN prescribing has been shown to reduce inappropriate use, decrease prescribing errors, lower the rate of overfeeding, and decrease associated costs of providing PN.[23] Standardizing the PN ordering process (ie, electronic order set or form) for prescribers can also reduce the variation commonly seen in nutrient dosing formats (eg, amount/day, amount/liter, percent final concentration of macronutrient).[41]

ASPEN has also developed standardized competencies as follows:

> The prescriber may be certified as a nutrition support clinician or other related nutrition board certification. If not certified in nutrition support, the prescriber should complete a didactic/interactive course such as the ASPEN PN Order Writing Workshop or a facility/organization developed program for initial competency. The prescriber will complete at least 10 PN orders for the initial competency evaluation (via patient case scenarios and actual patients) under the supervision of an experienced preceptor. These cases should reflect the spectrum of medical and nutrition conditions, body weights, and age range. The prescriber should follow these patients and modify daily PN orders over a period of several days. This allows demonstration of the ability to modify PN orders as needed for changing clinical conditions. For annual or every other year competency reevaluation, completion of ongoing continuing education requirements on nutrition support combined with PN order assessment of at least 5 cases or patients should be reviewed using the PN Order-Writing Competency Tool.[41]

Reviewing the PN Order

Healthcare professionals who prescribe PN often have inconsistent or no formal training in nutrition support.[42] Reports to the USP medical reporting program and Institute of Safe Medication Practices MedMarx system of medication errors suggest that this inexperience often leads to errors in writing PN orders, which results in the need to clarify the order or resolve omitted nutrients.[43] The ASPEN guidelines note, "The clinician and compounding pharmacist shall assess the PN formulation to determine whether its contents are within an acceptable standard range based on the specific patient population (eg, adult or pediatric). They shall also assess whether a clinical disease state or condition warrants a dose outside the standard range."[17]

Review of a zinc dose compared with the standard dose based on a patient's weight might have prevented the overdose in the case referred to earlier.[37] Errors are common when PN is prescribed, especially those related to transcription (ie, re-entering a PN order from a paper order or electronic medical record to an ACD).[12] ACDs have safeguards programmed into the software that alerts the pharmacist when a dose is outside an acceptable range, and these can be customized to a specific patient population receiving PN. Despite the availability of this safety feature, it is surprisingly not used often or bypassed by untrained pharmacy staff.[37]

PN is a multicomponent product and is therefore prone to problems of nutrient omission, compatibility, and stability.[42] The following are ASPEN guidelines pertinent to these issues:

> The calorie, protein, fluid, electrolyte, vitamin, trace element and medication content are reviewed for each and every PN prescription to assure that a complete and balanced nutrient formulation is provided. Balanced is defined as the presence of the proper proportion of calories, protein, fluid, electrolytes, vitamins, and trace elements to assure adequate use by and assimilation into the body. Each of the PN components should be assessed for appropriateness of dose and for the potential of a compatibility or stability problem. Any dose of a nutrient outside a normal range that is not explained by a specific patient condition or history shall be questioned and clarified before the PN is compounded.[17]

Pharmacists and pharmacy technicians must follow a standardized process for PN order review to safely prepare these complex formulations for IV administration. ASPEN has developed these standardized competencies for PN order review due to the lack of formal pharmacy training programs (no accredited residency programs), reduced number of board-certified nutrition support pharmacists in positions overseeing the PN process, and pharmacy technician shortages:

> The pharmacist should be board-certified, preferably as a nutrition support pharmacy specialist. An alternative is to have a board-certified nutrition support pharmacy specialist on staff who develops and oversees competencies for colleagues in the organization who review and prepare PN. If not board-certified in nutrition support, the pharmacist shall complete a didactic/interactive course such as the ASPEN professional development material (e.g., Interdisciplinary Review Course, Nutrition Support Fundamentals and Review Course, the module-based Self-Assessment program, or any of a number of on-demand webinars) in addition to the ASHP resources for

sterile compounding. An alternative course would be a facility or organizationally developed program for initial competency. The pharmacy technician should be certified and receive in-depth training in PN preparation to include the following: proper personal hygiene and protective equipment; cleaning of the ACD and compounding environment; setup and verification of the ACD and individual components; review formulation, label, and select appropriate bag; scan and check barcodes, pump admixture, or activate multichamber bag; be familiar with dosing differences between PN components intended for neonatal, pediatric, and adult patients, as institutionally appropriate; verify ingredients, including those that require manual admixture; safely combine components of PN, including the manual addition of ingredients; affix patient-specific label, auxiliary labels; store properly; and inventory management for individual PN components. Pharmacist shall review at least 10 PN orders for the initial competency evaluation (via patient case scenarios and actual patients) under the supervision of an experienced pharmacy preceptor. Pharmacist and pharmacy technician shall prepare at least 10 PN orders for each patient population managed by the organization (e.g., adult, pediatric, or neonate). For annual competency, completion of ongoing continuing education requirements on nutrition support should be combined with the following: PN order assessment of at least 2 cases or patients reviewed using the PN Order Review Competency Tool or PN preparation of at least 2 population-specific PN orders using the PN Preparation Competency Tool.[25]

Labeling PN

The PN safety consensus recommendations state that a standardized ordering format includes a standardized sequence of ingredients with standard units, which means labels will have all the PN ingredients listed in the same sequence and same units of measure as the PN order.[22] The pharmacy-generated PN label then becomes a vital tool for other pharmacists, pharmacy technicians, and nurses to compare the PN ingredients and rate of IV administration against the original order. The following guideline addresses this importance. "The PN label is compared with the PN order and for beyond-use date before administration."[17]

ACDs can produce a PN label in accordance with the ASPEN safe practice guidelines and consensus recommendations. The standardized PN ordering format must be used with the necessary information (eg, PN ingredients ordered in amounts per day for adults and amounts per kilogram per day for pediatric and neonatal patients) for the PN label to be programmed into the ACD. Consistency between the PN order and the label facilitates final review by the nurse (or caregiver/patient) before administration of the sterile IV preparation.

PN Compounding

Pharmacists and pharmacy technicians involved in the direct compounding of PN must demonstrate initial and biannual proper aseptic technique according to USP Chapter <797> standards for CSPs.[21] ASPEN PN safety consensus recommendations state that pharmacy technicians must be certified by the Pharmacy Technician Certification Board if they are involved in PN compounding.[22] An initial and annual compounding competency test for pharmacy staff members must include common PN calculations for all age populations, compounding of PN base solutions, preparing dilutions (eg, PN product shortage, glucose or electrolyte laboratory analysis), aseptic technique manipulations for a Category 2 CSP, proficient use of ACD technology for PN preparation, and the ability to identify PN incompatibilities.[22]

Standardized, Commercially Available Multichamber PN Bags

Given the complexities of prescribing PN and limited healthcare prescriber PN training, pharmaceutical companies developed commercially available multichamber PN bags for clinical use. These are generally available for peripheral and central venous administration and are intended to meet the daily maintenance nutritional requirements of a specific patient population, including 2-in-1 and 3-in-1 PN formulations with varying final concentrations of each macronutrient (eg, amino acids, dextrose, ILE) with or without electrolytes. ASPEN clinical guidelines suggest commercially available multichamber PN bags be considered as an option for an institution to best meet their patient needs alongside customized compounded PN.[23] These products are often used at smaller healthcare organizations (ie, less than 200 beds) because they require minimal compounding and are useful if the pharmacy is not fully compliant with USP Chapter <797> or outsourcing of PN is not available. Ideally, an appropriately trained nutrition support clinician should assist in making the determination if commercially available multichamber PN bags are appropriate for the facility's patient population.

The primary drivers to use standardized, commercially available multichamber PN are determining a desired clinical outcome (eg, artificial nutrition for a nonmalnourished patient with a postoperative ileus unable to consume an oral diet [eg, *Nil per os* or NPO] at hospital day 7), safety of utilizing such a system (eg, minimal compounding required), and overall costs. Compared to compounded customized PN, a study estimated approximately 15 PN patients need to use commercially available multichamber PN bags a day to break even with costs.[44] However, another study has shown that commercially available multichamber PN bags are less expensive when compared to compounded customized PN.[45] The primary advantages of using the commercially available multichamber PN bags includes fewer compounding steps, up to a 2-year shelf-life if not removed from external overwraps, and pharmacy time savings of up to 60 minutes per PN bag compared with a compounded customized PN (see **Box 22-1**).[46] Fluid restriction, severe electrolyte abnormalities or hyperglycemia, and acute liver or kidney injury are the primary reasons to avoid using these commercially available multichamber PN bags in complicated hospitalized patients requiring PN.

1. Properly trained pharmacist reviews and verifies the PN order for appropriateness for the given patient.
2. Prepare and print PN label with PN order that has undergone an independent trained pharmacist double-check.
3. Review PN components for completeness of materials (including sterile syringes and needles if manual additives are needed) required, including tubing for ACD.
4. Following USP standards, complete hand hygiene, garbing, and gloving.
5. Collect all individual PN components for ACD in clean room.
6. Perform disinfection process of ACD and laminar flow hood.
7. Power up the ACD and follow instructions on touch screen.
8. Perform load-cell verification with calibration weight of ACD.
9. Perform aseptic completion of line setup process and introduction of individually barcoded components to ACD.
10. Pharmacist completes verification of ACD setup to specified standards (eg, verify any syringe contents and used vials). Repeat verification during replacement of each ingredient during compounding.
11. Attach a sterile calibration bag to the ACD and labeled "Not for Human Use" with system calibration completed via touch screen. Then the pharmacy technician and pharmacist sign the daily ACD setup report.
12. Apply printed label to empty, appropriately sized PN bag. Scan the barcode to verify the correct PN formulation.
13. Empty labeled PN bag is connected to the ACD (eg, load cell) and pharmacist verifies it is the correct PN formulation.
14. Pharmacist ensures inclusion of all required components available in ACD, then disconnect the PN bag from the ACD.
15. Weigh PN bag and approve as per quality control weight standards.
16. Prepare any manually added individual components (ie, below minimal volume of ACD delivery or PN product on drug shortage). A trained pharmacist verifies it. Then the pharmacy technician introduces it to the PN bag and seals the cap.
17. Apply appropriate auxiliary label (eg, "Refrigerate") to PN bag. Labeling quality control is complete after independent trained pharmacist double-checks it with the original PN order.
18. Store PN bag at appropriate refrigerated temperature prior to delivery with 1.2 micron in-line filter for nursing use.
19. Power down ACD once all PN compounding is completed. Then remove and discard all tubing daily.
20. Clean all components of the ACD.

Example process when using 2-in-1 (amino acids/dextrose/sterile water for injection) PN formulations.

1. Review and verification of PN order with ILE for appropriateness for given patient by a trained pharmacist.
2. Prepare and print ILE label with PN order that has undergone an independent trained pharmacist double-check.
3. Collect appropriately sized ILE bag (eg, 100, 250, 500 mL).
4. Apply printed label to ILE bag. Have an independent trained pharmacist double-check with original PN order to verify all labeling information is correct.
5. Place ILE bag with PN bag prior to delivery with 1.2 micron inline filter for nursing use.

Example process when using standardized, commercially available multichamber PN formulation.

1. Review and verify PN order for appropriateness for given patient by a trained pharmacist.
2. Prepare and print PN label with PN order that has undergone an independent trained pharmacist double-check.
3. Collect appropriate commercial PN product and volume based on the PN label.
4. Verify commercial PN product's expiration date, remove any packaging overwrap, and inspect for any defects (eg, broken seal, leaking, or color changes).
5. Follow manufacturer's recommendations on breaking seals between chambers to ensure uniformity of mixing.
6. Prepare any manually added individual components (eg, multivitamins, trace elements, regular human insulin). A trained pharmacist verifies it and the pharmacy technician introduces it to PN bag, then the cap is sealed.
7. Apply appropriate auxiliary label (eg, "Refrigerate") to PN bag and complete labeling quality control after independent trained pharmacist double-checks with original PN order.
8. Store PN bag at appropriate refrigerated temperature prior to delivery with 1.2 micron inline filter for nursing use.

BOX 22-1. Example of standardized workflow process with ACD setup for PN compounding

ACD = automated compounding device; ILE = intravenous lipid emulsion; PN = parenteral nutrition.

Customized PN

In the United States, PN is generally compounded to a patient's needs by using defined standard formulations for the given institution (preferred) or specifically formulated from individual components. When PN is custom compounded as a 3-in-1 formulation for a given patient, the PN clinical guidelines recommend maintaining final concentrations of amino acids ≥ 4%, dextrose ≥ 10%, and ILE ≥ 2% for stability reasons (ie, at room temperature or refrigeration according to USP standards).[23] ASPEN guidelines for compounding PN with ACDs were adapted from the ASHP guidelines for use of ACDs.[14;15;17] The ASPEN guidelines relate to the pharmacist's responsibility to perform specific functions such as the following (Box 22-1):

- Perform checks of the final preparation to verify compounding accuracy by ensuring that data entered into the compounder are correct, the stations contain the correct ingredients, and the correct quantities of ingredients were used in compounding.
- Periodically observe the operation of the device to ensure it is working properly.

Input of the correct formula into the compounder is critical because electronic systems of ordering PN seldom easily interface with the ACD computer.[10;11;42] Vanek et al. have suggested that all ACDs should be fully integrated with the electronic health record and provide clinical decision support for prescribers and verifying pharmacists.[47] Ensuring correct ingredients are in place is also important because it has been reported that the barcode system used to verify the identity of products on ACD stations may be bypassed.[19] Driscoll et al. reported a quality control process to verify the accuracy of the volume transfer by the ACD by using a pharmaceutical balance to weigh the vials used in compounding before and at the end of the daily preparation of PNs. This is to ensure there are no errors in volume transfers of critical ingredients, such as potassium.[48] This procedure was initiated because it was felt that weighing the final product was insufficient to detect improper compounding of potentially harmful ingredients, such as potassium. In their example, a 2-L PN having an acceptable 5% error could have up to 100 mL of excess volume. If this entire volume was potassium at a concentration of 2 mEq/mL, administration of the PN could result in a potassium overdose. ASHP recommends that the amount pumped for each ingredient should be verified.[14;15]

ASPEN safe practices for PN states the following:

> Manufacturers of automated methods of PN compounding shall provide an additive sequence that ensures the safety of the compounding device. This compounding sequence should be reviewed with the manufacturer of the parenteral nutrient products used by the institution. As most institutions in the United States are represented by buying groups with many participants, such buying groups should not only ensure the safety and support of the ACD, but should avoid splitting PN contracts (mixing brands of amino acids, dextrose and ILE) unless such combinations have adequate physicochemical data that ensures the stability, compatibility and safety of the final formulations commensurate with the data for single source PN products.[17]

This practice was recommended after the Food and Drug Administration sent out a safety alert due to two patient deaths associated with a PN compounding error that occurred when the brand of amino acids products was changed.[31;49] The compounding sequence was not correct using the new product, which resulted in precipitation of calcium and phosphate. The PNs contained ILE (ie, milky white appearance), so pharmacy and nursing staff could not visualize the dibasic calcium phosphate precipitate at dispensing or while these were administered to several patients.

Pharmacists are responsible for assessing calcium and phosphate solubility during the verification and compounding of PN orders. However, the interaction between calcium and phosphate is complex and affected by several parameters, including the final concentrations of amino acids, dextrose, phosphate and calcium, as well as the form of calcium salt used with the gluconate salt being preferred.[17] The temperature of the PN formulation can also influence calcium and phosphate solubility with higher temperatures (beyond room temperature), creating more interaction and a greater risk of incompatibility as demonstrated with venous access device occlusion due to calcium phosphate precipitation from a patient's body temperature.[50] The pH of the final PN formulation is also an important consideration as a more acidic pH allows for greater amounts of calcium and phosphate. Unfortunately, a more acidic PN formulation can present problems if compounded as a 3-in-1 since ILE has a pH of 6 to 9. ILE do not possess pH buffering capacity, and the oil-in-water emulsion is more likely to crack or separate phases at a pH below 5.5.[51] According to correspondence from Tom Westerkamp, MS, RPh (January 2012), an example of how to use calcium and phosphate solubility for a specific commercially available amino acids product used in compounding PN is provided in **Figure 22-1**.

Gravity custom compounding of PN is discouraged because it is labor intensive and prone to mistakes in preparation. Error rates were reported between 5.3% and 47.2%.[19] Fortunately, only a small subset of hospitals with less than 200 beds routinely gravity compound PN.[4;6] Few resources exist for the proper order of mixing a PN formulation, as many publications do not explicitly describe their methods of admixture for 2-in-1 or 3-in-1 formulations. **Table 22-1** provides basic gravity and ACD order of mixing for PN formulations. Note that phosphate is provided early in the sequence, while calcium is always added later to prevent potential precipitation.[48;52–54] Also note that at any point in the compounding sequence, the total volume of the PN at the time of calcium addition when phosphate salts are (eg, sodium phosphate, potassium phosphate) present determines the actual solubility. The software configuration of the commercially available ACDs provides an order of

1. Determine final PN volume including electrolytes (L)
2. Determine final amino acids concentration (%)
3. Determine final dextrose concentration (%)
4. Determine final calcium gluconate concentration (mEq/L)
5. Determine final phosphate concentration (mmol/L)
6. Use the most appropriate compatibility curve listed below based upon the final concentrations of amino acids and dextrose (use most conservative estimate)

   Amino Acids Solution that contains:

   88 mEq Acetate/L

   40 mEq Chloride/L

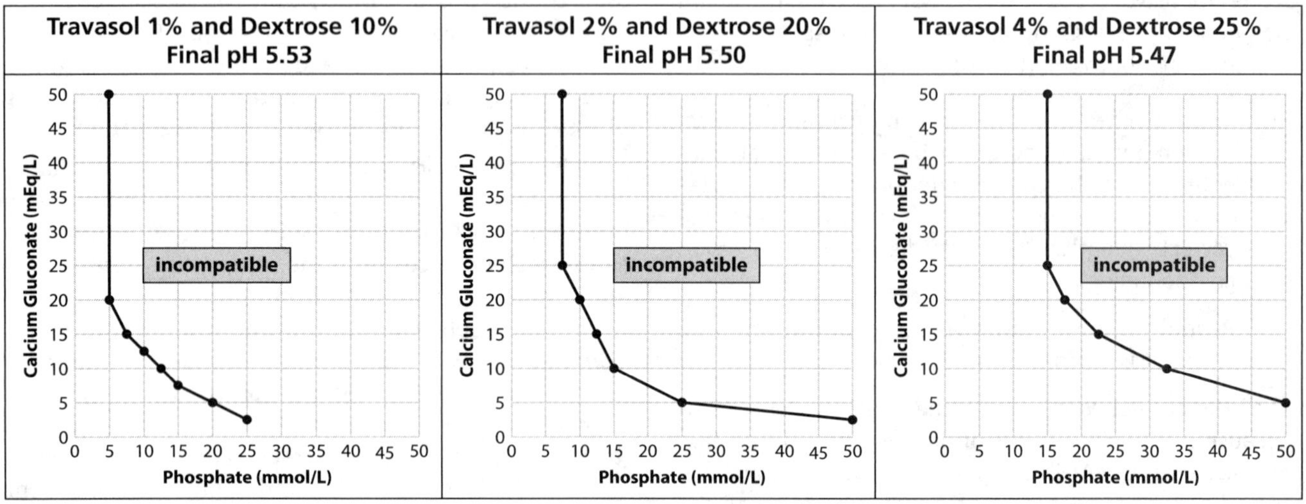

FIGURE 22-1. Determination of calcium phosphate compatibility in PN solutions containing travasol 10%

Information is based on stability at room temperature for 24 hours. Areas indicated as incompatible concentrations were based on visual inspection and microscopic analysis. PN = parenteral nutrition.

Source: Adapted from personal correspondence with Tom Westerkamp, MS, RPh at Baxter Healthcare Corporation in January 2012.

mixing that should only be adjusted based on manufacturer's recommendations or specific testing of the ACD within your own institution for safety.

The most relevant ASPEN guideline when considering the use of gravity compounding is the following:

> If the manual method currently in use at an institution has not been recently reviewed, or if the contract with a particular manufacturer of macronutrients is about to change, then a review of the compounding method is strongly recommended. This review shall include an evaluation of the most current literature as well as consultation with the manufacturer when necessary.[17]

Other important factors to consider in the compounding of PN are storage time, light exposure, and the temperature it is kept at prior to IV administration. Vitamin A decomposition occurs in the presence of light (eg, sunlight). Patient morbidity has been reported when homecare pharmacists have added IV multivitamins to home PN formulations for a week or more instead of before each daily infusion as is recommended.[55] Current beyond-use dating for PN at a controlled room temperature of 20 to 25°C is 30 hours or less, and it can last up to 10 days if it is refrigerated between 2 and 8°C.[21] PN is not recommended to serve as a vehicle for nonnutrient medications unless their addition to the PN is supported by pharmaceutical data. The data must describe the compatibility and stability of the additive medication, the final preparation under conditions of typical use, and clinical data confirming the expected therapeutic actions of the medication.[23]

Quality Assurance

ASPEN guidelines provide several methods to ensure accurate compounding by ACDs.[17] Gravimetric analysis is most frequently used. The final product is weighed and compared with an expected weight. As mentioned earlier, when applied specifically to the total final PN volume, the accuracy of individual ingredient transfer is not assessed. Individual monitoring using a gravimetric method for certain additives, such as potassium and phosphate salts, is recommended and may be accomplished within the compounding facility daily.

Chemical analysis has also been used to measure the dextrose concentration in the final preparation. Dextrose concentration may be measured directly in the final PN formulation.

TABLE 22-1. Parenteral Nutrition Order of Mixing

Gravity Compounding		
2-in-1 Formulation[52]	3-in-1 Formulation[53]	Automated Compounding Device[48]
1. Amino acids	1. Amino acids	1. H_2 antagonist
2. Dextrose	2. Dextrose	2. Sodium phosphate
3. Sterile water for injection	3. Sterile water for injection	3. Potassium phosphate
4. Sodium and/or Potassium phosphate	4. Sodium and/or Potassium phosphate	4. Potassium chloride
5. Sodium chloride and/or acetate	5. Sodium chloride and/or acetate	5. Sodium chloride
6. Potassium acetate and/or chloride	6. Potassium acetate and/or chloride	6. Potassium acetate
7. Trace elements	7. Magnesium sulfate or chloride	7. Sodium acetate
8. Magnesium sulfate or chloride	8. Multivitamins	8. Sterile water for injection
9. Calcium gluconate	9. Trace elements	9. Amino acids
10. Multivitamins	10. Calcium gluconate	10. Lipid emulsion
	11. Lipid emulsion	11. Amino acids
		12. Dextrose
		13. Magnesium sulfate
		14. Zinc chloride
		15. Multivitamins
		16. Calcium gluconate
		17. Sterile water for injection
		18. Trace elements
		19. Sterile water for injection

Potassium acetate followed by Magnesium Sulfate may form Potassium sulfate.[54]

Source: Based on Zhang Y, Xu Q, Trissel LA, et al. Physical compatibility of calcium acetate and potassium phosphates in parenteral nutrition solutions containing aminosyn II. *Int J Pharm Compd.* 1999;3(5):415–420. https://pubmed.ncbi.nlm.nih.gov/23985768/; Trissel LA, Gilbert DL, Martinez JF, et al. Compatibility of medications with 3-in-1 parenteral nutrition admixtures. *JPEN.* 1999;23(2):67–74. doi:10.1177/014860719902300267.; Ambados F, Brealey J. Precipitation of potassium sulphate during TPN solution admixture. *Aust J Hosp Pharm.* 1998;28:444.; Driscoll DF, Bacon M, Provost PS, et al. Automated compounders for parenteral nutrition admixtures. *JPEN.* 1994;18(4):385–386. doi:10.1177/014860719401800427.

The accuracy of the assay is dependent on proper dilution techniques because the concentration of glucose in PN samples is outside the limits of the assay used for analysis of biologic fluids. This also applies to PN samples for potassium, phosphorus, and other electrolytes. If institutional laboratory procedures are to be used for PN quality control, the procedure must comply with USP requirements for the assay.[21]

Refractometric analysis may be used as an indirect measure of glucose content. This method requires adequate staff training (ie, accuracy of the procedure improves with experience and training). Because it is based on how light is refracted as it passes through the PN, it cannot be used for PN that contains ILE.

Drug shortages of PN components have been evaluated since single dose vials attached to the ACD must be used within 12 hours after accessing according to USP standards, and this may further contribute to PN product waste. Hutchinson et al. performed an observational study of the sterility of 32 pooled samples of single dose vial additives for PN.[56] They found zero failed sterility samples after the single dose vials remained attached to the ACD for a mean time of 23.8 hours.[56]

In-process testing of PN is recommended and may be done before, during, or after PN compounding.[17] For example, the amount of the stock potassium chloride bottle used in compounding may be determined by gravimetric methods at several times during the day, and then compared with the amount predicted to be used based on the content of the PNs compounded to that point of the compounding process. This requires the number of patients who received a portion of the stock from the container be properly recorded so that the PN can be remade if an accuracy problem is identified. Another check of the decision support software is entering an extraordinary amount of ingredient to determine if an alert is provided or if a hard stop functions properly. A *hard stop* is a command that does not allow a PN to be compounded when certain conditions are met or not met. For example, the software must be programmed such that the PN is not able to be compounded if a 1,000-fold overdose of an additive is entered. There are several practice guidelines related to quality control in ASPEN safe practice guidelines. The most pertinent practice states that "end-product testing of PN formulations prepared with ACDs is recommended to verify compounding accuracy."[17]

COMPOUNDING ACCURACY

USP Chapter <797> provides methods to ensure volume accuracy of ACD compounding using sterile water for injection and gravimetric accuracy by testing the ACD balance with weights that represent the amounts likely to be compounded by the ACD.[20;21] A variety of ACDs are available for compounding with each device offering different options.

- Apex Compounding System (B. Braun Medical Inc.) is a 26-lead set device with a minimal volume of 0.2 mL with the following delivery accuracy of ± 10% or 0.03 mL, whichever is less at ≤ 1 mL and ≥ 0.2 mL; ± 3% at > 1 mL; Dextrose ± 6% at > 1 mL.[57]
- Pinnacle TPN Management System (B. Braun Medical Inc.) is a 6- to 9-lead set device with a minimal volume of 5 mL.[58]
- Exactamix (Baxter Healthcare Corporation) is a 12- or 24-lead set device with a minimal volume of 0.2 mL with the following delivery accuracy of ± 0.03 mL at 0.2 mL; ± 0.03 mL at 0.4 mL; ± 0.06 mL at 1 mL; ± 5% at 10 mL and greater.[59]

The manufacturers of PN ACDs provide an accuracy level (eg, within 5% to 15%) of the volume delivered. The pharmacy staff utilizing these devices must know how frequently this accuracy is achieved.[59;60] The volume of ingredient used to compound a sterile preparation influences ACD accuracy. The minimal volumes are mentioned above with each of the ACDs. Crill et al. identified problems with PN compounding using small volumes accurately.[61] Additive volumes in amounts less than 1 mL had the greatest variation in measured content. To assure ACD accuracy during compounding, the ACD needs to be able to perform adequate quality checks, interpret its own reports, and establish volume limits that may be compounded.

Precision of the device is also important because daily use will contribute to wear and potential failure of parts in the machine.[62] Issues for stand-alone ACDs are accuracy checks, qualitative and quantitative chemical testing for their CSPs, and cleaning and disinfecting the ACDs. Manufacturer recommendations about these issues must be followed until independent studies are done to validate manufacturer claims and methods. USP Chapter <797> recommends maintaining a daily record of accuracy assessments and reviewing the results periodically (eg, weekly) over time.[20;21] By checking for accuracy, cumulative errors can be identified before they become clinically significant.

USP Chapter <797> outlines the compounding environment, policy and procedures, staff training, and environmental monitoring requirements for sterile compounding. It is not clear what impact ACD hardware has on the effectiveness of the laminar airflow workbench. The ACD presence may alter the environment's ability to minimize or eliminate microbial or particulate contamination (ie, from turbulence) in the compounding environment. Sterility testing of the final preparation is not usually done because content and integrity of the compounded PN preparation would be compromised. The technique of culturing the compounded PN preparation may be faulty and result in microbial contamination. Contamination of a product compounded by an ACD is possible. Chung and Head found that 5 of 40 (12.5%) TNAs compounded using an ACD that had the transfer set and individual component (eg, amino acids, dextrose, ILE) containers left overnight had microbial contamination with either a *Bacillus* species or coagulase-negative staphylococci.[63] Extending the use of the transfer set to 48 hours would have reduced cost, but, as a result of the findings, the authors recommended following the manufacturer guidelines for the device and changing the transfer set and component containers daily. This emphasizes the importance of following manufacturer recommendations for safe use of an ACD in PN compounding.

OUTSOURCING PARENTERAL NUTRITION

ASHP has published guidelines on the outsourcing of CSPs to allow institutions to strategically evaluate the best way to provide IV medications in today's economy with USP standards.[64] Approximately one fifth of hospital pharmacies outsource their production of PN, with larger hospitals more than doubling that amount based on the 2014 and 2017 ASHP surveys.[4;6] Drug shortages related to PN products over the last 15 years could be a major reason for institutions to outsource their PN production, as obtaining specific PN components can be difficult or impossible depending on hospital bed size and PN usage patterns. Additionally, it may be a way to manage or reduce labor costs and facility remodeling to meet USP standards while still providing quality assurance for the end product. Outsourcing facilities generally provide healthcare organizations with quarterly reports on their performance and quality assurance surrounding the CSPs they provide. Contracts for outsourcing may be done on an annual or multiple-year basis, often reflecting changes in pricing for specific products (eg, PN and any technology updates in ACDs needed for their production).

SUMMARY

PN is one of the most complex CSPs prepared within healthcare organizations. ACD technology and use of standardized, commercially available multichamber PN bags have significantly improved the efficiency, workload, and accuracy of compounding PN formulations. Errors in PN compounding have been the result of brand product differences (eg, amino acids products), miscalculations, incorrect transcription into an ACD, bypassing barcode safety features designed to ensure the proper product is placed correctly on the ACD compounding stations, and not using ACD software (eg, gravity compounding). PN guidelines and standards have been developed to assist the pharmacy staff in establishing a safe system of prescribing, order review and verification, and compounding. It is strongly recommended that these PN guidelines and standards, as well as ACD manufacturer suggested use, be evaluated and followed at every facility. A PN quality assurance program must be in place to ensure sterile, accurate compounding with trained pharmacy staff and provide continual, individual PN review for quality control assessing patient safety.

REFERENCES

1. Driscoll DF. Stability and compatibility assessment techniques for total parenteral nutrition admixtures: setting the bar according to pharmacopeial standards. *Curr Opin Clin Nutr Metab Care*. 2005;8(3):297–303. doi:10.1097/01.mco.0000165009.24202.64.
2. Pedersen CA, Schneider PJ, Scheckelhoff DJ. ASHP national survey of pharmacy practice in hospital settings: monitoring and patient education-2012. *Am J Health Syst Pharm*. 2013;70(9):787–803. doi:10.2146/ajhp120777.
3. Pedersen CA, Schneider PJ, Scheckelhoff DJ. ASHP national survey of pharmacy practice in hospital settings: prescribing and transcribing-2013. *Am J Health Syst Pharm*. 2014;71(11):924–942. doi:10.2146/ajhp140032.
4. Pedersen CA, Schneider PJ, Scheckelhoff DJ. ASHP national survey of pharmacy practice in hospital settings: dispensing and administration-2014. *Am J Health Syst Pharm*. 2015;72(13):1119–1137. doi:10.2146/ajhp150032.
5. Pedersen CA, Schneider PJ, Scheckelhoff DJ. ASHP national survey of pharmacy practice in hospital settings: monitoring and patient education-2015. *Am J Health Syst Pharm*. 2016;73(17):1307–1330. doi:10.2146/ajhp160081.
6. Schneider PJ, Pedersen CA, Scheckelhoff DJ. ASHP national survey of pharmacy practice in hospital settings: dispensing and administration-2017. *Am J Health Syst Pharm*. 2018;75(16):1203–1226. doi:10.2146/ajhp180151.
7. Pedersen CA, Schneider PJ, Ganio MC, et al. ASHP national survey of pharmacy practice in hospital settings: prescribing and transcribing-2019. *Am J Health Syst Pharm*. 2020;77(13):1026–1050. doi:10.1093/ajhp/zxaa104.
8. Pedersen CA, Schneider PJ, Ganio MC, et al. ASHP national survey of pharmacy practice in hospital settings: dispensing and administration-2020. *Am J Health Syst Pharm*. 2021;78(12):1074–1093. doi:10.1093/ajhp/zxab120.
9. Schneider PJ, Pedersen CA, Ganio MC, et al. ASHP national survey of pharmacy practice in hospital settings: clinical services and workforce–2021. *Am J Health Syst Pharm*. 2022;79(18):1531–1550. doi:10.1093/ajhp/zxac147.
10. Boullata JI, Guenter P, Mirtallo JM. A parenteral nutrition use survey with gap analysis. *JPEN*. 2013;37(2):212–222. doi:10.1177/0148607112464781.
11. Vanek VW, Ayers P, Charney P, et al. Follow-up survey on functionality of nutrition documentation and ordering nutrition therapy in currently available electronic health record systems. *Nutr Clin Pract*. 2016;31(3):401–415. doi:10.1177/0884533616629619.
12. Sacks GS, Rough S, Kudsk KA. Frequency and severity of harm of medication errors related to the parenteral nutrition process in a large university teaching hospital. *Pharmacotherapy*. 2009;29(8):966–974. doi:10.1592/phco.29.8.966.
13. Dickson LB, Somani SM, Herrmann G, et al. Automated compounder for adding ingredients to parenteral nutrient base solutions. *Am J Hosp Pharm*. 1993;50(4):678–682. **https://pubmed.ncbi.nlm.nih.gov/8470683/**.
14. American Society of Health-System Pharmacists. ASHP guidelines on the safe use of automated compounding devices for the preparation of parenteral nutrition admixtures. Developed through the ASHP council on professional affairs and approved by the ASHP board of directors on April 27, 2000. *Am J Health Syst Pharm*. 2000;57(14):1343–1348. doi:10.1093/ajhp/57.14.1343.
15. Iredell B, Mourad H, Nickman NA, et al. ASHP guidelines on the safe use of automated compounding devices for the preparation of parenteral nutrition admixtures. *Am J Health Syst Pharm*. 2022;79(10):730–735. doi:10.1093/ajhp/zxac004.
16. Raebel MA, McDonald JB. Twenty-four-hour single-container system for parenteral nutrient admixtures. *Am J Hosp Pharm*. 1985;42(6):1355–1358. https://pubmed.ncbi.nlm.nih.gov/3925769/.
17. Mirtallo J, Canada T, Johnson D, et al. Safe practices for parenteral nutrition. *JPEN*. 2004;28(6):S39–S70 [published correction appears in *JPEN*. 2006; 30:177]. doi:10.1177/0148607104028006s39.
18. Candy TA, Schneider PJ, Pedersen CA. Impact of United States pharmacopeia chapter 797: results of a national survey. *Am J Health Syst Pharm*. 2006;54:904–912. doi:10.2146/ajhp050447.
19. Flynn EA, Pearson RE, Barker KN. Observational study of accuracy in compounding i.v. admixtures at five hospitals. *Am J Health Syst Pharm*. 1997;54(8):904–912. doi:10.1093/ajhp/54.8.904.
20. USP <797> Pharmaceutical compounding—sterile preparations. In: *2020: USP Compounding*

Compendium. Rockville, MD: The United States Pharmacopeial Convention. doi:10.31003/USPNF_M99925_06_01.

21. USP <797> Pharmaceutical compounding—sterile preparations. In: *2023: USP Compounding Compendium*. Rockville, MD: The United States Pharmacopeial Convention. doi:10.31003/USPNF_M99925_07_01.

22. Ayers P, Adams S, Boullata J, et al. A.S.P.E.N. parenteral nutrition safety consensus recommendations. *JPEN*. 2014;38(3):296–333. doi:10.1177/0148607113511992.

23. Boullata JI, Gilbert K, Sacks G, et al. A.S.P.E.N. clinical guidelines: parenteral nutrition ordering, order review, compounding, labeling, and dispensing. *JPEN*. 2014;38(3):334–377. doi:10.1177/0148607114521833.

24. Ayers P, Adams S, Boullata J, et al. A.S.P.E.N. parenteral nutrition safety consensus recommendations: translation into practice. *Nutr Clin Pract*. 2014;29(3):277–282. doi:10.1177/0884533614531294.

25. Boullata JI, Holcombe B, Sacks G, et al. Standardized competencies for parenteral nutrition order review and parenteral nutrition preparation, including compounding: the ASPEN model. *Nutr Clin Pract*. 2016;31(4):548–555. doi:10.1177/0884533616653833.

26. Deng Y, Lin AC, Hingl J, et al. Risk factors for i.v. compounding errors when using an automated workflow management system. *Am J Health Syst Pharm*. 2016;73(12):887–893. doi: 10.2146/ajhp150278.

27. Cohen MR. Safe practices for compounding of parenteral nutrition. *JPEN*. 2012;36(2)(suppl):14S–19S. doi:10.1177/0148607111435332.

28. Institute for Safe Medication Practices. Another tragic parenteral nutrition compounding error. *ISMP Medication Safety Alert*. 2011;16:1–2.

29. Knowles JB, Cusson G, Smith M, et al. Pulmonary deposition of calcium phosphate crystals as a complication of home total parenteral nutrition. *JPEN*. 1989;13(2):209–213. doi:10.1177/0148607189013002209.

30. Hill SE, Heldman LS, Goo EDH, et al. Fatal microvascular pulmonary emboli from precipitation of a total nutrient admixture solution. *JPEN*. 1996;20(1):81–87. doi:10.1177/014860719602000181.

31. Shay DK, Fann LM, Jarvis WR. Respiratory distress and sudden death associated with receipt of a peripheral parenteral nutrition admixture. *Infect Control Hosp Epidemiol*. 1997;18(12):814–817. **https://pubmed.ncbi.nlm.nih.gov/9442405/**.

32. Reedy JS, Kuhlman JE, Voytovich M. Microvascular pulmonary emboli secondary to precipitated crystals in a patient receiving total parenteral nutrition: a case report and description of the high-resolution CT findings. *Chest*. 1999;115(3):892–895. doi:10.1378/chest.115.3.892.

33. Robinson RG, Fawcett CA, van Rij AM. Multiple central venous line occlusions following an error in parenteral nutrition formulation. *Aust N Z J Surg*. 1986;56(4):347–349. doi:10.1111/j.1445-2197.1986.tb06161.x.

34. Gupta N, Hocevar SN, Moulton-Meissner HA, et al. Outbreak of *Serratia marcescens* bloodstream infections in patients receiving parenteral nutrition prepared by a compounding pharmacy. *Clin Infect Dis*. 2014;59(1):1–8. doi:10.1093/cid/ciu218.

35. Moulton-Meissner H, Noble-Wang J, Gupta N, et al. Laboratory replication of filtration procedures associated with *Serratia marcescens* bloodstream infections in patients receiving compounded amino acid solutions. *Am J Health Syst Pharm*. 2015;72(15):1285–1291. doi:10.2146/ajhp150141.

36. Driscoll DF, Ling PR, Quist WC, et al. Pathological consequences from the infusion of unstable lipid emulsion admixtures in guinea pigs. *Clin Nutr*. 2005;24(1):105–113. doi:10.1016/j.clnu.2004.07.022.

37. Institute for Safe Medication Practices. Fatal, 1000-fold overdoses can occur, particularly to neonates, by transposing mcg and mg. *ISMP Medication Safety Alert*. 2007;12:1–4.

38. Mistry P, Smith RH, Fox A. Patient safety incidents related to the use of parenteral nutrition in all patient groups: a systematic scoping review. *Drug Saf*. 2022;45(1):1–18. doi:10.1007/s40264-021-01134-3.

39. Trissel LA, Gentempo JA, Saenz LM, et al. Effect of two work practice changes on the microbial contamination rates of pharmacy-compounded sterile preparations. *Am J Health Syst Pharm*. 2007;64(8):837–841. doi:10.2146/060199.

40. Barrocas A, Schwartz DB, Bistrian BR, et al. Nutrition support teams: institution, evolution, and innovation. *Nutr Clin Pract*. 2023;38(1):10–26. doi:10.1002/ncp.10931.

41. Guenter P, Boullata JI, Ayers P, et al. Standardized competencies for parenteral nutrition prescribing: the American society for parenteral and enteral nutrition model. *Nutr Clin Pract*. 2015;30(4):570–576. doi: 10.1177/0884533615591167.

42. Seres D, Sacks GS, Pedersen CA, et al. Parenteral nutrition safe practices: results of the 2003 American society for parenteral and enteral nutrition survey. *JPEN*. 2006;30(3):259–265. doi:10.1177/0148607106030003259.

43. Storey MA, Weber RJ, Besco K, et al. Evaluation of parenteral nutrition errors in an era of drug shortages. *Nutr Clin Pract*. 2016;31(2):211–217. doi:10.1177/0884533615608820.

44. Bozat E, Korubuk G, Onar P, et al. Cost analysis of premixed multichamber bags versus compounded parenteral nutrition: breakeven point. *Hosp Pharm*. 2014;49(2):170–176. doi:10.1310/hpj4902-170.

45. Turpin RS, Canada T, Liu FX, et al. Nutrition therapy cost analysis in the US: pre-mixed multi-chamber bag vs compounded parenteral nutrition. *Appl Health Econ Health Policy*. 2011;9(5):281–292. doi:10.2165/11594980-000000000-00000.

46. Blanchette LM, Huiras P, Papadopoulos S. Standardized versus custom parenteral nutrition: impact on clinical and cost-related outcomes. *Am J Health Syst Pharm*. 2014;71(2):114–121. doi:10.2146/ajhp120733.

47. Vanek VW, Ayers P, Kraft M, et al. A call to action for optimizing the electronic health record in the parenteral nutrition workflow. *Am J Health Syst Pharm*. 2018;75(18):1400–1420. doi:10.2146/ajhp180276.

48. Driscoll DF, Bacon M, Provost PS, et al. Automated compounders for parenteral nutrition admixtures. *JPEN*. 1994;18(4):385–386. doi:10.1177/014860719401800427.

49. Lumpkin MM. Safety alert: hazards of precipitation associated with parenteral nutrition. *Am J Hosp Pharm*. 1994;51(11):1427–1428. **https://pubmed.ncbi.nlm.nih.gov/7942876/**.

50. Robinson LA, Wright BT. Central venous catheter occlusion caused by body-heat-mediated calcium phosphate precipitation. *Am J Hosp Pharm*. 1982;39(1):120–121. **https://pubmed.ncbi.nlm.nih.gov/6798866/**.

51. Driscoll DF, Bhargava HN, Li L, et al. Physicochemical stability of total nutrient admixtures. *Am J Health Syst Pharm*. 1995;52(6):623–634. doi:10.1093/ajhp/52.6.623.

52. Zhang Y, Xu Q, Trissel LA, Baker MB. Physical compatibility of calcium acetate and potassium phosphates in parenteral nutrition solutions containing aminosyn II. *Int J Pharm Compd*. 1999;3(5):415–420. **https://pubmed.ncbi.nlm.nih.gov/23985768/**.

53. Trissel LA, Gilbert DL, Martinez JF, et al. Compatibility of medications with 3-in-1 parenteral nutrition admixtures. *JPEN*. 1999;23(2):67–74. doi:10.1177/014860719902300267.

54. Ambados F, Brealey J. Precipitation of potassium sulphate during TPN solution admixture. *Aust J Hosp Pharm*. 1998;28:444.

55. National Advisory Group on Standards and Practice Guidelines for Parenteral Nutrition. Safe practices for parenteral nutrition formulations. *JPEN*. 1998;22(2):49–66. **https://pubmed.ncbi.nlm.nih.gov/9527961/**.

56. Hutchinson HM, Sayre BE, Prettyman T, King E. Evaluating sterility of single dose vials on an automated compounding device. *Hosp Pharm*. 2017;52(4):286–293. doi:10.1310/hpj5204-286.

57. APEX compounding system. B. Braun Medical Inc. **https://www.bbraunusa.com/en/products-and-therapies/nutrition-therapy/pn-360/apex/apex-compounding-system.html**. Accessed January 23, 2023.

58. PINNACLE TPN management system. B. Braun Medical Inc. **https://www.bbraunusa.com/en/products/b4/pinnacle-tpn-managementsystem.html**. Accessed January 23, 2023.

59. EXACTAMIX compounder. Baxter Healthcare Corporation. **https://hospitalproducts-site.baxterdigital.net/sites/g/files/ebysai2186/files/2020-06/53007410_LABEL_EM2400_Win10.pdf**. Accessed January 23, 2023.

60. Fishwick JJ, Murphy CC, Riesenberg MC, et al. Weight-based accuracy of parenteral nutrient solutions prepared with an automated compounder. *Am J Health Syst Pharm*. 1997;54(6):678–679. doi:10.1093/ajhp/54.6.678.

61. Crill CM, Hak EB, Helms RA. Accuracy of parenteral nutrition solutions compounded with automated systems and by hand. *Am J Health Syst Pharm*. 2005;62(22):2345–2348, 2348. doi:10.2146/ajhp050322.

62. Driscoll DF. Delivery of nutritional therapy: quality assurance of automated compounding devices. *Nutrition*. 1996;12(9):651–652. doi:10.1016/s0899-9007(96)00185-2.

63. Chung K, Head G. Microbiologic quality-control study for the purpose of extending the use of transfer sets on the automix 3 + 3 and micromix automated total nutrient admixture compounding pumps. *JPEN*. 2005;29(2):118–124. doi:10.1177/0148607105029002118.

64. American Society of Health-System Pharmacists. ASHP guidelines on outsourcing sterile compounding services. *Am J Health Syst Pharm*. 2015;72(19):1664–1675. doi:10.2146/sp150024.

23

PEDIATRIC COMPOUNDING

Kathleen M. Gura

INTRODUCTION

The number of new medications marketed in the United States is constantly on the rise. In most cases, however, despite their unique needs, these new medications are not specifically approved by the U.S. Food and Drug Administration (FDA) for pediatric use, and they are typically not available in a suitable dosage form for pediatric patients. Approximately 20% of currently available medications are specifically approved for use with the pediatric population.[1] Furthermore, of those drugs receiving FDA approval since 2007, only 33.8% of the pediatric postmarketing studies mandated by the Pediatric Research Equity Act have been completed. Only 41.2% of the drug labels included any pediatric data.[2] Despite not being labeled for use in children, there is often a very real need for these therapies. The off-label use of medications is common in pediatric patients. Compounded formulations have an important role, especially in the treatment of infants and young children (those less than 6 years of age) or patients who require tailored doses based on body size, weight, and vascular access.

The fixed doses and concentrations intended for adults are often not appropriate for use in younger patients. Because these formulations are typically more suitable for adults, additional manipulations are needed. In fact, The Joint Commission suggests that the pharmacy prepare patient-specific, unit-dose pediatric medications instead of using a commercially available adult concentration to reduce the risk of pediatric medication errors and adverse events.[3] This chapter will focus on the issues surrounding the provision of parenteral medications to the neonatal, infant, and pediatric patient, with special emphasis on the neonate. In addition to specific compounding considerations, other aspects, such as standardization, product selection, and drug delivery systems, will also be addressed.

CHALLENGES IN DRUG DELIVERY

Concentration Considerations

Intravenous (IV) medications not approved for infants and young children are often not available in low concentrations that allow for the accurate and precise measurement of small doses. For example, the lowest commercially available concentration of enoxaparin is 100 mg/mL. If the dosing in an infant is 1.7 mg/kg, the volume of medication to be given to a one kilogram neonate is 0.017 mL, which is not possible to measure even when using a 1 mL tuberculin syringe. It is well known that there is great risk of errors occurring when measuring doses whose final volume is less than 0.1 mL. Such measuring errors with potent medications, like morphine and digoxin, have led to fatal outcomes in pediatric patients.[4;5]

One common approach to measure these small doses more accurately is to dilute the more concentrated medications intended for adults. There are numerous pitfalls associated with altering an adult formulation for use in infants and children. Often, there are insufficient data to support the assigned beyond-use dating of compounded formulations, and there is the inherent risk of error whenever such compounding is done. The diluted drug's stability and sterility may not be known. Furthermore, diluted medications may be stable for varying periods of time, and dilutions derived from multidose vials can lead to lower than desired concentrations of any present preservatives.

Routes of Delivery

Intravenous

Although the IV route is the preferred method of drug delivery in critically ill neonates (ie, birth to one month old), special attention must be paid to avoiding excessive fluid. In comparison with the 100 mL/hour infusion rates used

DOI 10.37573/9781585286492.023

in adults, full-term infants (gestational age ≥ 38 weeks) may only receive 10 to 20 mL/hour, and premature infants (gestational age < 37 weeks) receive only 3 to 5 mL/hour.[6]

A typical infant has a total circulating blood volume of approximately 75 to 80 mL/kg, while a neonate has 85 to 90 mL/kg, and adults have 65 to 70 mL/kg.[7] Thus, in contrast to the adult 0.5 to 1 mL/kg/hr fluid infusion rates, an older child may need about 1 to 2 mL/kg/hr while a 1 kg preterm requires as much as 8 mL/kg/hr.[8]

Obtaining vascular access in infants (1 month to 2 years) and children (2 to 12 years) is often a complicated process. Infants have poor vascular system integrity, reduced vascular diameter, and decreased perfusion, all of which can lead to endothelial damage during catheter insertion.[9] For these reasons, it is often difficult to find veins viable for IV access, especially in critically ill children. In active children, peripheral catheters are more likely to become dislodged, resulting in the IV being replaced more frequently. In comparison with adults, infants and small children have smaller peripheral veins, more subcutaneous (sub-Q) fat, are prone to vasoconstriction, and are much less likely to remain still during a painful procedure or infusion of acidic medications (eg, potassium, lidocaine). Multiple attempts at placing an IV catheter is harmful to pediatric patients for many reasons, including pain, stress, disruption of the skin's integrity, and increased risk of infection.

Scalp Vein Catheters

In addition to the more traditional peripheral and central venous catheters used in adults and older children, several other access routes are available for small children and infants. Scalp veins should only be used once other alternative access routes are exhausted. Scalp veins provide a secondary option for peripheral intravascular access in small children and infants because there is minimal sub-Q fat and no flexible joint, which means less movement. These differences reduce the chance of catheter dislodgement, which is a common occurrence with IV catheters placed in the arms or legs. Cannulation of the scalp vein is indicated in any patient who requires intravascular access for the administration of medications or fluids, and it helps preserve the vessels of the arms and legs for peripherally inserted central catheters.[10]

When inserting the catheter, care must be taken to avoid placing the scalp vein catheter near sites of superficial skin injury or infection. In most cases, at least partial shaving of the infant's head is necessary. It may take 6 to 12 months for hair to grow back properly, which may be upsetting to the parents. Hematoma is the most common complication.[11] One of the most limiting factors associated with scalp vein catheters is the risk of infiltration of the sub-Q tissue with IV medication or fluids, as it may cause superficial blistering, deep tissue necrosis, or tissue calcification, especially if calcium-containing fluids are used.[12] For these reasons, many centers do not allow the administration of vesicants or irritants (including parenteral nutrition [PN] or calcium containing fluids) through scalp catheters.

TABLE 23-1. Examples of Uses of Umbilical Vein and Artery Catheters

Umbilical Vein Catheters	Umbilical Artery Catheters
• Venous blood sampling	• Arterial blood gas sampling
• Emergency parenteral access for resuscitation medications, and fluids	• Continuous blood pressure monitoring
• Exchange transfusion(s)	• Exchange transfusion(s)
• Monitoring of central venous pressure	• Infusion of maintenance and resuscitation fluids
• Vascular access in low-birth-weight infants	

Umbilical Catheters

Another access site unique to the neonate involves the umbilical vein and arteries. The umbilical stump typically contains three vessels (ie, one umbilical vein, two umbilical arteries) that may also be used to administer maintenance fluids and medications. The umbilical vein is usually the largest of the three vessels, and, for the first few days of life, it can be used as an access site in neonates.[12] For venous access, the catheter tip should enter into the umbilical vein and end in the inferior vena cava. The catheter tip should be at the level of the inferior vena cava next to the diaphragm. An abdominal x-ray is used to confirm placement. Like other vascular access sites, umbilical venous catheters can be used for fluid and medication administration. Limitations to umbilical artery catheterization include clinical conditions, such as necrotizing enterocolitis, omphalocele, or gastrochisis.[12] **Table 23-1** describes the typical uses of umbilical vein and artery catheters.

Intramuscular Injections

Other routes of parenteral drug administration also have limitations when used in infants and young children. For example, in adult patients, the relatively large surface area and bulk of the gluteal muscles make it the preferred site for an intramuscular (IM) injection (see **Table 23-2** for information on age, site, maximum volume, and needle size). Because most adult patients cooperate during the process, it also allows for accurate identification of landmarks, so as to avoid the sciatic nerve. In infants less than 12 months of age, the anterolateral thigh is the preferred site for IM injection.[13] Medications are injected into the bulkiest part of the vastus lateralis thigh muscle, which is the junction of the upper and middle thirds of this muscle. In preterm infants, the preferred injection site is the middle third of the anterior aspect of the thigh, lateral from the midline (ie, rectus femoris muscle). To avoid the risk of sciatic nerve damage from gluteal injection, IM injections should not be given in the buttocks in preterm infants and neonates.[13] Using the vastus lateralis muscle avoids the risk of sciatic nerve damage. Also, the vastus lateralis muscle offers a larger muscle mass than the gluteal region, and therefore has reduced risk

TABLE 23-2. Volume Limits and Preferred Injection Sites for Intramuscular Injections by Age

Age	Maximum Volume	Needle	Preferred Site	Comments
Preterm babies (< 37 wk gestation) up to 2 mo of age; and/or very small infants	0.5 mL per injection site	25 gauge 5/8 in (16 mm)	Vastus lateralis The middle third of the anterior aspect of the thigh lateral from the midline (ie, rectus femoris muscle)	In neonates and infants, do not use the deltoid muscle. It is not developed enough to absorb medication adequately. IM injections should not be given in the buttocks in preterm infants and neonates.
Large infant	1 mL	23 or 25 gauge, 1 in (25 mm)	Vastus lateralis	If two IM injections are being administered, one medication should be injected into the right thigh and the other into the left thigh.
School-age child	1 mL	25 or 26 gauge Deltoid: 5/8-1 in (16–25 mm) Any other site except deltoid: 1-1 ¼ in (25–31 mm)		
Older child with well-developed muscle mass	2 mL No more than 1 mL given at the deltoid site	22-25 gauge Deltoid: 5/8-1 ¼ in (16-31 mm)		
Adult	2 mL in the deltoid and thigh muscles and up to 5 mL in the gluteus maximus Preferably no more than 1 mL should be given at the deltoid site	22–25 gauge Deltoid: 5/8-1 ½ in (16-38.1 mm) Ventrogluteal: 1 ½ in (38.1 mm)		Suggested needle lengths based on patient weight: *< 60 kg:* 5/8 in (16 mm) *60-70 kg:* 1 in (25 mm) *Women 70-90 kg and men 70–118 kg:* 1–1 ½ in (25-38.1 mm) *Women > 90 kg and men > 118 kg:* 1 ½ in (38.1 mm)

IM = intramuscular.

Source: Adapted with permission of Hughes WT. Complication resulting from an intramuscular injection. *J Pediatr.* 1967;70(6):1011–1013. doi:10.1016/s0022-3476(67)80283-x and Lippert WC, Wall EJ. Optimal intramuscular needle-penetration depth. *Pediatrics.* 2008;122(3): e556–e563. doi:10.1542/peds.2008-0374.

of severe local reactions. The deltoid in infants is not bulky enough to sufficiently absorb IM medications. The volume of the IM injection should not be more than 1 mL (0.5 mL if given into the deltoid muscle). In some cases, depending on the volume of the medication and the age of the patient, it may be necessary to divide the dose into two injections. If two IM injections are being administered, one medication should be injected into the right thigh and the other into the left thigh.[14]

Subcutaneous Injections

Sub-Q injections are frequently used in neonates, but absorption rates are variable. Neonates have far less fat as a percentage of body weight than adequately nourished older infants and children. Thus, medications given via sub-Q injections may be more rapidly absorbed. Thermoregulation of neonates (particularly newborns) is very dependent on external factors. Cold ambient temperatures or hypothermic conditions can also impair sub-Q absorption.[12] Typically, sub-Q injections are given into the thigh of infants or deltoid area of older children beneath skin and fat but above muscle. When faster absorption of the medication is required, the abdominal site may be used. The abdominal site is located just above and below the waist. This area is less impacted by muscle activity or movement. Care must be taken to avoid the area around the umbilicus/navel. The maximum volume of a sub-Q injection is usually 1.5 mL.[12]

Recently, continuous subcutaneous infusions (CSCI) have become a popular alternative to the IV route for infusing fluids in situations where obtaining IV access is difficult.[15] The medication is administered via an angiocatheter or butterfly needle into the fatty tissue under the skin, and it is absorbed systemically. In comparison with the IV route, it is considered to be safer to use CSCI because it has a lower risk of infection and no risk of air embolus. Access sites used for CSCI may last up to 72 hours or longer if there are no local reactions. Fluid can be delivered via CSCI using gravity at a rate of 1 mL/min at one site. If two sites are used, up to 3 L of fluid can be delivered through two separate sites over 24 hours.[15]

If a large volume of fluid is to be infused, the hypodermoclysis technique is often used. This is a method of infusing fluid into sub-Q tissue space that requires the use of hyaluronidase. In this case, an enzyme has been used to enhance fluid absorption from sub-Q tissue.[16] It is frequently used in geriatric and palliative care populations, but it is gaining popularity in pediatric patients.[16] Usual sites for hypodermoclysis include the abdomen, upper chest, above the breast, over an intercostal space, and the scapular area, although the thighs and the outer aspect of the upper arm have been used in bedridden patients.[16]

Hyaluronidase decreases the viscosity of the connective tissue through temporary lyses of the normal interstitial barrier, which increases the diffusion of the subcutaneously infused fluid up to 5-fold faster than if no enzyme is used.[17] One approach involves adding 150 units of hyaluronidase to each liter of fluid that is to be infused, and using an additional 75 units of hyaluronidase that is injected into each clysis site through short latex tubing near the needle.[15] Others suggest that, after securing the catheter, 1 mL (150 units) of hyaluronidase should be injected through the device, followed immediately by initiation of fluid infusion.[17] Hyaluronidase is available as a recombinant human preparation, or it is derived from animal sources.[18]

CSCI sites have been reported to last up to four days.[17] Studies involving insulin delivered via CSCI have shown variability in the onset insulin action and its duration of action over the life of the infusion set.[18] CSCI rehydration therapy is contraindicated in patients showing signs of circulatory failure, heart disorders, severe dehydration, shock, hypocoagulation, in any situation requiring more than 3 L/24 hours or careful fluid titration (eg, heart failure or renal failure), and in patients without intact skin sites.[17] It should not be used in patients with hypernatremia, those with serum osmolality greater than 300 mOsm/kg, evidence of fluid overload, or a blood urea nitrate/serum creatinine ratio greater than 25.[19]

Fluids infused via CSCI often include isotonic solutions that are typically used in IV replacement therapy, such as normal saline and lactated Ringer's solution.

Intraosseous Injections

The intraosseous (IO) route is an alternative for patients with difficult venous access, and it is often used in the emergency setting.[20] The marrow cavity within the bone provides noncollapsible vascular access, as blood flows from the medullary venous sinusoids into the central venous sinus, and then drained into the central venous circulation. The IO route is a rapid method of delivering crystalloids, colloids, medications, and blood products into the systemic circulation in a safe and reliable manner. It may be used in adults, children, infants, or newborns in any clinical situation where vascular access is emergently needed and peripheral access is not an option. Although relatively safe, IO is not without risk. Contraindications to using the IO route include ipsilateral fracture of the extremity (may increase risk of compartment syndrome and extravasation), previous placement in the same leg or site (because the old puncture site may allow for extravasation into soft tissue compartments), osteogenesis imperfecta and osteopetrosis (IO puncture may result in fracture), and presence of an infection at the proposed puncture site due to the risk of seeding infection.

Powered needle insertion devices are used to establish access within the bone, although spinal needles are often used in neonates. In infants and children, because of its flat wide surface and a thin layer of overlying tissue, the proximal tibia is the preferred insertion site, and the distal femur and distal tibia can also be used.[21] There are no limitations on the volume or type of fluid that can be infused via the IO route. The rules that guide practitioners in the administration of fluids and medications through the central venous access devices may be used, although many limit IO infusion to only isotonic fluids. Complications (eg, fracture, osteomyelitis) associated with the IO route are rare, especially if the correct techniques are followed and frequent assessment of the needle's position within the bone is performed.[22] Concerns of bone growth from insertion do exist, although there is no evidence to date in animal or clinical studies.[23] A recent retrospective study suggests that intraosseous complications may be underreported, and rates may be higher than previously reported.[24] Compartment syndrome can occur. This can be prevented by avoiding the use of excessive force while inserting the intraosseous cannula and by using a specifically designed fixation devices.[25]

Intradermal Injections

Intradermal (ID) injections involve the injection of small amounts of fluid (0.01 to 0.05 mL) into the dermis, which is located between the epidermis and the hypodermis. It is often done as part of a diagnostic procedure or in the administration of regional anesthetics. The injection is given in an area where the hair and skin are sparse, usually on the inner part of the forearm, although the upper chest, upper back, and back of upper arm have also been used. A 25-gauge needle, about 1 cm long, is generally used and is inserted at a 10- to 15-degree angle to the skin. In comparison with sub-Q and IM routes, the ID route has the longest absorption time. Given that the body's reaction to substances administered via the ID route is more easily visible because it is closer to the surface, the ID route is used for sensitivity tests, such as the Mantoux tuberculin and allergy tests.[26]

Ommaya Reservoir

Ommaya reservoirs are quarter-sized, soft, plastic, dome-shaped vascular access devices in which the catheter tip lies in one lateral ventricle that is attached to a reservoir that is surgically implanted under the scalp. It is used to deliver medications (eg, chemotherapy) into the cerebrospinal fluid (CSF) or to aspirate CSF, such as in cases of hydrocephalous. There are no age restrictions on the use of the device, although complications appear to be higher in premature infants.[27] One of the main benefits of this device is that medications are delivered directly into the CSF, and complications associated with lumbar puncture are avoided and patient comfort is improved.

Intrathecal Injections

Intrathecal (IT) delivery involves the injection of a medication into the spinal canal or into the subarachnoid space so that it reaches the CSF. It has been used to deliver spinal anesthesia, chemotherapy, and pain therapies. The IT route has also been used to deliver antimicrobials, as in the case of postneurosurgical infections. Like most parenteral medications, IT formulations are sterile isotonic drug solutions. The volume of IT injections ranges from 0.5 mL to 5 mL.[28] This can be a problem when attempting to solubilize lipophilic medications. Solubility can be improved by using the water-soluble salt form of the medication (eg, gentamicin sulfate) or by the use of buffers. To ensure the final product is sterile, in addition to adhering to strict aseptic technique during the compounding process, the medication is filtered at the time of administration using a 0.2 µm filter. IT injections must also be preservative free. Preservatives, such as benzyl alcohol and parabens, can cause inflammation of the arachnoid membrane and nerve damage.[29] Excipients, buffers, solubility enhancers, and even the medication itself can result in neurotoxicity. If possible, IT injections should contain as few excipients as possible, and the active medication should be evaluated for its propensity of causing neurotoxicity.

Minimizing Injection Pain

Minimizing injection pain is a major concern. Reducing the "pinch and burn" and giving the child a nearly pain-free experience can result in improved satisfaction for both the patient and the practitioner. For example, Laursen et al. noted that the perception of pain associated with sub-Q injections is multifactorial and includes the pH of the medication, temperature, injection volume, tonicity, the injection technique, the speed of injection, the needle size, the anatomic site, the child's characteristics, and the frequency of administration.[30] Ideally, the osmolality is 240 to 460 mOsm/kg, and the pH should normally be around 5 to 8.[31]

Buffers are often used to improve the pH of a medication as a way to reduce pain. Lidocaine 1% with 1:100,000 epinephrine normally has a pH of 4.2, but when buffered with sodium bicarbonate in a 10:1 dilution, it is superior to its unbuffered equivalent, as the pH is raised to more physiologic pH 7.4.[32]

The use of topical anesthetics, such as lidocaine and prilocaine 2.5%/2.5% cream, has been used to attenuate injection site pain. These agents are applied 60 to 120 minutes prior to the injection. When used to blunt the pain associated with an IV cannula insertion, however, it may hinder the procedure, as there is a biphasic vasoactive response that follows its application with initial vasoconstriction, which may make it difficult to establish access.[33] Ice or ethyl chloride spray can also be used, and they have a faster onset of action than topical anesthetics.[32;34] More recently, jet-injected lidocaine has been shown to be superior to vapocoolant spray in reducing venipuncture pain in children.[35] This is a form of needle-free local anesthesia that is administered through a special syringe (ie, J-Tip). J-Tips utilize a cartridge of compressed carbon dioxide to drive buffered lidocaine into the skin, but it may frighten some children, as it does so with a loud pop. In comparison with other techniques, the biggest advantage of using the J-Tip device is its immediate effect.

In infants less than 6 months of age, oral 24% sucrose solution has been used to decrease pain during painful or stressful procedures.[36] Studies have shown that it can decrease crying, heart rate, and pain when given prior to a painful procedure. It can only be given orally and should not be given via feeding tube. Although not fully understood, the proposed mechanism of action is thought to involve the activation of the endogenous opioid system through taste that provides natural analgesia.[36]

Distraction techniques during the administration of an injection are another way of decreasing pain. These include talking with the patient, having the patient look away, playing background music, or simply suggesting that the procedure is painless or has minimal pain.[37]

IMPACT OF EXCIPIENTS

When evaluating various parenteral medications intended for neonates and infants, the types of excipients present are a major consideration. Excipients are typically considered to be therapeutically inactive components of a medication that serve important roles as solvents, diluents, and preservatives. In general, although problematic excipients are known, safe exposure limits for neonates, infants, and children are not well established. For example, critically ill neonates, especially those receiving medications by continuous infusion, are at risk for exposure to toxic doses of benzyl alcohol, propylene glycol, and other excipients during routine medication administration (see **Table 23-3** and **Table 23-4**). In their review of inactive ingredients, the American Academy of Pediatrics (AAP) recommends mandatory labeling of inactive ingredients for all prescription and over-the-counter

TABLE 23-3. Examples of Parenteral Medications That May Contain Benzyl Alcohol

• Aminophylline
• Bacteriostatic sodium chloride 0.9% for injection
• Bacteriostatic sterile water for injection
• Cyanocobalamin
• Dexamethasone
• Diazepam
• Doxapram
• Enalaprilat
• Folic acid
• Heparin sodium
• Lidocaine
• Lorazepam
• Methylprednisolone acetate injectable suspension
• Pancuronium bromide
• Triamcinolone acetonide injectable suspension

TABLE 23-4. Examples of Parenteral Medications Containing Propylene Glycol

• Diazepam
• Digoxin pediatric
• Etomidate
• Fenoldopam
• Hydralazine
• Lorazepam
• Multivitamins (adult)
• Phenobarbital
• Phenytoin
• Sulfamethoxazole–trimethoprim

products.[38] A retrospective cohort study in Denmark assessed the impact of the total amount of excipient exposure administered to poly-medicated infants and children five years of age and younger. The study found that tolerance limits for ethanol and propylene glycol are commonly exceeded in poly-medicated patients due to the cumulative effects of these excipients.[39]

Benzyl Alcohol

Benzyl alcohol is an aromatic alcohol typically used in a concentration of 0.9% as a bacteriostatic preservative in multidose vials. Commonly used products that contain this preservative include bacteriostatic sodium chloride and sterile bacteriostatic water for injection. The toxic effects associated with benzyl alcohol (eg, respiratory failure, vasodilation, hypotension, convulsions, and paralysis) are well described.[40] Little is known, however, about the toxic effects or levels of benzyl alcohol in neonates, especially in sick premature infants. Normally, benzyl alcohol is rapidly oxidized to benzoic acid, conjugated with glycine in the liver, and excreted as hippuric acid. In the premature infant, however, this metabolic pathway is not fully developed. Any benzyl alcohol that was metabolized to benzoic acid is not able to be hepatically conjugated so it accumulates, resulting in metabolic acidosis.[41] In 1982, this common excipient was blamed for neonatal gasping syndrome and the deaths of 16 premature babies. The infants received it as an excipient in the flush solutions used to keep their IV catheters patent.[41] The neonatal gasping syndrome consists of hypotension, bradycardia, gasping respiration, hypotonia, progressive metabolic acidosis, seizures, and cardiovascular collapse, and it can be fatal.[42]

Benzyl alcohol toxicity has also been linked with the increased frequency of cerebral intraventricular hemorrhages and mortality reported in very low birth weight (VLBW) infants (weight < 1,000 g) who received flush solutions preserved with benzyl alcohol.[43] An increased incidence of developmental delay and cerebral palsy was also noted in this VLBW patient population, suggesting a secondary adverse effect of benzyl alcohol.[44] Similar toxicities of benzyl alcohol were described in a case report involving a 3,350 g infant who received 32 to 105 mg/kg/day.[45] Due to the risk of fatal toxic reactions arising from exposure to benzyl alcohol in excess of 90 mg/kg/day, the European Medicines Agency recommends that benzyl alcohol containing products not be used at all in premature babies or neonates and be limited in infants and children up to 3 years of age.[46]

Propylene Glycol

Propylene glycol is a colorless, odorless liquid used in numerous pharmaceutical, cosmetic, and food products. It is a frequently used excipient present in many parenteral medications as a drug solubilizer. Propylene glycol is used as stabilizer for vitamins and as a water-miscible cosolvent. Hyperosmolarity, lactic acidosis, seizures, and renal and hepatic toxicity have been linked with propylene glycol exposure.[47;48]

Toxicity is generally thought to be due to an accumulation of propylene glycol with plasma osmolar changes as one of the first signs. In most individuals, propylene glycol clearance is a combination of hepatic metabolism (alcohol dehydrogenase, 55%) to lactate and pyruvate through the tricarboxylic acid cycle or the glycolytic pathway followed by renal elimination (glomerular filtration rate, 45%).[49] However, this same process does not occur in neonates whose immature hepatic pathways and renal elimination capacity results in faster accumulation of propylene glycol and subsequent toxicity.[50] In fact, this hepatic enzyme pathway does not attain full adult activity until 12 to 30 months of age. In comparison with an elimination half-life of 2 to 5 hours in adults, neonates can have a propylene glycol half-life as long as 10 to 40 hours.[51;52] Because of the nonspecific nature of this clinical syndrome, the diagnosis of propylene glycol toxicity relies heavily on laboratory studies. The most common laboratory determinations include serum lactate and pyruvate concentrations as well as serum osmolality profile with a definitive diagnosis based on serum propylene glycol levels. Although many forms of metabolic acidosis are characterized by an abnormal anion gap, the accumulation of lactate, pyruvate, or exogenous toxins, such as propylene glycol, often produces an anion gap greater than 12 mmol/L.[53] In 1974, the World Health Organization (WHO) set an arbitrary limit of 25 mg/kg/day for orally ingested propylene glycol in adults.[54] In premature infants, propylene glycol toxicity has been reported following exposure of up to 3,000 mg/day.[51;55]

Other Considerations

Pharmacists cannot assume that if an excipient is generally recognized as safe (GRAS) by the FDA, it can be safely used in infants. In addition to the two aforementioned examples, several preterm infants died after receiving a formulation of vitamin E injection that contained polysorbate 80, a commonly used excipient that is considered GRAS.[56] It is the responsibility of the pharmacist to know which excipients are present in a particular parenteral product and whether it is suitable for use in the full- and preterm infant.[56]

Infection control practices may also vary in the pediatric population for similar reasons. Although conventional infection control measures used in adult patients are commonly used in infants and children, some limitations do exist when caring for the premature infants. For example, chlorhexidine gluconate is a commonly used topical antiseptic that is recommended by the Centers for Disease Control and Prevention (CDC) for skin cleansing before central venous catheter insertion in adults and children. However, due to limited safety data, its use is not recommended in children less 2 months old.[57] Trace amounts of chlorhexidine can be absorbed through the skin after a single bath in adults and term neonates without a negative outcome.[57] Following the finding in the 1970s that a similar phenol topical antiseptic, hexachlorophene, was also absorbed through the skin of neonates and resulted in vacuolar encephalopathy, similar concerns were raised with the use of chlorhexidine in the newborn.[58] Both of these agents are phenol derivatives, whereas hexachlorophene is a chlorinated bisphenol, and chlorhexidine is a chlorinated cationic biguanide. As a result of these differences in chemical structure, hexachlorophene is bacteriostatic with a slow onset of action that is only effective against gram-positive bacteria, while chlorhexidine is bactericidal with a more rapid onset of action and is effective against both gram-positive and gram-negative organisms. When used as directed, both products also leave a residue on the skin. Although there is limited evidence suggesting the safety of chlorhexidine in term infants, there are also limited data regarding the safety of its use in preterm infants. Preterm infants, especially those younger than 32 weeks gestation, have immature skin with increased permeability, underdeveloped neurologic systems, and metabolic limitations resulting in decreased drug clearance, which might predispose them to a higher rate of adverse reactions similar to that seen with hexachlorophene.

To date, skin toxicity remains a significant area of concern in preterm, low birth weight infants exposed to chlorhexidine, with the most common toxicity being skin burns.[59] In this population, skin burns can lead to hypothermia, excessive water loss, sepsis, and renal failure. Several studies have reported detectable chlorhexidine concentrations in the blood of preterm infants younger than 32 weeks gestation after skin exposure.[60] The clinical significance of detection remains unknown, as there are no established values for what is considered to be a safe concentration of chlorhexidine in the blood. Blood chlorhexidine concentrations appear to correlate with the strength of topical chlorhexidine solution used, as neonates exposed to 1% solutions had significantly higher blood concentrations of chlorhexidine compared with neonates exposed to 0.25% and 0.5% solutions. There are no reports of adverse health consequences as a result of such absorption in neonates.[60] In vitro and various animal studies, however, suggest there is still a potential risk of neurotoxicity. For these reasons, it is still suggested that chlorhexidine use be avoided in preterm infants, especially those younger than 32 weeks gestation and within the first 2 weeks of life.[57;60]

STORAGE CONTAINER CONSIDERATIONS

Plastic or Polyvinyl Chloride Toxicity

In addition to excipient and volume differences, care must be taken when selecting the proper container material for storing a compounded parenteral medication for a child. Certain plasticizers and contaminants can be detrimental to growing children. For example, the use of plastic containers and infusion sets containing diethylhexyl phthalate (DEHP) should be minimized whenever possible. DEHP is an industrial additive plasticizer found in polyvinyl chloride (PVC). Phthalates and their derivatives have been used since the 1930s in the manufacturing of plastic products to improve their flexibility and increase overall product durability.[61] The WHO International Agency for Research on Cancer (IARC) has classified these products as groups 2B or 3, as they could be teratogenic, carcinogenic, or result in reproductive toxicity.[62] The upper tolerable concentration of DEHP intake has been set by the FDA to be 0.6 mg/kg/day for PN exposures and 0.04 mg/kg/day for enteral nutrition.[63] In sick neonates, PN infusion systems have been shown to be one of the most important sources of DEHP load. Despite having a rapid turnover (half life < 24 hours), DEHP and its metabolites are regularly detected in human body fluids, such as plasma, urine, amniotic fluid, and breast milk.[64] In critically ill term and premature infants, DEHP has shown to increase oxidative stress and toxicity with PN infusion sets, and containers containing DEHP having been implicated as contributing factors.[65;66] One recent study demonstrated that phthalate exposure decreases pulmonary function and increases airway inflammation in asthmatic children.[67]

The physicochemical properties of the infusate are important factors in determining the risk of DEHP exposure. DEHP is not covalently bound to the plastic matrix, and it is able to release from PVC containers and tubing and leach into lipid containing fluids as it is infused into the patient.[63] One study attempted to assess the potential role of the type of lipid emulsion on the degree of DEHP leaching from PVC tubing.[68] Using PVC-based administration sets, six commercially available IV fat emulsions and their oil base components were left in direct contact. The amount of DEHP leached was measured using liquid chromatography. After 24 hours, depending on oil type, DEHP leaching varied significantly (P = .0000152). Olive-oil-based emulsions leached the most DEHP (65.8 mcg/mL IV fat emulsion), followed by the fish-oil-based emulsions (37.8 mcg/mL). Soybean-oil-based emulsions had the least DEHP leaching (19.6–27.8 mcg/mL).

With the increased availability of DEHP-free containers and infusion sets and the potential complications related with this plasticizer, practitioners should attempt to utilize DEHP-free products whenever possible. If no suitable alternative is available, efforts should be made to limit the duration of patient exposure.[63]

Glass and Aluminum Contamination

Plasticizers are not the only container related issue faced by pediatric practitioners. Glass containers also present their own unique problems. Glass containers may increase aluminum contamination simply because all the materials used to manufacture pharmaceutical containers contain some aluminum, either as a constituent (eg, aluminum oxide) or as an impurity. Pharmaceutical grade glass can contain as much as 6% aluminum of the total glass mass.[69]

Premature infants and patients with renal failure are at greater risk for aluminum toxicity because of their reduced capacity for renal aluminum elimination. It has been estimated that less than 0.5% of ingested aluminum is absorbed.[70] Parenterally infused aluminum, however, bypasses any protective barriers and directly enters the blood. Patients receiving long-term PN are at risk of developing osteomalacia and hypochromic microcytic anemia. Premature infants are further at risk for developing neurologic damage, such as depressed Bayley's neurodevelopmental scores.[70] Bishop et al. first reported the negative effects of aluminum contamination on infant neurodevelopment.[71] Neonates were randomized to receive either high aluminum load (eg, 45 mcg/kg/day) or aluminum depleted (eg, 4–5 mcg/kg/day) PN regimens. Infants in both groups receiving PN for less than 10 days had similar Bayley Mental Development Index scores. At 18 months old, however, infants who received the higher aluminum load had lower scores on the Bayley Mental Development Index than those who had received the aluminum-depleted solutions.

Although great emphasis has been placed on the extent of aluminum containments present in ingredients used to formulate PN, excipients present in other parenterals can also increase the aluminum burden that a child can be exposed to. For example, morphine and ranitidine contain phosphate; citrate is present in amikacin and dexamethasone; and gentamicin and dobutamine contain disodium edetate that also binds to aluminum, which enhances its extraction from the medication containers.[72] Other medications, such as furosemide and aminophylline, contain lower aluminum levels because they only consist of the pure drug and no problematic excipients.[72] Moreover, further dilution of a medication to allow for a more accurate measurement of the intended dose may actually increase the aluminum content, as some of the diluents used (eg, 0.9% sodium chloride, dextrose 10%) may also contribute to the overall aluminum load.[73]

Aluminum is also used intentionally in some vaccines as an adjuvant to increase the immune response to the vaccine. Adjuvants allow for lesser quantities of the vaccine and fewer doses. Low amounts of aluminum adjuvants are used in some vaccines (eg, diphtheria, tetanus, hepatitis A, hepatitis B, pneumococcal, and some *Haemophilus influenza* type b), but they are not used in the live viral vaccines (eg, rotavirus and measles/mumps/rubella/varicella).[74] The Center for Biologics Evaluation and Research regulates the amount of aluminum allowed in vaccines. The current limit for the amount of aluminum in the recommended individual dose of biological products, including vaccines, is within 0.85 to 1.25 mg.[74] In 2000, the National Vaccine Program Office (NVPO) determined that no changes to vaccine recommendations were necessary based on aluminum content.[75] Similarly, after reviewing the evidence, the WHO Global Advisory Committee on Vaccine Safety determined that no changes are needed to their vaccine policies.[76] **Table 23-5** lists the aluminum content in vaccines available at the time of publication. COVID-19 vaccines that have been authorized for emergency use in the United States do not contain any aluminum.[77] A recent FDA study has shown that the risk to infants posed by the total aluminum exposure received from the entire recommended series of childhood vaccines over the first year of life is extremely low.[74]

In addition to dilution and container issues, administration methods can also significantly contribute to aluminum loading (see **Table 23-6**). According to de Oliveria et al., approximately 60% of aluminum is already present in commercial products, while the remaining aluminum load is the result of preparation and administration methods.[73] De Oliveria et al. demonstrated that syringes and infusions sets used in the compounding and administration of a parenteral medication could increase the aluminum load. Furthermore, these same authors reported that simply rinsing the burettes and infusion sets with sterile water for injection prior to infusing the medication could potentially decrease the overall aluminum burden.[73] These additional sources of aluminum, however, are difficult to avoid. Although these contributions from administration methods are small, they can be significant contributions when added to what is already present in the commercial medications, making it difficult to accurately determine what a patient may potentially receive.

TABLE 23-5. Aluminum Content of Routine Infant and Pediatric Vaccines

Immunization ID	Product Name	Manufacturer	Aluminum Content (mg/dose)
COVID-19	Comirnaty	Pfizer-BioNTech	0
	Spikevax	Moderna	0
DTaP	Daptacel	Sanofi Pasteur	0.33
	Infanrix	GlaxoSmithKline	0.625
DT	Diphtheria and tetanus toxoid	Sanofi Pasteur	≤ 0.17
Influenza	Fluzone	Sanofi Pasteur	0
Hib (PRP-T)	Haemophilus B (ActHib)	Sanofi Pasteur	0
	Hiberix	GlaxoSmithKline	0
	Pedvax HIB	Merck	225
IPV	IPOL	Sanofi Pasteur	0
MMR	MMR II	Merck	0
Diph/HepB/pert-acel/polio/tet	Pediarix	GlaxoSmithKline	≤ 0.85
DTaP-Hib-IPV	Pentacel	Sanofi Pasteur	0.33
PCV13	Prevnar 13	Pfizer	0.125
HepB	Recombivax HB	Merck	0.5
	Energix-B	GlaxoSmithKline	0.25
ROTA	RotaTeq	Merck	0
Hepatitis A pediatric vaccine	VAQTA	Merck	0.225
	HAVRIX	GlaxoSmithKline	0.25
Varicella zoster virus VZV	Varivax	Merck	0

Source: Centers for Disease Control and Prevention (CDC). Vaccine excipient and media summary: excipients included in U.S. vaccines, by vaccine. https://www.cdc.gov/vaccines/pubs/pinkbook/downloads/appendices/b/excipient-table-2.pdf. Published November 1, 2021. Accessed April 4, 2023.

TABLE 23-6. Contribution of Each Compounding and Administration Method That Adds to the Total Amount of Aluminum Present in a Parenteral Medication*

Factor	% Contribution
Administration set	9%
Bag compounding	35%
Commercial additives	56%

*For more information, see reference 73.

COMPOUNDING PN FOR NEONATAL AND PEDIATRIC PATIENTS

In addition to the calcium and phosphorus compatibility issues (see **Table 23-7**), other compounding factors have been the focus of recent attention in hopes of preventing PN-related complications in neonates. These factors include minimizing aluminum exposure, protecting the solutions from light, and avoidance of DEHP containing materials. Premature infants and children with intestinal failure have immature or diminished antioxidant defenses that render them more susceptible to oxidant stress, which can influence the selection of many PN additives. Practitioners responsible for overseeing the compounding of PN solutions

TABLE 23-7. Factors Affecting Calcium and Phosphorus Solubility

• Calcium and phosphate salt concentrations
• Magnesium content
• Order of mixing
• pH of final solution
• Temperature
• Time
• Type and quantity of amino acids used

for neonates must be familiar with the differences in additive formulations and the impact that any potential product substitution may pose to this fragile population. In times of shortages, a proactive approach to conserve and prioritize supplies for neonates requiring PN and being aware of expert opinions and guidelines as the drug shortages crisis continues are necessary. For example, the American Society for Parenteral and Enteral Nutrition (ASPEN) provides guidelines for the use of PN additives in times of shortages in their publications and on their website (www.nutritioncare.org).

Total Nutrient Admixtures

Total nutrient admixtures (TNAs), also called 3-in-1 solutions, are PN solutions in which the lipid emulsion has been mixed with other ingredients to form one solution. The 3 refers to amino acid, dextrose, and lipid. A TNA provides the PN solution in a single bag as opposed to the traditional system, in which the lipid emulsion is administered as a bag or syringe via a separate line that is co-administered with the amino acid dextrose solution. Unfortunately, the necessary characteristics that allow for a stable TNA (eg, higher pH, low concentrations of calcium and phosphorus salts) make them unsuitable for neonates, infants, and small children. The high content of divalent ions (eg, calcium, magnesium) can further reduce particle zeta potential, resulting in coalescence. Also, the high concentrations of calcium and phosphorus typically present in a neonatal PN increase the risk of precipitation that cannot be detected in a TNA. In addition to electrolyte considerations, the pH of the pediatric amino acid solutions, especially when cysteine (L-cysteine) is added, can decrease the pH significantly and destabilize the lipid emulsion. In home care, where longer beyond-use dating is needed, the use of a dual chamber bag, where the lipid emulsion is separated from the other components until the time of administration, should also be considered to optimize stability. Practitioners must remember, however, that once the two chambers are mixed, the conventional TNA stability limits must be followed. Based on these issues and the limited amount of stability data, ASPEN recommends that 2-in-1 PN formulations be used in neonatal and infant patients and that lipids be infused separately.[78] Furthermore, ASPEN's clinical guidelines for ordering, compounding, labeling, and dispensing PN strongly discourages providing calcium and phosphate on alternate days in PN because it can result in significant urinary losses of both minerals on each day.[79]

Multivitamins

In the United States, several widespread shortages of parenteral multivitamins resulting in reports of symptomatic thiamine deficiency have stressed the importance of vitamins in patients receiving PN.[80] Even in adults, fatal vitamin deficiencies have been reported in patients receiving PN without vitamins in as short a time as a few weeks. In comparison with adult products, the pediatric versions of multivitamins contain higher amounts of vitamins K and D and lower amounts of B vitamins (see **Table 23-8**).[81–83] In the event of a parenteral multivitamin shortage, it is imperative that patients receive adequate thiamine with dextrose infusions to avoid metabolic lactic acidosis. Adult parenteral multivitamins should never be used in neonates because the propylene glycol and polysorbates contained in many of these products could be toxic.[84] Moreover, adult multivitamin products contain less vitamin D and K, and they may increase the risk of metabolic bone disease in pediatric patients on long-term PN therapy. Neonates who must receive PN without conventional pediatric parenteral multivitamins should always receive parenteral thiamine in the PN at a dose of 0.03 mg/kg/day.[85]

Amino Acids

The essential amino acids in PN include isoleucine, leucine, lysine, methionine, phenylalanine, threonine, tryptophan, and valine. In the premature infant, however, additional amino acids may be considered conditionally essential, as these neonates have a limited ability to synthesize them. These amino acids include cysteine, glutamine, glycine, histidine, taurine, and tyrosine.[86] The ideal mixture of amino acids for PN in premature infants is still unknown. Amino acid solutions have been designed to meet the protein requirements of premature infants based on the composition of breast milk. There are different amino acid solutions available for PN administration in premature infants that vary in composition of specific amino acids and concentration of protein (from 40%–53%). For example, because of difficulties in solubility, cysteine and tyrosine are not present in all products, nor do all products contain the amino acids taurine and glutamic acid.[86] These pediatric solutions, when compared with standard amino acid formulations originally designed for adults, result in a more balanced plasma amino acid pattern and improved neonatal growth, as evidenced by increased weight gain and net nitrogen retention.[87] In addition to different amino acid composition, most conventional amino acid solutions intended for use in adults and older children have a higher pH than those products intended for younger children. This can impact the solubility of calcium and phosphorus salts, such as decreased solubility if a higher pH product is substituted. Therefore, in times of shortages of conventional amino acid products, pediatric products should not be used for adult patients, and standard adult amino acid products should not be substituted for use in the neonate.

Cysteine (L-Cysteine)

Neonates are at risk of growth failure and metabolic derangements if they fail to receive adequate L-cysteine. In this population, supplementation with L-cysteine improves glutathione synthesis.[88] Glutathione is synthesized in the liver from the amino acids cysteine, glycine, and glutamine. It is a major intracellular antioxidant whose primary function is to protect cells from free radical damage, such as the damage that results from peroxides. Manufacturer dosage guidelines recommend that patients receiving a pediatric amino acid solution should be supplemented with L-cysteine at a dose of 40 mg/g amino acid, although doses as low as 20 mg/g may be just as effective.[89] Recently, a new formulation of cysteine hydrochloride has recommended doses as low as 7 mg/g amino acid for pediatric patients 12 to 17 years of age and 22mg/g amino acid for preterm infants, neonates, and children less than 12 years of age.[90]

Unlike multivitamins and amino acid products, when the L-cysteine has gone into a shortage situation, there is no substitute. In such situations, dose conservation measures should be used. In full-term infants, there is no need to supplement PN with L-cysteine, provided the infant receives at least 3 g/kg/day protein as adequate methionine (the precursor to L-cysteine) is provided when using commonly prescribed pediatric amino acid solutions. In times of shortage, L-cysteine should only be used in PN solutions for neonates less than 1 kg or for neonates weighing greater than 1 kg who are at high risk for L-cysteine deficiency, such as those who are septic or postsurgical.[89]

Trace Elements

In the first two weeks of life, the only trace element recommended from the first day of PN therapy is zinc.[91] During the last trimester of pregnancy, two thirds of zinc stores are transferred from the mother to the fetus.[92] Due to their lack of adequate tissue stores, along with increased urine zinc losses and increased catabolic needs, extremely premature neonates require 400 mcg/kg/day. Over 300 metabolic processes require zinc as a cofactor, and this trace element is essential for immune function, gene expression, growth, and the synthesis of nucleic acids and protein.[93] In infants receiving zinc-free PN, zinc levels decline dramatically, resulting in a deficiency that is associated with cutaneous changes, immunologic impairment, growth failure, and impaired wound healing.[93]

Pediatric trace metal combination products commonly added to PN solutions contain zinc, copper, manganese, and chromium. Although typically added on initiation of PN, the other trace elements contained in these combination products are not necessary until after 2 weeks of age. For this reason, some practitioners prefer to add trace elements to PN using individual additives rather than a single combination product.

Selenium is a component of glutathione peroxidase, which is protective against free radical injury. It is necessary for the formation of selenoproteins, which are essential antioxidants in skin that also have a role in keratinocyte growth and viability. Thus, like zinc, selenium deficiency can also cause cutaneous changes. All premature infants are born selenium-deficient, as placental transfer of selenium typically occurs after the 36th week of gestation.[94] Within weeks of birth, regardless of gestational age, neonates receiving selenium-free PN will rapidly deplete any existing selenium stores.[95] To achieve serum concentrations similar to a healthy breastfed infant, premature infants receiving PN should receive 3 mcg/kg/day of selenium. Failure to do so places premature infants who are selenium-deficient at risk for developing bronchopulmonary dysplasia due to exposure to high levels of oxygen that result in oxidative stress.[94]

Aluminum Contamination and FDA Mandate

As previously mentioned, aluminum exposure is a potential risk in all patients receiving prolonged courses on PN. In July 2004, the FDA issued a mandate that required manufacturers to include the aluminum content on the label of additives commonly used in compounding PN solutions. The amount of aluminum provided by PN should be less 5 mcg/kg/day, which is the threshold that the FDA deems safe.[96]

Calcium gluconate salts are a major source of aluminum contamination in PN patients. Because calcium gluconate salts are a large source of contamination, neonates are at risk of developing toxicity due to their high calcium requirements coupled with renal immaturity.[97] In response to the findings of potential adverse neurodevelopment associated with aluminum exposure, the use of calcium chloride in PN solutions has been re-evaluated. Calcium chloride salts are inherently less contaminated, and, in theory, could be used as an alternative to calcium gluconate salts. However, this could predispose patients, especially infants, to a potentially greater risk of developing metabolic acidosis due to the increased chloride load. Koo and colleagues suggest that using a 50% calcium gluconate and 50% calcium chloride mix in conjunction with the use of potassium and sodium acetate salts in place of sodium and potassium chloride could minimize this risk.[98] Calcium and phosphorus solubility would still be a concern, as calcium chloride salts have a higher degree of dissociation. Thus, less than optimal calcium and phosphate intake would still be problematic. This risk can be minimized if calcium chloride salts are used with an organic phosphate salt (eg, sodium glycerophosphate pentahydrate). However, these organic phosphate salts are expensive and are not available in many countries.[99]

The FDA has set an upper limit of 25 mg of aluminum per liter as the allowable amount for large volume parenterals (LVPs) utilized in PN compounding. To date, no acceptable upper limits have been established for small volume parenterals (SVPs). For those SVPs containing more than 25 mg/L, the exact amount of aluminum must be noted on the product label.

TABLE 23-8. Comparison of Pediatric and Adult Parenteral Multivitamin Products

Product	Supplier	A (international units)	B_1 (mg)	B_2 (mg)	B_6 (mg)	B_{12} (mcg)	Biotin (mcg)	C (mg)	Folic Acid (mcg)
Pediatric (< 11 yr old)									
Infuvite pediatric (per 5 mL)	Baxter	2,300	1.2	1.4	1	1	20	80	140
Adolescents and Adults (> 11 yr old)									
Infuvite adult (per 10 mL)	Baxter	3,300	6	3.6	6	5	60	200	600
Cernevit*	Baxter	3,500	3.51	4.14	4.53	6	69	125	414

*Not currently available in the United States.

Source: Based on Infuvite Pediatric [package insert]. Deerfield, IL: Baxter Healthcare Corporation; July 2014. https://www.accessdata.fda.gov/drugsatfda_docs/label/2014/021646s014lbl.pdf., Infuvite Adult [package insert]. Deerfield, IL: Baxter Healthcare Corporation; November 25, 2002. https://www.accessdata.fda.gov/drugsatfda_docs/label/2004/21163s011lbl.pdf., and Cernevit [package insert]. Deerfield, IL: Baxter Healthcare Corporation; April 1999. https://www.accessdata.fda.gov/drugsatfda_docs/label/1999/20924lbl.pdf.

D (international units)	E (international units)	K (mcg)	Niacinamide (mg)	Dexpanthenol (mg)	Excipients
Pediatric (< 11 yr old)					
400	7	200	17	5	Polysorbate 80 Anhydrous citric acid Sodium citrate Sodium hydroxide Hydrochloric acid Mannitol
Adolescents and Adults (> 11 yr old)					
200	10	150	40	15	Polysorbate 80 Propylene glycol Anhydrous citric acid Sodium citrate Sodium hydroxide Hydrochloric acid
220	11.2	NA	46	17.25	Glycine Glycocholic acid Lecithin (soybean) Sodium hydroxide Hydrochloric acid

To determine the potential patient exposure to aluminum, the following calculations are used.[100]

1. First, using the information contained in the package insert or on the product label, convert the aluminum content from mg/L to mg/mL. Note that for calculation purposes, unless otherwise stated in the package insert or on the product label, all LVPs use the value of 25 mg/L, while the actual content on the product label is used to calculate the aluminum for all SVPs unless the content is less than 25 mg/L, in which case 25 mg/L is used for the calculations.
2. Second, for each ingredient in the PN solution, multiply the volume of each additive by its respective aluminum content as calculated in step one.
3. Third, determine the entire aluminum content of the solution by totaling the individual aluminum contribution for each additive as determined in step two.
4. Fourth, divide the total aluminum content by the patient's weight to determine the mg/kg/day. Ideally, the target aluminum content should be less than 5 mg/kg/day, the level deemed safe by the FDA.

Figure 23-1 provides an example of a theoretical aluminum load calculation.

Since the implementation of the FDA mandate, it has been difficult to incorporate the maximum allowable limit into clinical practice due to limitations in current product formulations. At present, there are few options available to reduce the aluminum load in PN.[70] One option is to replace potassium phosphate with sodium phosphate salts that have considerably less aluminum. Furthermore, not all ingredients (eg, heparin, albumin, and insulin) that are frequently added to PN solutions are required to list their aluminum content on their label, which makes it even more difficult to accurately calculate potential aluminum exposure. A significant reduction in aluminum exposure in neonates receiving PN can be achieved by using the least contaminated products that are commercially available. Until more products contain low aluminum contamination and until labeling requirements are expanded for more products to note aluminum content, minimizing aluminum exposure from PN will continue to remain a challenge.

Ambient Light

When PN is exposed to ambient light, lipid peroxides and hydrogen peroxide are generated. This phenomenon was first reported in the early 1980s when it was observed that light exposure might cause vitamin instability, but most practitioners still choose not to cover solutions, especially if the multivitamins are added immediately prior to infusing.[101] Approximately 50% of the hydrogen peroxide production is reduced when the entire solution and delivery system (eg, amino acid and dextrose bag, lipid syringe, and tubing) is protected from ambient light.[102]

Multivitamins, however, are not the only component of PN that may be affected by light. The amino acids tryptophan and tyrosine undergo photo-oxidation to form

FIGURE 23-1. Example Calculation of Aluminum Load

AG is a 1-month-old, 5-kg female infant ordered to receive PN ~500 mL/day.
Total aluminum content per infused volume is 144.4 mcg (based on label information).
The theoretical aluminum load is 144.4 mcg ÷ 5 kg = 29 mcg/kg/day.

PN Composition (per day)			
Dextrose	72 g	Amino acids	10 g
NaCl	15 mEq	KCl	15 mEq
Calcium gluconate	10 mEq	KPhos	5 mmol
Magnesium sulfate	2.5 mEq	Trace elements	1 mL
MVI pediatric	5 mL		

Determine Total Aluminum Intake:

Additive	**Volume**	**Aluminum**	**Additive**	**Volume**	**Aluminum**
Dextrose 70%	103 mL	2.575 mcg	AA 10% TrophAmine	100 mL	2.5 mcg
NaCl 4 mEq/mL	3.75 mL	0.094 mcg	KCl	7.5 mL	0.75 mcg
Calcium gluconate	20 mL	101.12 mcg	KPhos	1.7 mL	28.22 mcg
Magnesium sulfate	0.63 mL	0.002 mcg	Trace elements	1 mL	2.5 mcg
MVI pediatric	5 mL	0.21 mcg	Sterile water for injection	257 mL	6.425 mcg

MVI = multivitamin for infusion; PN = parenteral nutrition.

free radicals with hepatotoxic properties.[102;103] Riboflavin appears to facilitate the photo-oxidation process by serving as a photosensitizing agent.[104] Other amino acids, such as methionine, histidine, and cysteine, are also susceptible. In addition to its impact on vitamins and amino acids, phototherapy might cause significant peroxidation in IV fat emulsions, resulting in the formation of cytotoxic triglyceride hydroperoxides.[105] Lipid hydroperoxides could theoretically cause pulmonary vasoconstriction via an interference with endogenous prostaglandin synthesis. It has been recommended by some that fat emulsion containers be covered with aluminum foil or supplemented with sodium ascorbate prior to light exposure.[106] However, results from a study on a large cohort of premature infants demonstrated no beneficial effect of partial light protection of PN on clinically relevant outcomes. This study did not provide complete protection against ambient light, therefore, further investigation is warranted.[107] Until recently, with conflicting data and a lack of risk associated by protecting PN solutions from light, the choice remained one of risk to benefit, with many neonatal intensive care units (NICUs) opting to cover PN solutions, as it may confer some benefits without the risk of undue harm.

In July 2019, the Pharmacovigilance Risk Assessment Committee (PRAC) of the European Medicines Agency revisited this topic. PRAC issued recommendations specific to products used in PN containing amino acids and/or lipids with regards to light exposure and the clinical impact of ambient light on neonates and children below 2 years of age that receive them.[108] In their review of literature, members of PRAC reported adverse outcomes in neonates receiving PN solutions with or without lipids that were not light protected. The committee recommended that manufacturers provide supplemental information to clinicians and to revise their labeling and package leaflets to recommend that, when used in neonates and children younger than two years old, PN and lipid infusions should be protected from ambient light (both the bag and the infusion set) until administration is complete, as peroxides and other degradation products could be generated that are detrimental to this vulnerable population.

DEHP Toxicity

As previously discussed, preterm neonates and critically ill infants experience increased oxidative stress and toxicity due to DEHP exposure. PN infusion sets and containers containing DEHP have been implicated as contributing to this risk.[65;66] Changing to PVC-free infusion systems has been shown to reduce the incidence of cholestatic liver disease.[109] In this study of 76 patients, one group (n = 30) received PN through PVC administration, while a second group (n = 46) had their PN infused through PVC-free tubing. The use of PVC infusion sets correlated strongly with the development of cholestasis (P = .0004). Based on these findings, DEHP-free containers and infusion sets should be used whenever possible to minimize risk. Interestingly, although contact time was reduced, cyclic infusion of PN did not appear to decrease the risk of phthalate exposure.[110]

Repackaging of Lipid Emulsions Into Syringes

For patient safety and cost savings, IV lipid emulsions (ILE) are often repackaged from the manufacturer's original container into syringes for use with the neonates and infants. Additionally, a recent ILE shortage has caused many centers to repackage ILE into syringes to conserve supplies. Despite this widespread practice among pediatric practitioners, repackaging ILE into syringes remains controversial, as it has been shown to be prone to microbial contamination.[111–113] In the United States, the products currently available are in 100, 250, and 500 mL containers. These are not suitable for neonates who typically receive doses of 10 to 20 mL per day. Whenever the original manufacturer's container is used in a neonate, the infant is put at risk for an infusion-related error. Errors in administration of ILE are a leading cause of medication errors among pediatric patients. One MEDMARX study reported errors involving ILE in 54 out of 173 hospitals (30%) between January 1, 2000 and December 31, 2005.[114;115] In most instances, such errors are a result of a tubing connection error, device failure, or human error involving misprogramming the infusion pump (eg, switching the infusion rate of the PN and the ILE). Such errors can result in a rapid infusion of the ILE, causing hypertriglyceridemia, which resolves on discontinuation of the ILE infusion. In other cases, more serious complications, such as metabolic acidosis, respiratory failure, and even death, have been associated with rapid infusion of an ILE.[116;117]

For the aforementioned reasons, it is common practice to dispense small doses of ILE in syringes. Since 1996, the CDC has recommended a 12 hour hang time for ILE that are infused separately from the dextrose and amino acid solution.[57] In infants, ILE are typically infused over 24 hours, and this can be accomplished by dividing the total daily dose into two containers that are replaced every 12 hours. The practice of repackaging ILE is not without its own risk, however. Lipid emulsions can become contaminated during the repackaging process, predisposing the patient to a nosocomial infection.[118–123] Unlike TNAs or dextrose and amino acid solutions that have sufficient hypertonicity that can suppress microbial growth, separate ILE infusions are more susceptible to supporting bacterial and fungal growth. Typical contaminants that are known to flourish in ILE include *Escherichia coli*, *Staphylococcus epidermidis*, diphtheroids, micrococci, *Malassezia furfur*, and *Candida albicans*. In one study, Obayashi and colleagues demonstrated that single-use packages of ILE that were inoculated with the opportunistic bacteria *Serratia marcescens* and *Burkholderia cepacia* exhibited considerable microbial growth.[119] Although the use of bacteria-eliminating 0.2-µm inline filters is often considered a preventative measure for IV fluids, they are not an option when dealing with ILE. Unlike crystalloids, due to the size of the fat globules present in the ILE, it is not possible to infuse these products through 0.2-µm inline filters without disrupting the emulsion.[124;125] At best, ILE can be infused through filters with a larger 1.2-µm pore size, which can trap particulate matter, yeast, and molds but do not eliminate bacteria.[125]

Lipid repackaging studies to date have been flawed, as it has not been possible to determine the point where the contamination of the syringe occurred (at the time of repackaging or during the administration process).[111;112] Cultures were performed on samples of residual ILE in syringes that were obtained from patients after the completion of the infusion.[111;112] Moreover, samples were not cultured in real time. Often, syringes were collected from patients and refrigerated overnight prior to being sent to the laboratory for culturing, adding another potential variable to interpreting the findings.[111] Since the implementation of USP Chapter <797> Pharmaceutical Compounding—Sterile Preparations and the CDC recommendations for a 12 hour hang time, there have not been any reported cases of outbreaks of sepsis in patients due to extrinsic contamination of parenteral lipid emulsions due to repackaging into syringes.

The decision to repackage fat emulsions into syringes still remains a clinical quandary, with many NICUs opting to utilize syringes to minimize the risk of accidental rapid infusion and conserve supplies in times of shortage.[125] Furthermore, if repackaging is done, it must be done in strict accordance with USP Chapter <797>.[126;127] Conversely, if lipid emulsions are infused directly from the manufacturer's source container, care must be taken to ensure that accidental rapid infusion and overdose do not occur. Regardless of which method of delivery is used, the source container (eg, syringe or original manufacturer's container) must be changed every 12 hours after initial entry.

Automated Compounding Devices: Template Safety Considerations

Although the benefits of PN are significant, any error that occurs with this complex therapy is an opportunity for serious harm. The use of specialized software and automated compounding devices is supposed to decrease calculation and compounding errors associated with this high-risk therapy, but it has not eliminated them and may have created new opportunities for error. ASPEN encourages the use of a total daily dose when prescribing nutrients for adult PN and daily weight-based doses (mg/kg/day) when prescribing nutrients for pediatric PN. This method of PN ordering, in contrast to per liter prescribing, supports the use of a 24 hour nutrient infusion system.[79]

Inappropriate dosing of nutrients, order entry errors, and compounding errors have all been associated with adverse outcomes and death in patients receiving PN. In one case, a keystroke error resulted in the death of a six-week-old infant who received a 60-fold overdose of sodium when a technician entered the prescribed dose of calcium (982 mg) into the mEq field for sodium.[128] Dose range alerts may not be present in PN order processing software to prevent such errors. Templates are typically developed to be used to standardize the way PN orders are processed and labeled within the software system. Often, due to variations in prescribing methods, special neonatal, pediatric, and adult templates are created, reflecting the weight-based versus daily dosing of macro- and micronutrients in the different age groups. Errors have occurred when the wrong template has been used. To avoid such errors, the templates should be standardized in a way that matches the format used when entering the orders into the pharmacy computer and automated compounding device. Standardization is required for the units of measure for each nutrient and the order in which each ingredient is prescribed and entered.[129] A recent report using failure and effects analysis reported that among all phases of the neonatal PN prescribing, preparing, and dispensing process, the one associated with the most failures occurred when the pharmacist transcribed the PN order into the order processing software, probably due to the numerous calculations, additive selection, and compatibility considerations.[130] Pharmacists must understand the limitations of the systems used and use checklists to reduce errors at the most critical steps before they reach the patient.

PARENTERAL MEDICATION SAFETY ISSUES UNIQUE TO THE PEDIATRIC PATIENT

It has been reported that the medication error rate for pediatric patients is three times greater than that for adults.[131] As mentioned previously, due to the available concentrations of many parenteral medications, it is often difficult to control the rate of drug delivery. In pediatric patients in particular, it is difficult to provide small doses accurately and in a consistent manner. Over 40 years ago, Leff and Roberts reported that syringe pump infusion and manual retrograde administration techniques were both safe and reliable methods of providing accurate parenteral drug delivery in this population.[132] Others, such as Nahata et al., found significant differences in serum concentration of tobramycin when different infusion methods were used.[133] Location of administration ports and methods of delivery resulted in substantial differences in the peak serum concentrations and the time required to achieve these peaks after infusion of tobramycin using different devices.[133] Similar findings were reported by Sherwin et al. who showed that gentamicin delivery may reach only 80% of the intended dose after 1 hour in a term infant and only 60% in an extremely low birth weight neonate due to the dead space in tubing coupled with reduced infusion rates.[134] Improper priming of tubing can also contribute to the loss of the intended dose.

Furthermore, in comparison with infusion rates used in adult patients, small changes in specific gravity can impact the amount of drug delivered when infused at slower rates typically used in a neonate. Medications with higher specific gravities can become trapped in the reservoirs of the infusion system (eg, filters, drip chambers, tubing).[135] Tubing diameter, the presence of extension sets, and priming volumes of filters can further alter delivery rates. When a medication is co-administered into another fluid, the potential for retrograde flow of the medication and poor mixing with the carrier fluid can result in erratic drug concentrations.[136]

Even the choice of carrier fluid to co-administer a medication can be significant in the neonate. For example, the co-administration of the antibiotic ceftriaxone with calcium containing IV fluids (eg, LR, D5LR, D5R, PN) can lead to potentially fatal lung and kidney damage due to precipitation reactions in the neonate. In a case series, nine infants had an adverse event related to the co-administration of ceftriaxone with a calcium-containing carrier fluid, seven of which were fatal.[137] Factors that contributed to developing this life-threatening adverse drug reaction included the use of ceftriaxone at dosages higher than those approved by the FDA, IV push administration, and giving the total daily dosage as a single infusion. Based on these cases, the product labeling has been updated to caution practitioners regarding the use of this antibiotic in neonates.

It is imperative that pharmacists become familiar with the impact of the design and limitations of these infusion devices and the impact of carrier fluids as they relate to drug delivery methods. Furthermore, they should know how differences in infusion methods can impact the proper interpretation of pharmacokinetic data and predispose infants and children to adverse effects associated with medications with a narrow therapeutic index. Even the selection of ancillary devices, such as syringe caps, must be carefully evaluated as potential choking hazards before including in hospital inventory.[138]

Storage and Dispensing Considerations

Suresh et al. reported that more than 50% of NICU medication errors were due to incorrect dispensing and administration, compared with less than 30% due to incorrect ordering and transcription.[139] To help minimize this risk, special attention should be made when designing cleanrooms and storage areas for parenteral medications intended for use in the neonate. Due to the wide variety of dosage forms and concentrations of many commonly used parenteral medications, the opportunity for dispensing errors is great. In many cases, different concentrations of the same medication are packaged in visually similar containers.[140] Care should be taken to avoid placing visually similar medications intended for neonates next to products and compounded preparations used in adults. For example, in one series describing medication errors, caffeine citrate (used to treat apnea of prematurity) was placed next to the headache treatment caffeine benzoate, infant strength sodium bicarbonate 4.2% injection was adjacent to the more concentrated 8.4% adult sodium bicarbonate injection, and the 10 mg/mL pediatric gentamicin next to the 40 mg/mL adult strength product. In each instance, an infant received the incorrect product or dose because of the similar appearance of the agents.[141] As part of the pharmacy's corrective action plan, the storage area in the cleanroom was reorganized. Specially marked shelving section segregated neonate only medication from the rest of the stock. According to the authors, because this simple change was made, no further dispensing errors involving adult and neonatal medication mix-ups have been observed at their institution.

Standardization Issues

Due to their diverse needs, manipulation of parenteral medications intended for infants and child is common. This practice, however, increases the risk for error and adverse patient outcomes.[142] The Institute of Medicine recommends that hospitals "implement standard processes for medication doses, dose timing, and dose scales in a given patient care unit."[143]

Rule of 6

For many years, it was common practice to prescribe critical care infusions in pediatric patients using the "Rule of 6." This weight-based approach involved individually compounding unique concentrations of critical care medications. The infant's weight (in kg) was multiplied by 6, and the calculated value was added as milligrams of drug to 100 mL of fluid. This concentration allowed a flow rate of 1 mL/hr to deliver 1 mcg/kg/min, making dosage changes easily accomplished. Because this practice results in variable concentrations, it makes it impossible to utilize standard concentrations for high-alert medications, which has been a Joint Commission National Patient Safety Goal.[144] In fact, a calculation error related to the use of this method may have contributed to an infant's death when it led to a misplaced decimal point that resulted in a 10-fold overdose of dopamine.[145] According to the National Patient Safety goals, prescribers should order critical care infusions using standard concentrations and vary the infusion rate in order to change the dose of medication delivered.[144]

ROLE OF INFORMATION SUPPORT

Creating a culture of safety is constantly evolving. Pediatric-specific decision support software and devices are improving but are still not at an optimal state. With the publication of AAP's article "Prevention of Medication Errors in the Pediatric Inpatient Setting," the need for computerized provider order entry (CPOE) systems requires robust decision support to be safe and effective.[146] Some decision support rules for drug and dosing schedules and CPOE systems are commercially available for children. However, most of these systems still require the institution's further modification to be clinically useful.[147] Order sets, templates, reminders, and clinical practice guidelines embedded within these information systems improve adherence to best practice and a more standardized approach to care. Other technological solutions used in the adult setting have been applied to the pediatric environment. Barcoding has been used to compare identification bands with medications and blood products before administration.[148] Other enhancements include patient-specific spreadsheets that can calculate emergency medication dosing sheets for bedside posting, which can be linked to a patient's most recent weight.[149] Despite these advantages, some limitations to technological support still remain, including ease of use, staff acceptance, cost, software integration into pre-existing facility informatics systems, the increase in new types of errors post implementation, and ability to address only a fraction of potential medication errors.[150]

Smart Pump Technology and Standardization

Switching to standard concentrations that can be used on smart syringe pumps has been shown to be an effective way to decrease the risk of compounding errors. Furthermore, use of these devices has resulted in improved documentation of medication errors and decreases in calculation and administration errors.[142] Implementing smart pumps that include a NICU medication and concentration library core offers an additional layer of safety. Conventional infusion technologies depend on the practitioner accurately programming the device and another individual performing a second independent double check of the pump settings. Errors could still occur because of human factors (eg, lack of knowledge about dose limits), system factors (eg, failing to perform the second check), or organizational factors (eg, multiple handoffs without proper communication).[151] Smart pumps incorporate sophisticated computer decision-making support, and they can store medication information (medication library), make calculations, and check entered information against pre-established dosage parameters that can be tailored for the neonate and pediatric patient population. In one pediatric study, upon implementation of smart pumps, there was a 73% decrease in infusion-related incident reports.[152]

In addition to standard doses and concentration limits, minimum and maximum administration guidelines can be defined as volume over time (eg, mL/hr) or dose per infant weight (eg, mcg/kg/min). Limits can be programmed as soft stops or hard stops. Based on these parameters, alerts can be fired if the entered dose is outside the minimum or maximum dose range.[153] Clinicians can override a soft limit warning, but a hard limit warning will require some corrective action to be taken before proceeding with administering the medication. Although the primary emphasis on preventing IV errors is often on doses that exceed maximum limits, low concentration soft alerts may be misinterpreted as being similar to low dose alerts, which also leads to significant errors.[153] In one case, a patient was prescribed IV insulin (regular) 12.5 units/hour. The pharmacy dispensed a standard insulin infusion of 100 units/100 mL (1 unit/mL). The nurse misprogrammed the pump, failing to select the standard insulin concentration and instead used a custom concentration option to enter the incorrect concentration of 5 units/100 mL (0.05 units/mL), which resulted in the pump delivering the insulin at a rate of 250 mL/hour. The entire bag containing 100 units of insulin infused in approximately 20 minutes.

Despite the improvements in drug delivery, the use of smart pumps do not prevent specific types of errors and have created new ones.[154] **Table 23-9** summarizes the types of errors associated with smart infusion pumps.

TABLE 23-9. Examples of Smart Infusion Pump Errors*

Error Type	Examples	Contributing Factors
Administration	• Drug not given • Incorrect route • Wrong drug • Wrong method of administration • Wrong patient	• Communication • Human factors • Name confusion • Packaging and design flaws • System-related
Drug library	• Drug library bypassed; infuse over time mode used • Drug library inadequate • Wrong library selected	• Communication • Human factors • Name confusion • Packaging and design flaws • System-related
Lack of documentation	• No order placed for administered medication • Verbal orders never documented for infused medication	• Communication • Human factors • System-related
Programming	• Incorrect concentration selected • Incorrect patient weight input • Wrong dose programmed • Wrong rate programmed • Wrong volume programmed	• Communication • Human factors • Name confusion • Packaging and design flaws • System-related
Other	• Infusion tubing switched • Wrong syringe size	• Human factors • Packaging and design flaws

*For more information, see reference 154.

TABLE 23-10. Recommendations for Safe Preparation of IV Admixtures for Neonates and Children*

• Standardize the concentrations used
• When preparing intravenous fluids, use one consistent formula or standard concentration (ie, not the Rule of 6)
• Use commercially available preparations whenever possible
• Minimize the need to prepare infusions on the patient care unit
• Have pharmacy on site to prepare all neonatal/pediatric infusions if commercial products are not available
• Independently double check all neonatal and pediatric IV admixtures before dispensing and administering

IV = intravenous.
*For more information, see reference 155.

Other Safety Initiatives or Considerations

Numerous approaches have been implemented to improve the safety of the provision of medications to neonates and children (see **Table 23-10**).[153] One approach is to develop algorithms that compare the ordered dose of a medication or IV fluid with the actual dose administered. Li et al. developed a series of novel computerized algorithms to identify medication administration errors within the electronic health record of all neonatal patients treated in a level four NICU.[156] A neonatologist developed the dosing limits utilized in the algorithms that were based on standard of care practices. The authors reported that error rates were higher for medications that were adjusted frequently and fluids administered concurrently. The algorithms identified many previously unidentified errors, demonstrating significantly better sensitivity (82% versus 5%) and precision (70% versus 50%) than conventional incident reporting.[156]

In May of 2016 ASHP, in conjunction with the Pediatric Pharmacy Advocacy Group, the Institute for Safe Medication Practices, and the Association for the Advancement of Medical Instrumentation, announced the launch of Standardize 4 Safety, a 3-year, multidisciplinary initiative focused on creating and promoting national standard concentrations for both IV and oral liquid medications.[157] Funded through the FDA's Safe Use Initiative, Standardize 4 Safety seeks to reduce errors associated with IV and oral liquid medications as well as improve continuity of the medication use process for patients through transitions of care. The project is an effort to reduce preventable harm from medications by creating and facilitating public and private collaborations with the healthcare community. Standard concentrations of commonly used parenteral medications have been created as guidelines.[158] As these are not mandatory, the hope is that healthcare systems will voluntarily adopt them as an error prevention strategy for patient safety.

SUMMARY

Because many medications used in neonates and children are used off-label, it is important for practitioners to consider the risk and benefits of each (ie, compounding or switching to an alternative age), how the routes of delivery vary, the methods used to administer these medications, and how the composition of the medications (ie, commercial products or compounded preparations) can impact safe drug delivery to this vulnerable population. Specialized resources (see **Suggested Reading**) should be consulted to guide clinicians in determining the most appropriate therapy and the optimal method to safely deliver it.

SUGGESTED READING

- Corkins MR. *The ASPEN Pediatric Nutrition Support Core Curriculum*. 2nd ed. Rockville, MD: The American Society for Parenteral and Enteral Nutrition; 2015.
- Corkins MR. *The ASPEN Pediatric Nutrition Support Handbook*. 2nd ed. Rockville, MD: The American Society for Parenteral and Enteral Nutrition; 2015.
- The Johns Hopkins Hospital, Kleinman K, McDaniel L, Molloy M. *The Harriet Lane Handbook*. 22nd ed. Philadelphia, PA: Elsevier; 2021.
- Phelps SJ, Hagemann TM, Lee KR, Thompson AJ. eds. *Pediatric Injectable Drugs: the Teddy Bear Book*. 11th ed. Bethesda, MD: American Society of Health-System Pharmacists; 2018.
- Institute for Safe Medication Practices. Guidelines for sterile compounding and the safe use of sterile compounding technology. **https://www.ismp.org/resources/guidelines-sterile-compounding-and-safe-use-sterile-compounding-technology**. Published May 4, 2022. Accessed April 3, 2023.
- Taketomo CK, Hodding JH, Kraus DM, eds. *Pediatric & Neonatal Dosage Handbook: an Extensive Resource for Clinicians Treating Pediatric and Neonatal Patients*. 28th ed. Hudson, OH: Lexicomp/Wolters Kluwer; 2021.
- Thomson Reuters Clinical Editorial Staff. *Neofax*. Whippany, NJ: PDR Network; 2019.

REFERENCES

1. Food and Drug Administration (FDA). Drug research and children. **https://www.fda.gov/Drugs/ResourcesForYou/Consumers/ucm143565.htm**. Published May 4, 2016. Accessed September 8, 2023.
2. Hwang TJ, Orenstein L, Kesselheim AS, et al. Completion rate and reporting of mandatory pediatric postmarketing studies under the US Pediatric Research Equity Act. *JAMA Pediatr*. 2019;173(1):68–74. doi:10.1001/jamapediatrics.2018.3416.

3. Preventing pediatric medication errors. *Sentinel Event Alert*. 2008;11(39):1–4.

4. Puntis JW. Morphine overdose in a newborn and the search for the third order 'why?'. *J Clin Forensic Med*. 1999;6(2):109–112. doi:10.1016/s1353-1131(99)90209-2.

5. Franke HA, Woods DM, Holl JL. High-alert medications in the pediatric intensive care unit. *Pediatr Crit Care Med*. 2009;10(1):85–90.doi: 10.1097/PCC.0b013e3181936ff8.

6. National Clinical Guideline Centre. IV fluids in children: intravenous fluid therapy in children and young people in hospital. *NICE Guideline*. December 2015;29. **https://www.ncbi.nlm.nih.gov/books/NBK338141/**.

7. Mohanharjai M. Fluid and electrolyte concepts in newborns. *Med J Armed Forces India*. 2002;58(2):182–183. doi:10.1016/S0377-1237(02)80075-2.

8. Figaji AA. Anatomical and physiological differences between children and adults relevant to traumatic brain injury and the implications for clinical assessment and care. *Front Neurol*. 2017;8:685. doi:10.3389/fneur.2017.00685.

9. Gura KM. Is there still a role for peripheral parenteral nutrition? *Nutr Clin Pract*. 2009;24(6):709–717. doi:10.1177/0884533609351318.

10. DeLemos C, Abi-Nader J, Akins PT. Use of peripherally inserted central catheters as an alternative to central catheters in neurocritical care units. *Crit Care Nurse*. 2011;31(2):70–75. doi:10.4037/ccn2011911.

11. Means SW, Spampinato MV, Rao AG, Hill JG. Preterm infant with subdural hematoma from malpositioned scalp intravenous catheter. *Adv Neonatal Care*. 2011;11(4):251–254. doi:10.1097/ANC.0b013e31822565b4.

12. Stovroff M, Teague WG. Intravenous access in infants and children. *Pediatr Clin North Am*. 1998;45(6):1373–1393, viii vii. doi:10.1016/s0031-3955(05)70095-x.

13. Hughes WT. Complication resulting from an intramuscular injection. *J Pediatr*. 1967;70(6):1011–1013. doi:10.1016/s0022-3476(67)80283-x.

14. Lippert WC, Wall EJ. Optimal intramuscular needle-penetration depth. *Pediatrics*. 2008;122(3):e556–e563. doi:10.1542/peds.2008-0374.

15. Berger EY. Nutrition by hypodermoclysis. *J Am Geriatr Soc*. 1984;32(3):199–203. doi:10.1111/j.1532-5415.1984.tb02002.x.

16. Farrand S, Campbell AJ. Safe, simple subcutaneous fluid administration. *Br J Hosp Med*. 1996;55(11):690–692. **https://pubmed.ncbi.nlm.nih.gov/8793132/**.

17. Spandorfer PR. Subcutaneous rehydration: updating a traditional technique. *Pediatr Emerg Care*. 2011;27(3):230–236. doi:10.1097/PEC.0b013e31820e1405.

18. Vaughn DE, Muchmore DB. Use of recombinant human hyaluronidase to accelerate rapid insulin analogue absorption: experience with subcutaneous injection and continuous infusion. *Endocr Pract*. 2011;17(6):914–921. doi:10.4158/EP11297.RA.

19. Lybarger EH. Hypodermoclysis in the home and long-term care settings. *J Infus Nurs*. 2009;32(1):40–44. doi:10.1097/NAN.0b013e3181922552.

20. Johnson M, Inaba K, Byerly S, et al. Intraosseous infusion as a bridge to definitive access. *Am Surg*. 2016;82(10):876–880. **https://pubmed.ncbi.nlm.nih.gov/27779964/**.

21. Engle WA. Intraosseous access for administration of medications in neonates. *Clin Perinatol*. 2006;33(1):161–168, ix. doi:10.1016/j.clp.2005.11.006.

22. Horton MA, Beamer C. Powered intraosseous insertion provides safe and effective vascular access for pediatric emergency patients. *Pediatr Emerg Care*. 2008;24(6):347–350. doi:10.1097/PEC.0b013e318177a6fe.

23. Brickman KR, Rega P, Schoolfield L, et al. Investigation of bone developmental and histopathologic changes from intraosseous infusion. *Ann Emerg Med*. 1996;28(4):430–435. doi:10.1016/s0196-0644(96)70010-0.

24. Hallas P, Brabrand M, Folkestad L. Complication with intraosseous access: scandinavian users' experience. *West J Emerg Med*. 2013;14(5):440–443. doi:10.5811/westjem.2013.1.12000.

25. Turner J, Thies KC. Intra-osseous-access-associated lower limb compartment syndrome in a critically injured paediatric patient. *Eur J Anaesthesiol*. 2018;35(12):981–983. doi:10.1097/EJA.0000000000000873.

26. Kränke B, Aberer W. Skin testing for IgE-mediated drug allergy. *Immunol Allergy Clin North Am*. 2009;29(3):503–516. doi:10.1016/j.iac.2009.04.003.

27. Jian L, Hang-song S, Zheng-lang L, et al. Implantation of Ommaya reservoir in extremely low weight premature infants with posthemorrhagic hydrocephalus: a cautious option. *Childs Nerv Syst*. 2012;28(10):1687–1691. doi:10.1007/s00381-012-1847-0.

28. Olmos-Jiménez R, Espuny-Miró A, Cárceles Rodríguez C, Díaz-Carrasco MS. Practical aspects of the use of intrathecal chemotherapy. *Farm Hosp*. 2017;41(01):105–129. doi:10.7399/fh.2017.41.1.10616.

29. Munir MA, Krishnan S, Ahmad M. A simple technique to reduce preservative/excipient related neurotoxicity of intrathecal (spinal) drugs. *Anesth Analg*. 2000;90(3):767–768. doi:10.1097/00000539-200003000-00055.

30. Laursen T, Hansen B, Fisker S. Pain perception after subcutaneous injections of media containing different buffers. *Basic Clin Pharmacol Toxicol*. February 2006;98(2):218–221.

31. Usach I, Martinez R, Festini T, Peris JE. Subcutaneous Injection of Drugs: Literature Review of Factors Influencing Pain Sensation at the Injection Site. *Adv Ther*. 2019;36(11):2986–2996. doi:10.1007/s12325-019-01101-6.

32. Strazar AR, Leynes PG, Lalonde DH. Minimizing the pain of local anesthesia injection. *Plast Reconstr Surg*. 2013;132(3):675–684. doi:10.1097/PRS.0b013e31829ad1e2.

33. Bjerring P, Andersen PH, Arendt-Nielsen L. Vascular response of human skin after analgesia with EMLA cream. *Br J Anaesth*. 1989;63(6):655–660. doi:10.1093/bja/63.6.655.

34. Fossum K, Love SL, April MD. Topical ethyl chloride to reduce pain associated with venous catheterization: a randomized crossover trial. *Am J Emerg Med*. 2016;34(5):845–850. doi:10.1016/j.ajem.2016.01.039.

35. Lunoe MM, Drendel AL, Levas MN, et al. A randomized clinical trial of jet-injected lidocaine to reduce venipuncture pain for young children. *Ann Emerg Med*. 2015;66(5):466–474. doi:10.1016/j.annemergmed.2015.04.003.

36. Barr RG, Young SN, Wright JH, et al. "Sucrose analgesia" and diphtheria-tetanus-pertussis immunizations at 2 and 4 months. *J Dev Behav Pediatr*. 1995;16(4):220–225. **https://pubmed.ncbi.nlm.nih.gov/7593655/**.

37. Birnie KA, Noel M, Chambers CT, et al. Psychological interventions for needle-related procedural pain and distress in children and adolescents. *Cochrane Database Syst Rev*. 2018;10(10):CD005179. doi:10.1002/14651858.CD005179.pub4.

38. American Academy of Pediatrics Committee on Drugs. "Inactive" ingredients in pharmaceutical products: update (subject review). *Pediatrics*. 1997;99(2):268–278. doi:10.1542/peds.99.2.268.

39. Valeur KS, Hertel SA, Lundstrøm KE, Holst H. The cumulative daily tolerance levels of potentially toxic excipients ethanol and propylene glycol are commonly exceeded in neonates and infants. *Basic Clin Pharmacol Toxicol*. 2018;122(5):523–530. doi:10.1111/bcpt.12950.

40. Centers for Disease Control (CDC). Neonatal deaths associated with use of benzyl alcohol—United States. *MMWR*. 1982;31(22):290–291. **https://pubmed.ncbi.nlm.nih.gov/6810084/**.

41. Gershanik J, Boecler B, Ensley H, et al. The gasping syndrome and benzyl alcohol poisoning. *N Engl J Med*. 1982;307(22):1384–1388. doi:10.1056/NEJM198211253072206.

42. Gershanik JJ, Beecher B, George W, et al. Gasping syndrome: benzyl alcohol poisoning. *Clin Res*. 1981;29:895a.

43. Jardine DS, Rogers K. Relationship of benzyl alcohol to kernicterus, intraventricular hemorrhage, and mortality in preterm infants. *Pediatrics*. 1989;83(2):153–160. **https://pubmed.ncbi.nlm.nih.gov/2783624/**.

44. Benda GI, Hiller JL, Reynolds JW. Benzyl alcohol toxicity: impact on neurologic handicaps among surviving very low birth weight infants. *Pediatrics*. 1986;77(4):507–512. **https://pubmed.ncbi.nlm.nih.gov/2421231/**.

45. Anderson CW, Ng KJ, Andresen B, Cordero L. Benzyl alcohol poisoning in a premature newborn infant. *Am J Obstet Gynecol*. 1984;148(3):344–346. doi:10.1016/s0002-9378(84)80086-1.

46. European Medicines Agency (EMA). Questions and answers on benzyl alcohol in the context of the revision of the guideline on 'excipients in the label and package leaflet of medicinal products for human use' (CPMP/463/00). **https://www.ema.europa.eu/docs/en_GB/document_library/Scientific_guideline/2014/02/WC500162032.pdf**. Published January 23, 2014. Accessed September 8, 2023.

47. MacDonald MG, Getson PR, Glasgow AM, et al. Propylene glycol: increased incidence of seizures in low birth weight infants. *Pediatrics*. 1987;79(4):622–625. **https://pubmed.ncbi.nlm.nih.gov/3822682/**.

48. Zar T, Graeber C, Perazella MA. Recognition, treatment, and prevention of propylene glycol toxicity. *Semin Dial*. 2007;20(3):217–219. doi:10.1111/j.1525-139X.2007.00280.x.

49. Allegaert K. Propylene glycol in neonates: never prescribed, frequently administered, hardly evaluated. *J Clin Toxicol*. 2012;2:e113.

50. Kulo A, de Hoon JN, Allegaert K. The propylene glycol research project to illustrate the feasibility and difficulties to study toxicokinetics in neonates. *Int J Pharm*. 2012;435(2):112–114. doi:10.1016/j.ijpharm.2012.05.014.

51. van de Lagemaat M, van de Pol LA, Zonnenberg IA, et al. MR spectroscopy shows pong propylene glycol half-life in neonatal brain. *Neonatology*. 2021;118(6):693–701. doi:10.1159/000519282.

52. Glover ML, Reed MD. Propylene glycol: the safe diluent that continues to cause harm. *Pharmacotherapy*. 1996;16(4):690–693. **https://pubmed.ncbi.nlm.nih.gov/8840379/**.

53. O'Donnell J, Mertl SL, Kelly WN. Propylene glycol toxicity in a pediatric patient: the dangers of diluents. *J Pharm Pract*. 2000;13:214–225.

54. WHO Expert Committee on Food Additives. *Seventeenth report of the Joint Food and Agriculture Organization: toxicological of certain food additives with a review of general principles and of specifications, technical report series no. 539*. Geneva: World Health Organization; 1974.

55. Valeur KS, Holst H, Allegaert K. Excipients in neonatal medicinal products: never prescribed, commonly administered. *Pharmaceut Med*. 2018;32(4):251–258. doi:10.1007/s40290-018-0243-9.

56. Alade SL, Brown RE, Paquet A Jr. Polysorbate 80 and E-Ferol toxicity. *Pediatrics*. 1986;77(4):593–597. **https://pubmed.ncbi.nlm.nih.gov/3960626/**.

57. O'Grady NP, Alexander M, Burns LA, et al. Summary of recommendations: guidelines for the prevention of intravascular catheter-related infections. *Clin Infect Dis*. 2011;52(9):1087–1099. doi:10.1093/cid/cir138.

58. Shuman RM, Leech RW, Alvord EC Jr. Neurotoxicity of hexachlorophene in the human: I. A clinicopathologic study of 248 children. *Pediatrics*. 1974;54(6):689–695. **https://pubmed.ncbi.nlm.nih.gov/4431666/**.

59. Chapman AK, Aucott SW, Milstone AM. Safety of chlorhexidine gluconate used for skin antisepsis in the preterm infant. *J Perinatol*. 2012;32(1):4–9. doi:10.1038/jp.2011.148.

60. Chapman AK, Aucott SW, Gilmore MM, et al. Absorption and tolerability of aqueous chlorhexidine gluconate used for skin antisepsis prior to catheter insertion in preterm neonates. *J Perinatol*. 2013;33(10):768–771. doi:10.1038/jp.2013.61.

61. Fischer CJ, Bickle Graz M, Muehlethaler V, et al. Phthalates in the NICU: is it safe? *J Paediatr Child Health*. 2013;49(9):E413–E419. doi:10.1111/jpc.12244.

62. International Agency for Research on Cancer (IARC). Di(2-ethylhexyl)phthalate (DEHP), 2000. **https://monographs.iarc.who.int/wp-content/uploads/2018/06/mono101-006.pdf**. Accessed September 8, 2023.

63. Food and Drug Administration (FDA). Safety assessment of di(2-ethylhexyl)phthalate (DEHP) released from PVC Medical Devices. **https://noharm-uscanada.org/sites/default/files/documents-files/117/Sum_FDA_Safety_Assess_DEHP.pdf**. Accessed July 29, 2023.

64. Silva MJ, Barr DB, Reidy JA, et al. Urinary levels of seven phthalate metabolites in the U.S. population from the National Health and Nutrition Examination Survey (NHANES) 1999-2000. *Environ Health Perspect*. 2004;112(3):331–338. doi:10.1289/ehp.6723.

65. Calafat AM, Needham LL, Silva MJ, Lambert G. Exposure to di-(2-ethylhexyl) phthalate among premature neonates in a neonatal intensive care unit. *Pediatrics*. 2004;113(5):e429–e434. doi:10.1542/peds.113.5.e429.

66. Shneider B, Cronin J, Van Marter L, et al. A prospective analysis of cholestasis in infants supported with extracorporeal membrane oxygenation. *J Pediatr Gastroenterol Nutr*. 1991;13(3):285–289. doi:10.1097/00005176-199110000-00008.

67. Kim YM, Kim J, Cheong HK, et al. Exposure to phthalates aggravates pulmonary function and airway inflammation in asthmatic children. *PLoS One*. 2018;13(12):e0208553. doi:10.1371/journal.pone.0208553.

68. Bagel S, Dessaigne B, Bourdeaux D, et al. Influence of lipid type on bis (2-ethylhexyl)phthalate (DEHP) leaching from infusion line sets in parenteral nutrition. *JPEN*. 2011;35(6):770–775. doi:10.1177/0148607111414021.

69. Bohrer D, Do Nascimento PC, Becker E, et al. Critical evaluation of the standard hydrolytic resistance test for glasses used for containers for blood and parenteral formulations. *PDA J Pharm Sci Technol*. 2004;58(2):96–105. **https://pubmed.ncbi.nlm.nih.gov/15113075/**.

70. Gura KM. Aluminum contamination in parenteral products. *Curr Opin Clin Nutr Metab Care*. 2014;17(6):551–557. doi:10.1097/MCO.0000000000000091.

71. Bishop NJ, Morley R, Day JP, et al. Aluminum neurotoxicity in preterm infants receiving intravenous-feeding solutions. *N Engl J Med*. 1997;336(22):1557–1561. doi:10.1056/NEJM199705293362203.

72. Bohrer D, Bertagnolli DC, de Oliveira SM, et al. Drugs as a hidden source of aluminium for chronic renal patients. *Nephrol Dial Transplant*. 2007;22(2):605–611. doi:10.1093/ndt/gfl569.

73. de Oliveira SR, Bohrer D, Garcia SC, et al. Aluminum content in intravenous solutions for administration to neonates: role of product preparation and administration methods. *JPEN*. 2010;34(3):322–328. doi:10.1177/0148607110362531.

74. Mitkus RJ, King DB, Hess MA, et al. Updated aluminum pharmacokinetics following infant exposures through diet and vaccination. *Vaccine*. 2011;29(51):9538–9543. doi:10.1016/j.vaccine.2011.09.124.

75. Eickhoff TC, Myers M. Workshop summary. Aluminum in vaccines. *Vaccine*. 2002;20(suppl 3):S1–S4. doi:10.1016/s0264-410x(02)00163-9.

76. World Health Organization (WHO). Global Advisory Committee on Vaccine Safety, 20-June 21, 2002. *Wkly Epidemiol Rec*. 2022;77(47):389–394.

77. Ciapponi A, Bardach A, Mazzoni A, et al. Safety of components and platforms of COVID-19 vaccines considered for use in pregnancy: A rapid review. *Vaccine*. 2021;39(40):5891–5908. doi:10.1016/j.vaccine.2021.08.034.

78. Mirtallo J, Canada T, Johnson D, et al. Task Force for the Revision of Safe Practices for Parenteral Nutrition: safe practices for parenteral nutrition. *JPEN*. 2004;28:S39–S70.

79. Boullata JI, Gilbert K, Sacks G, et al. A.S.P.E.N. clinical guidelines: parenteral nutrition ordering, order review, compounding, labeling, and dispensing. *JPEN*. 2014;38(3):334–377. doi:10.1177/0148607114521833.

80. Hahn JS, Berquist W, Alcorn DM, et al. Wernicke encephalopathy and beriberi during total parenteral nutrition attributable to multivitamin infusion shortage. *Pediatrics*. 1998;101(1):E10. doi:10.1542/peds.101.1.e10.

81. Infuvite Pediatric [package insert]. Deerfield, IL: Baxter Healthcare Corporation; July 2014. **https://www.accessdata.fda.gov/drugsatfda_docs/label/2014/021646s014lbl.pdf**. Accessed April 4, 2023.

82. Infuvite Adult [package insert]. Deerfield, IL: Baxter Healthcare Corporation; November 25, 2002. **https://www.accessdata.fda.gov/drugsatfda_docs/label/2004/21163s011lbl.pdf**. Accessed April 4, 2023.

83. Cernevit [package insert]. Deerfield, IL: Baxter Healthcare Corporation; April 1999. **https://www.accessdata.fda.gov/drugsatfda_docs/label/1999/20924lbl.pdf**. Accessed April 4, 2023.

84. MacDonald MG, Fletcher AB, Johnson EL, et al. The potential toxicity to neonates of multivitamin preparations used in parenteral nutrition. *JPEN*. 1987; 11(2):169–171. doi:10.1177/0148607187011002169.

85. Hanson C, Thoene M, Wagner J, et al. Parenteral nutrition additive shortages: the short-term, long-term and potential epigenetic implications in premature and hospitalized infants. *Nutrients*. 2012;4(12):1977–1988. doi:10.3390/nu4121977.

86. Mitton SG. Amino acids and lipid in total parenteral nutrition for the newborn. *J Pediatr Gastroenterol Nutr*. 1994;18(1):25–31. doi:10.1097/00005176-199401000-00004.

87. Helms RA, Christensen ML, Mauer EC, Storm MC. Comparison of a pediatric versus standard amino acid formulation in preterm neonates requiring parenteral nutrition. *J Pediatr*. 1987;110(3):466–470. doi:10.1016/s0022-3476(87)80519-x.

88. Viña J, Vento M, García-Sala F, et al. L-cysteine and glutathione metabolism are impaired in premature infants due to cystathionase deficiency. *Am J Clin Nutr*. 1995;61(5):1067–1069. doi:10.1093/ajcn/61.4.1067.

89. Plogsted S, Cober P, Gura KM, et al. Parenteral nutrition L-cysteine product shortage considerations. *Nutr Clin Pract*. 2015;30(4):579–580. doi:10.1177/0884533615593604.

90. ELCYS. (cysteine hydrochloride) [package insert]. Lenoir, NC: Exela Pharm Sciences, LLC; April 2019.

91. Greene HL, Hambidge KM, Schanler R, Tsang RC. Guidelines for the use of vitamins, trace elements, calcium, magnesium, and phosphorus in infants and children receiving total parenteral nutrition: report of the Subcommittee on Pediatric Parenteral Nutrient Requirements from the Committee on Clinical Practice Issues of the American Society for Clinical Nutrition. *Am J Clin Nutr*. 1988;48(5):1324–1342. doi:10.1093/ajcn/48.5.1324.

92. Burjonrappa SC, Miller M. Role of trace elements in parenteral nutrition support of the surgical neonate. *J Pediatr Surg*. 2012;47(4):760–771. doi:10.1016/j.jpedsurg.2012.01.015.

93. Centers for Disease Control and Prevention (CDC). Notes from the field: zinc deficiency dermatitis in cholestatic extremely premature infants after a nationwide shortage of injectable zinc - Washington, DC, December 2012. Erratum in: *MMWR*. 2013; 62:196. *MMWR*. 2013;62(7):136–137. **https://pubmed.ncbi.nlm.nih.gov/23425963/**.

94. Peirovifar A, Gharehbaghi MM, Abdulmohammad-Zadeh H, et al. Serum selenium levels of the very low birth weight premature newborn infants with bronchopulmonary dysplasia. *J Trace Elem Med Biol*. 2013;27(4):317–321. doi:10.1016/j.jtemb.2013.03.006.

95. Klinger G, Shamir R, Singer P, et al. Parenteral selenium supplementation in extremely low birth weight infants: inadequate dosage but no correlation with hypothyroidism. *J Perinatol*. 1999;19(8 Pt 1): 568–572. doi:10.1038/sj.jp.7200273.

96. Food and Drug Administration (FDA). CFR—Code of federal regulations title 21. **https://www.accessdata.fda.gov/scripts/cdrh/cfdocs/cfcfr/cfrsearch.cfm?fr=201.323**. Accessed September 8, 2023.

97. Hall AR, Arnold CJ, Miller GG, et al. Infant parenteral nutrition remains a significant source for aluminum toxicity. *JPEN*. 2017;41(7):1228–1233. doi:10.1177/0148607116638056.

98. Koo WW, Kaplan LA, Horn J, et al. Aluminum in parenteral nutrition solution—sources and possible alternatives. *JPEN*. 1986;10(6):591–595. doi:10.1177/0148607186010006591.

99. Gura KM. Aluminum contamination in products used in parenteral nutrition: has anything changed? *Nutrition*. 2010;26(6):585–594. doi:10.1016/j.nut.2009.10.015.

100. Gura KM, Puder M. Recent developments in aluminium contamination of products used in parenteral nutrition. *Curr Opin Clin Nutr Metab Care*. 2006;9(3):239–246. doi:10.1097/01.mco.0000222106.07924.7f.

101. Robinson DT, Ayers P, Fleming B, et al. Recommendations for photoprotection of parenteral nutrition for premature infants: An ASPEN position paper. *Nutr Clin Pract*. 2021;36(5):927–941. doi:10.1002/ncp.10747.

102. Shattuck KE, Bhatia J, Grinnell C, Rassin DK. The effects of light exposure on the in vitro hepatic response to an amino acid-vitamin solution. *JPEN*. 1995;19(5):398–402. doi:10.1177/0148607195019005398.

103. Bhatia J, Moslen MT, Kaphalia L, et al. Glutathione and tissue amino acid responses to light-exposed parenteral nutrients. *Toxicol Lett*. 1992;63(1):79–89. doi:10.1016/0378-4274(92)90110-6.

104. Laborie S, Lavoie JC, Chessex P. Paradoxical role of ascorbic acid and riboflavin in solutions of total parenteral nutrition: implication in photoinduced peroxide generation. *Pediatr Res*. 1998;43(5):601–606. doi:10.1203/00006450-199805000-00007.

105. Neuzil J, Darlow BA, Inder TE, et al. Oxidation of parenteral lipid emulsion by ambient and phototherapy lights: potential toxicity of routine parenteral feeding. *J Pediatr*. 1995;126(5 Pt 1):785–790. doi:10.1016/s0022-3476(95)70412-4.

106. Laborie S, Lavoie JC, Pineault M, et al. Protecting solutions of parenteral nutrition from peroxidation. *JPEN*. 1999;23(2):104–108. doi:10.1177/0148607199023002104.

107. Sherlock R, Chessex P. Shielding parenteral nutrition from light: does the available evidence support a randomized, controlled trial? *Pediatrics*. 2009;123(6):1529–1533. doi:10.1542/peds.2008-1865.

108. European Medicines Agency (EMA). PRAC recommendations on signals. **https://www.ema.europa.eu/en/documents/prac-recommendation/prac-recommendations-signals-adopted-8-11-july-2019-prac-meeting_en.pdf**. Published August 5, 2019. Accessed September 8, 2023.

109. von Rettberg H, Hannman T, Subotic U, et al. Use of di(2-ethylhexyl)phthalate-containing infusion systems increases the risk for cholestasis. *Pediatrics*. 2009;124(2):710–716. doi:10.1542/peds.2008-1765.

110. Kambia N, Dine T, Gressier B, et al. Strong variability of di(2-ethylhexyl)phthalate (DEHP) plasmatic rate in infants and children undergoing 12-hour cyclic parenteral nutrition. *JPEN*. 2013;37(2):229–235. doi:10.1177/0148607112450914.

111. Crill CM, Hak EB, Robinson LA, Helms RA. Evaluation of microbial contamination associated with different preparation methods for neonatal intravenous fat emulsion infusion. *Am J Health Syst Pharm*. 2010;67(11):914–918. doi:10.2146/ajhp090199.

112. Reiter PD. Sterility of intravenous fat emulsion in plastic syringes. *Am J Health Syst Pharm*. 2002;59(19):1857–1859. doi:10.1093/ajhp/59.19.1857.

113. Ebbert ML, Farraj M, Hwang LT. The incidence and clinical significance of intravenous fat emulsion contamination during infusion. *JPEN*. 1987;11(1):42–45. doi:10.1177/014860718701100142.

114. Hicks RW, Becker SC, Chuo J. A summary of NICU fat emulsion medication errors and nursing services: data from MEDMARX. *Adv Neonatal Care*. 2007;7(6):299–308, quiz 309–310. doi:10.1097/01.ANC.0000304969.23837.95.

115. Chuo J, Lambert G, Hicks RW. Intralipid medication errors in the neonatal intensive care unit. *Jt Comm J Qual Patient Saf*. 2007;33(2):104–111. doi:10.1016/s1553-7250(07)33012-2.

116. Heyman MB, Storch S, Ament ME. The fat overload syndrome. Report of a case and literature review. *Am J Dis Child*. 1981;135(7):628–630. doi:10.1001/archpedi.1981.02130310034012.

117. Wesson DE, Rich RH, Zlotkin SH, et al. Fat overload syndrome causing respiratory insufficiency. *J Pediatr Surg*. 1984;19(6):777–778. doi:10.1016/s0022-3468(84)80367-x.

118. Surmont I, Gavilanes A, Vandepitte J, et al. Malassezia furfur fungaemia in infants receiving intravenous lipid emulsions. A rarity or just underestimated? *Eur J Pediatr*. 1989;148(5):435–438. doi:10.1007/BF00595906.

119. Obayashi A, Oie S, Kamiya A. Microbial viability in preparations packaged for single use. *Biol Pharm Bull*. 2003;26(5):667–670. doi:10.1248/bpb.26.667.

120. Swindell K, Lattif AA, Chandra J, et al. Parenteral lipid emulsion induces germination of Candida albicans and increases biofilm formation on medical catheter surfaces. *J Infect Dis*. 2009;200(3):473–480. doi:10.1086/600106.

121. McKee KT Jr, Melly MA, Greene HL, et al. Gram-negative bacillary sepsis associated with use of lipid emulsion in parenteral nutrition. *Am J Dis Child*. 1979;133(6):649–650. doi:10.1001/archpedi.1979.02130060089023.

122. Jarvis WR, Highsmith AK, Allen JR, et al. Polymicrobial bacteremia associated with lipid emulsion in a neonatal intensive care unit. *Pediatr Infect Dis*. 1983;2(3):203–208. doi:10.1097/00006454-198305000-00006.

123. de Beaufort AJ, Bernards AT, Dijkshoorn L, et al. Acinetobacter junii causes life-threatening sepsis in preterm infants. *Acta Paediatr*. 1999;88(7):772–775. doi:10.1080/08035259950169080.

124. Worthington P, Gura KM, Kraft MD, et al. Update on the Use of Filters for Parenteral Nutrition: An ASPEN Position Paper. *Nutr Clin Pract*. 2021;36(1):29–39. doi:10.1002/ncp.10587.

125. Cober MP, Gura KM, Mirtallo JM, et al. ASPEN lipid injectable emulsion safety recommendations part 2: Neonate and pediatric considerations. *Nutr Clin Pract*. 2021;36(6):1106–1125. doi:10.1002/ncp.10778.

126. USP <797> Pharmaceutical compounding—sterile preparations. In: *2022: USP Compounding Compendium.* Rockville, MD: United States Pharmacopeial Convention; November 1, 2022. **https://doi.org/10.31003/USPNF_M99925_06_01**.

127. Omran EA, Eisa FF, Bakr WMK. Microbial contamination of neonatal injectable lipid emulsions at 12 and 24 hours' infusion time with evaluation of infection control measures. *J Pediatr Pharmacol Ther*. 2020;25(1):53–60. doi:10.5863/1551-6776-25.1.53.

128. Grissinger, M. Another tragic parenteral nutrition compounding error. *P T*. 2014; 39:810,822.

129. Grissinger M. Mismatched prescribing and pharmacy templates for parenteral nutrition lead to data-entry errors. *P T*. 2015;40(6):349–350. **https://pubmed.ncbi.nlm.nih.gov/26045641/**.

130. Arenas Villafranca JJ, Gómez Sánchez A, Nieto Guindo M, et al. Using failure mode and effects analysis to improve the safety of neonatal parenteral nutrition. *Am J Health Syst Pharm*. 2014;71(14):1210–1218. doi:10.2146/ajhp130640.

131. Kaushal R, Bates DW, Landrigan C, et al. Medication errors and adverse drug events in pediatric inpatients. *JAMA*. 2001;285(16):2114–2120. doi:10.1001/jama.285.16.2114.

132. Leff RD, Roberts RJ. Methods of intravenous drug administration in the pediatric patient. *J Pediatr*. 1981;98(4):631–635. doi:10.1016/s0022-3476(81)80782-2.

133. Nahata MC, Powell DA, Durrell DE, et al. Effect of infusion methods on tobramycin serum concentrations in newborn infants. *J Pediatr*. 1984;104(1):136–138. doi:10.1016/s0022-3476(84)80612-5.

134. Sherwin CM, Medlicott NJ, Reith DM, et al. Intravenous drug delivery in neonates: lessons learnt. *Arch Dis Child*. 2014;99(6):590–594. doi:10.1136/archdischild-2013-304887.

135. Rajchgot P, Radde IC, MacLeod SM. Influence of specific gravity on intravenous drug delivery. *J Pediatr*. 1981;99(4):658–661. doi:10.1016/s0022-3476(81)80287-9.

136. Leff RD, Johnson GF, Erenberg A, et al. Evaluation of an extension set for intermittent intravenous drug delivery to infants. *Am J Hosp Pharm*. 1985;42(6):1358–1362. **https://pubmed.ncbi.nlm.nih.gov/4014253/**.

137. Bradley JS, Wassel RT, Lee L, et al. Intravenous ceftriaxone and calcium in the neonate: assessing the risk for cardiopulmonary adverse events. *Pediatrics*. 2009;123(4):e609–e613. doi:10.1542/peds.2008-3080.

138. Botash AS. Syringe caps: an aspiration hazard. *Pediatrics*. 1992;90(1 Pt 1):92–93. **https://pubmed.ncbi.nlm.nih.gov/1614787/**.

139. Suresh G, Horbar JD, Plsek P, et al. Voluntary anonymous reporting of medical errors for neonatal intensive care. *Pediatrics*. 2004;113(6):1609–1618. doi:10.1542/peds.113.6.1609.

140. Stavroudis TA, Miller MR, Lehmann CU. Medication errors in neonates. *Clin Perinatol*. 2008;35(1):141–161, ix. doi:10.1016/j.clp.2007.11.010.

141. Sauberan JB, Dean LM, Fiedelak J, et al. Origins of and solutions for neonatal medication-dispensing errors. *Am J Health Syst Pharm*. 2010;67(1):49–57. doi:10.2146/ajhp090122.

142. Mackay MW, Cash J, Farr F, et al. Improving pediatric outcomes through intravenous and oral mediation standardization. *J Pediatr Pharmacol Ther*. 2009;14(4):226–235. doi:10.5863/1551-6776-14.4.226.

143. Kohn LT, Corrigan JM, Donaldson MS. *To err is human: building a safer health system*. Washington, DC: National Academy Press; 2000.

144. The Joint Commission. Strategies for phasing out the rule of six. *The Source*. 2004; 8(2):5–5(1).

145. Institute for Safe Medication Practices (ISMP). Avoid preparing infusions using the rule of 6 or Broselow tape. *ISMP Medication Safety Alert*. 2005;10:4.

146. American Academy of Pediatrics, Committee on Drugs and Committee on Hospital Care. Prevention of medication errors in the pediatric inpatient setting. *Pediatrics*. 1998;102(2 Pt 1):428–430. **https://pubmed.ncbi.nlm.nih.gov/9685445/**.

147. King WJ, Paice N, Rangrej J, et al. The effect of computerized physician order entry on medication errors and adverse drug events in pediatric inpatients. *Pediatrics*. 2003;112(3 Pt 1):506–509. doi:10.1542/peds.112.3.506.

148. Hardmeier A, Tsourounis C, Moore M, et al. Pediatric medication administration errors and workflow following implementation of a bar code medication administration system. *J Healthc Qual*. 2014;36(4):54–61, quiz 61–63. doi:10.1111/jhq.12071.

149. Vaidya V. CPOE revisited: a computerized calculator for continuous medication infusions. *Pediatr Crit Care Med*. 2006;7(3):282–283. doi:10.1097/01.PCC.0000216666.33255.9D.

150. Mir C, Gadri A, Zelger GL, et al. Impact of a computerized physician order entry system on compliance with prescription accuracy requirements. *Pharm World Sci*. 2009;31(5):596–602.doi:10.1007/s11096-009-9306-z.

151. Asdigha MN. Improving safety throughout the medication use process in a neonatal intensive care unit. *Hosp Pharm*. 2006;41:1067–1075.

152. Larsen GY, Parker HB, Cash J, et al. Standard drug concentrations and smart-pump technology reduce continuous-medication-infusion errors in pediatric patients. *Pediatrics*. 2005;116(1):e21–e25. doi:10.1542/peds.2004-2452.

153. Institute for Safe Medication Practices (ISMP). Smart pump custom concentrations without hard "low concentration" alerts can lead to patient harm. **https://www.ismp.org/resources/smart-pump-custom-concentrations-without-hard-low-concentration-alerts-can-lead-patient**. Published May 31, 2018. Accessed September 8, 2023.

154. Kirkendall ES, Timmons K, Huth H, et al. Human-Based Errors Involving Smart Infusion Pumps: A Catalog of Error Types and Prevention Strategies. *Drug Saf*. 2020;43(11):1073–1087. doi:10.1007/s40264-020-00986-5.

155. Levine S, Cohen MR. Preventing medication errors in pediatric and neonatal patients. Cohen MR, ed. *Medication errors*. 2nd ed. Washington, DC: American Pharmacists Association; 2007:481.

156. Li Q, Kirkendall ES, Hall ES, et al. Automated detection of medication administration errors in neonatal intensive care. *J Biomed Inform*. 2015;57:124–133. doi:10.1016/j.jbi.2015.07.012.

157. American Society of Health-System Pharmacists (ASHP). Standardize 4 safety. **https://www.ashp.org/pharmacy-practice/standardize-4-safety-initiative**. Accessed September 8, 2023.

158. American Society of Health-System Pharmacists (ASHP). ASHP Pediatric IV continuous infusion guidelines. **https://www.ashp.org/-/media/assets/pharmacy-practice/s4s/docs/Proposed-Standard-Concentrations-Pediatric-IV-Continuous-for-public-comment.ashx**. Published February 2019. Accessed September 8, 2023.

24

ALLERGENIC EXTRACTS

Mary C. McManamon and Matthew Madurski

INTRODUCTION

The prevalence of allergic disease and hypersensitivity is widespread across the globe, affecting people of all ages, genders, and nationalities. The World Allergy Association estimates that 30% to 40% of the world's population is affected by allergic rhinitis, allergic conjunctivitis, allergic asthma, or insect allergies. These numbers increase when considering food-related allergies and occupational and environmental causes of allergic reaction.[1] Allergies can lead to a myriad of reactions in patients, ranging from the onset of asthma to secondary effects, such as sinusitis, the formation of nasal polyps, conjunctivitis, otitis media with effusion, upper respiratory infections, breathing through the mouth, and sleep disorders.[1] In severe cases, some allergy patients experience significant reactions, including bronchospasm, laryngeal edema, hypotension, and fatal anaphylaxis.[1]

Patients who suffer allergy-related ailments can successfully control or eliminate the effects of allergic reactions by avoiding the source of the allergy or through medications. Several pharmacotherapeutic classes alleviate the symptoms associated with allergic reactions (eg, antihistamines, corticosteroids, decongestants, bronchodilators, anticholinergics, monoclonal antibody therapy, or other systemic medications).[1] While medications may benefit patients in this population, there are others who need additional treatments to alleviate or eliminate their symptoms. In these instances, subcutaneous allergy immunotherapy (SCIT) is an additional option.[2]

This chapter discusses the decision-making process involved in the creation of allergenic immunotherapy regimens and how these regimens are initiated and maintained. Sections are devoted to the selection and types of extracts used in immunotherapy treatments, the regulatory requirements for compounding allergenic extracts, and the proper storage and use of completed SCIT prescription sets.

ALLERGENIC IMMUNOTHERAPY REGIMENS

Over the past half century, many studies demonstrated success in treating allergic rhinitis, allergic conjunctivitis, allergic asthma, and stinging insect hypersensitivity with allergy immunotherapy.[2] Allergy immunotherapy has been shown to decrease asthma symptoms and medication use in allergic asthma patients, including children and adults.[3] This is accomplished by compounding therapeutic preparations extracted from materials at the source of patient immune responses (eg, pollens, mold cultures, dust mites, animal dander, and insects). These are generally prepared as stock solutions of proteins or glycoproteins extracted from source materials that are then added in sufficient quantities to a specific patient's immunotherapy treatment vial.[2]

The U.S. Food and Drug Administration (FDA) policy for the mixing, diluting, and repackaging of biologic products includes the preparation of SCIT from licensed allergenic extracts as prescribed to an individual patient. These prescription sets of extracts are defined as "vials or sets of vials of premixed licensed standardized and nonstandardized allergenic extracts for subcutaneous immunotherapy diluted with an appropriate diluent prepared by a licensed physician for an individual patient according to instructions from a valid prescription."[4] The FDA policy sets certain conditions for the preparation of these products[4]:

- The prescription set is prepared from FDA-licensed allergenic extracts and diluents that are sterile, pharmaceutical grade, and otherwise appropriate for such use.
- The prescription set is prepared in a physician's office, state-licensed pharmacy, federal facility, or outsourcing facility.
- Each prescription set is distributed only after the receipt of a valid prescription for an identified,

DOI 10.37573/9781585286492.024

individual patient (including a written order or notation in a patient's chart in a healthcare setting) directly from the prescribing practitioner or patient.

- The prescription set is prepared in a way that does not conflict with approved labeling of the licensed biological products that are part of the prescription set.
- The beyond-use date (BUD) for the prescription set is no later than the earliest expiration date of any allergenic extract or any diluent that is part of the prescription set, and the BUD does not exceed 1 year from the date the prescription set is mixed or diluted.
- The prescription set is prepared in accordance with the following:
    - If the prescription set is prepared in a state-licensed pharmacy, federal facility, or in a physician's office, it is prepared in accordance with *United States Pharmacopeia* (USP) Chapter <797>, except the BUD is as specified in the bullet referencing allergenic extract expiration.[5]
    - If the prescription set is prepared in an outsourcing facility, it is prepared in accordance with applicable current good manufacturing principles (CGMP) requirements, except the BUD follows the rules as specified in the bullet referencing allergenic extract expiration.
- The prepared prescription set is not sold or transferred by an entity other than the entity that prepared the prescription set. For purposes of this condition, a sale or transfer does not include administration of a prescription set in a healthcare setting.
- The prescription set is distributed only in states in which the facility preparing the prescription set meets all applicable state requirements.

With all of these considerations in mind, a physician chooses an immunotherapy regimen and determines which extracts should be included in a preparation based on skin testing results or serum immunoglobulin E (IgE) antibodies. Based on a patient's reactions to testing and local and regional allergens, a series of injections are ordered that build up to what is called a *maintenance dose*, which is the dose that provides therapeutic efficacy without significant adverse reactions. Some patients may not tolerate the maintenance dose, but they may achieve symptom control at a lower dose that can be determined through a build-up phase. During build up, patients receive injections of the maintenance dose of extracts diluted by factors of 10 for concentrations of 1:10,000 to 1:10, ending, in most cases, with the 1:1 maintenance dose.[2]

During the build-up phase, injections are usually given one to three times a week over a 3- to 6-month period, depending on individual patient response. Once a patient reaches their 1:1 maintenance dose at the end of the build-up phase, they continue to receive injections every two to four weeks. With this type of immunotherapy, improvement is generally noted within 1 year of starting treatment. If no improvement is seen, additional considerations are made to determine regimen adherence and ensure patients limit exposure to specific allergens. If there is no clear explanation for lack of success with immunotherapy, it may be best to consider other treatment options.

Depending on a patient's circumstances, they may opt into cluster or rush immunotherapy regimens, which can be used to achieve maintenance dosing more rapidly if patients are unable to adhere to a traditional injection regimen due to scheduling issues, inability to visit a physician office regularly, or some other reason. Cluster immunotherapy is an accelerated dosing schedule in which the patient receives two or three injections of increasingly concentrated doses in one visit. Visits occur one to two times per week. The maintenance dose is usually reached within 4 to 8 weeks as opposed to 3 to 6 months. Rush immunotherapy is an accelerated dosing schedule in which increasing doses are given every 15 to 60 minutes over 1 to 3 days until the target dose is achieved. The maintenance dose is achieved even more rapidly than in cluster dosing. However, there is a higher incidence of local and systemic reactions with this dosing schedule.[2]

Another regimen exists for patients who need venom immunotherapy for stinging insects. In this case it uses a build-up phase and dilute dosing comparable to allergenic extract therapy. The build-up phase for venoms is typically eight weeks with weekly injections. Some rush protocols achieve target dose in a few weeks, and ultra-rush protocols can achieve target dosing within a few days.[7] While dilutions for venom extracts can be as low as 1:100,000, the starting dose can be as high as 1:100 in some patients, thus allowing the maintenance dose to be achieved more rapidly. The typical maintenance dose for venom immunotherapy is 100 or 300 mcg for mixed vespid (three-insect combinations). This dose is given every four to eight weeks to maintain clinical efficacy.[2;6;7]

There are instances where dosing should be adjusted during immunotherapy build up. One situation is if a patient misses an appointment for immunotherapy. Although there is no one clear standard for how to decrease dosing, dosing adjustments are recommended for gaps in treatment longer than 14 days.[2] Dose adjustment should also be considered for large, localized reactions and systemic reactions.[2] Although local reactions are generally not a predictor for future systemic reactions, it is not uncommon to see a decrease in dosing after a local reaction.[8] A large localized reaction is usually considered to be larger than the palm of the patient's hand. If a systemic reaction occurs, the provider may choose to decrease the dose and proceed more slowly or they may choose to discontinue treatment altogether.[2] Clinicians should consider adjusting the dose during the maintenance phase when a new maintenance vial is mixed. Since extracts can lose potency over time, a newly mixed vial may be more potent, so it could cause a reaction.[9]

ALLERGENIC EXTRACT PRESCRIPTION SETS

Once a therapy regimen is determined, physicians order build-up and maintenance doses using combinations of different extracts in one or more vials and then are diluted to the appropriate starting concentration. This series of doses is the allergenic extract prescription set.

Selection of Extracts

Treatment extract choices are based on patient symptom history, skin test results, and or serum specific IgE antibodies. Patients should not be treated solely based on IgE test results. Treatment must also be based on positive skin tests or positive symptom history due to exposure. A patient's regional location and environment impacts extract choice because the inclusion of allergens they do not have antibodies against can cause new sensitization to that allergen.[9]

Immunotherapy extracts are either standardized or nonstandardized. Standardized extracts are approved by the FDA. Standardized extracts and their labeled potency are listed below.

- Epithelia: Cat hair and pelt are measured in bioequivalent allergy unit (BAU)/mL.
- Dust mites: While there are several species of dust mite, typical immunotherapy is limited to the two most common species of house dust mites, *Dermatophagoides farinae* and *Dermatophagoides pteronyssinus*.[2] Dust mites are measured in allergy units (AU)/mL.
- Pollen: Standardized pollens include short ragweed (measured in weight/volume [w/v]) and grasses (eg, Bermuda, Kentucky, perennial ryegrass, orchard, Timothy, meadow fescue, redtop, and sweet vernal grass), which are measured in BAU/mL.
- Hymenoptera venoms (eg, mixed vespids and winged insects): The extracts available for stinging insects include honeybee, wasp, yellow jacket, yellow hornet, and white-faced hornet. There is also a mixed vespid formulation available, which is a combination of the three insects in the family *Vespidae* (yellow jacket, yellow hornet, and white-faced hornet). All of the venoms are measured in mcg/mL.

Nonstandardized extracts can be produced and sold in multiple different concentrations and measurements. Due to the variability between manufacturers, it is important to confirm that the goal treatment dose is used to accurately calculate the amount of extract to be given.[10] Nonstandardized extracts include the following:

- Molds and fungi: These extracts include common indoor and outdoor mold species, such as *Cladosporium, Penicillium, Aspergillus, and Alternaria*. They are commonly measured in w/v or protein nitrogen units (PNU)/mL.[2]
- Animal danders: The most common nonstandardized animal extract is dog epithelia measured in w/v. Other animals include mouse, horse, rat, guinea pig, cattle, and so on. While it is best to remove household exposure during SCIT treatment, eliminating exposure to common house pets may be difficult or impossible. Patients can still receive treatments for these types of allergies even with a pet living in the home.[9]
- Miscellaneous: There are several extracts that fall outside of the above classifications (eg, cockroaches and fire ants). Cockroach exposure is linked to asthma, especially in inner city children.[11;12] There are limited studies demonstrating efficacy of cockroach immunotherapy in controlling asthma, but recent research shows more promise.[11]

Some insect and fungi extracts are high in proteolytic enzymes and should not be mixed with tree, grass, and weed extracts because they can cause decreased potency of the other extracts contained in the mix. The effect on other extracts varies, but pollens tend to be affected more than other extracts. Increasing the glycerin concentration to 50% can increase the stability of these combinations. The best practice is to refer to specific manufacturer recommendations in these combinations because the proteolytic concentration can vary. Lowest compatibility is reported in combinations of insects, such as cockroach or molds with pollen extracts. Dust mites generally maintain potency in combination with insects and mold as long as glycerin concentrations are greater than 10%.[6;13;14]

Selection of Diluents

There are three standard diluents used in the compounding of allergenic extract vials.

- Phenolated normal saline (NSP): This diluent contains 0.4% phenol, which acts as a bacteriostatic preservative. Any allergenic extract or immunotherapy vial that does not contain 50% glycerin must contain phenol to ensure maintenance of sterility. Even though it is an effective preservative, phenol can break down allergen proteins more quickly than other diluents.[6;9]
- Human serum albumin in normal saline (NS/HSA): This diluent typically contains 0.03% human serum albumin (HSA), 0.9% sodium chloride, and 0.4% phenol. HSA protects against protein breakdown usually seen with phenol, which makes it a preferred base solution for patient immunotherapy prescription sets and the preferred diluent for intradermal testing kits and insect venom reconstitutions and dilutions. HSA can also be less irritating than diluents containing glycerin. HSA acts as a stabilizer, which helps prevent adherence of allergens

to the glass vial. HSA is not, however, a preservative. Therefore HSA diluents still typically contain 0.4% phenol.[2-4;6-8]

- Glycerin: This diluent is commonly used in mass-produced allergen extracts. It is very stabilizing and helps ensure allergen potency while also providing a preservative effect. At high concentrations, glycerin can cause injection site pain, so it is often used as a diluent for bulk extracts from the manufacturer but not as a diluent for patient vials. As a result, maintenance vials that contain no diluent are likely to contain 50% glycerin, so any administration dose above 0.2 mL can result in increased pain during injection.[6;9]

Calculations for Extract Amounts in Maintenance Vials

The amount of extract to be added to the maintenance vial differs for each type of extract, which is based on a probable effective dose range. To calculate the amount of extract in a maintenance vial, it is assumed that the target maintenance dose is 0.5 mL of the maintenance vial. Based on this, a calculation should be performed with the equation $V_1C_1=V_2C_2$, with V_1 representing the final volume of the maintenance vial, C_1 representing the desired dose of extract per mL of maintenance vial, V_2 representing the volume of extract to be added to the maintenance vial, and C_2 representing the available extract concentration. This equation should be repeated for all extracts added to the vial, and then add up the total extract volume. The difference between desired final maintenance volume and the amount of extract added is equal to the amount of diluent to add to the vial.[2;15]

An example using this formula is as follows:

- V_1 = 5 mL
- C_1 = 2,000 BAU/mL
- V_2 = volume of extract needed (solve for this)
- C_2 = 10,000 BAU/mL
- $5 \times 2{,}000 = V_2 \times 10{,}000$
- $V_2 = (5 \times 2{,}000)/10{,}000 = 1$ mL

In this example, 1 mL of extract is needed to get a targeted dose of 2,000 BAU/mL, which equals a dose of 1,000 BAU/0.5 mL in each injection the patient receives from the maintenance vial. If no additional extracts are added, then 1 mL of extract is mixed with 4 mL of diluent to get a final volume of 5 mL for the maintenance treatment vial.

There is no uniform standard volume for producing allergenic immunotherapy extract vials. Instead, they are often determined by physician preference and prepared based on institution-specific compounding standards. Whatever the volume, however, it is rare for the extracts alone to reach the specified total volume for maintenance extract vials. This, along with the serial dilution process, necessitates the use of diluents.

Preservative Requirements and Beyond-use Dating

With the stabilizing and preservative effect of 50% glycerin, bulk extracts diluted in 50% glycerin can have a 6-year expiration from the time of extraction, 3 years for manufacturer storage, and up to 3 years expiration on the vial once shipped. A 10% glycerin diluent is available as a base solution for patient prescription sets, but total glycerin concentration should be considered when using 10% glycerin as a base to avoid patient pain and discomfort.[2-4;6-8]

All final preparations must contain a concentration of at least 0.25% phenol to maintain sterility. If the phenol concentration is less than 0.25%, the preparation must include at least 20% glycerin. Because bulk stock solutions of extracts contain 50% glycerin and standard diluents contain 0.4% phenol, it is not difficult to achieve these parameters when using the recommended extracts and diluents.[6]

The BUD of compounded extract vials should be based on manufacturer recommendations. BUDs should never exceed the expiration of any stock allergen extracts or diluents used to compound the product. In general, a longer BUD can be assigned for higher concentrations because the phenol and glycerin concentrations are higher. More dilute vials contain lower concentrations of the preservatives and are therefore assigned shorter BUDs. Based on recommendations from the manufacturer of each specific diluent, the maximum BUDs are as follows:

- 1:10 to 1:5,000 w/v, 1,000 to 20,000 PNU/mL, 500 AU/mL and stronger, and 1,000 BAU/mL and stronger are good for 1 year. This typically includes 1:1 maintenance vials and 1:10 dilutions.[9]
- 1:50,000 w/v and weaker, less than 1,000 PNU/mL, less than 500 AU/mL, and less than 1,000 BAU/mL are assigned 3 to 6 months for expiration. This typically includes 1:100, 1:1,000, and 1:10,000 dilutions.[9]
- Buffered saline with phenol typically loses potency faster than HSA diluents and should be considered in determining the BUD.[9]
- Reconstituted venoms are good for 6 or twelve months under refrigeration at a concentration of 100 mcg/mL and depending on manufacturer guidelines listed in the package insert.[9]
    - 1 to 10 mcg/mL concentrations are good for 1 month.
    - 0.1 mcg/mL venoms are good for 14 days.
    - All concentrations less than 0.1 mcg/mL are good for 24 hours.

PREPARATION OF ALLERGENIC EXTRACTS

USP Chapter <797> Requirements

USP Chapter <797> standards outline the requirements for personnel training and competency, garbing, facilities, and cleaning of the compounding area.[5]

Competencies

As with the compounding of all sterile products, personnel who compound allergenic extracts must meet certain requirements. Regular media fill and gloved fingertip testing must be completed and passed annually to demonstrate proper sterile technique. Anyone who has not compounded allergen extracts in 6 months should demonstrate knowledge in core competencies before compounding again. USP Chapter <797> notes that "annual personnel training and competency must be documented. Personnel must demonstrate knowledge and competency in these procedures by passing written or electronic testing before they can be allowed to compound allergenic extract prescription sets."[5]

Personnel Hygiene and Garbing

Before beginning compounding of allergen immunotherapy prescription sets, personnel must perform hand hygiene and garbing procedures according to facility standard operating procedures (SOPs). The minimum garb requirements include the following[5]:

- Low-lint garment enclosed at the neck with sleeves that fit snugly around the wrists (eg, gowns or coveralls)
- Low-lint, disposable covers for head that cover the hair and ears and, if applicable, disposable cover for facial hair
- Face mask
- Sterile, powder-free gloves

Compounding personnel must also rub sterile 70% isopropyl alcohol (IPA) onto all surfaces of the gloves and allow them to dry thoroughly throughout the compounding process.[5]

Facilities[5]

The compounding process must occur in an International Organization for Standardization Class 5 primary engineering control (PEC) or in a dedicated allergenic extracts compounding area (AECA). The PEC or AECA used to compound prescription sets must be located away from unsealed windows, doors that connect to the outdoors, and traffic flow, all of which may adversely affect the air quality. Neither a PEC nor an AECA may be located where environmental control challenges (eg, restrooms, warehouses, or food preparation areas) can negatively affect the air quality. The PEC or the work surfaces in the AECA must be located at least 1 meter away from any sinks. The impact of the activities conducted around or adjacent to the PEC or AECA must be considered carefully when designing such an area.

- If used, the PEC must be certified every 6 months.
- If used, a visible perimeter must establish the boundaries of the AECA.
    - Access to the AECA during compounding must be restricted to authorized personnel.
    - During compounding activities, no other activity is permitted in the AECA.
    - The surfaces of walls, floors, fixtures, shelving, counters, and cabinets in the AECA must be cleanable.
    - Carpet is not allowed in the AECA.
    - Surfaces should be resistant to damage by cleaning and sanitizing agents.
    - The surfaces in the AECA upon which the allergenic extract prescription sets are prepared must be smooth, impervious, free from cracks and crevices, and made of nonshedding material to allow for easy cleaning and disinfecting.
    - Dust-collecting overhangs such as utility pipes, ledges, and windowsills, should be minimized. If overhangs or ledges are present, they must be easily cleanable.
    - The AECA must be designed and controlled to provide a well-lit working environment with temperature and humidity controls for the comfort of compounding personnel wearing the required garb.

Cleaning and Disinfecting[5]

- All interior surfaces of a PEC must be cleaned and disinfected daily and when surface contamination is known or suspected. Apply sterile 70% IPA to the horizontal work surface between each prescription set.
- All work surfaces in an AECA where direct compounding occurs must be cleaned and disinfected daily and when surface contamination is known or suspected. Apply sterile 70% IPA to the horizontal work surface between each prescription set.
    - If present, walls, doors, and door frames within the perimeter of the AECA must be cleaned and disinfected monthly and when surface contamination is known or suspected.
    - Ceilings within the perimeter of the AECA must be cleaned and disinfected when visibly soiled and when surface contamination is known or suspected.

- Vial stoppers on packages of conventionally manufactured sterile ingredients must be wiped with sterile 70% IPA. Critical sites that are wiped must be allowed to dry before they are used to compound allergenic extract prescription sets.

Vial Preparation

Most allergenic extract compounding begins with the preparation of the 1:1 maintenance vial, which contains the most concentrated solution of extracts and diluents. From this vial, further dilutions can be made. Vial volumes vary depending on individual institutional requirements. For the purposes of this example, a 5 mL total volume is used (see **Figure 24-1** for sample labeling schematics).

Preparations must occur in the following order:

1. Prepare the 1:1 maintenance vial by combining the prescribed extracts into a sterile empty vial and adding sufficient diluent to reach a 5 mL total volume. Invert the vial several times to mix.
2. Following the preparation of the 1:1 maintenance vial, a set of serial 10-fold dilutions can be compounded from the maintenance vial. Withdraw 0.5 mL from the maintenance vial, inject it into a vial containing 4.5 mL of selected diluent, and invert it several times to mix. This is the 1:10 dilution vial.
3. To make the 1:100 dilution, remove 0.5 mL from the 1:10 vial and inject it into a second vial containing 4.5 mL of diluent to make a 1:100 dilution. Continue in this fashion until the desired final concentration is reached.[6]

When preparing dilutions, there are two syringe techniques to consider:

- New syringe method: With each new dilution, discard syringe used after injecting 0.5 mL of the more concentrated dilution into the vial containing 4.5 mL of diluent. Use a new syringe to draw up 0.5 mL for the subsequent vial.[6]
- Mix and rinse method: Use a single syringe when diluting from 1:1 to the desired final concentration. With this method, after injecting 0.5 mL extract from the maintenance vial into the vial containing 4.5 mL diluent, the syringe must be flushed three times to rinse, and the vial must be inverted before drawing up 0.5 mL to be injected for the next dilution.[6]

After preparation of a prescription set, vials should be visually inspected for particulate matter, color of solution (eg, 1:1 should be the darkest and solution should get progressively lighter with each dilution), fill volume of vial, and integrity of the vial, including checking for cracks, stopper issues, and so on.[6]

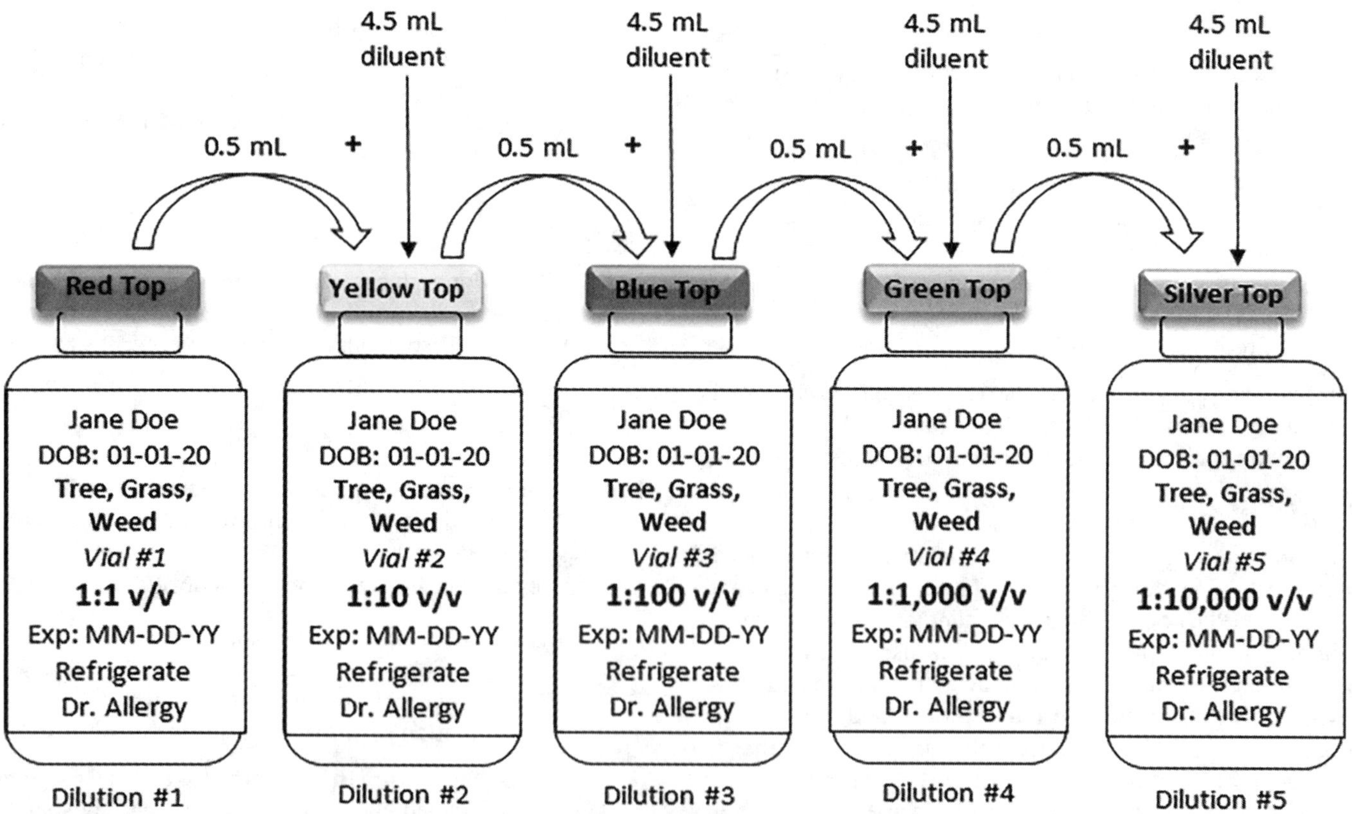

FIGURE 24-1. Sample dilution and vial labeling schematic

Source: Adapted with permission of the Cleveland Clinic Department of Pharmacy.

Vial Labeling, Coding, and Documentation

Each allergenic extract preparation follows certain required criteria for information on the label and color-coding individual vials based on dilution. Each label requires the following information[5]:

- Patient name
- Type and dilution of each vial and vial number
- BUD
- Storage conditions

Recommended information to include on the label to increase patient safety is as follows (see Figure 24-1 for an example):

- Date of birth
- Ordering physician
- Categories of extracts used (eg, trees, grasses, weeds)
- Assigned internal identification number

Standard allergenic extract dilution vials are available with color-coded tops. Color coding of vials is based on dilution as follows:

- 1:1 maintenance vial = Red
- 1:10 dilution vial = Yellow
- 1:100 dilution vial = Blue
- 1:1,000 dilution vial = Green
- 1:10,000 dilution vial = Silver

If color label printing is available, it is helpful to include the dilution color on the label as well.

As with any CSP, compounding of allergenic extract prescription sets is documented in a compounding record (CR) that must include the following information[5]:

- Name, strength or activity, and dosage form of the CSP
- Date and time of preparation of the CSP
- Assigned internal identification number (eg, prescription, order, or lot number)
- A method to identify the individuals involved in the compounding process and individuals verifying the final CSP
- Name of each component
- Vendor, lot number, and expiration date for each component for CSPs prepared for more than one patient and for CSPs prepared from nonsterile ingredients
- Weight or volume of each component
- Strength or activity of each component
- Total quantity compounded
- Final yield (eg, quantity, containers, number of units)
- Assigned BUD and storage requirements
- Results of quality control procedures (eg, visual inspection, filter integrity testing, pH testing)

Vial Storage

In general, all allergenic extract vials (bulk extract vials and compounded allergenic extracts) are stored refrigerated between 2°C and 8°C. Excursions from refrigeration should be limited. For example, a testing tray should not be left at room temperature all day when the vials are not being used. They should be returned to the refrigerator whenever possible to reduce loss of potency.[2;9] Potency loss can be due to heat sensitive protein degradation and activation of proteases, which degrade proteins.[6;16]

SUMMARY

The process of prescribing and administering allergenic immunotherapy treatments is complex. It involves coordination between prescribing physicians and those tasked with compounding allergenic extract vials. Attention must be paid to proper aseptic technique and color-coding conventions to ensure safe and effective preparations. When administered properly, immunotherapy treatments can provide relief to the millions of people worldwide who have immune-mediated reactions to common environmental allergens.

REFERENCES

1. Pawankar R, Holgate ST, Canonica GW, et al., eds. *WAO White Book on Allergy: Update 2013*. Milwaukee, Wisconsin: World Allergy Organization; 2013: 11–117. **https://www.worldallergy.org/UserFiles/file/WhiteBook2-2013-v8.pdf**. Accessed April 7, 2023.
2. Cox L, Nelson H, Lockey R, et al. Allergen immunotherapy: a practice parameter third update. *J Allergy Clin Immunol*. 2011;127(1 Suppl):S1–S55.
3. Tosca MA, Olcese R, Licari A, et al. Allergen immunotherapy and asthma. *Pediatr Allergy Immunol*. 2020;31(suppl 24):46–48. doi:10.1016/j.jaci.2010.09.034.
4. U.S. Department of Health and Human Services (HHS), U.S. Food and Drug Administration (FDA). *Mixing, Diluting, or Repackaging Biological Products Outside the Scope of an Approved Biologics License Application: Guidance for Industry*. Washington, DC: U.S. Department of Health and Human Services,

U.S. Food and Drug Administration; January 2018. **https://www.fda.gov/regulatory-information/search-fda-guidance-documents/mixing-diluting-or-repackaging-biological-products-outside-scope-approved-biologics-license**. Accessed April 15, 2023.

5. USP <797> Pharmaceutical compounding—sterile preparations. In: *2023: USP Compounding Compendium.* Rockville, MD: United States Pharmacopeial Convention; November 1, 2023: Issue 1. **https://doi.org/10.31003/USPNF_M99925_07_01**.
6. Nelson M, Cox L. Allergen immunotherapy extract preparation manual. *AAAAI Practice Management Resource Guide*. 2014 ed. Milwaukee, WI: American Academy of Allergy Asthma & Immunology: 2014. **https://www.aaaai.org/Aaaai/media/MediaLibrary/PDF%20Documents/Practice%20Management/PM%20Resource%20Guide/Ch-9-Allergen-Immunotherapy-Extract-Preparation-Manual-correction-July-19-12.pdf**. Accessed August 18, 2023.
7. Gruzelle V, Mailhol C, Waters DW, et al. Clinical utility of rush venom immunotherapy: current status. *J Asthma Allergy*. 2020;13:1–10. doi:10.2147/JAA.S200917.
8. Coop CA, Tankersley MS. Dose adjustment practices among allergists for local reactions to immunotherapy. *Ann Allergy Asthma Immunol*. 2007;99(1):77–81. doi:10.1016/S1081-1206(10)60625-4.
9. *Stallergenes Greer Allergy Immunotherapy Compendium*. 2nd ed. Cambridge, MA: Stallergenes Greer; 2016:1–200.
10. Daigle BJ, Rekkerth DJ. Practical recommendations for mixing allergy immunotherapy extracts. *Allergy Rhinol (Providence)*. 2015;6(1):1–7. doi:10.2500/ar.2015.6.0111.
11. Bassirpour G, Zoratti E. Cockroach allergy and allergen-specific immunotherapy in asthma: potential and pitfalls. *Curr Opin Allergy Clin Immunol*. 2014;14(6):535–541. doi:10.1097/ACI.0000000000000106.
12. Gruchalla RS, Pongracic J, Plaut M, et al. Inner City Asthma Study: relationships among sensitivity, allergen exposure, and asthma morbidity. *J Allergy Clin Immunol*. 2005;115(3):478–485. doi:10.1016/j.jaci.2004.12.006.
13. Esch RE. Allergen immunotherapy: what can and cannot be mixed? *J Allergy Clin Immunol*. 2008;122(3):659–660. doi:10.1016/j.jaci.2008.07.018.
14. Plunkett G. Update: stability of allergen extracts to establish expiration dating. *Curr Opin Otolaryngol Head Neck Surg*. 2016;24(3):261–269. doi:10.1097/MOO.0000000000000248.
15. Hoover H, Leatherman B, Ryan M, et al. Evidence-based dosing of maintenance subcutaneous immunotherapy: a contemporary review of state-of-the-art practice. *Int Forum Allergy Rhinol*. 2018;8(7):806–816. doi:10.1002/alr.22118.
16. Mustillo P, Martin B, Oppenheimer J, et al. *Allergen Immunotherapy Extract Preparation*. Arlington Heights, IL: American College of Allergy, Asthma & Immunology; October 2019.

25

RADIOPHARMACEUTICALS

George H. Hinkle

INTRODUCTION

Radiopharmaceuticals (radioactive drugs) consist primarily of two components. The first component is the chemical responsible for biodistribution or specific localization properties after patient administration. The second is the radionuclide that is transported to the organs or tissues by the chemical carrier. The combination of a unique chemical with a diagnostic radionuclide allows for detection or imaging of various diseases. When combined with a therapeutic radionuclide, the targeting of disease sites with the cellular destruction properties of radiation provides a therapeutic approach for treatment of benign and malignant diseases.

Medically useful radionuclides are chosen because their nuclear decay properties are considered ideal for either diagnosis or therapy. Short *half-lives*, the time required to reduce the radioactivity by one-half, are considered a primary driver of radionuclide selection. Three commonly used diagnostic radionuclides, ^{123}I, ^{99m}Tc and ^{68}Ga, have physical half-lives of 13 hours, 6 hours, and 68 min, respectively. The goal of using short half-life radionuclides requires the radiolabeling procedure (combining the chemical carrier with the radionuclide), patient administration of the final product, and completion of the diagnostic procedure to be completed within a few minutes to hours. Because most radiopharmaceuticals are injectables, the combining of the different chemicals with a variety of radionuclides for the final preparation of a number of radiopharmaceuticals must be completed using sterile techniques.

RADIOPHARMACEUTICALS: A UNIQUE CLASS OF DRUGS

A few unit-dose radiopharmaceuticals, typically with longer half-lives, are obtained from manufacturers in ready-to-inject forms that require removal from a sterile vial and measuring the quantity of radioactivity prior to patient administration. This practice is commonplace with a variety of injectable nonradioactive drugs. Workers involved in on-site sterile compounding of radiopharmaceuticals must possess an understanding of radiopharmaceutical chemistry, radiation safety, and sterile compounding practices. Compounding activities may involve the use of radionuclide generators as the source of radionuclides. This is a requirement for short half-life radionuclides, such as ^{99m}Tc (6 hours), ^{82}Rb (75 seconds) and ^{68}Ga (68 minutes), due to the need for an on-site source to meet daily patient needs. It is common for pharmacies to use commercially available nonradioactive sterile kits for compounding using radionuclide generator eluates. More unique compounding activities may involve radiolabeling of human blood products (ie, erythrocytes, leukocytes, platelets), dilution of manufacturer's multidose vials, preparation of patient-specific doses, and using nonsterile components for compounding single-use doses of commercially unavailable radiopharmaceuticals. These activities occur in an environment where aseptic technique must be followed to ensure patient safety. Additionally, they must adhere to radiation safety requirements for the protection of workers and the general public.

MICROBIAL RISK ASSOCIATED WITH RADIOPHARMACEUTICALS AS COMPOUNDED STERILE PREPARATIONS

When compounding using only sterile components, specific procedures are followed to ensure final product sterility. Compounding with nonsterile components requires achievement of a sterile product at the end of the process. The majority of radiopharmaceutical preparations involve the manipulation of sterile components in closed, sterile containers obtained from reputable manufacturers. Because most radionuclides used to prepare radiopharmaceuticals

DOI 10.37573/9781585286492.025

have short half-lives (decay quickly), radiopharmaceuticals are short-lived compounded sterile preparations (CSPs). Patient administration and expiration times are typically within a few hours of compounding, which requires routine preparation throughout the day. Radiopharmaceutical manufacturers supply multiple-dose vials (kits), which contain all of the nonradioactive ingredients used in the preparation of the final product. Short half-life radionuclides are then added to the sterile closed container (usually a 10 mL glass vial). This practice for compounding radiopharmaceutical CSPs, which adheres to manufacturer directions and conforms to quality assurance requirements (eg, expiration time, environmental controls) describes the common radiopharmaceutical preparation in nuclear pharmacies. An example of this is the routine preparation of ^{99m}Tc radiopharmaceutical kits. These preparations must be completed by qualified personnel in an International Organization for Standardization (ISO) Class 5 laminar air flow workbench (LAFW), which is located in an ISO Class 8 buffer area. They must meet other restrictions if dispensed as single dosages, including volume (≤ 15 mL) and expiration times (≤ 18 h). See Chapter 7 for details on ISO Classes.

The ^{99}Mo and ^{99m}Tc radionuclide generator system providing sterile, pyrogen-free ^{99m}Tc for radiopharmaceutical compounding must be eluted according to manufacturer's instructions and applicable regulations. This elution (removal of the ^{99m}Tc radionuclide from the generator system) must be completed in an ISO Class 8 environment.[1] Proper storage of the generator between elution includes the use of the manufacturer-provided elution needle protective cover, which contains preservatives for maintenance of sterility throughout the two-week shelf life of the generator. Storage and elution of radionuclide generators in an ISO Class 8 or cleaner air environment reduces the chance of the radionuclide generator system or the eluted radionuclide in solution being contaminated with microbes.

Some nuclear medicine procedures require the use of adjunctive medications or interventional agents for pharmacologic effects to enhance or improve the diagnostic quality of the nuclear medicine study. Although some hospitals prefer these nonradioactive drugs be dispensed from the hospital's pharmacy, the nuclear pharmacy providing radiopharmaceutical CSPs often prepares and dispenses these ancillary drugs. Sterile compounding and the preparation and dispensing of nonradioactive drugs are subject to USP Chapter <797> and USP Chapter <795> standards.[1]

Radiolabeling blood cells for (eg, white blood cells [WBC], red blood cells [RBCs], and platelets) diagnostic imaging is often prepared in and dispensed from nuclear pharmacies. Blood products are a biohazard, so radiolabeling blood cells with radionuclides must be isolated from other sterile compounding functions within a nuclear pharmacy. Guidelines for handling blood products should be established to prevent cross-contamination of other products and to protect nuclear pharmacy personnel from potential infectious organisms in infected blood.

U.S. PHARMACOPEIAL CONVENTION STANDARDS

With the introduction of USP Chapter <797> Pharmaceutical Compounding—Sterile Preparations in 2004, healthcare professionals were provided standards that describe compounding for the entire spectrum of sterile preparations for patient use. USP Chapter <797> specifies that sterile compounding pertains to all pre-administration manipulations (eg, preparation, storage, and transport) of CSPs.[2] In 2008, a revision of USP Chapter <797> was published that includes a section on radiopharmaceuticals as CSPs, which details standards for radiopharmaceuticals and nonradioactive drugs dispensed by nuclear pharmacies.[2] Application of practice standards described in USP Chapter <797> helped ensure the aseptic processing of radiopharmaceuticals and other parenteral medications dispensed from nuclear pharmacies. The majority of hospitals and clinics that use radiopharmaceuticals for diagnosis and therapeutic procedures outsource the compounding of radioactive drugs to commercial nuclear pharmacies. Since the introduction of USP Chapter <797>, The Joint Commission and other accrediting bodies expanded on the safe use of drugs to include radiopharmaceuticals. As part of the responsibilities assumed by accredited institutions to meet medication management standards, departments of pharmacy must take steps to properly manage the use of radiopharmaceuticals. In addition to assessment of facilities, equipment, personnel, training, and regulatory compliance, the overall review of a commercial nuclear pharmacy providing unit-dose radiopharmaceuticals to the institution must include compliance with sterile compounding standards.[3] Sterile compounding standards in USP general chapters apply to all places (eg, hospitals, clinics, pharmacies, physician offices) and all healthcare personnel (eg, pharmacists, pharmacy technicians, nurses, physicians) involved in the preparation, storage, manipulation, and transportation of compounded sterile preparations. Nuclear medicine technologists and nuclear medicine facilities are also included.

Achieving the goals of USP Chapter <797> while maintaining good radiation safety practices provides additional challenges involving the design and layout of nuclear pharmacies, use of required radiation shielding devices and instruments for the measurement of radioactivity, and observation of mandated radiation safety practices seemingly contradictory to sterile compounding procedures.

When USP Chapter <797> was first published, nuclear medicine professionals required to follow the same standards were faced with a number of challenges unique to the compounding of radiopharmaceuticals. The primary issue involved the use of radiation shielding and radiation measuring instrumentation in the same environment where sterile compounding took place. The incorporation of required radiation safety standards into aseptic handling scenarios described in USP Chapter <797> was unclear. Lack of specific guidance for sterile compounding of radioactive drugs led to confusion about the interpretation of standards by nuclear pharmacies, nuclear medicine professionals, and inspectors using USP Chapter <797> standards as direction.

USP CHAPTER <825>: DEVELOPMENT

Activities during the 2016 revision of USP Chapter <797> provided opportunities to address the many disconnects between practice and standard guidance. USP solicited comments from stakeholders, which exemplified the inability to combine USP Chapter <797> standards for sterile compounding with the radiation safety procedures and short half-life decay properties of the radiopharmaceuticals necessary for clinically useful times of a few minutes to hours. Review of written comments and follow-up meetings with nuclear pharmacies and other nuclear medicine professionals led USP to develop a new general chapter, which specifically addresses sterile compounding of radiopharmaceuticals. The Expert Panel on Radiopharmaceuticals used USP Chapter <797> for the basis of aseptic handling and sterile compounding, but they included changes that allowed a clear understanding of compliance activities for practitioners and inspectors. USP Chapter <825> Radiopharmaceuticals—Preparation, Compounding, Dispensing, and Repackaging now delineates compounding activities specific for radiopharmaceuticals and provides standards associated with these activities that, unlike USP Chapter <797>, balance radiation risks with aseptic handling practices.[1] Concentrating on radioactive drugs, USP Chapter <825> includes sections unique to short half-life radiopharmaceuticals and radiolabeling of patient blood components (RBCs, WBCs and platelets). The chapter also includes standards for the preparation and compounding of radioactive CSPs and for ensuring the sterility of the final radioactive preparation.

USP CHAPTER <825>: SCOPE, GOALS, AND OBJECTIVES

USP Chapter <825> provides standards for the preparation, compounding, dispensing, and repackaging of sterile and nonsterile radiopharmaceuticals included in the practice of pharmacy and medicine. It applies to all practice settings where activities involving radiopharmaceuticals occur, including nuclear pharmacies, nuclear cardiology imaging clinics, and nuclear medicine departments of hospitals. It also applies to all individuals involved in the preparation, compounding, dispensing and repackaging of radiopharmaceuticals, including pharmacists and physicians who hold authorized user regulatory status and those working under their supervision, such as pharmacy technicians, nuclear medicine technologists, residents, and student and trainees. However, USP Chapter <825> standards are not applicable to manufacturing activities involving U.S. Food and Drug Administration (FDA)-approved or investigational radiopharmaceuticals. USP Chapter <823> Radiopharmaceuticals for Positron Emission Tomography (PET)—Compounding, Investigational, and Research Uses supersedes USP Chapter <797> and USP Chapter <825> for guidance involving PET radiopharmaceuticals. Upon release of a PET radiopharmaceutical as a finished drug product from the commercial manufacturing facility, further handling, manipulation of unit doses from a vial, and use of the product is considered compounding activities and subject to standards in USP Chapter <797> and USP Chapter <825>. Nuclear medicine departments and nuclear cardiology imaging clinics involved in patient administration of unit dose radiopharmaceuticals with no additional manipulation after receipt are not subject to USP standards other than ensuring that the nuclear pharmacy outsourcing facility is compliant.[1]

The creators of USP Chapter <825> started with existing documents (USP Chapter <797> and other standards), regulatory guidance (ie, form the Nuclear Regulatory Commission, FDA, state boards of pharmacy), and other radiopharmaceutical handling guidelines from the American Pharmacists Association. Revised and edited material from these sources and other additional content formed the basis for minimum standards for the preparation, compounding, dispensing and repackaging of sterile and nonsterile radiopharmaceuticals. Consequently, USP Chapter <825> standards describing facilities and engineering controls, personnel qualifications, training and hygiene, cleaning and disinfecting, and air and surface monitoring procedures mostly parallel those found in USP Chapter <797>.

Facilities and Engineering Controls

USP Chapter <825> includes a description of the facility layout and environmental controls for classified areas and the segregated radiopharmaceutical processing area (SRPA). Like most areas where sterile compounding is performed, potential microbial contamination is present in the air of the compounding environment and on the surfaces used to complete the compounding process in a nuclear pharmacy. The compounding nuclear pharmacist must keep in mind that every surface and critical site exposed to ambient air is coated with layers of particulates that are loaded with viable microbes.

Although the entire nuclear pharmacy should be clean, it is important to understand the need for the area where radiopharmaceuticals are compounded to be cleaner than offices, conference rooms, bathrooms, packaging areas for unit-dose radiopharmaceuticals, radioactive waste storage areas, and supply rooms. There are many ways to design or remodel a nuclear pharmacy to meet requirements for CSPs used in the practice of nuclear medicine. Designers must keep radiation safety conditions in mind to limit radiation exposure of personnel. This can be achieved by segregating areas containing large quantities of radioactive materials away from areas where staff spend the majority of their work day.

Nuclear pharmacy design has limited access to areas where radioactive materials are handled and stored to comply with radiation safety regulations. Unrestricted areas include offices, restrooms, and employee lounge and eating areas without radiation safety restrictions. Portions of the nuclear pharmacies where radioactive materials are handled or stored (ie, restricted areas) require limited access to those properly trained in the safe use of radioactive materials. USP Chapter <825> requires personnel entering and working in restricted areas where sterile compounding of radiopharmaceuticals takes place to be properly trained and qualified for aseptic processing. In addition to the requirements for radiation safety training, nuclear pharmacy personnel involved in the preparation of CSPs must receive training, testing, and documentation of aseptic techniques.

The layout of a nuclear pharmacy where sterile preparations are compounded includes areas designated for specific functions. The sterile compounding area is located in a secondary engineering controlled (SEC) environment away from other work areas not used for aseptic processing. Isolation of the sterile compounding area to limit access by nuclear pharmacy staff not involved in aseptic transfer procedures reduces the introduction of microbial containing particulates into the sterile compounding area. The isolated sterile compounding area of the nuclear pharmacy should be separate from the remainder of the facility by a door or clear lines of demarcation on the floor. This area must be kept free of any items exposed to a patient care or treatment area of the hospital or clinic. USP Chapter <825> requires sterile compounding to take place in a properly maintained LAFW (ISO Class 5) as the primary engineering control (PEC), which is located within an ISO-classified buffer room with an anteroom or a SRPA in order to minimize the risk of microbial contamination.[1]

Maintenance of a Clean Environment

Important contributors to successful aseptic compounding are cleaning and disinfecting to minimize microbial growth on surfaces used during sterile compounding. Written procedures must describe the frequency and methods for cleaning and disinfection of facilities, LAFW surfaces, radiation barriers, and critical sites on any other components used. USP Chapter <825> prescribes minimum frequency for cleaning and disinfection of sterile compounding areas.[1]

The cleaning regimen should ensure that established limited microbial growth standards are maintained at all times. All cleanable surfaces of the laminar airflow compounding and dispensing area must be sanitized at the beginning of each shift using a residue-free agent, such as sterile 70% isopropyl alcohol (IPA). Floors must be mopped daily, beginning with the cleanest areas where the LAFWs are located, and then proceeding through the buffer and anterooms before finishing with the remainder of the nuclear pharmacy's restricted area. Before entering a controlled area, washing hands with soap and water followed by the use of residue-free antiseptics to decontaminate exposed areas of skin is the standard for all personnel. Care must be taken when bringing items into the sterile compounding areas required for completion of tasks. Objects that shed particulates, such as pencils, boxes, paper towels, and cotton balls, should be eliminated from the list of items allowed in the areas. Items required for radiopharmaceutical sterile compounding and dispensing, such as syringe shields, syringe holders, and other radiation protection devices, must have their surfaces cleaned with a sterilant before entering a controlled area. Table 5 of USP Chapter <825> includes cleaning and disinfecting regimens for various surfaces of the nuclear pharmacy.[1]

A large amount of particulate matter is shed by people working in the compounding area. This includes fibers from clothing, spray and particulates from sneezing, coughing, or talking, as well as shed skin cells. These particulates carry viable microbes that can contaminant the area and products. To control particulates in the area and prevent microbial contamination, careful cleansing of hands and arms followed by donning of clean room garb is required. Gloved hands should be sanitized using sterile 70% IPA just before and during the time working in the LAFW. Although gloves have been sanitized, they are not sterile, even immediately after spraying with alcohol. They become less so with each item touched. It is therefore important to avoid touching critical areas, such as vial septa, bare needles, and open syringe tips. Clean, low-shedding laboratory coats with fitted cuffs, gloves, and sleeves must be donned in the buffer area and worn while working in the laminar airflow hoods.

Studies have shown that airborne microbes are spread in air on the surfaces of dust particles, dried flakes of skin, and droplets of saliva expelled from the mouth. These particulates will settle out of the air onto the surfaces of LAFWs, sterile syringes, needles, and other items within the direct compounding area. Providing quality air that contains a minimal number of particulates within the direct compounding area drastically reduces the chances of microbial contamination of sterile compounded radiopharmaceuticals. An l-block shield, which reduces personnel exposure to ionizing radiation, also serves as a barrier to shield the product from particles that might be expelled while talking or breathing as work is performed in the LAFW.

LAFWs are designed to minimize airborne contamination from contacting critical sites that may lead to failure of aseptic processes. The vertical LAFW is preferred for radiopharmaceutical manipulations.[1] Movement of high-efficiency particulate air (HEPA)-filtered air is from the top of the unit, which passes downward through the work area and exits through small holes at the back, sides, and front of a stainless steel work space. This vertical movement of air is preferred because the placement of a lead-glass radiation shield or other protective devices to limit radiation exposure to the worker causes minimal disruption of airflow compared with a horizontal laminar airflow hood (**Figure 25-1**).

Established standards require semiannual certification of LAFW performance. In the certification process, the LAFW is tested to ensure the HEPA filter removes particles greater than 0.3 microns and that no significant areas of the filter are blocked, which prevents the flow of the air. LAFWs must have an air velocity of 90 feet per minute (± 20%) with a minimum of 30 air changes per hours (ACPH) for ISO Class 7 and 20 ACPH for ISO Class 8 areas.[1] The hood should run continuously, except for during required maintenance. If the hood is turned off, it must run for at least 30 minutes and then be cleaned before use. The use of sterile 70% IPA with

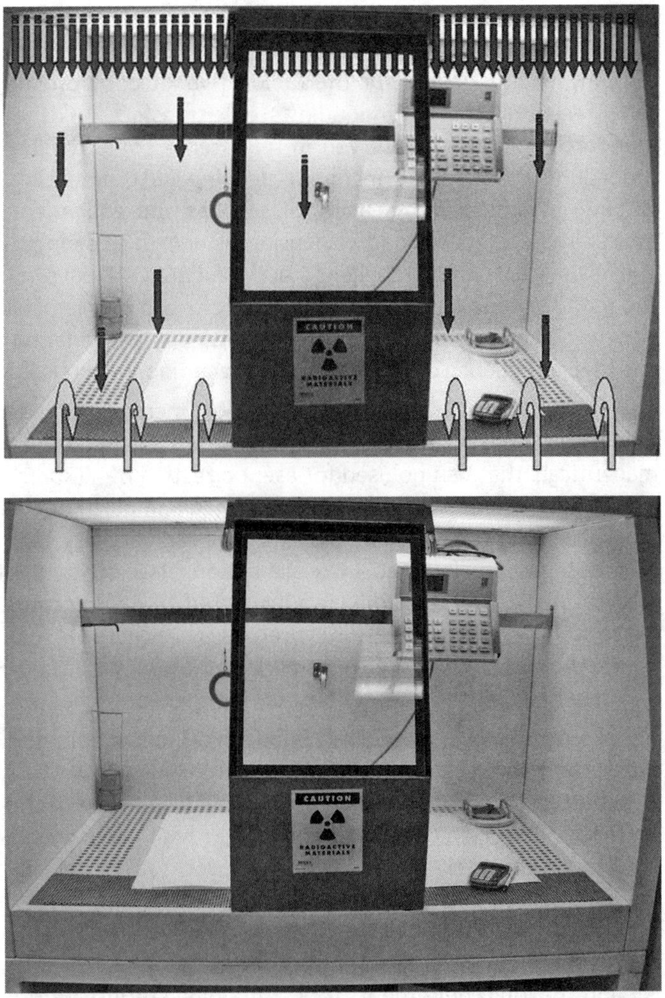

FIGURE 25-1. The movement of air within a vertical laminar airflow workbench with lead-glass radiation barrier in place

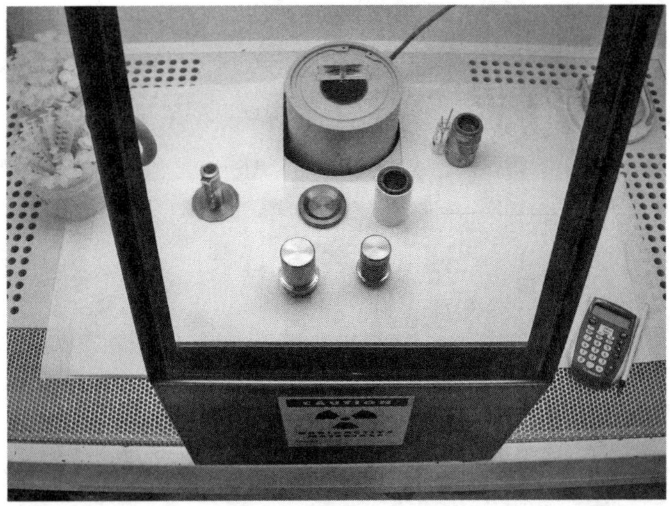

FIGURE 25-2. Placement of items in a laminar airflow workbench required for radiopharmaceutical compounding and dispensing

a clean nonshedding cloth is recommended for cleaning. The surfaces of the hood should be wiped from back to front and from top to bottom, progressing from the cleanest area to the potentially least clean area. Alcohol should never be sprayed into the hood while it is operating. This could cause damage to the HEPA filter when spray droplets are pulled into the filter.

Nuclear pharmacy personnel must receive proper training for the aseptic preparation and dispensing of radiopharmaceuticals in a LAFW. To begin, personnel should check that only the materials, supplies, and equipment needed to complete the work are placed within the hood. This will ensure minimal disruption of the laminar airflow. An example of proper placement of items needed for compounding and dispensing is shown in **Figure 25-2**. The lead-glass l-block at the front of the hood is required to reduce the radiation exposure of the nuclear pharmacy staff. At the center, near the back of the workspace, is the dose calibrator required to measure radioactivity in the multidose vial and unit dose syringes as the radiopharmaceutical is prepared and dispensed. Other items include syringe shields, vial shields, long-handle tongs to move radioactive materials and eliminate direct touching with fingers, syringes, and a calculator for use during compounding. The work surface should be covered with nonshedding, absorbent paper to absorb any radioactive spills that may occur. Care should be taken to minimize the number of air vent holes covered when cutting and placing the absorbent paper.

Proper aseptic technique includes working inside the LAFW in the rectangular area enclosed by the air vent holes in the surface of the hood. This avoids working in the area where clean air blowing down from the HEPA filter and room air mix at the face of the hood. While working in the hood, it is important to prevent obstacles, such as equipment, from blocking the path of clean air. Anything in the path of the clean air could shed particles or cause eddies in the airflow that might introduce particulates onto the surface of an exposed needle or vial septum.

Vial shields containing radioactivity are commonly inverted and placed on the surface of the hood to further reduce radiation exposure of nuclear pharmacy staff. Care must be taken not to place it directly on absorbent paper, which could be a source of particles on the vial septum surface. Rather, it should be placed on a clean tungsten disk or another hard, nonshedding, clean surface.

When entering the vial with the needle, the vial shield and syringe should be held horizontally or perpendicular to laminar airflow, as shown in **Figure 25-3**. This ensures clean air is blowing past the critical site where the needle punctures the vial septum and minimizes particulates blowing past that area.

Personnel Training and Evaluation of Aseptic Compounding Techniques

Creating a clean environment and the adoption of sterile preparation procedures only yield the expected results

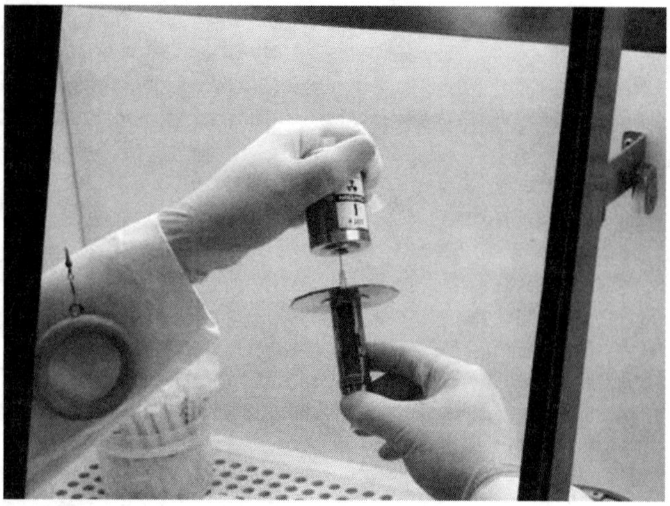

FIGURE 25-3. Proper technique used to withdraw patient dosage from a compounded radiopharmaceutical

if nuclear pharmacy personnel involved in the process are properly trained and sufficiently motivated to do their best job. Initial training, continuing education experiences, and laboratory exercises that test the staff's aseptic technique must be documented and reviewed by nuclear pharmacy administrative staff. In addition to formal training, there should be an oral and or written assessment of understanding of materials and information. Additionally, experiential training in aseptic techniques must be evaluated using a media fill challenge test. A minimum acceptable instruction includes basic aseptic technique and blood-borne pathogen training.

Individuals entering the sterile compounding area must be properly garbed. They must also maintain proper personal hygiene to minimize the risk of microbial contamination of the environment and the compounded radioactive drugs. Nuclear pharmacy personnel involved in the preparation of sterile radiopharmaceuticals that are not for immediate use must prove initial and ongoing competency in the following categories:

- Aseptic technique training with a documented assessment
- Garbing and hand hygiene
- PEC cleaning and disinfecting
- Gloved fingertip and thumb sampling
- Media fill testing

Assessment of sterile compounding techniques by simulated media fill is a required task for nuclear pharmacy staff to be able to complete in order to work in a real nuclear pharmacy and for validation of aseptic procedures. The media fill challenge test simulates sterile manipulations conducted daily in a nuclear pharmacy, including kit preparation and dispensing unit dosages from multidose vials. Microbial growth medium, such as Soybean-Casein Digest Medium (SCDM), is substituted for the radioactive kit components to represent normal compounding sterile transfers. All other standard procedures observed in real sterile compounding procedures are observed, including cleaning and disinfection, garbing, assembly and cleaning of supplies and equipment, aseptic manipulations, and dispensing of unit-dose syringes. The vials filled in this challenge are incubated 14 days for the required time period and inspected for signs of microbial growth. Successful completion of the training, examination, and media challenge demonstrate aseptic compounding skills.[1]

The FDA published a guidance document describing media fill validation of aseptic preparations of PET radiopharmaceuticals that can be used for aseptic testing of all radioactive drugs.[4] This media fill test uses media in place of the radiopharmaceutical kit components and radioactivity. The unit dosages are injected into incubation vials containing growth media, and then the vials incubated 14 days according to standard protocols. This procedure is conducted in four replicates throughout the work period, introducing fatigue and other factors that may appear during the work schedule.

If outsourced, the administration of sterile compounded radiopharmaceuticals to patients occurs miles from and hours after the compounding, testing, and dispensing of the unit-dose drug. The responsibility for training individuals involved in the packaging, handling, transportation, delivering, and storing of radiopharmaceuticals falls on the nuclear pharmacy leadership. A clear understanding of the importance of producing a sterile, injectable radiopharmaceutical and the job requirements for maintaining sterility before administration to patients leads to greater personnel commitment to institutional recommended practices.

Expiration (End-of-use Dating) of Radiopharmaceuticals

Radiopharmaceutical CSPs using manufacturer-provided sterile components follow the use-by times (expiration times) assigned by the manufacturer, which are also indicated in the prescribing information. For example, ^{99m}Tc must be used (patient administration) within six hours after preparation. ^{99m}Tc radiolabeled drugs dispensed in unit-dose syringes for patient administration from multidose radiopharmaceutical vials, which are prepared under USP Chapter <825> guidelines, assume use-by time dating indicated by the manufacturer's recommendations for that particular radiopharmaceutical kit.

USP Chapter <825> standards allow for the assignment of beyond-use dating (BUD) that can extend the expiration times of prepared radiopharmaceuticals based on the risk of microbial contamination during compounding actions. The assignment of BUDs for radiopharmaceuticals longer than the manufacturer's recommended use-by time must be reinforced by assessments that measure quality and purity, including sterility, radiochemical and radionuclide purity, and product-specific properties. Table 7 of USP Chapter <825> provides BUD values for manipulations and preparation conditions for radiopharmaceuticals.[1]

USP CHAPTER <825>: RADIOPHARMACEUTICAL-SPECIFIC STANDARDS

The differences found in USP Chapter <825> are reflective of the unique properties of radioactive drugs. The chapter emphasizes the importance of following good radiation safety practices while being attentive to the time element for the clinical use of radiopharmaceuticals, and details how to balance this with aseptic handling practices.

Radiation Safety Considerations

USP Chapter <825> recognizes the proper handling of radiopharmaceuticals to ensure worker and general public safety is considered when compounding sterile radiopharmaceuticals. The guiding principles of radiation safety, including time, distance, shielding, and contamination control, are addressed in the new standard. In addition, it includes directions from practitioners for balancing aseptic handling practices with radiation safety considerations. To meet radioactive contamination control guidelines, USP Chapter <825> specifically addresses the need for inclusion of absorbent pads in ISO Class 5 hoods, the use of vertical air flow hoods, and the handling of sharps during radiopharmaceutical compounding. Placement of radiation measuring instrumentation needed during compounding activities in ISO Class 5 hoods is also included in the USP Chapter <825> standard.[1]

Immediate Use of Sterile Radiopharmaceuticals

USP Chapter <825> allows for the preparation, including minor deviations, of a radiopharmaceutical dosage for a single patient using sterile components available from a radiopharmaceutical manufacturer (FDA-approved radiopharmaceutical kit). Emergency (after-hours) preparation of a single dose for a patient administration within an hour period and discarding the remaining material qualifies as an immediate use radiopharmaceutical preparation.[1]

Radiopharmaceuticals for immediate use are often prepared in hospitals or imaging centers and nuclear medicine practices where engineering controls (ie, LAFWs) are the exception. Requirements for the ambient atmosphere for areas where immediate use preparations are compounded includes a nonpatient care space free from clutter and low traffic patterns during radioactive drug preparation.[1]

Nuclear medicine personnel involved in sterile compounding of radiopharmaceuticals for immediate use are not required to complete aseptic qualifications, including aseptic technique training and assessment. However, they should have basic aseptic technique and blood-borne pathogen training, which is typically included in nuclear medicine technology education programs.[1] Additionally, precautions related to personal hygiene include instructions for hand washing and garbing before beginning sterile preparation activities. These differ from the hand hygiene and garbing for traditional radiopharmaceutical compounding in SRPA spaces.[1]

Environment for Preparation of Immediate Use of Sterile Radiopharmaceuticals

USP Chapter <825> provides guidance for facilities, such as the hot lab found in nuclear medicine practices with a SRPA, where clean rooms or PECs are not available. A room with an ambient air environment lacking PECs and SECs is typically a nonpatient care space that is free from clutter and has low traffic patterns during preparation of radioactive drugs for immediate use. Although the area for sterile preparation is not a SRPA, the area must be functionally separate from any nonsterile activities while sterile compounding is occurring. If the area is used for nonsterile activities (radiolabeling food for gastric studies), it must be cleaned and the countertop/lab bench space where the radiolabeling will occur disinfected. Strict adherence to aseptic technique and observation of shortened use (patient administration and or discarding) time is also essential given the lack of engineering controls.[1]

Preparation of Radiolabeled Blood Components

Diagnostic studies utilizing radiolabeled autologous red blood cells, leukocytes, and platelets have been a mainstay of nuclear medicine imaging for decades. A number of different compounding procedures can be used to provide a radiolabeled blood component for a specific diagnostic study.

While observing safe practices to guard against infection from blood-borne pathogens, the individual involved in the preparation of the radiolabeled blood components must use aseptic technique to prevent the introduction of microbes into the preparation prior to patient administration. Equally important is the prevention of cross-contamination of another patient's blood sample, nonblood related radiopharmaceutical, equipment, supplies, and areas where compounding is handled. USP Chapter <825> special precautions for the preparation of radiolabeled blood components for nonimmediate use include the separation of areas where blood components are handled from areas where preparation of traditional radiopharmaceuticals are conducted. Handling of blood components in an ISO Class 5 biological safety cabinet (BSC) located in an ISO Class 7 buffer area must follow specific guidelines. These guidelines state that only one patient's blood sample can be in the hood at a time, and that it is required to clean and disinfect the hood and reusable equipment prior to starting another blood radiolabeling procedure.

Equipment, such as centrifuges, dose calibrator, vial and syringe shields, disposable tubes, syringes, needles, and other consumables required for handling blood components during the radiolabeling procedure should be located in the ISO Class 7 buffer area. This helps avoid the need for leaving the area after hand hygiene and garbing is completed before entering. All disposable items should be removed from the ISO Class 5 BSC, and reusable equipment must be cleaned and disinfected after each radiolabeled blood procedure prior to further use. The final radiolabeled blood preparation should be administered as soon as possible upon completion. It cannot be used later than six hours after collection of the whole blood sample from the patient.

Preparation of Radiolabeled Red Blood Cells for Immediate Use

USP Chapter <825> provides guidance for the preparation of radiolabeled red blood cells for immediate use by describing the required dedicated space and equipment for blood handling and radiolabeling. Although radiolabeling in ambient environments with no controlled air exchange or engineering controls is allowed, the dedicated space, often located in a nuclear medicine hot lab, must be removed from high traffic and patient care areas, and be separated with controlled access throughout the radiolabeling procedure. Recommended cleaning and disinfecting procedures must be used to clean the area and reusable equipment (eg, dose calibrator, vial and syringe shields) before and after radiolabeling. Requirements for hand hygiene and garbing for immediate use preparations must be followed. The final radiolabeled red blood cell preparation should be administered as soon as possible after completion of radiolabeling. It cannot be administered later than one hour after the critical site of the vial used for radiolabeling is exposed to ambient air.

USP CHAPTER <825>: ENFORCEABILITY

USP Chapter <825> was developed based on public health need. The chapter provides quality standards and guidance to those involved in the preparation, compounding, dispensing, and packaging of radiopharmaceuticals. Since its publication date of December 1, 2020, USP Chapter <825> is informational only. It is not regarded as official guidance until other USP guidelines are met. Regulatory agencies (eg, Centers for Medicare & Medicaid Services, FDA, Boards of Pharmacy) and accreditation organizations (The Joint Commission) are using an early adoption of revised standard notices to begin inspections with USP Chapter <825> standards as guidance.[5]

SUMMARY

The U.S. market for radiopharmaceuticals is projected to rise from $4.8 billion (42 million patient dosages) in 2021 to $7.5 billion in 2026 (over 60 million patient dosages).[6] The expansion of radiopharmaceutical usage is sustained by the increasing prevalence of cancer and cardiovascular diseases, generating new applications and advancement of both diagnostic and therapeutic radioactive drugs. The majority of radiopharmaceutical dosages are prepared by nuclear pharmacists completing sterile manipulations of commercially available components. The 2008 revision of USP Chapter <797> provided guidance applicable to radiopharmaceuticals compounded in nuclear pharmacy practice with the goal of safeguarding the aseptic processing of radiopharmaceuticals. Achieving the goals of USP Chapter <797> while retaining established radiation safety practices proved to be a challenge. The design and layout of a nuclear pharmacy compounding space, incorporation of required supplies and equipment, and observation of mandated radiation safety practices were not addressed in the standards intended for traditional pharmacy compounding activities.

USP Chapter <825> Radiopharmaceuticals—Preparation, Compounding, Dispensing, and Repackaging was developed to address the many disconnects between the compounding of sterile and nonsterile radiopharmaceuticals and standard guidance. Specific guidance for sterile compounding of radiopharmaceuticals found in USP Chapter <825> address the lack of explicit guidance for radiopharmaceuticals in USP Chapter <797>. USP Chapter <825> provides nuclear pharmacy and nuclear medicine professionals with clear direction for compounding sterile and nonsterile radiopharmaceuticals with standards that create a balance between good radiation safety practices and aseptic handling standards. Those responsible for the supervision of medications in hospital settings now have clear direction for the management of radioactive drug use in the institution.

REFERENCES

1. USP <825> Radiopharmaceuticals preparation, compounding, dispensing, and prepackaging. In: *United States Pharmacopeia 42nd Revision -National Formulary*. 37th ed. Rockville, MD: United States Pharmacopeial Convention; 2019.

2. USP <797> Pharmaceutical compounding: Sterile Preparations. In: *United States Pharmacopeia* 39th *Revision - National Formulary*. 34th ed. Rockville, MD: United States Pharmacopeial Convention; 2016.

3. American Society of Health-System Pharmacists. ASHP Guidelines on Outsourcing Sterile Compounding Services. **https://www.ashp.org/-/media/assets/policy-guidelines/docs/guidelines/outsourcing-sterile-compounding-services.ashx**. Accessed January 9, 2023.

4. U.S. Food and Drug Administration (FDA). Guidance media fill for validation of aseptic preparations for positron emission omography (PET) drugs. **https://www.fda.gov/media/81974/download**. April 2012. Accessed January 9, 2023.

5. 3.10 Applicability of Standards. In: *USP 32: General notices and requirements: applying to standards, tests, assays, and other specifications of the United States Pharmacopeia*. **https://www.uspnf.com/sites/default/files/usp_pdf/EN/USPNF/generalNoticesandRequirementsFinal.pdf**. Accessed January 9, 2023.

6. Nuclear Medicine Market by Type – Global Forecast to 2026. *Markets and Markets.* **www.marketsandmarkets.com/Market-Reports/radiopharmaceuticals-market-417.html**. Accessed July 31, 2023.

BIOLOGICALS, BIOSIMILARS, AND VACCINES

26

Hallie Barr and Ben Lopez

INTRODUCTION

Biological agents are used for the prevention, treatment, and cure of disease in humans. The term *biological* is used to distinguish agents isolated from natural sources and laboratory-produced versions of natural sources from chemically produced low molecular medications. Biological agents are difficult to identify or characterize, resulting in rigorous production processes. Robust oversight of biological agent manufacturing is required because standard chemical and molecular biology techniques may not detect changes to the biological molecule that could significantly alter the safety or efficacy profile. Within the U.S. Food and Drug Administration (FDA), the Center for Biologics Evaluation and Research (CBER) and the Center for Drug Evaluation and Research (CDER) regulate the development, manufacturing, approval, access, and the safe and effective use of biologics within humans. The CDER regulates monoclonal antibodies (MABs), cytokines, immunomodulators and proteins, including recombinant versions. The CBER regulates vaccines, cellular products, gene therapy, allergenic extracts, antivenins, blood, and blood components.[1] These agents represent an array of products with many applications in medicine including cytokines, gene therapy, MABs, and the immunomodulator bacillus Calmette-Guérin (BCG).

The scope of this chapter encompasses the safe handling of commonly prepared therapeutic biological agents within an institutional or specialized compounding pharmacy. There is no single, comprehensive guidance that describes the risks and mitigations associated with handling biological agents in the health-system setting. Additionally, as with conventional drugs, considerations for compounding biologics differ depending on the characteristics of each agent. Concepts from at least three references can be reviewed to develop procedures related to safe handling of biological agents: Biosafety in Microbiological and Biomedical Laboratories (BMBL), National Institutes of Health (NIH) Guidelines for Research Involving Recombinant or Synthetic Nucleic Acid Molecules, and United States Pharmacopeia (USP) Chapter <800> Hazardous Drugs—Handling in Healthcare Settings.[2-5]

While these references are individually comprehensive, there are some limitations when applying them to compounding of biological agents. BMBL and the NIH Guidelines were developed to guide basic-sciences research and thus have limitations when applied to pharmacy compounding. Conversely, the mitigations described within USP Chapter <800> were developed within the National Institute for Occupational Safety and Health (NIOSH) hazardous drug framework, and as such excludes most biological agents from its scope.

TYPES OF BIOLOGICAL AGENTS

Vaccines

Vaccines are biological agents that strengthen the immune system to target certain infectious causes of disease. Vaccines have been developed against both viral and bacterial causes of infection. Vaccines that target specific viruses have proven to reduce the risk of certain types of cancer (eg, Human Papillomavirus 9-valent Vaccine, Recombinant).[6] During the SARS-CoV-2 (COVID-19) pandemic, novel vaccines were developed using a lipid-encapsulated viral spike protein mRNA. It is important to note that these mRNA vaccines do not contain viral material and can be treated as nonhazardous. Many vaccines are made with live or inactivated viruses and bacteria; therefore, each product should have an individualized approach to handling if sterile compounding is necessary.

Cytokines

Cytokines are proteins produced by white blood cells (WBCs) that are involved with signal transduction pathways within the human body.[7] There are three types of therapeutic cytokines: interferons, interleukins, and hematopoietic growth factors. Interferons and interleukins activate specialized WBCs to enhance the body's natural immune response.[7] Hematopoietic growth factors stimulate the proliferation

DOI 10.37573/9781585286492.026

of the bone marrow in the setting of neutropenia and anemia.[8] Cytokines are used therapeutically in the treatment of cancer, hepatitis, neutropenia, anemia, and multiple sclerosis. To date, cytokines have not been considered hazardous according to NIOSH.

Monoclonal Antibodies

Monoclonal antibodies (MABs) are used to treat cancer as well as autoimmune, cardiac, neurological, and infectious diseases. MABs are not conventional cytotoxic agents because they do not damage the genetic material of cells directly or indirectly. MABs have several mechanisms of action. In general, these agents typically bind a specific antigen, and the effect may be either an enhanced or suppressed immune response. In targeted therapy, MABs interact with specific molecules that interfere with tumor growth and progression. For example, MABs like rituximab stimulate an immune response by targeting proteins present on the surface of cancer cells that are not present on healthy cells. Other MABs suppress immune response by binding to proinflammatory agents, thereby disabling receptor binding and the subsequent downstream response.[9]

MABs' low risk of occupational exposure is attributed to their large molecular structure and poor absorption via dermal, mucosal, and inhalation exposure.[9] Nonconjugated MABs, with the exception of pertuzumab, have been excluded from the NIOSH 2016 hazardous drug list and can be handled as nonhazardous agents.[2] MABs, when coupled with a chemotherapeutic agent (eg, ado-trastuzumab emtansine) or a radioactive substance, must be handled as hazardous drugs. MABs developed in the future must be assessed for potential risk of occupational exposure.

Cellular and Gene Therapy

Cellular and gene therapy is a rapidly evolving area that includes products like cancer vaccines, cellular immunotherapies and human gene therapies. Cellular therapies largely represent autologous and allogeneic forms of various cells used to treat or cure disease. Gene therapy is the introduction of genetic material into an individual or modification to an individual's genetic material to achieve a therapeutic outcome.[10] Cellular and gene therapy research encompasses the investigation of treatments for a diverse range of diseases including cancer, acquired immunodeficiency syndrome, cystic fibrosis, Parkinson disease, cardiovascular disease, arthritis, and many others. Gene therapy uses viral and nonviral vectors to recognize certain cells and insert genetic material into the cells. Viral vectors are predominately used in research for intracellular delivery. Oncolytic viruses (OVs) are made from many different DNA and RNA viruses. OVs' mechanism of action begins by specifically infecting tumor cells, replicating, and destroying cancer cells while leaving the normal cells undamaged. In addition, OVs also create an immunological response to both itself and the infected tumor.[11] Talimogene laherparepvec is an oncolytic herpes virus for the treatment of advanced, inoperable melanoma. Cellular therapy can become gene therapy through the ex vivo introduction of genetic alterations that allow a cell to express a specific receptor or protein. One example is tisangenlecluecel, an autologous T-cell therapy that is genetically modified ex vivo to produce a chimeric antigen receptor (CAR), allowing the CAR T-cell to target and kill CD19 expressing cancer cells. More novel gene therapies utilize viral vectors to introduce normal copies of genes that have been mutated in patients with inherited diseases such as beta thalassemia and spinal muscular atrophy. Gene therapy presents a widely expanding field of therapeutics with the potential to cure debilitating diseases, but also brings challenges and questions related to their oncogenesis and genotoxicity to the healthcare worker handling these products. Additionally, pharmacies may not have the experience handling cellular-based therapies and may need to develop policies and procedures that specifically address their handling and rigorous record-keeping requirements. Some cell therapies are delivered from the manufacturer in a ready-to-use dosage form; however, some may require manipulation and should be handled as biohazardous when performing sterile compounding in a pharmacy setting.

Immunomodulators

BCG is an attenuated strain of *Mycobacterium bovis*. It was originally developed as a vaccine for the prevention of tuberculosis and is now an agent that is approved for cancer therapy. BCG is instilled intravesically for the treatment of bladder cancer, and it has a stimulatory effect on the immune system. The beneficial effect of BCG is believed to begin with a cascade of immunologic events causing the activation of T-cells, B-cells, macrophages, dendritic cells, and natural killer cells.[12]

BCG has a high risk for transmission. To avoid cross-contamination, other compounded sterile preparations (CSPs) should not be prepared in the same area where BCG is prepared, and proper decontamination/deactivation should occur after preparation. A separate room for BCG preparation is recommended. Healthcare workers have been infected or caused cross-contamination during the preparation and administration of the agent.[13] BCG is listed on the 2016 NIOSH hazardous drug list and must be handled following the standards in USP Chapter <800> Hazardous Drugs—Handling in Healthcare Settings.[3]

SAFE HANDLING OF BIOLOGICAL AGENTS

Risks Associated with Handling Biological Agents

Biological agents are diverse; as such, the following safe handling requirements will not apply evenly to all biological medications. It is important to develop a risk-based approach that incorporates all available information on each individual agent. One approach is to develop an algorithm that can aid a reviewer in determining the appropriate safety measures that should be implemented to protect healthcare workers while performing sterile compounding of biological agents.[14]

Biosafety Levels

Biological safety levels (BSLs) were originally established for the handling of biological agents in the laboratory setting. Biosafety is intended for the containment of hazardous biological agents.[5] Containment decreases exposure risk to personnel and prevents environmental contamination. There are four levels of containment, which are determined by biological agent risk groups (RGs) related to infectivity, severity of disease, and ease of transmission as well as the nature of the work conducted, origin of the microbe, the agent in question, and route of exposure.[5] Biological agents are classified in ascending risk groups from levels RG-1 to RG-4 which correspond with associated ascending containment strategies from BSL-1 to BSL-4. Increasing safety levels require progressively increased containment of the biologic agent. Each level increases protection for handling the biological agents (**Table 26-1**). At this time, biological agents prepared in the pharmacy are classified as BSL-1 or BSL-2.[5]

Determining Risk to Apply Appropriate Mitigations

Every medication on formulary must have its hazardous status reviewed in accordance with USP Chapter <800>. Medications that are added to formulary after the publication of the most recent NIOSH list must be evaluated against the NIOSH hazardous drug characteristics. However, biological agents may pose additional risks that are outside the NIOSH hazardous drug criteria. Thus, the BMBL's escalating risk groups and associated biosafety containment strategies designed for laboratories can be translated into mitigations for pharmacy compounding. This strategy is analogous to the assessment-of-risk process outlined in USP Chapter <800> and allows institutions to apply hazard mitigations in proportion to the biological agent's risk. Not all mitigations outlined in this section are required to be used for all biological agents.

Training

To promote safe handling of biological agents, employee training, competency, and proficiency must be established. All personnel involved in the handling of biological agents should be trained in safe handling principles including receiving, preparation, administration, and disposal of biological agents.[3]

The following topics should be included in training related to the safe handling of biological agents:

- The health risk of the biological agent
- Handling of biological agents for each job function
- Strict adherence to aseptic technique
- Correct use of safety equipment
- Standard operating procedure (SOP) for exposure
- Spill management
- Decontamination and cleaning
- Disposal[15]

Employees should demonstrate proficiency annually. Additional training is required for the addition of a new hazardous biological agent, change in safety equipment, or a major change in the SOP.

TABLE 26-1. Risk Group and Recommended Containment Strategies

Risk Group	Containment Strategy
Risk Group 1: Agents not associated with disease in healthy adult humans	Biosafety Level 1: A basic level of containment that relies on standard microbiological practices with no special primary or secondary barriers recommended, other than a sink for handwashing.
Risk Group 2: Agents associated with human disease that is rarely serious and for which preventive or therapeutic interventions are *often* available	Biosafety Level 2: Work with a broad spectrum of indigenous moderate-risk agents that are present in the community and associated with human disease of varying severity.
Risk Group 3: Agents associated with serious or lethal human disease for which preventative or therapeutic interventions may be available (high individual risk but low community risk)	Biosafety Level 3: Work with indigenous or exotic agents with a potential for respiratory transmission, and which may cause serious and potentially lethal infection.
Risk Group 4: Agents likely to cause serious or lethal human disease for which preventative or therapeutic interventions are not usually available (high individual risk and high community risk)	Biosafety Level 4: Work with dangerous or exotic agents that pose a high individual risk of life-threatening disease, which may be transmitted via the aerosol route and for which there is no available vaccine or therapy.

Source: Reprinted with permission of Blind JE, McLeod N, Campbell KJ. Viral-mediated gene therapy and genetically modified therapeutics: A primer on biosafety handling for the health-system pharmacist. *Am J Health-Syst Pharm.* June 2019;76(11):795–802. https://doi.org/10.1093/ajhp/zxz056.

Engineering Controls for Containment

Engineering controls for containment during sterile compounding of hazardous drugs are classified as primary, secondary, and supplementary levels of control. USP Chapter <800> outlines containment primary engineering controls (C-PEC) such as biological safety cabinets (BSCs) and containment secondary engineering controls (C-SECs) where such C-PECs are located.[3] Details regarding the specifications and setup for these engineering controls are available in USP Chapter <800>. It should be noted that the engineering controls described in USP Chapter <800> exceed the recommended containment for RG-1/BSL-1 biological agents. RG-2/BSL-2 agents that require manipulation or could aerosolize should be prepared within a biological safety cabinet located within an International Organization for Standardization (ISO) Class 7 buffer room with an ISO Class 7 anteroom. Access should be restricted to areas where RG-2/BSL-2 agents are prepared, and all areas where such agents are stored should have a universal biohazard sign visible.

Containment supplemental engineering controls such as closed-system drug transfer devices (CSTDs) are reasonable to consider when preparing or administering biological agents, although many manufacturers may not have data regarding compatibility. Other caveats regarding CSTDs are identified in USP Chapter <800> and should be reviewed carefully prior to use with biological agents.

Personal protective equipment (PPE) is another form of safety equipment. PPE used in combination with the BSC and/or compounding aseptic containment isolator (CACI) maintains an aseptic environment and offers greater protection for healthcare personnel. PPE includes shoe covers, head and facial hair covers, gown, sterile gloves, eye shields or safety goggles, and a respirator if necessary. For additional information about safety equipment, refer to Chapters 6, 13, and 27.[3,5,16]

SAFE HANDLING OF BIOLOGICAL AGENTS

BSL-1 and BSL-2 handling standards are described in the Centers for Disease Control and Prevention's (CDC's) BMBL publication.[5] The BMBL standards have been extrapolated to the pharmacy preparation standards of USP Chapter <797> and USP Chapter <800>. All biological agents prepared must comply with USP Chapter <797> (**Table 26-2**). BSL-2 agent preparation must comply with USP Chapter <797> and USP Chapter <800>. USP Chapter <800> describes safe handling of hazardous drugs from receipt of the biological agent to the disposal of the product. Pharmacy departments should develop and maintain policies and procedures specific to their institutions. These requirements are outlined below.[3,15,16]

Personal Protective Equipment

PPE is necessary for any sterile product preparation. Selection should take into consideration the type of preparation and the type of handling that will be conducted (ie, receiving, cleaning, decontamination, etc.).

The following PPE is needed to safely prepare biologics:

- Powder-free chemotherapy gloves that meet American Society for Testing and Materials standard D6978 or equivalent
- Disposable, impermeable gown with closure in the back, long sleeves, and tight-fitting cuffs
- Head and shoe covers
- Safety glasses/goggles if there is risk for spill or splashes; a face shield with safety goggles provides maximum protection

TABLE 26-2. Biological Safety Level Minimum Requirements

Level	Biological Agents	Handling Guidelines	Primary Engineering Control	Compounding Facility	Ante Area	Buffer Area
Biosafety Level 1	Not associated to consistently cause disease in healthy humans, minimal potential hazard to personnel and environment	USP Chapter <797>	LAFS, LAFW, or CAI personal protective equipment	Segregated compounding area or anteroom and buffer room	ISO Class 8 positive pressure	ISO Class 7 positive pressure
Biosafety Level 2	Agents associated with disease, moderate risk to personnel and environment	USP Chapter <797> USP Chapter <800>	Class II-A2 or II-B2 BSC, CACI personal protective equipment	Restricted entry, anteroom with segregated room	ISO Class 7 positive pressure	ISO Class 7 negative pressure

BSC = biological safety cabinets; CACI = compounding aseptic containment isolator; CAI = compounding aseptic isolator; ISO = International Organization for Standardization; LAFS = laminar airflow system; LAFW = laminar airflow workbenches

Source: Adapted with permission of Yarbro CH, Wujcik D, Gobel BH. *Cancer Nursing: Principles and Practice.* 6th ed. Burlington, MA: Jones & Bartlett Publishers; 2005:537.

- A properly fitted N95 respirator or a powered air-purifying respirator (PAPR) depending on the activity

Receiving

A designated area with neutral or negative pressure outside of the sterile compounding area must be available when receiving BSL-2 biological agents. PPE must be worn during unpacking, and the shipping container should be checked for damage or leakage. If the box is damaged, quarantine the container and transfer the product to a BSC. After the product is isolated, decontamination and disposal procedures should be followed. If there is risk of respiratory exposure, a cartridge-type respirator or PAPR should be worn. Following the disposal of the biological agent in a biohazard container, the unpacking area and BSC should be decontaminated and then disinfected before preparing other CSPs.

Storage

Biological agents must be stored at the manufacturer-specified temperatures. If a freezer or refrigerator is required for BSL-2 agents, it must be located in a negative pressure room with at least 12 air changes per hour. The temperature of the refrigerator or freezer must be monitored daily and alarmed to detect temperature fluctuations that may damage the product. Certain biological agents require storage in an ultralow freezer (–20°C or –70°C) that should be acquired before the receipt of the drug. Agents should not be refrozen once they are thawed.

Cleaning and Decontamination

In addition to the USP Chapter <797> requirements for cleaning and disinfection steps for sterile compounding, the biological agent must also be deactivated and the BSC surface decontaminated as outlined in USP Chapter <800>. The cleaning step occurs prior to compounding and physically removes contaminants. After cleaning is complete, the surface is disinfected to inactivate the micro-organisms.[16] After compounding deactivation renders the biological agent inactive, and decontamination removes the residue.[3] Most Environmental Protection Agency-approved disinfectants such as quaternary ammonium compounds are widely available in hospital settings. These agents are commonly used to chemically disinfect bacteria, fungi, and most viruses.[5] In the case of viral biological agents, an appropriate virucidal agent should be chosen for deactivation. It is essential to follow recommended contact times allowing the cleaning agent to remain wet on the surface for a period of time appropriate for the respective microorganism. Immediately following the dose preparation, the same deactivation, decontamination, cleaning, and disinfection steps should be repeated on the BSC surface.

Preparation

Care should be taken to avoid cross-contamination during the preparation of biological agents. Before preparation by a trained pharmacy employee, affix a biohazard warning sign on the entry door, and document the biosafety level, responsible investigator (if applicable), and emergency contact information in the event of a spill. It is important to follow the recommendations of the manufacturer for healthcare providers who are immunocompromised or otherwise who should not prepare or administer biologic agents. A segregated room with a designated BSC is preferred for BSL-2 agents. If more than one BSC is located in the same buffer room, only the biological agent should be prepared to prevent cross-contamination.[17] Proper cleaning and decontamination processes must be completed before compounding other preparations resumes. If possible, prepare intrathecal doses in a separate BSC from the one used to prepare BSL-2 agents.

Before compounding biologic preparations, proper hand hygiene and garbing requirements should be followed according to the requirements of USP Chapter <797>. A checklist should be created, and all the essential items needed for preparation should be gathered including syringes, needles, sterile wipes, disinfectant solution, disinfectant soaked wipes, biohazardous waste bag, and the biological product. The biohazard waste bag must remain inside the BSC during the entire preparation to allow for proper disposal of contaminated agents. Items should be wiped with sterile 70% isopropyl alcohol before placing them in the BSC. Carefully follow all manufacturer preparation instructions, and consider timing and logistical requirements for product thawing, if applicable.

Luer-lock syringes should be used to prevent possible disconnection of the needle from the syringe. A CSTD should be used to prepare the dose if compatibility and stability allows. If a CSTD cannot be used, equalize pressure in the vial to minimize the risk of aspirating the hazardous agent.

Disposal

Waste must be disposed of in a manner that ensures hazardous materials are contained. Place gown, outer gloves, and nonsharp disposal items into a biohazard bag or air-tight container located inside the BSC. The exterior surfaces of the waste bag/containers should be decontaminated before removal from the BSC. The bag/containers are then placed in a second air-tight container/bag labeled "biohazardous." Needles should not be bent, sheared, replaced in the needle sheath or guard, or removed from the syringe.[5] The syringes and vials must be placed in a puncture-proof air-tight container. Waste should be disposed of according to universal biohazard precautions and sent for incineration as soon as possible.

Transportation

For transporting biological agents within the health system, the dose should be double-bagged in a second air-tight container. The container should be labeled "biohazardous" and packed in a manner to prevent accidental spills or breakage. Spill kits are required to be carried during transportation of hazardous biological therapy. Because of the nature of these agents, they should be delivered for immediate administration and not stored on the nursing unit. A pneumatic tube system should not be used to transport the dose. For transport of hazardous biological therapy between facility buildings, an absorbent material should be placed in the second, leak-proof container in the case of breakage during transport. The outermost container should be rigid and labeled as "biohazardous."

Spills

A spill kit containing all necessary PPE, absorbent towels, prepared disinfectant, biohazard waste bags, and disposable cleaning supplies should be maintained at any institution that prepares and administers biological agents. The hospital's cleaning procedure and emergency contact number should also be available in the kit. All spills must be reported immediately to the pharmacy manager and documented.

If a spill occurs inside the BSC, the spill should immediately be covered with a wipe saturated with an appropriate deactivation agent for 30 minutes. Appropriate PPE must be worn, and the BSC should remain on during the spill cleaning. Once deactivation of the agent has occurred, decontaminate the BSC and place all items and PPE into a closed biohazard container for incineration. Needles and sharps should be discarded in an appropriate biohazard sharps container.

If a spill occurs outside the BSC, cover the spill with a wipe saturated with an appropriate deactivation agent for 30 minutes. Evacuate the area for 30 minutes to let any aerosols settle. After the allotted time, return to the spill wearing appropriate PPE and respiratory protection. The area should be cleaned, and all items and PPE should be placed into a closed biohazard container for incineration. Needles and sharps should be discarded in an appropriate biohazard sharps container.

SUMMARY

Biological agents have many therapeutic applications in healthcare and are classified as either BSL-1 or BSL-2. As the BSL risk increases, there is a need for increased containment of the agent to protect the healthcare personnel preparing the agent and the environment. To ensure compliance with USP Chapter <797> and USP Chapter <800>, adequate training, safety equipment, and appropriate facilities are required. With many new agents on the horizon, it is imperative for institutions to practice safe handling procedures during the receiving, storage, preparation, and disposal of biological agents.

REFERENCES

1. Transfer of biopharmaceutical (biologics) within FDA from CBER to CDER. Biopharma Website. **www.biopharma.com/CBERtoCDER.html**. Accessed August 31, 2023.
2. National Institute for Occupational Safety and Health (NIOSH). *NIOSH List of Antineoplastic and Other Hazardous Drugs in Healthcare Settings, 2016*. Cincinnati, OH: U.S. Department of Health and Human Services; 2016. **https://www.cdc.gov/niosh/docs/2016-161/pdfs/2016-161.pdf**. Accessed August 31, 2023.
3. USP <800> hazardous drugs—handling in healthcare settings. In: *2016: USP Compounding Compendium*. Rockville, MD: United States Pharmacopeial Convention; 2016.
4. U. S. Department of Health and Human Services (HHS). *NIH Guidelines for Research Involving Recombinant or Synthetic Nucleic Acid Molecules (NIH Guidelines)*. Bethesda, MD: National Institutes of Health; April 2019. **https://osp.od.nih.gov/wp-content/uploads/NIH_Guidelines.pdf**.
5. U.S. Department of Health and Human Services (HHS), Centers for Disease Control and Prevention (CDC), National institutes of Health (NIH). *Biosafety in Microbiological and Biomedical Laboratories*. 6th ed. Washington, DC: U.S. Department of Health and Human Services; Revised June 2020. **https://www.cdc.gov/labs/pdf/SF__19_308133-A_BMBL6_00-BOOK-WEB-final-3.pdf**.
6. Schmiedeskamp MR, Kockler DR. Human papillomavirus vaccines. *Ann Pharmacother*. 2006;40:1344–1352.
7. Schuster M, Nechansky A, Kircheis R. Cancer immunotherapy. *Biotechnol J*. 2006;1:138–147.
8. Vose JM, Armitage JO. Clinical applications of hematopoietic growth factors. *J Clin Oncol*. 1995;13:1023–1035.
9. King J, Alexander M, Byrne J, et al. A review of the evidence for occupational exposure risks to novel anticancer agents—a focus on monoclonal antibodies. *J Oncol Pharm Pract*. 2016;22:121–134.
10. Roth RI, Fleischer NM. Gene therapy: applications to pharmacy practice. *JAPhA*. 2002;42:692–698.

11. Singh PK, Doley J, Kumar GR, et al. Oncolytic viruses and their specific targeting to tumour cells. *Indian J Med Res*. 2012;136:571.

12. Yarbro CH, Wujcik D, Gobel BH. *Cancer Nursing: Principles and Practice*. 6th ed. Burlington, MA: Jones & Bartlett Publishers; 2005:537.

13. TICE® BCG [package insert]. Durham, NC: Merck Teknika LLC; 2022.

14. Blind JE, McLeod EN, Campbell KJ. Viral-mediated gene therapy and genetically modified therapeutics: a primer on biosafety handling for the health-system pharmacist. *Am J Health-Syst Pharm*. 2019;76(11): 795–802.

15. Health and Safety Authority. *Guidelines to the Safety, Health and Welfare at Work (Biological Agents) Regulations*. Dublin, Ireland: Health and Safety Authority; 2014.

16. USP <797> Pharmaceutical compounding—sterile preparations. In: *2016: USP 39–NF 34*. Rockville, MD: United States Pharmacopeial Convention; 2016.

17. Vulto AG, Stoner N, Balásová H. European Association of Hospital Pharmacists guidance on the pharmacy handling of gene medicines. *Eur J Hosp Pharm Pract*. 2007;13:29–39.

27

HANDLING AND COMPOUNDING OF HAZARDOUS DRUGS

Nicholas A. Link and Patricia A. Roberts

INTRODUCTION

Concern regarding the safety of workers handling hazardous drugs (HDs), specifically antineoplastic agents, surfaced in the 1970s when reports of second cancers in patients treated with these agents were coupled with the discovery of mutagenic substances in nurses who handled these drugs and cared for treated patients.[1–3] The nonspecific nature of the cytotoxic action of these drugs renders all cells at risk for DNA damage, patient and caregiver alike.

Evidence of Exposure and Adverse Effects

Exposure to HDs in the workplace has been associated with acute and short-term reactions. Anecdotal reports in early literature ranged from malaise and flu-like symptoms to hair loss, nail damage, and mucosal sores.[4–7] Reproductive studies on healthcare workers have shown increases in fetal abnormality, fetal loss, and fertility impairment.[8–11]

Increased incidence of cancers for these exposed groups has been investigated with varying success.[12;13] The small number of individuals available for study presents a dilemma for the statistician. Two recent and related studies, however, described evidence of drug uptake (drug being incorporated into workers' bodies) and chromosomal changes in workers exposed to workplaces contaminated with HD residue.[14;15] The DNA of exposed workers showed a statistically significant increased frequency of damage to chromosome 5 or 7 and an increased frequency of damage to chromosome 5 alone. As signature lesions in chromosomes 5, 7, and 11 have been shown to be associated with chemotherapy-treatment-related myelodysplastic syndrome and acute myeloid leukemia, these results provide additional evidence for harmful effects from occupational exposure to HDs.[16]

Much research has been done on healthcare workers regarding biomarkers of HD exposure (intact HD or a metabolite measured in the body, usually in urine samples) and biomarkers of effect, a measurable biochemical alteration within an organism (usually related to the genotoxic properties of HDs).[17–19] An early review noted that none of the then available biological and analytical methods were sufficiently reliable or reproducible for routine monitoring of HD exposure in the workplace.[17] A more recent review of studies extending through 2010 advocated using combinations of selected markers to validate protective measures and safety guidelines used in reducing exposure to HDs in healthcare workers.[19] Both reviews recommend more research be conducted on the important issue of healthcare worker exposure to HDs.

Workplace Contamination

A landmark multisite study in the United States and Canada published in 1999 examined workplace contamination with HDs compared to European sites.[20] This study found that in the U.S. 75% of compounding areas and 65% of patient administration areas were contaminated with measurable amounts of the marker HDs cyclophosphamide, fluorouracil, and ifosfamide. Substantial levels of contamination from the sampled HDs were detected on a variety of surfaces in pharmacy drug preparation areas and in drug administration areas. Despite efforts and strategies made public following the 1999 study (eg, National Institute for Occupational Safety and Health [NIOSH] 2004 HD alert and American Society of Health-System Pharmacists [ASHP] 2006 guidelines for HD handling), HD contamination within medication use areas of multiple U.S. and Canadian hospitals continued, as shown by articles published into the 2010s.[21–24] Results indicate that frequently touched surfaces, such as pens, door handles, and carts, have detectible HD residue.[24] Samples within the drug preparation areas resulted in the highest levels of HD contamination.[24] In the U.S. study, 60% of wipe samples taken tested positive for HD contamination and 3 of 68 healthcare worker urine samples were found positive for one of the tested medications.[23]

Note: The authors acknowledge Luci A. Power and Joseph W. Coyne who authored this chapter in the previous edition.

DOI 10.37573/9781585286492.027

Results from a study of 5842 HD wipe samples from 338 healthcare institution pharmacies retrieved between 2009 and 2015 revealed that the highest amount of positive samples were found closest to the compounding areas (biological safety cabinet [BSC] surfaces, airfoil, and the floor below the BSC).[25] The same study also demonstrated that additional areas outside the compounding space had HD contamination.[25] Notably, even with use of closed-system drug transfer device (CSTD) technology, all five drugs studied, paclitaxel, docetaxel, cyclophosphamide, ifosfamide, or fluorouracil, were still detected at levels as high as greater than 1,000 ng/ft^3 in some areas.[25] Routes of unintentional HD exposure to healthcare workers include dermal and mucosal absorption, inhalation, injection, and ingestion, which can occur in any step of the HD handling process from receipt to disposal.[26] Ultimately, these ongoing results justify that HD handling guidance and strategies are necessary to address contamination potential of healthcare workers despite technological advances in practice.

BEST PRACTICES, STANDARDS, AND REGULATIONS

There are multiple agencies and sources for best practices and standards regarding handling HDs to help protect healthcare workers. This section serves to summarize some of the important sources and their place in practice.

Occupational Safety and Health Administration

The Occupational Safety and Health Administration (OSHA) originally published federal guidelines for antineoplastic HDs in 1986.[27] Although OSHA covers mostly private sector employers and workers, Section 18 of the Occupational Safety and Health Act of 1970 encourages states to develop and operate their own job safety and health programs.[28] States are allowed to make regulations more stringent than federal mandates or add additional standards not addressed by federal OSHA standards. Several states have passed legislation that allows the state to regulate HDs. Both federal and state-specific guidelines (if applicable) for management of HDs can be found on OSHA's website.[29]

National Institute for Occupational Safety and Health: Hazardous Drug Working Group

NIOSH, as part of the Centers for Disease Control and Prevention (CDC), assembled a Hazardous Drug Working Group in 2000 to study HD contamination in the healthcare setting, assess possible health risks, and provide better guidance for safe handling. The Working Group published the 2004 NIOSH Alert *Preventing Occupational Exposure to Antineoplastic and Other Hazardous Drugs.*[21] The alert included an extensive literature background, detailed recommendations, modified HD criteria, and an appendix that is a compilation of lists of HDs.[21] The list was compiled from information submitted by institutions and by the Pharmaceutical Research and Manufacturers of America.[21] The 2016 list is the most recent edition, although a draft from 2020 is pending publication.[30;31] Readers should monitor the NIOSH webpage for updated NIOSH publications.[32]

USP Chapter <800> Hazardous Drugs—Handling in Healthcare Settings

On February 1, 2016, the U.S. Pharmacopeia (USP) published a new general chapter, Chapter <800> Hazardous Drugs—Handling in Healthcare Settings.[26] USP Chapter <800> standards apply to all healthcare personnel and all healthcare facilities where HDs are handled or manipulated, including their storage and distribution. Sections of USP Chapter <800> are provided verbatim in the following text to avoid possible misinterpretations of intent. This chapter is not intended to be a substitute for the provisions of USP Chapter <800>.

DEFINING HAZARDOUS DRUGS

HDs may include antineoplastic or cytotoxic drugs, biologic formulations, antiviral agents, immunosuppressive agents, and drugs that present reproductive risks. Research reports and guidelines have used various terms to define their concerns. The nonspecific and broad nature of potential health hazards that present a risk to workers handling certain drugs in healthcare settings was addressed in the 1990 ASHP *Technical Assistance Bulletin on Handling Cytotoxic and Hazardous Drugs.*[33] This was the first use of the term hazardous drug to convey an occupational exposure risk. ASHP selected this term to harmonize with the then newly released OSHA Hazard Communication Standard (HCS) that was originally finalized in 1994.[34]

HAZARDOUS DRUG CRITERIA

NIOSH HD List and USP Chapter <800>

NIOSH recommends standard precautions or universal precautions be taken in handling HDs. However, the NIOSH HD list contains many nonantineoplastic drugs and drugs in tablet and/or capsule form. NIOSH recognized that no single approach covers the diverse potential for occupational exposures to the drugs. Although NIOSH did not attempt to perform risk assessments on each drug or propose exposure limits, it has provided guidance for personal protective equipment (PPE) and ventilated engineering controls for the various scenarios in which a drug may be handled in healthcare settings.[30] This guidance may be found in Table 5 of the NIOSH 2016 HD list.[30] Future updates to this guidance will be found on the NIOSH webpage for NIOSH publications.[32]

The 2016 NIOSH approach involves three groups of drugs.[30]

Group 1. Antineoplastic drugs

Group 2. Nonantineoplastic drugs that meet one or more of the NIOSH criteria for an HD (including reproductive risk)

Group 3. Drugs that primarily pose a reproductive risk to people who are actively trying to conceive and those who are pregnant or breastfeeding (some of these drugs may be present in breast milk)

USP Chapter <800> has adopted the NIOSH HD criteria and list. Based on this list, USP Chapter <800> has specified containment requirements for the following[26]:

- Drugs on the NIOSH list that must follow the requirements.
    - Any HD active pharmaceutical ingredient.
    - Any antineoplastic HD requiring manipulation.
- Drugs on the NIOSH list that do not have to follow all the containment requirements if an assessment of risk is performed and implemented.
    - Any final dosage form of compounded HD preparations and conventionally manufactured HD products, including antineoplastic dosage forms that do not require any further manipulation other than counting or repackaging (unless required by the manufacturer).
- For dosage forms of other HDs on the NIOSH list, the facility may perform an assessment of risk to determine alternative containment strategies and work practices.

Minimum considerations for assessing alternative containment strategies for HDs through an assessment of risk must include the type of HD (antineoplastic, nonantineoplastic, reproductive risk only), dosage form, risk of exposure, packaging, and manipulation.[26] The assessment of risk must be reviewed by the facility every 12 months. Adherence to all HD containment strategies outlined by USP Chapter <800> is required if an assessment of risk is not performed.[26]

HAZARD COMMUNICATION

Policies and Procedures and Standard Operating Procedures

The OSHA HCS requires all HD worksites to have comprehensive hazard communication programs that include container labeling and other forms of warnings, safety data sheets (SDS), and employee training.[35] NIOSH and ASHP discuss safety programs that include standard operating procedures (SOPs) for the safe handling of HDs.[21;22;36] USP Chapter <800> requires that facilities handling HDs must incorporate the chapter's standards into their occupational safety plan.[26] The facility's program must include a list of HDs, facility and engineering controls, competent personnel, safe work practices, proper use of appropriate PPE, and policies for HD waste segregation and disposal.[26]

SOPs for the safe handling of HDs must be in place for all situations where they are in use throughout a facility. A comprehensive safety program must be developed that deals with all aspects of the safe handling of HDs. This program must have input from those representing all affected workers, such as pharmacy, nursing, medical staff, clinical support staff, housekeeping, transportation, maintenance, employee health, risk management, industrial hygiene, clinical laboratories, and safety.

Safety Data Sheets

A key element of the HCS comprehensive hazard communication program is the SDS formerly Material Safety Data Sheets (MSDS).[34;35] Employers are required to have an SDS available for all hazardous agents located in the workplace. A comprehensive safety program must include a process for monitoring and updating the SDS database. When an HD is purchased for the first time, an SDS must be requested and received from the drug's manufacturer or distributor. The SDS should define the appropriate handling precautions, including protective equipment, controls, and spill management, associated with the drug.

LABELING, RECEIVING, STORAGE, AND TRANSPORT

Labeling

No universal symbol or wording has been adopted for the labeling of HDs, their containers, or waste. Frequently, HDs are labeled with the universal biohazard symbol (see **Figure 27-1**), which is inaccurate. The biohazard

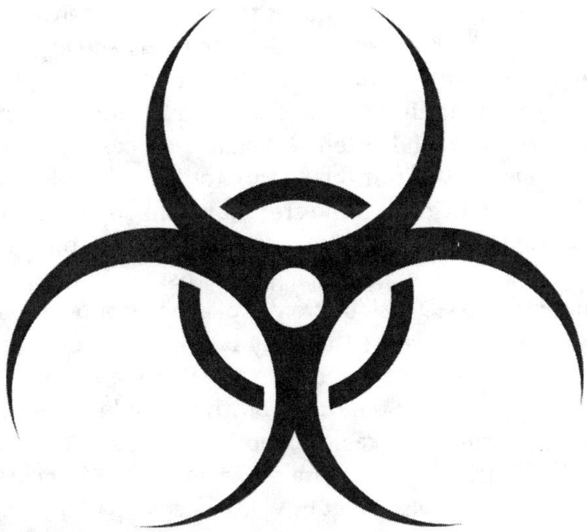

FIGURE 27-1. Biohazard symbol

This symbol is not appropriate for hazardous drugs.

symbol was developed to label biological materials that carry a significant health risk, including viral samples and used hypodermic needles (ie, a living hazard that may be decontaminated by disinfecting or autoclaving). As HDs cannot be decontaminated or deactivated by disinfection or autoclaving, the use of this symbol is misleading and should be avoided. This is especially critical with the development of certain therapies that contain biologicals that must be labeled as biohazards and handled and disposed of as blood-borne pathogens (eg, *Bacillus* Calmette-Guerin [BCG], talimogene laherparepvec).[37–39]

Once an authoritative body has selected a symbol or wording to denote an HD, this must be used to identify HDs and HD areas. USP Chapter <800> requires that identified HDs receive special handling precautions and be clearly labeled at all times during their transport.[26] The labeling process for compounded HDs must ensure contamination is not introduced into the non-HD handling areas.[26] HCS requires that workplace labels or other forms of warning are legible, in English, and prominently displayed on the container or readily available in the work area.[35] HCS allows languages in addition to English where needed. Prudent practice would be to label HDs at all times during their receipt, storage, handling, transport, and disposal to ensure proper handling throughout the HD's life cycle. Cartons of HDs transported from manufacturer or distributor should be labeled with an acceptable identifier to notify personnel receiving them to wear appropriate PPE when opening them. Drug packages, bins, shelves, and all storage areas of HDs should bear distinctive labels identifying them as requiring special precautions.

Receiving

Hazardous drug surface contamination has been found on pharmacy distributor shipping containers, posing a risk to healthcare workers receiving a hazardous drug order from the distributor.[40] In order to mitigate risk to healthcare workers, SOPs for the safe handling of HDs must begin from the receipt of the package from the manufacturer or distributor. USP Chapter <800> requires that entities receiving HDs must establish standard procedures for this activity. "HDs should be received from the supplier in impervious plastic to segregate them from other drugs and to allow for safety in the receiving and internal transfer process."[26] Sealing these drugs in plastic at the distributor level provides additional safety for workers who are required to unpack cartons. Unpacking shipping containers of HDs that may have been damaged in packing or shipping are a risk of exposure due to uncontained HD residue from broken vials or bottles and harm from broken glass that may be in the carton or container. Unpacking intact cartons can still be a risk because HD residue has been measured on the outside of HD vials and on the primary packaging of both injectable and oral formulations, including unit-dose packaging.[41–43] PPE, including chemotherapy gloves, must be worn when unpacking HDs.[26] A single pair of chemotherapy gloves is sufficient for unpacking an intact carton or container, and a "spill kit must be accessible in the receiving area."[26]

If the carton or container appears damaged, PPE appropriate for a spill should be donned. Because there may be no ventilation protection in the area where damaged containers are handled, the use of complete PPE, including a NIOSH-certified respirator, is recommended.[44] Surgical masks do not provide adequate protection from the harmful effects of these drugs.

USP Chapter <800> provides the following list of requirements for receiving and handling damaged HD shipping containers in a table format[26]:

- If the shipping container appears damaged:
  - Seal the container without opening it and contact the supplier.
  - If the unopened package is to be returned to the supplier, enclose the package in an impervious container and label the outer container "Hazardous."
  - If the supplier declines return, dispose of it as hazardous waste.
- If a damaged shipping container must be opened:
  - Seal the container in plastic or an impervious container.
  - Transport it to a containment primary engineering control (C-PEC) and place it on a plastic-backed preparation mat.
  - Open package and remove undamaged items.
  - Wipe the outside of the undamaged items with a disposable wipe.
  - Enclose the damaged item(s) in an impervious container and label the outer container "Hazardous."
  - If the supplier declines return, dispose of it as hazardous waste.
  - Deactivate, decontaminate, and clean the C-PEC, and discard the mat and cleaning disposables as hazardous waste.

Storage

HDs must be delivered to the HD storage area immediately after unpacking.[26] USP Chapter <800> requires that "HDs be stored in a manner that prevents spillage or breakage if the container falls but prohibits storing HDs on the floor. In areas prone to specific types of natural disasters (e.g., earthquakes), the manner of storage must meet applicable safety precautions, such as secure shelves with raised front lips."[26]

Multiple studies have shown that some HDs have sufficient vapor pressure that allows for volatilization at room temperature.[45–47] As this may present an additional exposure risk from inappropriate storage, antineoplastic HDs requiring manipulation other than counting and repackaging of the final dosage form must be stored in a containment area meeting the following storage guidelines[26]:

- Stored separately from non-HDs
- Stored in a manner that prevents contamination and personnel exposure
- Stored in an externally ventilated, negative pressure room with at least 12 air changes per hour (ACPH)
- Stored in the containment secondary engineering control (C-SEC)
- Refrigerated antineoplastic HDs stored in a dedicated refrigerator

USP Chapter <800> allows nonantineoplastic, reproductive risk only HDs and final dosage forms of antineoplastic HDs to be stored with other inventory if permitted by facility policy.[26]

Separation of HD inventory improves control and reduces the number of staff members potentially exposed to the danger. Additionally, HDs placed in inventory should be protected from potential breakage by storing in appropriately sized bins that properly contain all stock. Studies have reported contamination on the drug vial as well as pharmacy storage bins.[40–43] All staff members should wear American Society for Testing and Materials (ASTM) standard D6978 gloves when handling HD vials.[41–43] A manufacturing process has been reported that potentially reduces drug vial surface contamination, however, this process is patented and not widely used.[48]

Transport and Packaging

USP Chapter <800> requires the following:

> HDs that need to be transported must be labeled, stored, and handled in accordance with applicable federal, state, and local regulations. HDs must be transported in containers that minimize the risk of breakage or leakage. Pneumatic tubes must not be used to transport any liquid HDs or any antineoplastic HDs because of the potential for breakage and contamination.[26]

Sealed containers (eg, sealable plastic bags) are preferable to reduce contamination in the event of accidental dropping.

When compounded sterile preparations (CSPs) are distributed to locations outside the premises in which they are compounded, packing materials should be selected that maintain the product's physical integrity, stability, and sterility.[26] Packing should simultaneously protect personnel who transport packed CSPs from harm. "The entity must have written SOPs to describe appropriate shipping containers and insulating materials, based on information from product specifications, vendors, and mode of transport."[26] Labels and accessory labeling consisting of storage, disposal, and HD category information must be included for all transported HDs.[26] A spill kit should accompany delivery of injectable HDs to patient care areas even though they are transported in a sealable plastic bag or other protective container.[36]

ENVIRONMENT

HDs as CSPs are regulated by USP Chapter <797> and USP Chapter <800> for compounding environments.[26;49] USP Chapter <800> requirements for HD handling, storage, and compounding environments emphasize containment utilizing C-PECs (ie, the device in which compounding takes place) and C-SECs (the room in which the C-PEC is placed).[26] Specific discussion on the requirements of C-PECs and C-SECs for HD compounding are described at length in the corresponding chapters on primary and secondary engineering controls (Chapters 6 and 7, respectively).

Some areas are required to have negative pressure from surrounding areas to contain HDs and minimize risk of exposure.[26] Negative pressure is generally achieved through external ventilation (ie, exhausting to the outside). "Access to environments where HDs are handled must be restricted to authorized personnel to protect persons not involved in HD handling."[26] As with all environments where sterile products are compounded, eating, drinking, and the presence of food is prohibited due to the possibility of bringing microbial contamination into the compounding area.[49] Additional concerns for areas where HDs are compounded include unintentional contamination of food or drink with HD residue.

Because much of the compounding and administration of HDs throughout the United States is done in outpatient or clinic settings with the patients and their family members proximal to compounding, storage, and administration areas, care must be taken to minimize contamination and to maximize the effectiveness of cleaning (decontamination) activities. Design of these areas must include surfaces that are readily cleaned and decontaminated. Upholstered and carpeted surfaces must be avoided because they are not readily cleanable. Locating break areas and refreshment areas for staff, patients, and others away from areas of potential contamination is also critical in reducing unwanted exposure.[26]

PROTECTIVE EQUIPMENT

PPE includes items, such as gloves, gowns, respirators, goggles, and face shields, that provide a physical barrier from hazardous physical or chemical exposures. PPE is designed to be used in conjunction with engineering controls and safe work practices to protect individual workers while they are wearing it. PPE is not designed to reduce environmental contamination. PPE is advocated for all workers who perform any activities involving HDs.[21;26;36] Recent studies show the number of job categories potentially exposed to HDs extends beyond those that are directly involved with compounding and administration.[24;50–52] Thus, it is important to emphasize the use of PPE when handling HDs.

For compounding sterile doses of HDs, PPE must meet the requirements of USP Chapter <797> to maintain product sterility and the requirements of USP Chapter <800> to protect the worker.[26;49] Gowns, head and hair covers, two pairs of shoe covers, and two pairs of chemotherapy gloves are required for compounding sterile HDs.[26] USP Chapter <797> requires a surgical mask to be worn during sterile compounding.[49] For all other activities, a facility's SOP must describe the appropriate PPE to be worn based on its occupational safety plan and assessment of risk.[26] The NIOSH HD list contains a table of PPE and engineering controls for working with HDs in healthcare settings, which provides guidance for PPE use with each HD handling activity.[30] Consider all PPE worn when handling HDs to be contaminated with at minimum trace quantities of HDs. PPE must be placed in an appropriate waste container and further disposed of per local, state, and federal regulations.[26] Because vials may have significant HD residue on the outside and HD compounding transfers residue to gloves, the outside glove used to compound HD doses should be considered contaminated. NIOSH has created a workplace solution on PPE available on the NIOSH website.[53] PPE requirements for compounding sterile preparations that are not hazardous are further described in Chapter 13. The following section in this chapter elaborates on PPE use in compounding or handling HD CSPs and items considered contaminated.

Gloves and Best Practices

Gloves are essential for handling HDs. Studies on gloves indicate that many latex and nonlatex materials are effective protection against permeation from many HDs.[54–56] Most studies found permeability of gloves to HDs to be dependent on the drug, gloving material, thickness of gloves, and exposure time.

ASTM developed test standard D6978-05 (2013) for assessing the resistance of medical gloves to permeation by chemotherapy drugs.[56] Gloves that meet this standard earn the designation chemotherapy gloves. Gloves selected for use with HDs must meet this ASTM standard.[26] There is a second ASTM standard F739-99A, which uses a standard test method for permeation of liquids and gases through protective clothing materials under conditions of continuous contact.[56] In a recent report, it was noted that ASTM F739 has been used instead of the chemotherapy glove standard, ASTM D6978-05, to evaluate gloves.[56] The standard used to test the gloves should be listed on the glove box. NIOSH, ASHP, and USP state gloves should be tested to the ASTM D6978 standard.[21;22;26;36] Practitioners should be proactive, assess the standard of testing of the gloves being used for HD handling, and only use gloves appropriately tested to the ASTM D6978 standard.

Some antineoplastic HDs, such as carmustine and thiotepa, pass through gloving materials more rapidly than other drugs.[54] When handling HDs, double-gloving is suggested to provide more protection.[21;55] Wearing two pairs of gloves allows for removal of the outer glove while the skin of the hand and wrist is still covered. The inner glove should be worn under the cuff and the outer glove over the cuff to accomplish this. Changing the outer glove while retaining the inner glove during HD handling is a work practice that provides added protection against skin contact with HDs. During sterile compounding, the outer glove must be sterile. The outer glove may be wiped off with a sterile alcohol wiper to reduce any HD or microbial contamination on the glove. Ensure that a supply of sterile chemotherapy gloves is available near the C-PEC to allow for glove changing if needed.

USP Chapter <800> states the following[26]:

- Chemotherapy gloves should be worn for handling all HDs including nonantineoplastics and for reproductive risk only HDs.
- Chemotherapy gloves must be powder-free because powder can contaminate the work area and can adsorb and retain HDs.
- Gloves must be inspected for physical defects before use. Do not use gloves with pin holes or weak spots.
- Two pairs of chemotherapy gloves are required for compounding sterile HDs.
- When used for sterile compounding, the outer chemotherapy gloves must be sterile.
- Chemotherapy gloves should be changed every 30 minutes unless otherwise recommended by the manufacturer's documentation and must be changed when torn, punctured, or contaminated.
- Hands must be washed with soap and water after removing gloves.

Additional best practices for gloves include the following:

- Wear double gloves at all times when handling drug vials, including while performing inventory control procedures and when assembling HDs prior to compounding, because vials are known to have drug residue on the outside.[21]
- The use of two pairs of chemotherapy gloves is required for compounding as a work practice as well as for improved resistance to permeation.[21;55]
- Once compounding is completed, remove outer gloves and contain them in a disposal bag within the C-PEC. Discard as trace waste unless the gloves are heavily contaminated (ie, from a spill, leak or cleaning the C-PEC).[26]
- In the C-PEC, the inner glove is worn to affix labels and place the preparation into a sealable containment bag for transport. (*Note:* Transport bags must never be placed on the C-PEC work surface during compounding to avoid inadvertent contamination of the bag's outside surface and because the transport bag is nonsterile.)

- When removing the outer gloves, the contaminated glove fingers must only touch the outer contaminated surface of the glove, never the inner surface. If the inner glove becomes contaminated, both pairs of gloves must be changed.
- When removing any PPE, care must be taken to avoid putting contamination into the environment. Both the inner and outer gloves should be considered contaminated. Glove surfaces must never touch the skin or any surface that may be touched by the unprotected skin of others.
- Contain and dispose of contaminated inner and outer gloves as trace chemotherapy waste unless they are overtly contaminated (eg, from cleaning up a spill). Then dispose as hazardous waste.

Glove Practices in a Compounding Aseptic Containment Isolator

Compounding aseptic containment isolators (CACIs) are equipped with attached gloves or gauntlets. These gloves or gauntlets should be considered contaminated once the CACI has been used for compounding HDs. Contamination from the gloves or gauntlets may be transferred to the surfaces of all items within the cabinet. Gloves and gauntlets must be surface cleaned after compounding is complete. USP Chapter <800> and USP Chapter <797> require that the glove closest to the CSP during sterile compounding must be sterile.[26;49]

Gowns and Best Practices

Gowns or coveralls are worn during the compounding of sterile preparations to maintain sterility and protect the worker from the preparation.[26;49] The selection of gowning materials depends on the goal of the process. Chapter 13 reviews proper gowning technique and selection for non-HD sterile compounding. Personal protective gowns are recommended during the handling of HD CSPs to protect the worker from inadvertent exposure to extraneous drug residue on surfaces or generated during the compounding process. Guidelines for the safe handling of HDs recommend the use of gowns for compounding in a C-PEC, administration, spill control, and waste management to protect the worker from contamination by any residue generated during these processes.[21;22;36]

USP Chapter <800> specifies that a gown worn for HD protection must adhere to the following[26]:

- Gowns must be disposable and shown to resist permeability by HDs.
- Gowns must be selected based on the HDs handled. Disposable gowns made of polyethylene-coated polypropylene or other laminate materials offer better protection than those made of uncoated materials.
- Gowns must close in the back (ie, no open front), be long sleeved, and have closed cuffs that are elastic or knit.
- Gowns must not have seams or closures that can allow HDs to pass through.
- Gowns must be changed per the manufacturer's information on permeation of the gown. If no permeation information is available for the gowns used, change them every 2 to 3 hours or immediately after a spill or splash.
- Gowns used during HD handling must not be worn in areas without HDs in order to avoid spreading HD contamination and exposing other healthcare workers.
- Cloth laboratory coats, surgical scrubs, isolation gowns, or other absorbent materials are not appropriate protective outerwear when handling HDs because they permit the permeation of HDs, and they can hold spilled drugs against the skin, thereby increasing exposure. Clothing may also retain HD residue from contact and may transfer to other healthcare workers or various surfaces.

Washing of nondisposable clothing contaminated with HD residue should only be done according to facility policy, as drug residue may be transferred to other clothing. Potentially contaminated clothing must not be taken home under any circumstances. There are no specific standards for gowns or gowning materials to be tested for HD permeation. As a precaution, HD gowns should be coated and labeled to have permeability resistance to HDs per manufacturer testing.[26]

Studies on the effectiveness of disposable gowns in resisting permeation and penetration by HDs found variation in the protection provided by different available materials. In an evaluation of polypropylene-based gowns, it was found that polypropylene spunbond nonwoven material alone and polypropylene-polyethylene copolymer spunbond provided little protection against permeation by a battery of aqueous- and nonaqueous-based HDs.[57] Various constructions of polypropylene (eg, spunbond/meltblown/spunbond [SMS]) resulted in materials that are completely impermeable or only slightly permeable to HDs. It was noted that these coated materials are similar in appearance to several other nonwoven materials but perform differently. Workers could expect to be protected from exposure for up to 4 hours when using the coated gowning materials.[57] Similar findings in a study of 6 disposable gowning materials and 15 HDs have been reported.[58] Thus, justifying the need for HD gowns to be labeled as resistant to HD permeability.

Contamination of gowns during glove changes must be considered. If the inner pair of gloves requires changing, a gown change may be needed. Gowns should be removed carefully and properly disposed of as trace contaminated waste to avoid becoming a source of contamination to other staff and the environment.[21;26] Gowns used for cleaning or spill management and other uses may be more heavily contaminated. These gowns should be contained in sealable bags and discarded as bulk hazardous waste.

Additional best practices for gowns include the following:

- Wear protective gowns during compounding HDs, during administration, when handling waste from patients recently treated with HDs, and when cleaning up spills of HDs.[21;22;36]
- Wash hands after removing and disposing of the gown.

Compounding sterile HDs in an enclosed environment, such as a CACI, is not exempt from gown use.[49] Protective gown use is prudent because the process of handling drug vials and final preparations and accessing the isolator's pass-throughs may present an opportunity for HD contamination.

Additional Personal Protective Equipment

USP Chapter <797> defines required garbing for all personnel compounding sterile preparations.[49] Shoe and hair coverings must be worn during the sterile compounding process to minimize particulate contamination of the compounding environment and the sterile preparation.[49] With the potential for HD contamination on the floor in the compounding and administration areas, shoe coverings are also used as contamination control mechanisms.

> When compounding HDs, a second pair of shoe covers must be donned before entering the C-SEC and doffed when exiting the C-SEC. Outer shoe covers worn in HD handling areas must not be worn to other areas to avoid spreading HD contamination and exposing other health-care workers.[26]

Donning PPE for Sterile Compounding per USP Chapter <797>

Prior to entering the C-SEC, personnel shall don PPE in an order that reduces risk of contamination.[49] First, don two pairs of shoe covers, a head and facial hair cover (if needed), and a face mask. Then clean hands and forearms with soap and running warm water. Dry skin completely and then don a disposable HD gown. Don the inner glove (may be sterile or nonsterile and must be ASTM D6978 rated) and cover with the gown cuff. Sterile chemotherapy gloves are available inside the C-SEC adjacent to the C-PEC and should be the last item donned before compounding begins.[49] Further detail about donning PPE for sterile compounding is described in Chapter 13.

In addition to garb that is designed to maintain sterility, additional PPE may be needed to protect personnel.[26] Eye and face protection should be used whenever there is a possibility of exposure from splashing or uncontrolled aerosolization of HDs (eg, containing a spill or damaged shipping carton). Face shields in combination with goggles may be used to provide a full range of protection against splashes to the face and eyes. Although face shields provide improved skin protection, face shields alone do not provide full eye and face protection.[26;53] Similar circumstances warrant the use of a respirator. Surgical masks required in sterile compounding do not provide worker protection in these circumstances. All workers that utilize a respirator must be fit tested and trained to use the appropriate respirator according to OSHA respirator standards.[44] The appropriate size respirator must be available at all times.

Doffing and Disposal of Used PPE

In the doffing process, chemotherapy gloves worn during compounding must be carefully removed and discarded immediately into a waste container approved for trace contaminated waste inside the C-PEC, or it must be contained in a sealable bag for discarding outside the C-PEC.[26] Then, outer shoe covers and hair covers must be removed (while wearing gloves) when leaving the compounding area, and disposed of in the trace contaminated waste container before leaving the C-SEC. Shoe coverings that are overtly contaminated (eg, from spill cleanup) must be disposed as hazardous waste. The remaining steps of doffing PPE after compounding are described in Chapter 13 and are applicable to HD and non-HD compounding.

All PPE worn when handling HDs should be considered contaminated with at a minimum trace quantities of HDs.[26] PPE that was overtly contaminated (ie, during cleaning the C-PEC or from a spill) must be disposed of as hazardous waste. PPE must be placed in an appropriate waste container and further disposed of per local, state, and federal regulations.

WORK PRACTICES

With or without supplemental engineering controls, no ISO 5 C-PECs alone provide perfect containment of HD residues. Workers must recognize the limitations of the equipment and accommodate them with appropriate work practices.

Work Practices for Sterile Compounding of HDs

Work practices for the compounding of sterile HDs is essential to minimize contamination and maximize productivity. Personnel should be organized in their approach to compounding and collect all HDs and supplies needed to complete a sterile dose or batch, including the labels, prior to starting the preparation. Clean reusable bins are useful for transferring items into the C-SEC for compounding. Supplies and HDs for individual doses may be assembled and placed into separate bins prior to transfer to the C-SEC. Additional chemotherapy gloves may also be placed in the bins. This practice should eliminate the need to exit the Class II BSC or CACI once compounding has begun. Bins must be decontaminated and disinfected after being placed into the C-PEC prior to further use.

When working in a C-PEC, the following best practices should be considered:

- Do not place unnecessary items in the work area of the C-PEC.
- Do not overcrowd the C-PEC.
- Transport bags must never be placed in the C-PEC during compounding to avoid inadvertent HD contamination of the outside surface of the bag.
- Follow appropriate decontamination practices for all surfaces in the C-PEC and anything else exposed to HDs.
- Seal and then decontaminate surfaces of waste and sharps container before removing them from the C-PEC.
- Hands should be washed with soap and running water, and all PPE must be replaced after decontaminating the C-PEC and before beginning sterile compounding.
- Disinfection of all work surfaces in a C-PEC must occur per USP Chapter <797> standards (further described in Chapter 14).
- USP Chapter <800> notes that when compounding HD preparations in a C-PEC, a plastic-backed preparation mat should be placed on the work surface of the C-PEC.[26]
- The mat should be changed immediately if a spill occurs and regularly during use. It should be discarded at the end of the daily compounding activity. A large mat that might block the front or rear grilles must be avoided.
- Bottles, wipers, and waste containers left in the C-PEC should be considered potentially contaminated with HDs. Any items that are to be removed from the C-PEC must be contained in clean sealable bags prior to removal. These items may be cleaned, disinfected, and replaced in the C-PEC using clean gloves.

SUPPLEMENTAL ENGINEERING CONTROLS

USP Chapter <800> describes an adjunct control (also known as a containment supplemental engineering control) that provides additional levels of protection during compounding or administration of HDs.[26] The device most frequently discussed in this category is the *CSTD*, which is defined by NIOSH and USP Chapter <800> as a drug transfer device that mechanically prohibits the transfer of environmental contaminants into the system and the escape of hazardous drug or vapor concentrations outside the system.[21;26] USP Chapter <800> outlines a requirement that CSTDs be used for administering antineoplastic HDs, and that CSTDs should be used in the compounding process when the dosage form allows. CSTDs are not an alternative for PPE used in the compounding or administration of HD, nor are they an alternative for use of primary and secondary engineering controls in the compounding process.

In originally defining the CSTD, NIOSH did not specify design or performance criteria for what constitutes an effective CSTD.[21] In 2015, NIOSH published draft performance test protocols and vapor containment performance test protocols for CSTDs used during pharmacy compounding and administration, but the drafts have yet to be finalized.[59;60] A number of devices marketed as CSTDs have been around since 2004. The U.S. Food and Drug Administration (FDA) designated these devices as Class II medical devices not requiring premarket approval.[61] The FDA 510(k) process neither establishes independent performance standards for devices submitted as "substantially equivalent," nor does it test or approve these devices. Based on a successful review of the 510(k) submission, the FDA clears the new device for sale in the United States.[61] Many devices marketed for sterile compounding or administration have been cleared by the FDA 510(k) process under various product codes. Some devices marketed and used for HD compounding are not CSTDs by definition and may not be appropriate for HD use. The FDA created the product code ONB specifically for a closed antineoplastic and HD reconstitution and transfer system.[62] Although the FDA does not independently test applications under this code, the application process is more stringent for the manufacturer. Products that are marketed as CSTDs but have not been cleared by the FDA under Product Code ONB should not be considered CSTDs.

In the absence of a performance standard, some CSTDs have been shown in peer-reviewed studies to limit the potential of generating aerosols and reduce HD contamination in the workplace.[63–67] Despite all the published research, not all unique CSTDs have been studied, and no marker has been shown to be superior in measuring CSTD effectiveness or has been universally adopted. USP Chapter <800> states there is no certainty that all CSTDs will perform adequately unless the following occurs:

> Until a published universal performance standard for evaluation of CSTD containment is available, users should carefully evaluate the performance claims associated with available CSTDs based on independent, peer-reviewed studies and demonstrated containment reduction.[26]

The conclusion of USP is reinforced by the analysis of related CSTD literature.[68]

Additional best practices for CSTDs include the following:

- CSTDs known to be physically or chemically incompatible with a specific HD must not be used for that HD.

- When CSTDs are not able to be utilized, aseptic technique and negative pressure technique should be utilized during compounding practices.[22;36]
- Select a CSTD that has been evaluated by all potential users (pharmacy and nursing staffs), health and safety staff, and human factors staff if available for compatibility with work practices.
- NIOSH and ASHP recommend the use of a CSTD in conjunction with a complete HD safe handling program, including a C-PEC, PPE, and best work practices.[21;22;36]
- Select a CSTD that does not inhibit laminar flow when compounding or prevent clean air from reaching the critical sites of the CSTD, vials, or syringes during use with sterile products in an engineering control.
- CSTDs are not a substitute for good work practices or precleaning of HD vials.
- Select a CSTD system that reduces HD escape during all work practices (eg, vial transfer, syringe transfer, bag transfer, and HD transfer during administration).
- Select a CSTD that has a vial adaptor that locks onto the HD vial, has a syringe adaptor that locks onto the HD syringe, or provides an integrated syringe system and locks onto intravenous administration sets to prevent removal during or after administration. Removal of CSTD components allows leakage and transfer of contamination to the gloves of workers, to other work surfaces, and to the general environment.

TRAINING AND DEMONSTRATING COMPETENCE

All staff involved in compounding sterile HDs must be trained in the standard and stringent aseptic techniques necessary for working with HD CSPs.[26;49] Once trained, staff must demonstrate competence by an objective method and competency must be reassessed on a regular basis (see Chapters 3, 4, and 5 for details).[21;26]

USP Chapter <800> requires the following[26]:

- All personnel who handle HDs must be trained based on their job functions.
- Training must occur before the employee independently handles HDs.
- The effectiveness of training for HD handling competencies must be demonstrated by each employee.
- Personnel competency must be reassessed at least every 12 months.
- Personnel must be trained prior to the introduction of a new HD or new equipment and prior to a new or significant change in process or SOP.
- All training and competency assessment must be documented.

Additionally, USP Chapter <800> specifies the scope and focus of the training, which must include the following[26]:

- Overview of entity's list of HDs and their risks
- Review of the entity's SOPs related to handling of HDs
- Proper use of PPE
- Proper use of equipment and devices (eg, engineering controls)
- Response to known or suspected HD exposure
- Spill management
- Proper disposal of HDs and trace-contaminated materials

DEACTIVATING, DECONTAMINATING, CLEANING, AND DISINFECTING

Per USP Chapter <800>, "all areas where HDs are handled and all reusable equipment and devices must be deactivated, decontaminated and cleaned."[26] Written SOPs must be established that list the training requirements necessary for personnel, the agents used, the frequency, and documentation requirements for deactivation, decontamination, and cleaning.[26] Additionally, personnel completing these procedures must wear appropriate PPE that protects them from HD contamination and the cleaning agent used, which includes impermeable disposable gowns and two pairs of chemotherapy gloves, at minimum.[26]

The purpose of decontamination is to remove HD residue.[26] Multiple guidelines agree that decontamination of areas where HDs are stored, mixed, administered, or otherwise handled is critical to reduce the levels of HD residue on various surfaces.[21;22;26;36] USP Chapter <800> states that "decontamination occurs by inactivating, neutralizing, or physically removing HD residue from non-disposable surfaces and transferring it to absorbent, disposable materials (e.g., wipers, pads, or towels) appropriate to the area being cleaned."[26] It is preferred to deactivate or render inert a hazardous substance, but no single process has been found to deactivate all currently available HDs.[26;69;70] For C-PEC surfaces used in the sterile compounding of HDs, there is still a need for disinfection using sterile alcohol after decontamination.[26;49]

Decontamination should be conducted per manufacturer recommendations of the cleaning agents and surface, as some cleaning agents may damage surfaces. Researchers have shown that strong oxidizing agents, such as sodium hypochlorite and hydrogen peroxide, are effective deactivators of many HDs.[71–74] However, sodium hypochlorite can damage stainless steel surfaces, which is a common material used in cleanroom design and C-PECs, and additional steps may be necessary to neutralize the agent or remove it from the surface to prevent breakdown.[26;70]

A C-PEC must be decontaminated with appropriate solutions, then disinfected at least daily.[26] Decontamination of the work surface of the C-PEC must occur between compounding of different HDs in addition to any time a spill or voluntary interruption occurs.[26] The area under a C-PEC work tray requires at least monthly deactivation, decontamination, and cleaning.[26] Prior to accessing the work tray, all other C-PEC surfaces should be thoroughly decontaminated and cleaned. Respiratory protection may need to be donned because accessing the work tray compromises the containment of the device.[26]

It is important to note that despite decontamination agents and procedures being completed, it is possible for HD surface contamination to remain detectable on surfaces.[75] Thus, establishing the importance of properly utilizing PPE and executing all best practices in regard to HD handling is essential for decreasing the risk of any exposure to personnel.

Spill Control

Spill management and control is an important aspect of handling HD CSPs and manufactured HD vials. Per USP Chapter <800>, policies and procedures must be developed to attempt to prevent spills and outline the cleanup of HD spills. The SOPs must specify who is responsible for spill management, the type of PPE required for cleanup, and must address the size and scope of the spill.[26] Spill kits containing all of the materials needed to clean up HD spills should be assembled or purchased and be readily available in all areas where HDs are routinely handled. The SOP must outline where the kits are located and the spill kit's capacity.[26] Spills must be contained and cleaned up immediately by workers trained in spill management and the use of PPE and NIOSH-certified respirators.[26] Signs must be available to warn of restricted access to the spill area.[26] SOPs should describe how to establish access to workers trained to follow the OSHA Hazardous Waste Operations and Emergency Response Standard who may provide spill management in the event of a large spill.[76]

If a spill occurs, the circumstances and management of the spill must be documented.[26] Staff and nonemployees exposed to an HD spill should also complete an incident report or exposure form and report to the designated emergency service for initial evaluation per facility SOPs. All spill cleanup materials, including PPE utilized, must be disposed of as hazardous waste.[26] Appropriate methods of cleaning should follow the initial spill cleanup process.[36]

WIPE SAMPLING

Routine environmental wipe sampling for HD residue is recommended by USP Chapter <800> to survey HD surface contamination.[26]

When completed, USP Chapter <800> states surface wipe sample areas should include the following:

- Interior of the C-PEC and equipment contained in it
- Pass-through chambers
- Surfaces in staging or work areas near the C-PEC
- Areas adjacent to the C-PEC (eg, floors directly under the C-PEC, staging and dispensing area)
- Areas immediately outside the HD buffer room of the C-SCA
- Patient administration areas

Ultimately, the sampling practice can help reveal the effectiveness of CSTDs, C-PECs, decontamination practices, SOPs, and work practices of those handling HDs in sampled areas. This practice is a recommended addition to a comprehensive HD handling program.[77] However, there are currently no certifying agencies for vendors of wipe sampling kits and no standard for acceptable limits for HD surface contamination.[26;77]

Wipe sampling technology has evolved in recent past.[78] Historically limited to time- and resource-consuming analytical methods of gas chromatography, high performance liquid chromatography, and ultra-high performance liquid chromatography used in tandem with mass spectrometry, analytical methods have expanded to lateral flow immune assay, which can produce results in real time.[67;78] Currently, the principle of as low as reasonably achievable (ALARA) is recommended for evaluating and assessing HD handling practices from HD wipe sampling data with known limitations.[77]

CONTAINMENT AND DISPOSAL

USP Chapter <800> indicates that all personnel performing cleaning or waste removal in HD handling areas must be trained in appropriate procedures to prevent HD contamination and following all applicable local, state, and federal regulations.[26]

In 1976, the Environmental Protection Agency (EPA) enacted the Resource Conservation and Recovery Act (RCRA) to provide a mechanism for tracking hazardous waste from its generation to its disposal.[79] These regulations apply to pharmaceuticals and chemicals discarded by pharmacies, hospitals, clinics, and other commercial entities. In 2019, the EPA published the final rule titled "Management Standards for Hazardous Waste Pharmaceuticals and Amendment to the P075 Listing for Nicotine."[80] This final rule outlines requirement for healthcare facilities that are small quantity generators (SQGs) or large quantity generators (LQGs) of hazardous waste to follow subpart P of 40 CFR part 266 within the final rule for all hazard waste pharmaceuticals.[76;80]

Per the EPA final rule, a *hazardous waste pharmaceutical* is "a solid medication waste that is listed or exhibits hazardous characteristics (i.e. toxicity, corrosivity, ignitability, reactivity)."[80] For simplicity sake, if feasible, a facility may consider defining all pharmaceuticals as a hazard waste pharmaceutical and dispose of all agents (unless incompatible or metal containing) as hazardous waste.[81] For intents and purposes of this book's chapter, all drugs considered HD by NIOSH are considered hazardous waste due to toxicity potential. EPA guidance for pharmaceuticals must also be applied to partially filled containers, contaminated pharmaceutical spill cleanup materials, PPE, and electronic nicotine delivery systems.[80] The EPA no longer categorizes empty containers that once held hazardous pharmaceuticals as hazardous waste. However, OSHA and USP Chapter <800> continue to designate HD contaminated items, such as PPE, empty vials, and syringes used in HD compounding, be handled as trace waste.[26;81]

Best practices for defining hazardous drug waste and corresponding disposal SOPs include the following[81]:

- Separate streams of creditable waste, hazardous waste, incompatible metal bearing waste, and controlled substances.
- Develop a standard waste management chart.
- Partner with environmental services to sequester and dispose of nonpharmaceutical hazardous waste, such as cleaning agents.
- Develop a list of pharmaceutical agents that are hazardous and metal-bearing. Integrate this review into formulary addition and maintenance processes.
- Educate pharmacy and nursing staff on hazardous waste pharmaceuticals' disposal and container standards.

Once hazardous waste has been identified, it must be collected, stored, and transported according to specific EPA and Department of Transportation (DOT) requirements.[79;82] Properly labeled, leak-proof, and spill-proof containers of nonreactive plastic are required for areas where hazardous waste is generated. DOT Packing Group II containers are required for transportation.[83]

Only individuals who meet OSHA-mandated hazardous waste awareness training may transport the waste containers from satellite accumulation to the storage sites.[84;85] Hazardous waste must be properly manifested and transported by a federally permitted hazardous waste transporter to a federally permitted hazardous waste storage, treatment, or disposal facility.[76;82] A licensed contractor may be hired to manage the hazardous waste program. Investigation of a contractor, including verification of possession and type of license, should be completed and documented before a contractor is engaged.

SUMMARY

An effective safety program for the handling of sterile doses of HDs must encompass both HD preparation and worker protection. USP Chapter <800>, NIOSH, and OSHA have developed guidance for handling HDs in healthcare settings to improved worker safety. Technologies and regulations continue to be refined to support the safe handling of HDs, including improved storage, environment, engineering controls, monitoring practices, and work practices.

REFERENCES

1. Weisburger JH, Griwold DP, Prejean JD, et al. Tumor induction by cytostatics. The carcinogenic properties of some of the principal drugs used in clinical cancer chemotherapy; recent results. *Cancer Res.* 1975;52:1–17.
2. Harris CC. The carcinogenicity of anticancer drugs: a hazard in man. *Cancer*. 1976;37(2)(suppl):1014–1023. doi:10.1002/1097-0142(197602)37:2+<1014::aid-cncr2820370805>3.0.co;2-z.
3. Falck K, Gröhn P, Sorsa M, et al. Mutagenicity in urine of nurses handling cytostatic drugs. *Lancet*. 1979;1(8128):1250–1251. doi:10.1016/s0140-6736(79)91939-1bnbnbncv.
4. Ladik CF, Stoehr GP, Maurer MA. Precautionary measures in the preparation of antineoplastics. *Am J Hosp Pharm*. 1980;37:1184, 1186.
5. Crudi CB. A compounding dilemma: I've kept the drug sterile but have I contaminated myself? *NITA*. 1980;3:77–78.
6. Crudi CB, Stephens BL, Maier P. Possible occupational hazards associated with the preparation/administration of antineoplastic agents. *NITA*. 1982;5(4):264–265. **https://pubmed.ncbi.nlm.nih.gov/6922411/**.
7. Reynolds RD, Ignoffo R, Lawrence J, et al. Adverse reactions to AMSA in medical personnel. *Cancer Treat Rep*. 1982;66(10):1885. **https://pubmed.ncbi.nlm.nih.gov/6215121/**.
8. Hemminki K, Kyyrönen P, Lindbohm ML. Spontaneous abortions and malformations in the offspring of nurses exposed to anaesthetic gases, cytostatic drugs, and other potential hazards in hospitals, based on registered information of outcome. *J Epidemiol Community Health*. 1985;39(2):141–147. doi:10.1136/jech.39.2.141.
9. Valanis B, Vollmer W, Labuhn K, et al. Occupational exposure to antineoplastic agents and self-reported infertility among nurses and pharmacists. *J Occup Environ Med*. 1997;39(6):574–580. doi:10.1097/00043764-199706000-00013.
10. Valanis B, Vollmer WM, Steele P. Occupational exposure to antineoplastic agents: self-reported miscarriages and stillbirths among nurses and pharmacists. *J Occup Environ Med*. 1999;41(8):632–638. doi:10.1097/00043764-199908000-00004.

11. Fransman W, Roeleveld N, Peelen S, et al. Nurses with dermal exposure to antineoplastic drugs: reproductive outcomes. *Epidemiology*. 2007;18(1):112–119. doi:10.1097/01.ede.0000246827.44093.c1.

12. Skov T, Lynge E, Maarup B, et al. Risks for physicians handling antineoplastic drugs. *Lancet*. 1990;336(8728):1446. doi:10.1016/0140-6736(90)93148-i.

13. Skov T, Maarup B, Olsen J, et al. Leukaemia and reproductive outcome among nurses handling antineoplastic drugs. *Br J Ind Med*. 1992;49(12): 855–861. doi:10.1136/oem.49.12.855.

14. McDiarmid MA, Oliver MS, Roth TS, et al. Chromosome 5 and 7 abnormalities in oncology personnel handling anticancer drugs. *J Occup Environ Med*. 2010;52(10):1028–1034. doi:10.1097/JOM.0b013e3181f73ae6.

15. McDiarmid MA, Rogers B, Oliver MS. Chromosomal effects of non-alkylating drug exposure in oncology personnel. *Environ Mol Mutagen*. 2014;55(4):369–374. doi:10.1002/em.21852.

16. Pedersen-Bjergaard J, Andersen MK, Christiansen DH, et al. Genetic pathways in therapy-related myelodysplasia and acute myeloid leukemia. *Blood*. 2002;99(6):1909–1912. doi:10.1182/blood.v99.6.1909.

17. Baker ES, Connor TH. Monitoring occupational exposure to cancer chemotherapy drugs. *Am J Health Syst Pharm*. 1996;53(22):2713–2723. doi:10.1093/ajhp/53.22.2713.

18. Sessink PJM, Bos RP. Drugs hazardous to healthcare workers. Evaluation of methods for monitoring occupational exposure to cytostatic drugs. *Drug Saf*. 1999;20(4):347–359. doi:10.2165/00002018-199920040-00004.

19. Suspiro A, Prista J. Biomarkers of occupational exposure do anticancer agents: a minireview. *Toxicol Lett*. 2011;207(1):42–52. doi:10.1016/j.toxlet.2011.08.022.

20. Connor TH, Anderson RW, Sessink PJM, et al. Surface contamination with antineoplastic agents in six cancer treatment centers in Canada and the United States. *Am J Health Syst Pharm*. 1999;56(14):1427–1432. doi:10.1093/ajhp/56.14.1427.

21. National Institute for Occupational Safety and Health (NIOSH). *NIOSH Alert: Preventing Occupational Exposure to Antineoplastic and Other Hazardous Drugs in Health Care Settings*. Cincinnati, OH: NIOSH—Publications Dissemination; September 2004. **www.cdc.gov/niosh/docs/2004-165/**. Accessed January 4, 2023.

22. American Society of Health-System Pharmacists (ASHP). ASHP guidelines on handling hazardous drugs. *Am J Health Syst Pharm*. 2006;63:1172–1191.

23. Connor TH, DeBord DG, Pretty JR, et al. Evaluation of antineoplastic drug exposure of health care workers at three university-based US cancer centers. *J Occup Environ Med*. 2010;52(10):1019–1027. doi:10.1097/JOM.0b013e3181f72b63.

24. Hon C-Y, Teschke K, Chu W, et al. Antineoplastic drug contamination of surfaces throughout the hospital medication system in Canadian hospitals. *J Occup Environ Hyg*. 2013;10(7):374–383. doi:10.1080/15459624.2013.789743.

25. Salch SA, Zamboni WC, Zamboni BA, et al. Patterns and characteristics associated with surface contamination of hazardous drugs in hospital pharmacies. *Am J Health Syst Pharm*. 2019;76(9): 591–598. doi:10.1093/ajhp/zxz033.

26. USP <800> Hazardous drugs—handling in healthcare settings. In: *USP 43–NF 38*. Rockville, MD: United States Pharmacopeial Convention; 2020.

27. Occupational Safety and Health Administration (OSHA). *Guidelines for cytotoxic (antineoplastic) drugs*. Washington, DC: Occupational Safety and Health Administration, Office of Occupational Medicine; 1986:pub 8-1.1

28. Occupational Safety and Health Administration (OSHA). Section 18: state jurisdiction and state plans. In: Occupational Safety and Health Act of 1970 (OSH Act 1970).— **www.osha.gov/pls/oshaweb/owadisp.show_document?p_table=OSHACT&p_id=2743#18**. Accessed January 4, 2023.

29. Occupational Safety and Health Administration (OSHA). Hazardous Drugs. **https://www.osha.gov/hazardous-drugs**. Accessed January 4, 2023.

30. National Institute for Occupational Safety and Health (NIOSH). *NIOSH List of antineoplastic and other hazardous drugs in healthcare settings, 2016*. Cincinnati, OH: U.S. Department of Health and Human Services, Centers for Disease Control and Prevention, National Institute for Occupational Safety and Health; September 2016. **www.cdc.gov/niosh/docs/2016-161/default.html**. Accessed January 4, 2023.

31. National Institute for Occupational Safety and Health (NIOSH). *NIOSH List of antineoplastic and other hazardous drugs in healthcare settings, 2020*. Cincinnati, OH: U.S. Department of Health and Human Services, Centers for Disease Control and Prevention, National Institute for Occupational Safety and Health; 2020. **https://www.cdc.gov/niosh/docket/review/docket233c/pdfs/DRAFT-NIOSH-Hazardous-Drugs-List-2020.pdf**. Accessed August 18, 2023.

32. National Institute for Occupational Safety and Health (NIOSH). Workplace safety and health topics: hazardous drug exposures in healthcare. **https://www.cdc.gov/niosh/topics/hazdrug/default.html**. Accessed January 4, 2023.

33. American Society of Health-System Pharmacists (ASHP). ASHP technical assistance bulletin on handling cytotoxic and hazardous drugs. *Am J Hosp Pharm*. 1990;47(5):1033–1049. **https://pubmed.ncbi.nlm.nih.gov/2186621/**.

34. Occupational Safety and Health Administration (OSHA). Side-by-side comparison of OSHA's existing hazard communication standard (HCS 1994) vs. the revised hazard communication standard (HCS 2012). **https://www.osha.gov/hazcom/side-by-side**. Accessed January 4, 2023.

35. Occupational Safety and Health Administration (OSHA).Toxic and hazardous substances. 29 C.F.R. part 1910-1200. 2013. **www.osha.gov/pls/oshaweb/owadisp.show_document?p_table=STANDARDS&p_id=10099**. Accessed January 4, 2023.

36. Power LA, Coyne JW. ASHP guidelines on handling hazardous drugs. *Am J Health Syst Pharm*. 2018;75(24):1996–2031. doi:10.2146/ajhp180564.

37. Occupational Safety and Health Administration (OSHA). Bloodborne pathogens. 29 C.F.R. part 1910-1030. 2012. **www.osha.gov/pls/oshaweb/owadisp.show_document?p_table=STANDARDS&p_id=10051**. Accessed January 4, 2023.

38. TICE BCG (BCG Live) [prescribing information]. Roseland, NJ: Organon USA Inc.; February 2009. **www.fda.gov/downloads/BiologicsBloodVaccines/Vaccines/ApprovedProducts/UCM163039.pdf**. Accessed January 4, 2023.

39. IMLYGIC (talimogene laherparepvec) [prescribing information]. Thousand Oaks, CA: Amgen Inc.; February 2023.**http://pi.amgen.com/~/media/amgen/repositorysites/pi-amgen-com/imlygic/imlygic_pi.ashx**. Accessed July 29, 2023.

40. Redic KA, Fang K, Christen C, et al. Surface contamination of hazardous drug pharmacy storage bins and pharmacy distributor shipping containers. *J Oncol Pharm Pract*. 2018;24(2):91–97. doi:10.1177/1078155216679027.

41. Hedmer M, Georgiadi A, Bremberg ER, et al. Surface contamination of cyclophosphamide packaging and surface contamination with antineoplastic drugs in a hospital pharmacy in Sweden. *Ann Occup Hyg*. 2005;49(7):629–637. doi:10.1093/annhyg/mei042.

42. Schierl R, Herwig A, Pfaller A, et al. Surface contamination of antineoplastic drug vials: comparison of unprotected and protected vials. *Am J Health Syst Pharm*. 2010;67(6):428–429. doi:10.2146/ajhp080621.

43. Power LA, Sessink PJM, Gesy K, Charbonneau F. Hazardous drug residue on exterior vial surfaces: evaluation of a commercial manufacturing process. *Hosp Pharm*. 2014;49(4):355–362. doi:10.1310/hpj4904-355.

44. Occupational Safety and Health Administration (OSHA), U.S. Department of Labor. Respiratory protection. 29 C.F.R. part 1910.134. 1998. **www.osha.gov/pls/oshaweb/owadisp.show_document?p_table=STANDARDS&p_id=12716**. Accessed January 4, 2023.

45. Connor TH, Shults M, Fraser MP. Determination of the vaporization of solutions of mutagenic antineoplastic agents at 23 and 37°C using a desiccator technique. *Mutat Res*. 2000;470(1):85–92. doi:10.1016/s1383-5718(00)00105-4.

46. Kiffmeyer TK, Kube C, Opiolka S, et al. Vapor pressures, evaporation behavior and airborne concentrations of hazardous drugs: implications for occupational safety. *Pharm J*. 2002;268:331–337.

47. Larson RR, Khazaeli MB, Dillon HK. A new monitoring method using solid sorbent media for evaluation of airborne cyclophosphamide and other antineoplastic agents. *Appl Occup Environ Hyg*. 2003;18(2):120–131. doi:10.1080/10473220301435.

48. Power LA, Sessink PJ, Gesy K, et al. Hazardous drug residue on exterior vial surfaces: evaluation of a commercial manufacturing process. *Hosp Pharm*. 2014;49(4):355–362. doi:10.1310/hpj4904-355.

49. USP <797> Pharmaceutical compounding—sterile preparations. In: *USP NF 2023 Issue 1*. Rockville, MD: United States Pharmacopeial Convention; 2020.

50. Hon C-Y, Teschke K, Chua P, et al. Occupational exposure to antineoplastic drugs: identification of job categories potentially exposed throughout the hospital medication system. *Saf Health Work*. 2011;2(3): 273–281. doi:10.5491/SHAW.2011.2.3.273.

51. Hon CY, Teschke K, Shen H, et al. Antineoplastic drug contamination in the urine of Canadian healthcare workers. *Int Arch Occup Environ Health*. 2015;88(7):933–941. doi:10.1007/s00420-015-1026-1.

52. Hon CY, Teschke K, Demers PA, Venners S. Antineoplastic drug contamination on the hands of employees working throughout the hospital medication system. *Ann Occup Hyg*. 2014;58(6): 761–770. doi:10.1093/annhyg/meu019.

53. National Institute for Occupational Safety and Health (NIOSH). Personal protective equipment for healthcare workers who work with hazardous drugs. **www.cdc.gov/niosh/docs/wp-solutions/2009-106/pdfs/2009-106.pdf**. Published October 2008. Accessed August 18, 2023.

54. Wallemacq PE, Capron A, Vanbinst R, et al. Permeability of 13 different gloves to 13 cytotoxic agents under controlled dynamic conditions. *Am J Health Syst Pharm*. 2006;63(6):547–556. doi:10.2146/ajhp050197.

55. Landeck L, Gonzalez E, Koch OM. Handling chemotherapy drugs—Do medical gloves really protect? *Int J Cancer*. 2015;137(8):1800–1805. doi:10.1002/ijc.29058.

56. Connor TH, Power LA, Massoomi F, et al. Are gloves and gowns safe for handling chemotherapy? *Pharmacy Purchasing & Products*. **www.pppmag.com/download.php?file=documents/V12N1/pdfs/ppp_1501_ppe.pdf**. Accessed August 18, 2023.

57. Connor TH. An evaluation of the permeability of disposable polypropylene-based protective gowns to a battery of cancer chemotherapy drugs. *Appl Occup Environ Hyg*. 1993;8:785–789.

58. Harrison BR, Kloos MD. Penetration and splash protection of six disposable gown materials against fifteen antineoplastic drugs. *J Oncol Pharm Pract*. 1999;5:61–66.

59. National Institute for Occupational Safety and Health (NIOSH). A vapor containment performance protocol for closed system transfer devices used during pharmacy compounding and administration of hazardous drugs. **www.cdc.gov/niosh/docket/review/docket288/pdfs/a-vapor-containment-performance-protocol-for-closed-system-transfer-devices.pdf**. Accessed August 18, 2023.

60. National Institute for Occupational Safety and Health (NIOSH). A performance test protocol for closed system transfer devices used during pharmacy compounding and administration of hazardous drugs. **https://www.cdc.gov/niosh/docket/review/docket288a/pdfs/aperformancetestprotocolforclosedsystemtransferdevices.pdf**. Accessed August 18, 2023.

61. U.S. Food and Drug Administration (FDA), Center for Devices and Radiological Health. Premarket notification (510k) process. **www.fda.gov/medicaldevices/deviceregulationandguidance/howtomarketyourdevice/premarketsubmissions/premarketnotification510k/default.htm**. October 03, 2022. Accessed August 18, 2023.

62. U.S. Food and Drug Administration (FDA), Center for Devices and Radiological Health. Product code classification database: product code ONB. **www.accessdata.fda.gov/scripts/cdrh/cfdocs/cfPCD/classification.cfm?ID=ONB**. Accessed August 18, 2023.

63. Harrison BR, Peters BG, Bing MR. Comparison of surface contamination with cyclophosphamide and fluorouracil using a closed-system drug transfer device versus standard preparation techniques. *Am J Health Syst Pharm*. 2006;63(18):1736–1744. doi:10.2146/ajhp050258.

64. Clark BA, Sessink PJ. Use of a closed system drug-transfer device eliminates surface contamination with antineoplastic agents. *J Oncol Pharm Pract*. 2013;19(2):99–104. doi:10.1177/1078155212468367.

65. Bartel SB, Tyler TG, Power LA. Multicenter evaluation of a new closed system drug-transfer device in reducing surface contamination by antineoplastic hazardous drugs. *Am J Health Syst Pharm*. 2018;75(4):199–211. doi:10.2146/ajhp160948.

66. Forshay CM, Streeter SO, Salch SA, Eckel SF. Application of the 2015 proposed NIOSH vapor containment performance protocol for closed system transfer devices used during pharmacy compounding and administration of hazardous drugs. *J Oncol Pharm Pract*. 2019;25(5):1160–1166. doi:10.1177/1078155218787256.

67. Brechtelsbauer E. Identification and reduction of hazardous drug surface contamination through the use of a novel closed-system transfer device coupled with a point-of-care hazardous drug detection system. *Am J Health Syst Pharm*. November 12, 2022. Digital ahead of print.

68. McDiarmid MA, Polovich M, Power LA, et al. Published review of closed-system drug-transfer devices: Limitations and implications. *Am J Health Syst Pharm*. 2018;75(24):1982–1985. doi:10.2146/ajhp180631.

69. Roberts S, Khammo N, McDonnell G, Sewell GJ. Studies on the decontamination of surfaces exposed to cytotoxic drugs in chemotherapy workstations. *J Oncol Pharm Pract*. 2006;12(2):95–104. doi:10.1177/1078155206070439.

70. Queruau Lamerie T, Nussbaumer S, Décaudin B, et al. Evaluation of decontamination efficacy of cleaning solutions on stainless steel and glass surfaces contaminated by 10 antineoplastic agents. *Ann Occup Hyg*. 2013;57(4):456–469. doi:10.1093/annhyg/mes087.

71. Hansel S, Castegnaro M, Sportouch MH, et al. Chemical degradation of wastes of antineoplastic agents: cyclophosphamide, ifosfamide and melphalan. *Int Arch Occup Environ Health*. 1997;69(2):109–114. doi:10.1007/s004200050124.

72. Castegnaro M, De Méo M, Laget M, et al. Chemical degradation of wastes of antineoplastic agents. 2: Six anthracyclines: idarubicin, doxorubicin, epirubicin, pirarubicin, aclarubicin, and daunorubicin. *Int Arch Occup Environ Health*. 1997;70(6):378–384. doi:10.1007/s004200050232.

73. Contec Healthcare. Peridox RTU hazardous drug cleaning removal test report. **https://www.contecinc.com/hubfs/Website%20Assets/Product%20Center/Product%20Literature/Healthcare/Old%20Product%20Literature%20for%20TEMPORARY%20USE/peridox_rtu_hazardous-drug-cleaning-removal-test-summary.pdf?hsLang=en**. Accessed July 29, 2023.

74. Simon N, Guichard N, Odou P, et al. Efficiency of four solutions in removing 23 conventional antineoplastic drugs from contaminated surfaces. *PLoS One*. 2020;15(6):e0235131. doi:10.1371/journal.pone.0235131.

75. Arpino P, Yeomelakis J, Oommen A. Effectiveness of a decontamination procedure in a pharmacy buffer room contaminated by 5 antineoplastic agents. *Am J Health Syst Pharm*. 2020;77(24):2081–2088. doi:10.1093/ajhp/zxaa320.

76. United States Environmental Protection Agency (EPA). Code of Federal Regulation. General Requirements. 40 CFR Part 262.20 Subpart B. **https://www.ecfr.gov/current/title-40/chapter-I/subchapter-I/part-262/subpart-B/section-262.20**. Accessed January 2, 2023.

77. Connor TH, Zock MD, Snow AH. Surface wipe sampling for antineoplastic (chemotherapy) and other hazardous drug residue in healthcare settings: Methodology and recommendations. *J Occup Environ Hyg*. 2016;13(9):658–667. doi:10.1080/15459624.2016.1165912.

78. Connor TH, Smith JP. New approaches to wipe sampling methods for antineoplastic and other hazardous drugs in healthcare settings. *Pharm Technol Hosp Pharm*. 2016;1(3):107–114. doi:10.1515/pthp-2016-0009.

79. United States Environmental Protection Agency (EPA). The Resource Conservation and Recovery Act of 1976. U.S. Code Title 42. Chapter 82, Sections 6901–6992k. 1976. **www.epa.gov/laws-regulations/summary-resource-conservation-and-recovery-act**. Accessed January 2, 2023.

80. United States Environmental Protection Agency (EPA). Final rule: management standards for hazardous waste pharmaceuticals and amendment to the P075 listing for nicotine. 42 USC §6912, §6921-6924. 84 FR 5816. **https://www.federalregister.gov/documents/2019/02/22/2019-01298/management-standards-for-hazardous-waste-pharmaceuticals-and-amendment-to-the-p075-listing-for**. Accessed January 2, 2023.

81. Brechtelsbauer E, Shah S. Update on pharmaceutical waste disposal regulations: Strategies for success. *Am J Health Syst Pharm*. 2020;77(7):574–582. doi:10.1093/ajhp/zxz360.

82. U.S. Department of Transportation (DOT). Hazardous materials table, special provisions, hazardous materials communication, emergency response information, training requirements, and security plans. 49 CFR parts 172–172.123. **www.ecfr.gov/cgi-bin/text-idx?tpl=/ecfrbrowse/Title49/49cfr172_main_02.tpl**. Amended July 24, 2023. Accessed January 2, 2023.

83. Federal Motor Carrier Safety Association. How to comply with federal hazardous materials regulations. **www.fmcsa.dot.gov/regulations/hazardous-materials/how-comply-federal-hazardous-materials-regulations**. Updated July 18, 2022. Accessed January 2, 2023.

84. Occupational Safety and Health Administration (OSHA). Initial training. 29 CFR part 1910.120(e)(3)(i). **www.osha.gov/pls/oshaweb/owadisp.show_document?p_table=standards&p_id=9765**. Updated May 14, 2019. Accessed January 2, 2023.

85. Occupational Safety and Health Administration (OSHA). Hazardous waste operations and waste response. 29 CFR part 1910.120(q)(1–6). **www.osha.gov/pls/oshaweb/owadisp.show_document?p_table=standards&p_id=9765**. Updated May 14, 2019. Accessed January 2, 2023.

28

BATCH COMPOUNDING

Matthew M. Brown

INTRODUCTION

Batch compounding is the preparation of more than one compounded sterile preparation (CSP), as described in a master formulation record (MFR), in a single process that is expected to have uniform character and quality within specified limits.[1] The process may be simple (eg, dividing a single ingredient into multiple doses) or more complex (eg, combining multiple ingredients into a single product and then dividing it into multiple doses). Batch compounding should not be confused with batching the same drug for multiple patients if each is receiving an individualized, patient-specific dose. In this instance, each dose requires an individual compounding record. When batch compounding, each dose has the same container closure system, volume, and drug quantity and concentration. The process is performed following a MFR and must be documented on a compounding record. An example of batch compounding is preparing a standardized dose of a specific product to stock in anticipation of patient orders, such as antibiotic infusions or electrolytes. Alternatively, it could be multiple doses for a single patient at prescribed intervals, such as total parenteral nutrition (TPN) infusions for home infusion patients.

The compounding process may be sterile-to-sterile (ie, all components and starting supplies that come in contact with the final preparation are sterile) or nonsterile-to-sterile (ie, using nonsterile components or supplies in the compounding process before aseptic filtration or terminal sterilization). The process and compounding environment dictate the final beyond-use date (BUD) of the preparation. *United States Pharmacopeia* (USP) Chapters <797> and <795> provide a minimum set of standards for preparing CSPs and nonsterile preparations, respectively.[1;2]

REGULATORY CONSIDERATIONS FOR BATCH COMPOUNDING

In 2012, New England Compounding Center grievously injured 793 patients and killed 64 others across 10 states.[3] This event became a representation of the dangers of batch compounding without proper quality assurance activities and regulatory oversight. In response, Congress passed the Drug, Quality and Security Act (DQSA), which added 503B to the Food, Drug, and Cosmetic Act (FD&C). A 503A pharmacy operates as a traditional pharmacy, compounding products for an individual patient pursuant to a patient-specific prescription. State boards of pharmacy regulate 503A compounding. USP Chapter <797> and USP Chapter <795> set minimum standards for pharmacies operating under section 503A of the FD&C Act.[1;2;4] A 503B facility batches compound nonpatient-specific products for use in clinics or hospitals. The U.S. Food and Drug Administration (FDA) regulates 503B facilities, which must follow current good manufacturing practices (CGMP).

Facilities must be aware of the risks associated with batch compounding. Contamination or errors that occur while compounding a single product for an identified patient would, in theory, limit harm to a specific patient. In contrast, errors and contamination occurring during batch compounding have the potential to harm large numbers of patients, presenting a greater risk to the general public. Pharmacies engaging in batch compounding should carefully consider their internal quality assurance procedures, facilities, and regulatory requirements during process development.

Under section 503A of the FD&C, a pharmacist may only compound after the receipt of a valid patient-specific prescription; before receipt of a valid patient prescription based on an established provider, patient, and pharmacy relationship; or in limited quantities before the receipt of a valid patient-specific prescriptions.[4] FDA guidance for 503A pharmacies defines *limited quantity* as a 30-day supply as calculated by a documented 30-day usage period over the prior year as chosen by the compounder. Pharmacies may not distribute drugs compounded in advance until receipt of a valid, patient-specific prescription. "Restricting anticipatory compounding to limited quantities serves to limit the number of patients likely to be affected if there are drug product mix-ups or contamination."[5]

DOI 10.37573/9781585286492.028

In a hospital setting, there is often a need to have compounded preparations readily available for patients presenting critical needs. To meet this need, hospitals may batch compound and distribute products before receipt of a valid, patient-specific prescription, which is in violation of the prescription requirement for 503A pharmacies. As of this writing, the FDA has issued draft guidance for hospitals distributing compounded products prior to receiving a patient-specific prescription.[5;6]

- Drug product distribution is limited to facilities owned and controlled by the same entity that owns and controls the hospital pharmacy.
- Only patients within the owned and controlled healthcare facility may receive the products according to a patient-specific prescription or order.
- Compounding activities meet all other requirements outlined in the FD&C.

Hospitals that wish to distribute product across a broader geographic area, use sterility testing to extend BUDs, or compound nonpatient-specific products (eg, flush syringes administered without a patient order) should consider registering as a 503B facility.

MASTER FORMULATION RECORDS

A specific MFR must be developed to address desired attributes of the batched preparation (eg, final concentrations of ingredients, final pH, and osmolarity) and to ensure consistency and repeatability between batches. Required diluents, preservatives, and other excipients, antioxidants, chelating agents, and buffers should also be considered. A pharmacist must review the formulation to determine if the preparation meets formulation and stability requirements as well as physiologic norms for solution osmolarity and a pH appropriate for the intended route of administration. If used, procedures to calibrate or verify accuracy of equipment should be included. Additionally, all calculations required in compounding must be specified in the MFR. For example, the method for increasing the volume of a formula to allow for overfill must be indicated. An overfill factor may be specified so that calculations of required excess amounts are handled consistently for each ingredient.

MFRs must be written clearly and be easy to understand so personnel that follow procedures in the MFR can compound the batch preparation the same way each time. The order of addition of ingredients must be specified if a certain sequence is required (eg, calcium and phosphate or amino acids, dextrose, and lipids). A step-by-step procedure should be developed for all compounding activities, including in-process tests (eg, pH checks).

At a minimum, MFRs must include the following[2]:

- Name, strength or activity, and dosage form
- Ingredient identities and quality, including relevant characteristics (eg, purity grade, salt form, etc.)
- Type and size of container closure
- Complete instruction for preparation, including all equipment, supplies, compounding steps, and precautions
- Physical description of the final product
- BUD and storage requirements
- Stability reference to support selected BUD
- Quality control procedures
- Any information needed to complete the formulation (eg, pH adjustment, sterilization methods, etc.) and ensure repeatability

Prior to use, MFRs should be reviewed by at least two pharmacists to verify all calculations, information, and directions are correct. Pharmacies must have a document control process in place that documents revisions to the MFR.

Compounding and Batch Control Records

A compounding record documents the preparation of each CSP. In batch compounding, the MFR may be used to create the compounding record. To keep batches identical, all compounding activities must be reproduced uniformly by following the MFR, and activities and checks must be documented on the compounding record. See **Figures 28-1** and **28-2** for example MFR and compounding record templates, respectively.

A unique lot or control number must be assigned to each batch. A mechanism to generate and maintain lot numbers should be described in the facility standard operating procedures (SOPs). The batch control record can be a paper log that includes the assigned lot or control number, the date of compounding, the name of the compounded product, and any additional information required by the facility. It can also be maintained electronically or as part of an intravenous (IV) workflow system.

A compounding record must satisfy all USP quality control practices and include the following[1]:

- Name of the CSP, strength or activity, and dosage form
- Date and time of compounding
- Assigned lot or batch number
- Identification of individuals compounding and verifying the final product
- Name, strength or activity of ingredients or components, and chemical grades if pertinent
- Quantity of ingredients (weight or volume)
- Manufacturer's name or national drug code (NDC) number, lot numbers, and expiration dates of each component and ingredient

NAME OF PREPARATION (name, strength/activity, dosage form) ☐ USP monograph ☐ Assigned name
INGREDIENTS (name, strength/activity, quantity/amount)
CALCULATIONS ☐ Not applicable
EQUIPMENT
COMPATIBILITY AND STABILITY INFORMATION (including references, if available) ☐ Not applicable
MIXING AND PREPARATION INSTRUCTIONS (Include order and duration of mixing, temperature/other environmental controls, etc.)
CONTAINER AND CLOSURE TYPE (Note both storage and dispensing containers, if different.)
BUD ASSIGNED ☐ 12 hours ☐ 24 hours ☐ 4 days ☐ 10 days ☐ 45 days ☐ BUD assignment based on: ______________________ ☐ Other reference (list reference and note BUD): ______________________
PACKAGING/STORAGE REQUIREMENTS ☐ Refrigerate ☐ Freeze ☐ Protect from light
DESCRIPTION OF FINAL PREPARATION
SAMPLE LABEL
QUALITY CONTROL PROCEDURES AND EXPECTED RESULTS

BUD = beyond-use date.

FIGURE 28-1. Master formulation record template example

Source: Reprinted with permission of American Society of Health-System Pharmacists. Kienle PC. *The Chapter <797> Answer Book*. 2nd ed. Bethesda, MD: American Society of Health-System Pharmacists; 2023.

PREPARATION (name, strength/activity, dosage form):	Master Formulation Record
CALCULATIONS:	

INGREDIENT (name, strength/activity, dosage form)	AMOUNT (mL, g, etc.)	MFR	EXP DATE	LOT NUMBER

DATE AND TIME PREPARED:	Affix Label Here
CONTROL/RX/ORDER NUMBER:	
TOTAL QUANTITY COMPOUNDED:	
PHYSICAL DESCRIPTION:	
BEYOND-USE DATE:	
QUALITY CONTROL RESULTS (if applicable):	
Prepared by:	Checked by:

EXP = expiration, MFR = manufacturer

FIGURE 28-2. Compounding record template example

Source: Reprinted with permission of American Society of Health-System Pharmacists. Kienle PC. *The Chapter <797> Answer Book*. 2nd ed. Bethesda, MD: American Society of Health-System Pharmacists; 2023.

- Total quantity compounded
- Theoretical and final yield (eg, number of units)
- Assigned BUD and storage conditions
- Results of quality control procedures (eg, sterility testing, filter integrity testing, visual inspection, pH)
- Reference to the MFR
- Calculations

Compounding records may be paper-based or stored electronically in a pharmacy computer system with appropriate audit controls. Records must be kept organized and be easily retrievable. Using software that allows for barcode scanning of ingredients and photographic or gravimetric documentation of compounding can enhance the safety of the batch compounding process.[8] Each time a batch is compounded, a compounding record must be generated to document batch preparation and control.

Compounding records must include all quality control results, which may include sterility testing, content assays, filter integrity tests, biological indicator results, and visual inspection results. The theoretical yield of the batch (weight, volume, or units) must be specified on the compounding record. For frequently compounded batches, an anticipated yield may also be included. The actual yield also must be recorded. Discrepancies between theoretical or anticipated yields and actual yields must be investigated, and the results or corrective actions documented.

Compounding procedures must be checked and double-checked. Technicians must be adequately supervised by a licensed pharmacist in the compounding area. The pharmacist must check that correct ingredients are selected and that correct volumes or weights are added. Finally, the pharmacist must verify compounding accuracy and complete and record the results of all final release checks. When automated compounding devices (ACDs) are used, a pharmacist must verify the data entered into the ACD before compounding begins, and checks must verify the accuracy of ingredients delivered. The operator should periodically observe the automated compounding device during mixing to ensure its proper operation.[1] The expected weight based on the specific gravities of the ingredients and their respective volumes must be documented on the compounding record.

Other quality controls may be needed when multiple sterile ingredients are combined into a single sterile or nonsterile reservoir for subdivision into multiple units. Associated calculations must be performed and verified prior to the approval of the compounding record. Methods of sterilization and testing of preparations for sterility are discussed in Chapters 12 and 18. If there are doubts about whether a preparation has been properly prepared or sterilized, it must not be used.

In-process testing verifies the compounding environment and preparation meet established criteria during compounding. Sterile preparations must not be compounded in a buffer room that fails to meet environmental criteria. When the environment does not meet established criteria, the compounding of sterile preparations should immediately cease, and corrective action must be taken. Steps taken to correct the problem and their results must be documented.

In-process testing and checks may be as simple as visual inspections of physical properties (eg, color, odor, and clarity) or as complex as detailed chemical analyses for content. Checks for pH can easily be performed with a small, handheld meter. Verification of compounding device calibration (eg, repeater pump delivery volume or syringe volume) should occur prior to drug addition or filling operations.

INGREDIENT AND COMPONENT SELECTION

When appropriate and available, the compounding process should use FDA-approved commercial drug products.[1] Commercially manufactured drug products have been proven safe and effective by new drug application (NDA) or abbreviated new drug application (ANDA) processes. Drug manufacturers follow strict CGMP protocols, are regularly inspected by the FDA, and the final products are extensively tested for sterility and stability. Using commercially available sterile drugs prevents unnecessarily exposing patients to potentially ineffective or unsafe CSPs.[9]

Active pharmaceutical ingredients (APIs) used in CSPs must be accompanied by a certificate of analysis (COA) and meet the criteria in a USP monograph if one exists. COAs from FDA registered manufacturers of bulk drug substances establish that each lot received by the pharmacy meets USP monograph specifications.[1] If a USP monograph does not exist and the drug is not an FDA-approved drug, it must appear on the list of products approved by the FDA as acceptable for compounding. COAs should be kept per individual pharmacy or local board of pharmacy requirements on record retention.

When bulk ingredients are received without a COA from the manufacturer, they must be quarantined to prevent use until the manufacturer's COA can be obtained or assay testing is completed. If the pharmacy cannot perform assay tests, the material should be sent to a qualified laboratory.

PERSONNEL COMPETENCY

For sterile compounding, garbing competency, gloved fingertip and thumb testing, and media fill testing are the most critical validation processes for compounding competency. A media fill test is used to validate a sterilization or aseptic processing procedure. It ensures that engineering controls, personnel training, compounding procedure, and other processes result in a sterile product. Therefore, a media fill is required to mimic the most difficult processes in complexity and quantity. It is not appropriate to perform a media fill with 6 to 9 vials or 20 manipulations in a single IV bag and assume this demonstrates that personnel are competent enough to compound 250 syringes or fill 250 IV bags during a single batch session. For batch compounding, a failed media fill by a single compounder may indicate that a person needs additional training or practice with aseptic processes. Failed media fills by multiple personnel may indicate overly complex processes, SOP deficiencies, component sterility failure, or engineering control failure. Mitigating failure is critical for batch compounding, as deficiencies in the process have the potential to adversely affect many patients.

Sterility testing does not substitute for personnel competency evaluation of aseptic processing and does not guarantee that all articles in a batch are sterile. As USP Chapter <71> states, "These Pharmacopeial procedures (i.e, sterility tests) are not by themselves designed to ensure that a batch of product is sterile or has been sterilized. This is accomplished primarily by validation of the sterilization process or of the aseptic processing procedures."[10]

Equipment and Supplies Specifications

The MFR must specify all equipment, containers, and supplies needed for compounding. The brand name and model or item number of equipment and supplies must be listed as well as any applicable performance characteristics (eg, weight limits for scales). Specification of all details, such as lengths and diameters of tubing, ensures that the same items can be reordered if equipment malfunctions or supplies are depleted. For complicated equipment setups, a diagram can illustrate the proper sequence of assembly.

A pharmacy must ensure that equipment and devices used in compounding operate properly and are within acceptable tolerance limits. Records of equipment calibration, testing, maintenance, and cleaning should be kept on file. Routine maintenance checks should be performed as recommended by the equipment manufacturer. Each piece of equipment (scale, primary engineering control, pump, incubator, etc.) should have a dedicated record for the life of the equipment. This record should include installation qualifications, operational qualifications, validation studies, certifications, calibrations, routine or preventative maintenance records, and any troubleshooting or repair documentation.

Facility SOPs or the MFR must include requirements for cleaning and disinfecting the compounding area and equipment. All material and equipment kept in the compounding area must be easily cleanable. Requirements for packaging compounded preparations (eg, types of containers and methods of closure) should be included in the MFR. The final container for the sterile preparation must maintain its integrity (ie, sterility, identity, strength, quality, and purity) throughout the BUD.

Single-use sterile components purchased from licensed manufacturers should be used for any items that come in direct contact with sterile drug products or excipients. In-house preparation and sterilization of CSP supplies and components, such as syringes, tubing, filters, and vessels, is complicated, expensive, and introduces unnecessary risks to patient safety. For items used in presterilization mixing for nonsterile-to-sterile products, supplies that come into direct contact with the CSP must also be depyrogenated if appropriate.

Label

Labels must meet USP Chapter <797> or USP Chapter <795> labeling standards and any additional state defined requirements. A sample CSP label should be part of the MFR. Standardized label text must be developed for each commonly batched preparation to ensure consistency between batches. If compounding software that generates labels is not available, a pharmacist must verify that labels have the correct lot number, BUD, and storage conditions prior to printing and labeling. If preparations are compounded in advance, stored, and then dispensed to individual patients, both a preparation label and a final patient-specific label are required.

Visual Inspection

As a condition of release, each compounded unit should be inspected immediately after compounding against lighted white and black backgrounds for visible particulates or other foreign matter and proper fill volume. It is recommended that each product be observed for 5 seconds for each background. The final preparation must also be inspected for proper labeling, container leaks and integrity, and solution cloudiness, color, and volume. Defective preparations must immediately be discarded or marked and segregated to prevent their administration. When preparations are not distributed promptly after compounding, a predistribution inspection should be conducted because defects (eg, precipitation, cloudiness, and leakage) may develop.[1]

Compounding Accuracy

A pharmacist must verify that the preparation was compounded accurately with the correct ingredients, quantities, containers, and reservoirs. Any volume calibrations or syringe in-process checks must be verified on the compounding record along with any equipment calibration or verifications. Automated pump calibration must be verified before pumping and mixing. The volumes of each pumped ingredient must be checked to establish that the automated pump is within the accuracy limits set by the manufacturer.

Testing and Quarantine of Final Preparations

The MFR must list the appropriate checks and tests to ensure that batch CSPs are free from defects and meet all quality specifications. Sterile preparations must not be released until all quality specifications have been reviewed and all release requirements are met. Tests should include visual inspection and checks for compounding accuracy and formulation integrity (eg, sterility, pyrogenicity, and potency). End product sterility testing must be performed, and valid product stability documentation must be noted if required for the assigned BUD.[1] It is best practice to store quarantined products separate from other products to avoid dispensing a quarantined product prior to release. Segregation options include using color coded containers to store quarantined lots with seals or zip ties to prevent removal of product prior to release and having separate storage areas (eg, keeping totes with quarantined product locked in a segregated area).

IV Workflow and Compounding Software

If possible, electronic compounding software should be used. Software provides a multitude of benefits for compounders and patients. Most notably, barcode scanning can ensure that the proper product, component, or supply is selected. For sterile compounding, IV workflow software may be more appropriate for use. Compounding software can also ensure that MFRs meet all regulatory requirements, provide a mechanism to restrict access to modify the MFR based on user designation, and provide audit history. In the event of a recall, compounding software provides a quick and reliable method for finding impacted units and quickly alerting providers and patients if necessary. Many electronic medical record systems used by hospitals have compounding modules available. There are also multiple options available that are designed for hospital and retail settings.

SUMMARY

Batch compounding of CSPs requires strict adherence to procedure. Any failure in the process of compounding can lead to waste and pose a threat to patient safety. Batch compounding poses a much higher risk to the general public compared to patient specific compounding. Master formulation and compounding records establish a uniform approach to the compounding process, and utilization of compounding software can greatly improve patient safety.

REFERENCES

1. USP <797> Pharmaceutical compounding—sterile preparations. In: *2023: USP Compounding Compendium.* Rockville, MD: United States Pharmacopeial Convention; 2023: Issue 1. **https://doi.org/10.31003/USPNF_M99925_07_01**.
2. USP <795> Pharmaceutical compounding—non-sterile preparations. In: *2023: USP Compounding Compendium.* Rockville, MD: United States Pharmacopeial Convention; 2023: Issue 1. **https://doi.org/10.31003/USPNF_M99595_06_01**.
3. January 31, 2018: New England compounding center pharmacist sentenced for role in nationwide fungal meningitis outbreak [press release]. Boston, MA: U.S Department of Justice; January 31, 2018. **https://www.fda.gov/inspections-compliance-enforcement-and-criminal-investigations/press-releases/january-31-2018-new-england-compounding-center-pharmacist-sentenced-role-nationwide-fungal**. Accessed April 22, 2023.
4. U.S. Food & Drug Administration (FDA). United States CFR 21 USC § 353a. Pharmacy compounding. **https://uscode.house.gov/view.xhtml?hl=false&edition=prelim&path=%2Fprelim%40title21%2Fchapter9&req=granuleid%3AUSC-prelim-title21-section353a&num=0&saved=L3ByZWxpbUB0aXRsZTIxL2NoYXB0ZXI5%7CZ3JhbnVsZWlkOlVTQy1wcmVsaW0tdGl0bGUyMS1jaGFwdGVyOQ%3D%3D%7C%7C%7C0%7Cfalse%7Cprelim**. Accessed April 22, 2023.
5. U.S. Food & Drug Administration (FDA). *Prescription Requirement Under Section 503A of Federal Food, Drug, and Cosmetic Act: Guidance for Industry*. Silver Spring, MD: U.S. Food & Drug Administration; December 2016. **https://www.fda.gov/files/drugs/published/Prescription-Requirement-Under-Section-503A-of-the-Federal-Food–Drug–and-Cosmetic-Act-Guidance-for-Industry.pdf**. Accessed April 22, 2023.
6. U.S. Food & Drug Administration (FDA). *Hospital and Health System Compounding Under Section 503A of the Federal Food, Drug, and Cosmetic Act Guidance for Industry*. Silver Springs, MD: U.S. Food & Drug Administration; October 2021. **https://www.fda.gov/regulatory-information/search-fda-guidance-documents/hospital-and-health-system-compounding-under-section-503a-federal-food-drug-and-cosmetic-act**. Accessed April 22, 2023.
7. Kienle PC. *The Chapter <797> Answer Book*. 2nd ed. Bethesda, MD: American Society of Health-System Pharmacists; 2023.
8. Institute for Safe Medication Practices (ISMP). Guidelines for sterile compounding and the safe use of sterile compounding technology. **https://www.ismp.org/resources/guidelines-sterile-compounding-and-safe-use-sterile-compounding-technology**. Published May 4, 2022. Accessed April 28, 2023.
9. U.S. Food & Drug Administration. *Compounded Drug Products That are Essentially Copies of a Commercially Available Drug Product Under Section 503A of the Federal Food, Drug, and Cosmetic Act*. Silver Springs, MD: U.S. Food & Drug Administration; January 2018. **https://www.fda.gov/regulatory-information/search-fda-guidance-documents/compounded-drug-products-are-essentially-copies-commercially-available-drug-product-under-section**. Accessed April 22, 2023.
10. USP <71> Sterility tests. In: *USP: Compounding Compendium.* Rockville, MD: United States Pharmacopeial Convention; Official prior to 2013. **https://doi.org/10.31003/USPNF_M98810_01_01**.

29

DEALING WITH LATEX ALLERGIES

Lynda Kiliany

INTRODUCTION

The task of preparing compounded sterile preparations (CSPs) for patients with an allergy to latex proteins has been a topic that has caused pharmacy personnel much consternation and confusion for over three decades. Although latex-containing syringe plungers and injection port coverings on intravenous bags, bottles, and tubing sets were once a major concern in the pharmacy cleanroom, these products are now commonly manufactured without natural rubber. This leaves most of the attention in sterile compounding centered on how to deal with latex-containing vial stoppers. This chapter provides some background information on latex allergens, compares and contrasts different latex processing methods, describes the epidemiology and manifestations of a latex allergy, reviews the manufacture and functional testing of elastomeric vial stoppers, examines case reports linking latex-containing vial stoppers to symptoms of latex allergy, and discusses the merits of various methods used by pharmacy personnel to mitigate the perceived risk to patients.

HISTORY AND BACKGROUND OF LATEX USE

The use of rubber items has been traced as far back as 1600 BC in Mesoamerica where archeologists discovered artifacts, such as rubber balls and wooden tool handles, wrapped in rubber.[1] By the late 1700s, the dried latex was commonly called rubber because it effectively rubbed out pencil marks from paper.[2] In 1843, Charles Goodyear and Nathaniel Hayward discovered the process of vulcanization, which stabilized the rubber and led to widespread manufacturing of natural rubber materials.[1;2] The first patent for rubber surgical gloves was granted in 1878.[1] By the time World War I ended, surgeons had widely adopted the use of rubber gloves to prevent infection. However, the routine use of rubber gloves in other healthcare settings didn't become widespread until the advent of universal precautions in the late 1980s as a response to the AIDS epidemic.[1]

This chapter focuses on natural rubber products produced from the milky sap of the commercially grown rubber tree, *Hevea brasiliensis*, which is shown in **Figure 29-1**. This tree is cultivated primarily in tropical countries, including Malaysia, Thailand, and India.[1] The main constituents of *H. brasiliensis* sap are water and natural rubber (the polymeric hydrocarbon 1,4, *cis*-polyisoprene).[2;3] Several of the proteins in *Hevea* latex bind to immunoglobulin E (IgE) antibodies and are potent allergens.[3]

Latex and rubber are terms that are often used interchangeably. Both may be used to describe natural and synthetic materials. It is important to note that not all natural latex is *Hevea* latex. Another commercial source of natural rubber is the latex extracted from a guayule plant. Guayule is an evergreen shrub that is native to the southwestern United States and northern Mexico. Proteins from this plant have not shown cross-reactivity with *Hevea* latex allergens.[1;4] Products produced from guayule rubber are considered to be safe alternatives to *Hevea* latex products.[4] Latex may also describe a viscous emulsion that resembles natural rubber latex but is composed of synthetic polyisoprene, nitrile, neoprene, or other materials.[3] These synthetic rubbers do not contain antigenic proteins cross-reactive with *Hevea* latex. Interestingly enough, latex house paint contains no natural rubber latex and should not pose a problem to individuals sensitized to *Hevea* proteins.[5] (See **Table 29-1** for key latex terminology.)

IDENTIFICATION OF ALLERGENIC *HEVEA BRASILIENSIS* PROTEINS

Approximately 250 polypeptides have been identified in natural *Hevea* latex with at least 60 of these able to bind to IgE.[3] Of these, currently 15 have been registered by the International Nomenclature Committee of Allergens in the

Note: The author acknowledges Stephen K. Hetey who authored this chapter in the previous edition.

DOI 10.37573/9781585286492.029

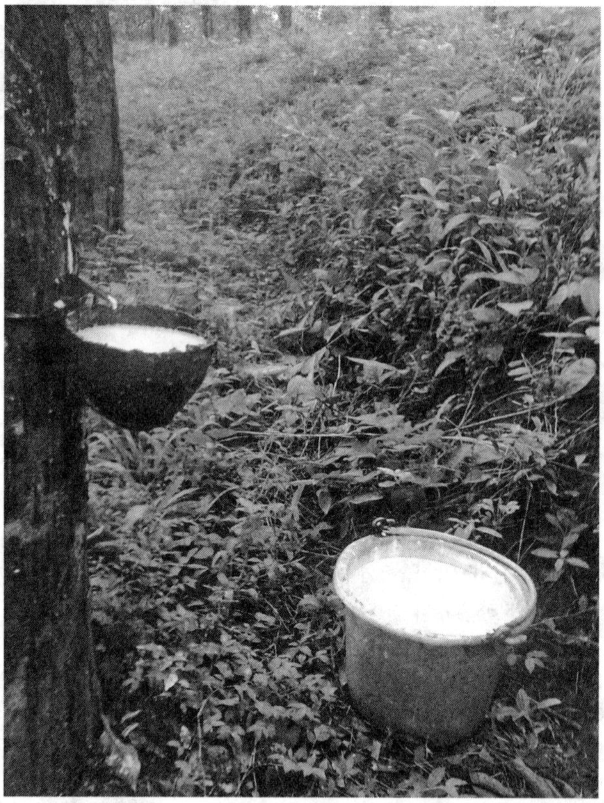

FIGURE 29-1. A filled cup of natural latex from a tapped rubber tree beside a bucket full of natural latex

Source: Reprinted with permission of Calicut, I. Tapped rubber tree. Wikimedia Commons. https://commons.wikimedia.org/wiki/File:Tapped_rubber_tree.jpg. Accessed September 8, 2023.

International Union of Immunologic Societies (IUIS).[3] The official designation is *Hevea brasiliensis* (Hev b), named for the species and genus of the plant, followed by numbers 1 through 15 for identification. Four *Hevea* proteins (Hev b 1, 3, 5, and 6.02) are used as indicator allergens for evaluating the allergen content in rubber products and detecting the presence of latex in the environment.[3;4] (See **Table 29-2** on page 385 for a comparison of the four latex indicator proteins.)

Latex sap is a heterogeneous fluid, hence, the latex proteins are not evenly dispersed within it.[8] Upon centrifugation, the latex sap fractions into three distinct layers, the rubber cream, the C-serum, and the B-serum. Only 1% to 2% of the fresh weight of *Hevea* latex is protein.[8] Approximately 70% of these proteins are soluble in water.[8]

The top layer, known as rubber cream, contains the water-insoluble particles of natural rubber. Two main allergenic proteins are associated with the surface of the rubber particles, Hev b 1 and Hev b 3.[3] These proteins are closely bound to the rubber particle, but a small amount of the protein can solubilize when the latex is ammoniated to prevent bacterial growth.[8] Ammoniated latex is used to manufacture dipped rubber products, such as medical gloves.[3] Sensitivity to Hev b 1 and Hev b 3 has been particularly associated with spina bifida patients. These patients were likely sensitized as a result of direct mucosal contact with products containing *Hevea* rubber while undergoing multiple surgeries and frequent bladder catheterizations.[3]

In contrast to the top layer, the middle layer (C-serum) and the bottom fraction (B-serum) contain mainly water-soluble proteins. The C-serum consists of the latex cytosol. Four recognized Hev b allergens (Hev b 5, 7, 8, and 9) are found within the C-serum.[3] The proteins contained

TABLE 29-1. Key Latex Terminology

Term	Definition
Dry natural rubber (DNR) process	A rubber manufacturing process using natural latex that has been acid coagulated into dry sheets or crumbled particles. The rubber undergoes prolonged treatment at high heat and is used to form solid rubber products by compression, molding, or extrusion.
Latex	Any polymer (natural or synthetic) in a water-based liquid or viscous state.
Latex allergy	An immune-mediated reaction to Hev b proteins associated with clinical symptoms.
Latex sensitization	The presence of immunoglobulin antibodies to Hev b protein without clinical manifestations.
Natural latex	A milky fluid consisting of very small rubber particles obtained from plants (usually *H. brasiliensis*) and dispersed in an aqueous medium.
Natural rubber	This includes all materials made from or containing natural latex. Products containing natural rubber may be produced by the dry natural rubber (DNR) or the natural rubber latex (NRL) process.
Natural rubber latex (NRL) process	A manufacturing process using a concentrated colloidal suspension of natural latex that has been ammoniated to prevent bacterial growth. Products are formed by dipping, extruding, or coating.

Hev b = *Hevea brasiliensis.*

Source: Based on Hamilton RG. Latex allergy: epidemiology, clinical manifestations, and diagnosis. In: Bochner BS, TePas E, eds. UpToDate. Waltham, MA: UpToDate; 2022. https://www.uptodate.com/contents/latex-allergy-epidemiology-clinical-manifestations-and-diagnosis. Updated November 22, 2021. Accessed April 26, 2022., U.S. Department of Health and Human services (HHS). *Guidance for Industry: User Labeling for Devices that Contain Natural Rubber (21 CFR 801.437); Small Entity Compliance Guide; Guidance for Industry.* The. Rockville, MD: U.S. Food & Drug Administration; April 1, 2003. https://www.fda.gov/media/71135/download. Accessed September 8, 2023, and Hepner DL, Castells MC. Latex allergy: an update. *Anesth Analg.* 2003;96(4):1219–1229. doi:10.1213/01.ANE.0000050768.04953.16.

in the B-serum function mainly as plant defense proteins.[8] Allergenic proteins found in the B-serum include Hev b 2, 4, 6.01/6.02, 7, 10, 11, and 13.[3] Hev b 2 is considered to be one of the most allergenic latex proteins in terms of IgE binding and skin reactivity.[8] This protein only solubilizes in solutions with a high salt content, thereby resisting removal with water during glove manufacturing but dissolving when the wearer's gloved hands perspire.[8]

LATEX PROCESSING METHODS

It is imperative to understand that the method of latex processing influences the protein content and the allergenicity of the resulting product.[9] Most harvested *Hevea* latex (90%) is acid coagulated into dry sheets or crumbled particles and used to manufacture molded rubber products including vehicle tires, shoe soles, vial stoppers, injection ports, and syringe plungers.[3;9] This dry natural rubber (DNR) processing method involves prolonged treatment at high temperatures, decreasing the finished product's allergenicity. The result of the DNR process is a solid rubber product. Solid natural rubber products contain low levels of latex allergens, consisting mainly of Hev b 1 and Hev b 3.[3]

In contrast to the DNR process, the natural rubber latex (NRL) process results in an ammoniated colloidal suspension that is used to form products by dipping, extruding, or coating.[9] This process is used to manufacture elastic rubber products, such as toy balloons, medical gloves, catheters, and condoms. Dipped rubber products, such as medical gloves, contain higher levels of latex allergens (Hev b 5, Hev b 6, and Hev b 13) than molded rubber products.[3] The majority of allergic reactions to *Hevea* latex occur as a result of exposure to dipped rubber products.[3]

Most DNR products have a protein content of less than 20 mcg/g, while medical gloves produced by the NRL process (dipping) have an average protein content of 700 mcg/g.[9] There can also be a wide variation in the latex content between gloves made by different manufacturers. Yunginger et al. showed protein content varied as much as 3,000-fold between different glove producers.[10]

In a particularly interesting study, Peixinho et al. tested 82 samples of surgical gloves and found a difference in allergen levels between the internal and external glove surfaces. Concentrations of Hev b 1 and Hev b 3 were higher on external glove surfaces, while concentrations of Hev b 5 and Hev b 6.02 were found to be higher on internal glove surfaces. This finding suggested a relationship between sensitization routes in different risk groups (ie, healthcare workers from exposure to the inner glove and spina bifida patients from contact exposure to the external glove surfaces during surgery).[11]

Donning powder (usually cornstarch) may be used in latex gloves to facilitate donning and doffing. Latex protein may adhere to this powder, producing a deadly dust that may distribute into the environment and cause allergic airway symptoms in sensitized individuals.[12] After many years of epidemiology work across the globe, scientists have concluded that the latex epidemic was caused by environmental contamination of aerosolized latex allergens carried on donning powder.[13] Because labeling alone could not mitigate the risk of illness or injury caused by the distribution of allergens from powdered gloves into the environment, the U.S. Food and Drug Administration (FDA) banned the sale of powdered medical gloves in 2017.[14] Avoiding powdered latex gloves and *Hevea* latex products in general is the most effective way to reduce exposure to *Hevea* latex allergens.[3]

CLINICAL MANIFESTATIONS OF *HEVEA* LATEX SENSITIVITY

The appearance of clinical symptoms following exposure to *Hevea* latex products depends on the route of exposure, the amount of allergen in the rubber-containing product, and the underlying mechanism of the reaction (ie, immune-mediated, cell-mediated, or irritant).[3] Two types of allergic reactions are of clinical concern with exposure to *Hevea* latex products, type I (IgE-mediated immediate-type hypersensitivity reactions) and type IV (T cell-mediated delayed hypersensitivity reactions).[15] Only type I reactions are allergic reactions to Hev b proteins.[3] The type IV reactions are allergic reactions to chemicals, such as rubber accelerators that are added during the manufacturing process.[3;15] Type I reactions are the least common reactions but may manifest with the most severe symptoms up to and including fulminant anaphylaxis.[12]

Type I reactions occur in two phases. On initial exposure, individuals are sensitized and produce IgE antibodies specific for Hev b. Upon re-exposure to latex, the latex-specific IgE antibodies located on the surfaces of mast cells are cross-linked by latex antigens, triggering the release of inflammatory mediators.[15] Clinical symptoms generally appear within minutes following re-exposure in a sensitized individual. Type I reactions to natural latex include the following:

- Allergic contact urticaria: Contact urticaria is the most common allergic reaction reported by healthcare workers using NRL gloves.[3] It appears as redness, pruritus, and wheal and flare reactions at the site where rubber contacts the skin of a sensitized individual, usually within 10 to 15 minutes of donning NRL gloves.[3;12] Sites other than the gloved hand can also exhibit urticaria if touched by the latex protein.[12] Contact urticaria symptoms may precede more severe allergic reactions.[12]
- Rhinitis, conjunctivitis, and asthma: Respiratory symptoms may occur in a latex-sensitized individual secondary to the inhalation of latex-laden donning powder in the environment. Sneezing, watery eyes, nasal congestion, runny nose, and asthma symptoms may be so severe that exposed workers may have to leave their place of employment if they cannot decrease or eliminate exposure.[3;12]

- Anaphylaxis: Life-threatening type I IgE-mediated reactions may occur during medical, dental, or surgical procedures and may present as cardiovascular collapse in anesthetized patients.[16] Latex-containing products that have been associated with anaphylaxis in the medical setting include surgical gloves, balloon-tipped catheters, condoms, and dental cofferdams.[3]

Type IV allergic reactions typically occur 24 to 96 hours after direct skin contact with a natural rubber product (eg, gloves, shoes, sporting equipment, and medical devices).[3] Type IV reactions to NRL medical gloves manifest as allergic contact dermatitis, which appears as an eczematous rash, often with vesicles.[3] Skin lesions may extend beyond the gloved hand.[12] The reaction is a response to chemicals added during the manufacturing process, not an allergy to Hev b protein.[3;12] Although it is not a reaction to Hev b allergens, the breakdown of the skin may increase the risk of IgE sensitization.[3]

Irritant contact dermatitis is a nonallergic reaction characterized by dry, crusted, and irritated skin. It may occur within minutes or hours following donning of gloves.[12] It is the most common complaint of individuals who wear gloves made from *Hevea* latex. It may also occur with synthetic gloves.[3] Clinical symptoms are a result of epidermal injury to areas under the glove and do not extend beyond the gloved area.[12] Symptoms may be compounded by sweating associated with occlusion from the glove, frequent hand washing, and use of chemical hand sanitizers.[3;12]

EPIDEMIOLOGY AND RISK FACTORS FOR LATEX ALLERGY

The first report of an anaphylactic reaction to surgical gloves was in 1984.[1] The epidemic of latex allergies started in the 1980s and extended into the 1990s. By 1991 in the United States, it was reported that 1 out of every 8 patients with spina bifida developed anaphylaxis during induction of anesthesia.[13] Most agree that the advent of universal precautions, which were introduced in response to the AIDS epidemic, played a key role in the sudden increase of identified latex allergies. Increased exposure to latex due to the increased use of powdered latex gloves led to increased sensitization rates. Some believe that the quality of latex gloves also decreased during this period. As manufacturers struggled to keep up with increased demand for their products, they stimulated trees for growth, tapped younger trees, and reduced customary storage periods and leaching steps. The changes in cultivation and processing methods were factors that may have contributed to a finished product with increased allergenic protein content.[1;3;13] A growing awareness of latex allergies may also have contributed to the large number of reported cases during that time.[1]

Risk factors that have been identified for the development of latex allergies include having a history of occupational exposure, multiple surgeries, and/or an atopic tendency.[3] The degree of exposure may be the most important risk factor for sensitization, but rates of sensitization may vary based on the route of exposure and the type and level of allergens present.[17] Water-soluble latex proteins are readily eluted on mucous and peritoneal membranes from contact with NRL gloves during medical, dental, or surgical procedures or by the inhalation of donning powder.[12] Direct mucosal and parenteral exposure are thought to pose the highest risk of anaphylaxis.[17]

Primary sensitization to latex may not always be a result of exposure to natural rubber.[8] Certain fruits show cross-reactivity with *Hevea* latex. This cross-reactivity is known as latex-food allergy syndrome or latex-fruit syndrome. Up to 50% of individuals who are allergic to latex may also be sensitive to certain fresh fruits.[4] Common fruits that have shown cross-reactivity to latex include kiwi, avocado, papaya, and banana (see Table 29-2).[2-4;8]

The frequency of latex sensitization in the general population is currently estimated to be less than 2%.[15] Occupations that have higher sensitization rates include healthcare workers sensitized before the introduction of powder-free latex gloves, rubber industry workers, and food handlers. The prevalence of latex allergies in occupationally exposed healthcare workers was estimated to be as high as 17% at its peak.[13] One patient population that had historically high rates of latex sensitization was children with spina bifida who were sensitized over multiple surgeries early in life and had frequent bladder catheterizations. Sensitization rates in this population have been reported to be as high as 69% because of direct internal or mucosal contact with natural rubber.[15] The good news is that latex avoidance strategies have been effective in reducing rates of primary latex sensitization in this group.[18]

DIAGNOSIS AND MANAGEMENT OF LATEX ALLERGIES

The diagnosis of latex allergy can be challenging and complicated because of the number of different allergenic proteins present in *H. brasiliensis*, each with different characteristics. Of the more than 250 identified proteins, at least 60 of these bind to IgE, but only 15 of the principle allergens have been given official numbers.[3] Different batches of latex can vary in allergy content, which is possibly due to normal seasonal variation in the *H. brasiliensis* tree as well as differences in collection and processing methods of the latex sap.[15] The sensitization and eliciting doses of each Hev b protein may differ according to the route of exposure. The dose of allergen that causes sensitivity may be different from the dose that elicits a response.[17]

Skin prick testing is generally the method of choice for confirming an allergy to latex. However, there is no commercially available skin test reagent for latex available in the United States at this time.[3;16] In the U.S., diagnosis is usually made based on clinical history in addition to serum testing for latex-specific IgE. These cannot be mutually exclusive since allergens elicit adverse effects in two stages

TABLE 29-2. Latex Indicator Proteins, Clinical Relevance, and Methods of Sensitization*

IUIS Code	Description	Solubility in Water	Latex Fraction	Cross-reactivity	Clinical Relevance	Method of Sensitization
Hev b 1	Rubber elongation factor	insoluble	Surface of large rubber particles	Papain, fig	Spina bifida patients	Direct mucosal exposure
Hev b 3	Small rubber particle protein	insoluble	Surface of small rubber particles	NA	Spina bifida patients	Direct mucosal exposure
Hev b 5	Acidic protein	soluble	C-serum	Kiwi	Glove allergenicity healthcare workers	Direct skin contact or inhalation of antigen attached to donning powder
Hev b 6.02	Hevein protein	soluble	C-serum	Avocado, banana, chestnut	Glove allergenicity healthcare workers	Direct contact with skin or inhalation of antigen attached to donning powder

Hev b = *Hevea brasiliensis*; IUIS = International Union of Immunologic Societies; NA = not applicable.

* Indicator proteins are used to assess allergen content in rubber products and latex allergens in the environment.

Source: Based on Raulf M. The latex story. *Chem Immunol Allergy.* 2014;100:248–255. doi:10.1159/000358863., Hamilton RG. Latex allergy: epidemiology, clinical manifestations, and diagnosis. In: Bochner BS, TePas E, eds. UpToDate. Waltham, MA: UpToDate; 2022. https://www.uptodate.com/contents/latex-allergy-epidemiology-clinical-manifestations-and-diagnosis Updated November 22, 2021. Accessed April 26, 2022., Hamilton RG. Latex allergy: management. In: Bochner BS, TePas E, eds. UpToDate. Waltham, MA: UpToDate; 2022. https://www.uptodate.com/contents/latex-allergy-management Updated January 8, 2020. Accessed March 25, 2022., and Yeang HY, Arif SA, Yusof F, et al. Allergenic proteins of natural rubber latex. *Methods.* 2002;27(1):32–45. doi:10.1016/S1046-2023(02)00049-X.

(ie, sensitization of the immunologically naïve individual followed by a response on repeated exposure).[17] Standardized skin tests, where available, are said to have high sensitivity (93%) and specificity (100%).[16] Serologic tests have lower sensitivities in the range of 70% to 80%.[16] Because of this lower sensitivity, 20% to 30% of latex-allergic patients may have a negative result.[16] Glove provocation tests may be employed when clinical suspicion is high but serologic testing is negative.[16] Nonstandardized, office-prepared reagents have been used but are not reliable in the potency or characterization of latex allergens present. Variations between testing methods and whether the testing reagent is standardized should be considered when one is evaluating published case reports or studies involving latex-containing vial stoppers.

Latex allergies cannot be cured, but they can be managed. Avoiding latex is the primary method of management.[4] Pharmacological prophylaxis in the acute care setting with antihistamines, steroids, or H-2 blockers is not recommended. These medications do nothing to change the fact that mast cells or basophils have become sensitized. In fact, their administration may blunt the early warning signs of anaphylaxis.[7] Individuals with a history of latex allergies should wear a medical alert bracelet and carry self-injectable epinephrine.[4] The use of immunotherapy has been limited by the frequency and severity of reactions to it.[4] Anti-IgE therapy is under investigation for latex allergies as an off-label treatment, but omalizumab treatment is costly and patients must have the appropriate body weight and total serum IgE levels to be candidates.[4]

ELASTOMERIC COMPONENTS USED IN PHARMACEUTICAL PACKAGING

Before discussing the case against latex-containing elastomeric components, their composition and manufacture must first be described. Vials containing parenteral dosage forms usually have closures known as stoppers or bungs.[19] The vial closure and the crimp form part of the container closure system. The stopper functions as a seal to protect the drug product from product loss and contamination caused by microbial or environmental contaminants.[20] The most commonly used type of vial stopper is composed of an elastomeric material. *Elastomers* are pliable polymers that can quickly return to their original state after being stretched.[21] Elastomers can be used for other pharmaceutical applications as well (eg, syringe plungers, needle shields, tip caps used for packaging prefilled syringes, and injection ports for flexible bags).[20]

The manufacturing process for natural rubber vial stoppers is a DNR process. It starts with weighing and mixing raw materials, which is followed by vulcanization. After vulcanization, the material is usually molded by compression. After molding comes coating, washing, and siliconization.[19] A typical vial stopper may be composed of 60% rubber, 30% fillers and pigments, 5% plasticizers, and 5% additional chemicals (eg, accelerators, activators, and antioxidants).[19] The rubber component may be natural rubber, but it is more commonly composed of a synthetic polymer such as butyl rubber or chlorobutyl rubber.[19] Butyl and halobutyl (ie, chlorobutyl, bromobutyl) elastomeric closures are particularly suited for long-term storage of pharmaceuticals because of their ability to maintain a protective headspace of inert gases over the product and prevent ingress of atmospheric oxygen and water vapor.[21] Elastomeric closures made from natural or synthetic polyisoprene rubber are excellent at resealing, making them suitable for multidose applications.[21] Halobutyls can also be blended with polyisoprene to take advantage of the positive properties of each and to balance out the negative.[21]

Elastomeric closures for injections must pass a variety of biological and physiochemical tests to determine their suitability for a particular application.[19-21] *United States Pharmacopeia* (USP) General Chapter <382> Elastomeric Component Functional Suitability in Parenteral Product Packaging/Delivery Systems is scheduled to become official in 2025.[20] This new chapter represents a paradigm shift by USP, switching the focus from testing individual elastomeric components by the supplier to the fitness of the entire container-closure system under the drug manufacturer's intended in-use conditions.[20] Pertinent to our topic is the discussion of functional testing of elastomeric closures on vial and bottle systems. These systems have elastomeric closures that are fitted and compressed onto the container flange opening and mechanically held in place by a seal component called a ferrule.[20]

Vial and bottle closures allow single or multiple penetrations by a hypodermic needle or a single penetration with a spike piercing device. Needle self-sealing capacity tests apply to multidose vials and packaging systems that must be accessed more than one time during dose preparation and subsequent administration to the patient. Needle puncture testing for product preparation is performed using an 18-gauge needle. Tests for subsequent product access are performed with 21-gauge needles unless otherwise specified.[20] However, both the needle chosen and the number of penetrations used in testing must simulate the most challenging intended-use conditions for the product.[20] Pharmacy personnel must bear in mind the manufacturer's design and testing when considering alternative means of vial access to avoid or minimize latex.

The FDA has not banned the use of natural rubber in the manufacture of medication vial stoppers. USP and the FDA considered a ban in the 1990s but found insufficient evidence to support a ban at that time.[9] Evidence gained since that time may support a different conclusion since the decision was based on failure to detect leached latex protein using the Lowry assay.[9;22] The Lowry assay is now considered to be not sensitive enough to detect low levels of latex protein.[9;22] Fortunately, recognition of latex allergies and the availability of suitable alternatives has resulted in fewer pharmaceuticals on the market manufactured with DNR vial stoppers. Most modern medication vial stoppers are now manufactured from synthetic rubbers.[19]

Evidence Against DNR Vial Stoppers

There is very little scientific evidence relating DNR vial stoppers to clinical allergic reactions. Most of the scientific literature is in the form of case reports published during the 1990s and early 2000s, some of which were later refuted upon receipt of additional information from the manufacturer.[9;23-26] Adding to the difficulty of establishing a causal relationship is the obvious risk of conducting a controlled study. This leads to the conclusion that the recommendation to remove a vial stopper to avoid latex is more based on theory than evidence-based science.[9] The case reports do, however, highlight the difficulty in obtaining reliable information on the DNR content of pharmaceutical products, even from the drug manufacturer.

The first anecdotal reports of latex reactions associated with DNR stoppers surfaced in the 1990s during the peak of the latex epidemic. Vassallo et al. reported an allergic reaction to methylprednisolone withdrawn from a vial stopper containing DNR.[23] The two-part vial was activated to mix the medication. Then, the outer rubber stopper was removed so that the medication could be drawn up into a glass syringe without having the needle pass through the vial stopper. Several minutes after the injection, the patient had marked erythema along the course of the corresponding vein. Sensitivity to latex particles in the methylprednisolone was presumed. Although the vial stopper had not been penetrated with a needle, the vial contents were in contact with the stopper during the mixing procedure. The patient had previously been tested for latex allergy by radioallergosorbent test (RAST) with a strongly positive result. The authors concluded that this was the first case of an allergic reaction to latex from the stopper of a medication vial.[23] After the publication of this report, the authors discovered that the vial stoppers were made with a synthetic butyl rubber rather than DNR.[24]

There have been several case reports involving insulin. Towse et al. described a local reaction at the site of a 24-year-old patient's insulin injection.[25] The patient was known to have had occupational exposure to latex gloves and was found to be seropositive for latex-specific IgE antibodies. Subsequent intradermal testing was performed using insulin diluent obtained from two manufacturers using two types of syringes. One insulin manufacturer indicated that their stoppers were made with synthetic butyl rubber. The other manufacturer used DNR in the stopper. Additionally, one syringe manufacturer indicated that natural rubber was used for the syringe plunger tip while the other manufacturer did not use natural rubber in their syringes. The patient had a positive response to the diluent drawn from the vial identified as having a DNR stopper (regardless of whether the vial septum was punctured with a needle) but not to the injection using components identified as being free of natural rubber. This suggested the presence of a latex allergen in the solution.[25] The patient was advised to use the insulin and syringes that did not contain DNR. Further communication by the MacCracken group with the insulin manufacturer, Eli Lilly, revealed that the vial top (stopper) of the insulin diluent vials, which had been previously identified as being latex-free by the Towse group, did contain 10% DNR.[26]

MacCracken et al. described a case involving a 13-year-old boy with a history of new-onset diabetes who experienced a local reaction at the site of an insulin injection.[26] The patient was known to have undergone many bladder repair surgeries and had experienced swollen lips after visiting the dentist, presumably due to the dentist's latex gloves. The patient was positive for latex-specific IgE antibodies. An investigative approach ensued using various insulins, syringes, and manipulation techniques. A dual-syringe technique was finally successful in preventing reactions. The dose was initially drawn up in one syringe and then transferred to a second syringe by removing the syringe plunger and injecting the insulin into the barrel of the second syringe. The plunger was replaced, and the injection was then given with the clean syringe that did not pierce the insulin vial top. The authors described the technique as inconvenient and costly, but the method did not require the removal of the insulin stopper.[26]

Hoffman reported a case involving a 6-year-old girl with insulin-dependent diabetes mellitus experiencing local reactions to her insulin injections.[27] A call to the insulin manufacturer revealed that the vial stopper did contain natural rubber. She did not react when the vial stopper was removed from the insulin vial before drawing up the dose. Eventually, she was successfully converted to an insulin pen. By using the pen, the needle entering the skin did not penetrate the rubber septum, although the needle entering the insulin cartridge did.[27]

Vaccines may be manufactured in vials with DNR stoppers, in prefilled syringes with a natural rubber sheath covering the needle, or in a prefilled syringe that has a natural rubber syringe plunger. Lear and English reported an anaphylactic reaction following the administration of a Hepatitis B Vaccine to a 44-year-old woman.[28] The vaccine was identified as having a natural rubber bung and was administered with a syringe having a natural rubber plunger. An intramuscular injection of the vaccine was subsequently administered to the patient with no reaction using a glass syringe from a vial with the rubber stopper removed. Latex particles transferred onto the needle were presumed to have caused the reaction.[28]

Russell et al. reviewed data from the Vaccine Adverse Event Reporting System (VAERS).[29] Reports submitted between January 1, 1991, and October 15, 2003, were queried using the search terms "latex" and "rubber." On review, only 147 reports (0.1%) out of 167,233 notifications mentioned latex allergy. Of the 147 reports, 28 developed a possible allergic event. Two patients required hospitalization but had a complete recovery. The majority of the cases (86%) were female. It was postulated that this may have been due to the prevalence of latex sensitization in healthcare workers, of which the majority were female. Besides possible contamination with latex, many vaccines contain other known allergens, including yeast proteins, egg proteins, and gelatin. Consequently, the authors concluded that it was impossible to implicate latex allergens as the sole cause of the reactions.[29]

Participants from the World Allergy Organization, the European Academy of Allergy and Clinical Immunology, the American Academy of Allergy, Asthma, and Immunology, and the American College of Allergy, Asthma, and Immunology formed a committee and subsequently published a consensus document in 2016 concerning allergic reactions to vaccines. The committee recognized that vaccines packaged with DNR latex posed a theoretical risk to latex-allergic patients, but they indicated that it would be difficult to elute latex allergens from these molded rubber products. They concluded by stating that allergic reactions to vaccines caused by latex in the vaccine packaging are exceedingly rare. Therefore, no special precautions, aside from administration of the vaccine wearing nonlatex gloves and the usual brief observation period following injection, are required when administering vaccines to latex-allergic patients.[30] The U.S. Centers for Disease Control and Prevention (CDC) publishes a list of vaccines indicating those that have latex content in their packaging. The CDC takes a more conservative approach, recommending that patients with severe anaphylactic reactions to latex avoid vaccines supplied in vials or syringes containing natural rubber.[31] For many of these vaccines, there are latex-free alternatives.

There was also a case reported in 2007 involving the administration of an intravenous lipid emulsion to an infant. The patient experienced a rash following the infusion. The pharmacist prepared subsequent doses by removing the latex-containing stopper from the bottle of lipids before withdrawing the dose, and the baby had no further reactions. The vial stopper was presumed to be the cause of the rash. A RAST test from the baby was negative, but this result was thought to be a false-negative result given that the RAST test for latex has a false-negative rate of at least 20%.[32]

The Rationale for Using Special Compounding Techniques

Special sterile preparation techniques used to prepare CSPs for latex-sensitive patients are theoretically based on two mechanisms with scant evidence to support either one. One theory proposes that latex proteins concentrate in the interior of the DNR stopper and are released at the time of needle puncture. Puncturing the closure may introduce rubber particles into the solution either by coring or shaving off small rubber particles during needle insertion or by surface contamination of the needle.[9] Following this line of thought, multiple needle punctures would increase the risk of releasing latex allergens into the vial contents. The other theory proposes that contamination occurs from the contact of the medication with surface proteins on the DNR stopper.[9] Since most latex proteins are water soluble, latex allergens could potentially leach into solutions stored under a latex-containing vial closure during manufacture, shipment, storage, and dose preparation.

Jones et al. investigated whether glutaraldehyde cross-linked (GAX) collagen contained latex allergens after storage in syringes with natural rubber syringe plungers.[33] The study consisted of both in vivo and in vitro testing. Forty-five healthy volunteer patients (who had been previously diagnosed with latex allergy) and 31 control subjects (not known to be latex allergic) were tested by skin prick using a panel of test extracts with positive and negative controls. The GAX-injectable collagen extracts were prepared from collagen solution stored for 3 months (short-term storage) and 45 months (long-term storage) in syringes with a natural rubber plunger. The 31 control subjects reacted to only the histamine control solution. Therefore, the investigators concluded that the test extracts did not contain irritants. Six of the 45 patients identified as having a latex allergy failed to react to a standardized latex test reagent or had uninterpretable skin tests. The remaining 39 patients were found to be highly reactive to the latex test reagent, but only one reacted to the collagen stored in a syringe with a rubber plunger. This patient did not react to collagen solution with no prior contact with a syringe plunger, suggesting that the reaction was not due to an irritant response. No latex protein was detected in vitro using a sensitive latex enzyme-linked immunosorbent assay for antigenic protein in either the short-term or long-term collagen solutions or the syringe plunger extracts. The investigators concluded that there may have been very low levels of latex in the collagen syringes that caused the patient to react.[33] However, they could not rule out that the patient may have reacted to other nonlatex proteins or chemical additives in the rubber.

To answer the question of whether removing a vial stopper reduces the latex content of an injectable product, Thomsen and Burke prepared 20 samples using a conventional aseptic technique, which involved a single needle puncture through vial stoppers containing 13% to 16% natural rubber with an 18-gauge needle.[34] Twenty samples were also prepared using a latex-precaution technique consisting of removing the vial stopper to avoid puncturing the stopper with a needle. One latex-contaminated positive control and five latex-free negative controls were prepared. All samples were prepared in a laminar airflow hood by an experienced pharmacy employee certified in aseptic technique by the pharmacy department. Samples were divided with one part sent to the institution's microbiology laboratory and the other to an outside laboratory for analysis of the latex allergen concentration. Samples were considered to be contaminated with latex allergen if the concentration of latex allergen exceeded the assay's 250 ng/mL limit of detection. Seventeen of the 45 test samples had 250 to 540 ng of latex allergen per milliliter. The breakdown according to the preparation method was not indicated. One of the vials prepared by removing the rubber stopper had microbial growth, a gram-positive coccus.[34] The investigators questioned whether the 17 samples contained latex since concentrations were close to the assay's limit of detection. Further laboratory analysis was performed. The samples were found to be at the detection limit due to ionic interference resulting from sodium chloride binding to the antibodies in the assay. Once this finding was considered, the samples were found to have no measurable allergen. Study limitations included the small sample size and the low sensitivity of the latex immunoassay.[34] The authors concluded that preparation by removing the vial stopper produced no detectable reduction in latex allergen concentration in the samples, and that any potential benefit achieved by removing the vial stopper had to be weighed against the risk of introducing problems with dilution, dosing errors, and contamination.[34]

Primeau et al. studied whether latex proteins leached into solutions through direct contact with rubber stoppers could produce skin reactions.[35] Their study was a blinded study with both in vitro and in vivo analysis. Five types of vial closures (1 made with 95% natural rubber, 1 with 66% natural rubber, and 3 made of synthetic rubbers) were coded A to E and inserted onto vials containing a phenol-saline-human serum albumin intradermal skin testing diluent. The vials were stored in an inverted position until their use within 9 months. Twelve to 24 hours before each study visit, a set of 5 vials was punctured 40 times with a 21-gauge needle while inverted. These solutions were denoted as 40P. Forty punctures were used to demonstrate a worst-case use condition as could be expected with a multidose vial. Solutions removed from nonpunctured vials were designated 0P. Eighteen latex-allergic subjects and 11 control subjects were recruited for the study. Study participants were evaluated for the presence of latex-specific IgE using the Pharmacia CAP system. Six of the latex-allergic subjects were excluded from the latex-allergy group due to positive intradermal skin tests from the negative control diluent.

The twelve remaining volunteers having latex allergy and 11 volunteers without latex allergy were subjected to intradermal skin tests using a solution from each of the 0P and 40P vials along with a saline negative control and a histamine positive control. Intradermal skin tests using vials A to E were negative in the subjects without latex allergy. Two subjects with latex allergy had a positive skin reaction to solutions from the 0P natural rubber closure vials. Five subjects with latex allergy experienced positive intradermal skin tests to the 40P solutions in one or both vials containing natural rubber stoppers. Seven of the 12 subjects with latex allergy did not display positive reactions to any of the solutions stored under DNR closures, including the subject with the highest latex-specific IgE level in the serum. Surprisingly, two of the five participants with skin reactions to solutions from vials with DNR closures had a positive intradermal test reaction to solution stored under a bromobutyl synthetic closure. However, the result was not reproducible.

In vitro analysis was also performed on the vial closures and solutions from each vial type. The five vial closures were each cut in half and 5 grams were extracted in a phosphate buffered saline solution before CAP inhibition analysis. In vitro testing confirmed the presence of latex allergen in extracts obtained from the cut natural rubber vial closures, although the level was very low. The cut synthetic closures had no detectable latex. No allergen was detected in vitro by the laboratory in any of the solutions stored in either the 0P or 40P vials A to E using a RAST inhibition assay with a limit of detection of 0.5 allergen units/milliliter.

The investigators concluded that latex allergens can be released into solutions stored in contact with natural rubber vial closures in sufficient quantity to provoke a response by intradermal testing.[35] This conclusion was surprising given that none of the solutions had detectable latex. However, the authors also noted that intradermal testing is at least a thousand times more sensitive than skin puncture testing and 100 times more sensitive than RAST inhibition analysis. The reactions to the bromobutyl closures were postulated to be caused by chemicals, such as accelerators added to the rubber during manufacture, although the authors noted that this theory needed study and there was no supporting data. The reactions of the excluded six participants to the negative control remained unexplained. The authors concluded that neither the popping-the-top method nor the single-stick rule used by many institutions for medication preparation removes the possibility of latex contamination resulting from direct contact of the medication with the nonpunctured DNR vial closure during storage.[35] Thus, neither method provides adequate protection for patients with a latex allergy. Limitations to this study include the small size and the unexplained fact that nearly as many latex-allergic participants (who were then excluded from further testing) reacted to the negative control solution as the number of participants who reacted to the vials with natural rubber closures.

This leaves us with a few case reports and small equivocal studies to support the necessity of using alternative preparation methods when preparing CSPs for latex-allergic patients. Most troubling is the failure to detect latex in any of the test solutions that precipitated a reaction in a study participant. Thus, it remains theoretically possible for latex allergens to be released into a pharmaceutical stored under a DNR vial stopper in sufficient quantity to provoke an allergic reaction, but it is not conclusively proven.[22]

Strategies Used to Avoid or Minimize Latex During Compounding of Sterile Preparations

The cornerstone of preventing allergic reactions in sensitized individuals is avoiding exposure to the offending agent. One method of avoiding latex has been called the catalog-avoidance approach.[22] This method of avoiding latex requires reviewing the medication inventory and keeping a record of the vials that contain natural rubber in their closures. With this method, some ask if the labor cost of maintaining an up-to-date library of latex-containing products is worth the benefit considering that less than 20% of medications are packaged with vial closures that contain latex.[22] Some institutions subscribe to a searchable, online latex drugs database to identify medications with vial stoppers made from natural rubber. While this database claims to list over 90% of available injectable products on the U.S. market, there may still be products encountered where no information is available about latex content, necessitating a call to the manufacturer.[36] Disadvantages to this method of avoiding latex include the potential for a lack of timely information available at the point of care, the manufacturer may not always give accurate information (as seen in the previous case reports), and there may not always be a suitable alternative for a medication manufactured with natural rubber in the vial stopper. In the case of maintaining an in-house database, the information must be continuously updated to be reliable.[9;22] In this era of drug shortages and multiple suppliers, keeping an accurate list could be an arduous task. Despite its limitations, when accurate information is available, avoiding pharmaceuticals packaged underneath DNR vial stoppers is the best approach to protect patients who are sensitized to *Hevea* latex.

Another method widely used by pharmacies attempting to avoid latex is known as the popping-the-top method of preparation.[9;22] This method involves removing the rubber stopper with a decapping tool or pliers to avoid having to puncture it with a needle. The theory behind this technique is that most of the allergenic proteins reside in the interior of the rubber rather than on the surface. Piercing the stopper allows these proteins to be released into the vial contents.[9] However, available studies do not support the removal of the vial stopper as an evidence-based strategy for avoiding or reducing latex.[9] This technique fails to address the potential for latex allergens to leach from the vial closure during shipping or storage.[22] Although USP Chapter <797> does not give specific recommendations for preparing CSPs for patients with a latex allergy, the practice of removing the vial stopper does not align well with good aseptic technique due to the possibility that microbial or particulate contamination may be introduced into the vial contents as the stopper is removed. If a decapping tool is used, it should be clean, rust-free, and properly sanitized before bringing it into the ISO Class 5 primary engineering control (PEC). Removing the stopper creates an open system somewhat similar to breaking an ampule. When removed under laminar airflow in the pharmacy by trained compounding personnel, followed by filtering the vial contents with a compatible 0.22-micron filter, the risk of introducing contamination into the final product is probably lessened but not eliminated.[9] At the point of care, this method cannot be endorsed or recommended.[35] Other disadvantages of using this technique include the difficulty of reconstituting and mixing sterile powders. Failure to achieve a uniform solution when dissolving a powder may result in the potential to cause dosing errors. There is also a potential for increased medication waste since the remaining drug will likely be discarded once the vial stopper is removed. Finally, the popping-the-top method cannot be used for hazardous medications since this would unnecessarily increase the exposure of the caregiver to hazardous agents. Given the lack of evidence that this method prevents clinical reactions in latex-sensitive patients, the popping-the-top method of preparation needs to be strongly discouraged.

There is no evidence that filtering solutions removed from vials with DNR stoppers during the preparation of the CSP will reduce or eliminate exposure to latex proteins.[37] Filtering may be expected to remove rubber cores and fragments, but it will not remove water-soluble latex proteins already in the solution. Stopper fragmentation or coring with subsequent injection of small fragments of rubber has been hypothesized as a mechanism for sensitization of patients to latex.[9] Subcutaneous injection of tiny fragments of DNR can be expected to occur frequently in diabetic patients injecting insulin from containers using DNR closures. However, there is no evidence of increasing sensitization to latex as a result.[9] But, even if DNR microemboli do not sensitize the patient to latex allergy, the risk to patients already sensitized is unknown.[9]

Asakura et al. found evidence of coring at a high frequency in insulin pen cartridges.[38] This study found evidence of rubber pieces that were at least 0.01 mm in size at a rate of 73% for the primary injection. Rubber fragments in both the primary and secondary injections were able to pass through a 31-gauge needle, indicating a possibility for microscopic rubber particles to be injected into the subcutaneous tissue. The insulin formulation used in the study had a dual-layer stopper composed of natural and butyl rubber. The authors stated concern that coring is a serious problem and recommended that the relationship between coring and latex allergy needed further study.[38] The Asakura study demonstrated that even a single puncture with a 31-gauge needle poses a significant risk of transferring rubber particles to the patient.[38]

Given the difficulty associated with cataloging medications packaged under DNR closures as well as the risks posed by removing vial stoppers, many institutions adopted a method for latex minimization called the single-stick rule, which is followed by patient observation.[9;22] This method assumes that latex protein distribution into the solution will be minimized while still maintaining a closed system to limit the potential of microbial or particulate contamination of the vial contents.[22] In this method, all vials are punctured only once with a needle. This method may be accompanied by a change to a new needle before the administration of the drug or preparation of the CSP. While the catalog-avoidance method puts the burden of labor on the pharmacy staff, the single-stick rule with observation places the burden on nursing. The key to this method's success is the observation of the patient with vital signs at 30-minute intervals for up to 2 hours post injection.[22] Reportedly, this method has been used successfully for years at The Johns Hopkins Hospital in Baltimore, Maryland.[22] Disadvantages to using this method of preparation include the difficulty of verifying that a compounder correctly applied this technique using remote pharmacy workflow verification systems and the potential increase in waste if the remaining vial contents cannot be used without a second withdrawal. Pharmacies taking this approach to manage latex allergies must consider whether a universal approach is truly required given that, as of 1997, no more than 20% of all medications are packaged with a DNR closure, and only a few patients may be sufficiently sensitized to have a systemic reaction.[22] Like the popping-the-top method, this approach does not take into consideration that latex may leach from the vial stopper during shipment or storage.[22] There is also the possibility of introducing latex contamination with a single puncture.

One method that has been recommended for withdrawing multiple doses from a vial without repeated punctures to the vial septum is to access the vial with a dispensing pin.[22] Dispensing pins come in a variety of designs and intended uses. Unfortunately, using a dispensing pin to comply with a single-stick rule cannot be considered a universal solution. Like all tools, dispensing pins must be used appropriately to prevent contamination of the CSP. Dispensing pins may ease withdrawal from a medication vial, but they typically make a larger hole in the vial septum than conventional needles. It is essential to use an appropriately sized pin to prevent coring of the rubber stopper and leaking of contents. Care must be taken to prevent the pin from sliding in and out of the vial stopper since slippage could increase contamination risk. Care must also be taken not to touch any critical sites when withdrawing multiple doses. Vials with dispensing pins inserted may not be removed from the ISO Class 5 PEC if they do not maintain container closure integrity (ie, remain closed). Dispensing pins may not be removed from a vial and reused. Pharmacies utilizing dispensing pins in the compounding lab must define proper use in their standard operating procedures, train staff appropriately, and evaluate whether staff are properly using these devices during media fill testing.

When considering the use of alternative preparation methods, the potential benefit of the method used to avoid latex must be weighed against the potential risk of causing harm to the patient. The popping-the-top method tips the scale to the side of risk due to the opportunity to cause harm if microbial or particulate contamination is introduced during the removal of the vial stopper. For this risk, no benefit is gained because the vial contents stored under a DNR stopper may still contain latex protein.[22] By comparison, the single-stick rule and observe method does not pose any increased risk to the patient from microbial or particulate contamination of the medication. It must be clear, however, that this method of preparation does not eliminate the risk of exposure to latex allergens, as it ignores the fact that latex allergens may theoretically leach into solutions stored in vials with DNR stoppers during manufacture, shipment, and storage. Single stick with observation may minimize the potential to introduce rubber particles into the solution by coring or fragmenting the stopper, but it does not eliminate it. See **Table 29-3** for a summary of methods used to avoid or minimize latex when compounding CSPs.

HEALTH-SYSTEM PHARMACY PRACTICES

The first published guidance for pharmacists preparing compounded sterile products for patients with latex allergy appeared in the *American Journal of Health-System Pharmacy* in 1998.[39] The author's recommendation to remove the vial stopper was wisely accompanied by a recommendation to filter the product with a 0.22-micron filter since stopper removal could increase the risk of bacterial contamination. Exceptions to filtering were made for products not compatible with filtration, such as suspensions. Thomsen and Burke published their work in the *American Journal of Health-System*

TABLE 29-3. Comparison of Latex Avoidance and Minimization Methods

Method	Avoids Latex	Minimizes Latex	Evidence-based
Catalog and avoid	Yes*	NA	Yes
Single-stick rule with observation	No	Theoretical	Anecdotal†
Popping-the-top method	No	Theoretical	No

NA = not applicable.

*Avoids latex when accurate information is available.

† Reported to be successful at The Johns Hopkins Hospital in Baltimore, Maryland.

Source: Based on Heitz JW, Bader SO. An evidence-based approach to medication preparation for the surgical patient at risk for latex allergy: is it time to stop being stopper poppers? *J Clin Anesth.* 2010;22(6):477–483. doi:10.1016/j.jclinane.2009.12.006. and Hamilton RG, Brown RH, Veltri MA, et al. Administering pharmaceuticals to latex-allergic patients from vials containing natural rubber latex closures. *Am J Health Syst Pharm.* 2005;62(17):1822–1827. doi:10.2146/ajhp050021.

Pharmacy in January of 2000.[34] They concluded that a latex minimization technique (popping-the-top rule) did not yield solutions with less latex allergen than those prepared with a single vial puncture. Another update on preparing medications for latex-allergic individuals was published in the September 2005 issue of the *American Journal of Health-System Pharmacy* by Robert Hamilton and his team.[22] Their recommendation had several parts. First, all at-risk patients had to be identified on admission with careful histories. The pharmacy had to follow a universal single-stick rule (ie, all vials, fluid bags, and bottles could be punctured only once and all unused medication had to be discarded). Labels on CSPs prepared for latex-allergic patients had to clearly state "latex precautions" to alert nursing staff of the need for additional monitoring. Finally, nurses had to monitor the patient (as required by the institution's policy) for signs and symptoms of a possible systemic reaction.[22]

A study published in 2006 indicated that there is generally a lack of consensus among pharmacy professionals and health-system pharmacies when compounding parenteral nutrition solutions for latex-allergic patients.[37] Of the 100 institutions surveyed (two from each state), 10% had a policy to remove vial stoppers, 5 institutions had a policy to allow 1 puncture through vial closures, and 1 institution allowed 20 punctures. One institution had a policy to use a 5-micron filter needle, presumably to remove rubber fragments but not latex protein. This study also highlighted a general unawareness of institutional policies concerning the preparation of injections for latex-allergic patients.[37] It also recognized the need for better allergy histories. The survey results showed that a majority of pharmacies used only information in the medical record to confirm a latex allergy. A clinical pharmacist familiar with the various presentations of latex sensitivity could assist the medical team in eliciting true allergies from the more common irritant contact dermatitis reactions.

Recognition of latex allergies has led many health systems to create latex-safe environments. Creating a latex-safe environment is a multidisciplinary approach that seeks to avoid latex allergen exposure.[4] Pharmacists managing cleanrooms must take care to assure that the sterile compounding areas are maintained as latex-safe environments to protect patients and caregivers. Only gloves made without NRL are appropriate for use in sterile compounding areas.[22] Care must also be taken to avoid hidden sources of NRL in other personal protective equipment or compounding supplies purchased for use in the cleanroom.

Two things are clear. First, any compounding strategy other than avoiding vials with stoppers made from DNR is at best a latex minimization strategy. Second, pharmacies using special preparation techniques to minimize latex allergens must not use misleading statements, such as "latex free" or "does not contain latex" on their prescription labels. The FDA issued a guidance document in 2014 recommending that terminology such as "latex-free" and "does not contain latex" should not be used by manufacturers because there is no analytical method that identifies all proteins in NRL and assures that there are no proteins or substances in natural rubber products that may lead to allergic reactions in patients.[40] Although this guidance does not target health-system pharmacies compounding sterile preparations, it does imply that using the term "latex-free" is not an accurate way of describing a preparation made using the single-stick rule or the popping-the-top methods of preparation because neither method assures the absence of latex allergens in the resulting CSP. A comment to follow latex precautions on the preparation label would be more suitable and alert nursing staff to closely monitor the patient upon administration of the CSP.[22]

Pharmacies adopting the single-stick rule with an observation approach as a method of latex minimization must do so in conjunction with a multidisciplinary team since this method depends on direct observation of the patient after the administration of the product.[22] Pharmacists participating in multidisciplinary committees dealing with latex allergies should also be familiar with applicable guidelines from other professional societies to avoid conflicting processes. For instance, in their 2018 revision of guidelines, the American Association of Nurse Anesthesiology (AANA) recommended that vials be punctured only one time.[41] The Association of Surgical Technologists (AST) also revised its best practices in 2018. AST guideline III specifically recommends against removing rubber stoppers, choosing instead to follow the single-stick method of vial access to reduce the incidence of coring and fragmentation of the vial stopper.[42] Both guidelines emphasize obtaining careful histories, creating latex-safe environments, and identifying medications and supplies containing natural rubber.

IMPORTANT POINTS TO CONSIDER

- Some latex proteins are water soluble and may be eluted into the vial contents during manufacture, shipping, and storage. Neither removing the stopper nor puncturing the stopper once removes this risk.[22]
- No pharmacy compounding method can remove *Hevea* latex from a pharmaceutical that is contaminated with latex allergens.
- There is no evidence that the popping-the-top method results in less latex protein contamination of the vial contents than puncturing the vial with a single needle puncture.[9;34]
- The avoidance of powdered latex gloves in hospitals has led to decreasing rates of latex sensitization in healthcare workers and patients who receive multiple surgeries.[3]
- Some early case reports implicating latex vial stoppers as the cause of an allergic reaction misidentified the medication stopper as natural rubber.[9]

SUMMARY

The risk of a pharmaceutical vial stopper causing clinical symptoms appears to be diminishing. This is due to decreased rates of latex sensitivity in the general population and the fact that only a minority of pharmaceutical products are now packaged using DNR in the stopper formulation. Avoidance remains the only sure method of preventing sensitization to *Hevea* protein or a reaction in a sensitized individual. Medications without DNR vial stoppers should be sourced whenever possible. Neither the popping-the-top nor the single-stick methods of preparation assure that there are no latex allergens in the resulting admixture if the medication is packaged with a DNR stopper.

Pharmacy staff should follow standard aseptic technique when preparing CSPs, taking care to use techniques that minimize rubber coring or fragmentation of the vial stopper for all patients (see **Table 29-4**).[43] At the point of care, the single-stick rule with observation method of minimizing latex exposure is an acceptable strategy since it aligns closely with the CDC's recommendation of one needle, one syringe, and one puncture for single-use vials in patient care areas to prevent microbial contamination.[44] Although the benefit of a single-stick rule as a latex minimization strategy is not clear, the method poses no additional risk to the patient. Clinicians should always be prepared for unexpected reactions following the injection of any medication regardless of the preparation method used. The ultimate solution for dealing with latex allergies is to ban *Hevea* latex from use in all drug packaging.[22]

TABLE 29-4. Prevention of Coring or Fragmentation of a Vial Stopper

Needle Selection	Techniques
Select thinner, higher gauge needles.	Puncture within the target circle (bull's eye) of the stopper.
Use needles only once.	Insert the needle using the anticoring technique.[a]
Use needles with a sharp point, not a blunt tip.	Do not twist or rotate needles during insertion.
Use needles with lubrication on the needle surface.	Minimize the number of punctures into a single stopper.

[a] The anticoring technique means to enter a vial with a needle in the following manner. Place the needle tip with the bevel facing up on the center of the vial stopper (inside of the bull's eye) with the needle shaft at an approximately 45-degree angle to the surface of the stopper. A slight downward pressure is placed on the needle as the angle is increased. The needle must enter the stopper at a 90-degree angle with the tip and heel entering the vial stopper at the same place. This prevents the coring of the vial stopper.

Source: Based on Côté S. Stopper functionality – key considerations. West Pharma Blog. https://www.westpharma.com/blog/2022/march/key-considerations-to-choose-rubber-stopper-for-vial-containment-system. March 24, 2022. Accessed September 8, 2023.

REFERENCES

1. Ownby DR. A history of latex allergy. *J Allergy Clin Immunol*. 2002;110(2)(suppl):S27–S32. doi:10.1067/mai.2002.125336.
2. Raulf M. The latex story. *Chem Immunol Allergy*. 2014;100:248–255. doi:10.1159/000358863.
3. Hamilton RG. Latex allergy: epidemiology, clinical manifestations, and diagnosis. In: Bochner BS, TePas E, eds. UpToDate. Waltham, MA: UpToDate; 2022. **https://www.uptodate.com/contents/latex-allergy-epidemiology-clinical-manifestations-and-diagnosis**. Updated November 22, 2021. Accessed September 8, 2023.
4. Hamilton RG. Latex allergy: management. In: Bochner BS, TePas E, eds. UpToDate. Waltham, MA: UpToDate; 2022. **https://www.uptodate.com/contents/latex-allergy-management**. Updated January 8, 2020. Accessed September 28, 2023.
5. Allergy L. American Academy of Allergy Asthma & Immunology website. **https://www.aaaai.org/conditions-and-treatments/library/allergy-library/latex-allergy**. Reviewed September 28, 2020. Accessed September 28, 2023.

6. U.S. Department of Health and Human services (HHS). *Guidance for Industry: User Labeling for Devices that Contain Natural Rubber (21 CFR 801.437); Small Entity Compliance Guide; Guidance for Industry*. The. Rockville, MD: U.S. Food & Drug Administration; April 1, 2003. **https://www.fda.gov/media/71135/download**. Accessed September 28, 2023.

7. Hepner DL, Castells MC. Latex allergy: an update. *Anesth Analg*. 2003;96(4):1219–1229. doi:10.1213/01.ANE.0000050768.04953.16.

8. Yeang HY, Arif SA, Yusof F, et al. Allergenic proteins of natural rubber latex. *Methods*. 2002;27(1):32–45. doi:10.1016/S1046-2023(02)00049-X.

9. Heitz JW, Bader SO. An evidence-based approach to medication preparation for the surgical patient at risk for latex allergy: is it time to stop being stopper poppers? *J Clin Anesth*. 2010;22(6):477–483. doi:10.1016/j.jclinane.2009.12.006.

10. Yunginger JW, Jones RT, Fransway AF, et al. Extractable latex allergens and proteins in disposable medical gloves and other rubber products. *J Allergy Clin Immunol*. 1994;93(5):836–842. doi:10.1016/0091-6749(94)90374-3.

11. Peixinho C, Tavares-Ratado P, Tomás MR, et al. Latex allergy: new insights to explain different sensitization profiles in different risk groups. *Br J Dermatol*. 2008;159(1):132–136. doi:10.1111/j.1365-2133.2008.08614.x.

12. Gawchik SM. Latex allergy. *Mt Sinai J Med*. 2011;78(5):759–772. doi:10.1002/msj.20281.

13. Kelly KJ, Sussman G. Latex allergy: where are we now and how did we get there? *J Allergy Clin Immunol Pract*. 2017;5(5):1212–1216. doi:10.1016/j.jaip.2017.05.029.

14. Devices B. Banned devices; powdered surgeon's gloves, powdered patient examination gloves, and absorbable powder for lubricating a surgeon's glove. Final rule. *Fed Regist*. 2016;81(243):91722–91731. **https://pubmed.ncbi.nlm.nih.gov/28030886/**.

15. Warshaw EM. Latex allergy. *Skinmed*. 2003;2(6):359–366. doi:10.1111/j.1540-9740.2003.02177.x.

16. Parisi CAS, Kelly KJ, Ansotegui IJ, et al. Update on latex allergy: new insights into an old problem. *World Allergy Organ J*. 2021;14(8):100569. doi:10.1016/j.waojou.2021.100569.

17. Poley GE Jr, Slater JE. Latex allergy. *J Allergy Clin Immunol*. 2000;105(6 Pt 1):1054–1062. doi:10.1067/mai.2000.106925.

18. Blumchen K, Bayer P, Buck D, et al. Effects of latex avoidance on latex sensitization, atopy and allergic diseases in patients with spina bifida. *Allergy*. 2010;65(12):1585–1593. doi:10.1111/j.1398-9995.2010.02447.x.

19. Sandle T. Closures for pharmaceutical preparations: a review of design and test considerations. *Biopharm Int*. 2012;25(12).

20. USP <382> Elastomeric component functional suitability in parenteral product packaging/delivery systems. In: *2023: USP Compounding Compendium*. Rockville, MD: United States Pharmacopeial Convention; December 1, 2023. **https://doi.org/10.31003/USPNF_M11355_03_01**.

21. Curry W, Conway S, Goodfield C, et al. Reducing the risk of contamination of sterile parenteral products via ready-to-use closure components. *AAPS PharmSciTech*. 2010;11(4):1572–1579. doi:10.1208/s12249-010-9531-8.

22. Hamilton RG, Brown RH, Veltri MA, et al. Administering pharmaceuticals to latex-allergic patients from vials containing natural rubber latex closures. *Am J Health Syst Pharm*. 2005;62(17):1822–1827. doi:10.2146/ajhp050021.

23. Vassallo SA, Thurston TA, Kim SH, et al. Allergic reaction to latex from stopper of a medication vial. *Anesth Analg*. 1995;80(5):1057–1058. doi:10.1097/00000539-199505000-00039.

24. Vassallo SA, Thurston TA, Kim SH, Todres ID. Response to Letters to the editor [letter]. Overreaction to latex allergy. *Anesth Analg*. 1997;84(2):468. **https://journals.lww.com/anesthesia-analgesia/fulltext/1997/02000/overreaction_to_latex_allergy.50.aspx**. Accessed August 25, 2023.

25. Towse A, O'Brien M, Twarog FJ, et al. Local reaction secondary to insulin injection. A potential role for latex antigens in insulin vials and syringes. *Diabetes Care*. 1995;18(8):1195–1197. doi:10.2337/diacare.18.8.1195.

26. MacCracken J, Stenger P, Jackson T. Latex allergy in diabetic patients: a call for latex-free insulin tops. *Diabetes Care*. 1996;19(2):184. doi:10.2337/diacare.19.2.184a.

27. Hoffman RP. Latex hypersensitivity in a child with diabetes. *Arch Pediatr Adolesc Med*. 2000;154(3):281–282. doi:10.1001/archpedi.154.3.281.

28. Lear JT, English JSC. Anaphylaxis after hepatitis B vaccination. *Lancet*. 1995;345(8959):1249. doi:10.1016/s0140-6736(95)92039-0.

29. Russell M, Pool V, Kelso JM, et al. Vaccination of persons allergic to latex: a review of safety data in the Vaccine Adverse Event Reporting System (VAERS). *Vaccine*. 2004;23(5):664–667. doi:10.1016/j.vaccine.2004.06.042.

30. Dreskin SC, Halsey NA, Kelso JM, et al. International Consensus (ICON): allergic reactions to vaccines. *World Allergy Organ J*. 2016;9(1):32. doi:10.1186/s40413-016-0120-5.

31. Latex in Vaccine Packaging. In: Hall E, Wodi AP, Hamborsky J, et al. *Epidemiology and Prevention of Vaccine-Preventable Diseases. The Pink Book: Course Textbook.* 14th ed. Washington, DC: Centers for Disease Control and Prevention; 2021. **https://www.cdc.gov/vaccines/pubs/pinkbook/downloads/appendices/b/latex-table.pdf**. Accessed May 30, 2023.

32. Wynn RJ, Boneberg A, Lakshminrusimha S. Unexpected source of latex sensitization in a neonatal intensive care unit. *J Perinatol*. 2007;27(9):586–588. doi:10.1038/sj.jp.7211793.

33. Jones JM, Sussman GL, Beezhold DH. Latex allergen levels of injectable collagen stored in syringes with rubber plungers. *Urology*. 1996;47(6):898–902. doi:10.1016/S0090-4295(96)00037-4.

34. Thomsen DJ, Burke TG. Lack of latex allergen contamination of solutions withdrawn from vials with natural rubber stoppers. *Am J Health Syst Pharm*. 2000;57(1):44–47. doi:10.1093/ajhp/57.1.44.

35. Primeau MN, Adkinson NF Jr, Hamilton RG. Natural rubber pharmaceutical vial closures release latex allergens that produce skin reactions. *J Allergy Clin Immunol*. 2001;107(6):958–962. doi:10.1067/mai.2001.115630.

36. Frequently Asked Questions. Latexdrugs.com Website. **http://latexdrugs.com/faq.html**. Accessed September 30, 2023.

37. Abd El-Atti S, Martinelli B, Yourich B, et al. Nationwide survey of hospital practices when compounding parenteral nutrition solutions in latex-allergic patients. *Nutr Clin Pract*. 2006;21(5):513–517. doi:10.1177/0115426506021005513.

38. Asakura T, Seino H, Nozaki S, Abe R. Occurrence of coring in insulin vials and possibility of rubber piece contamination by self-injection. *Yakugaku Zasshi*. 2001;121(6):459–463. doi:10.1248/yakushi.121.459.

39. Rice SP, Gutfeld MB. Preparation of latex-safe sterile products. *Am J Health Syst Pharm*. 1998;55(14):1462–1467, 1466–1467. doi:10.1093/ajhp/55.14.1462.

40. U.S. Department of Health and Human Services. Recommendations for Labeling Medical Products to Inform Users that the Product or Product Container is not Made with Natural Rubber Latex: Guidance for Industry and Food and Drug Administration Staff. U.S. Food & Drug Administration: Rockville, MD; December 2, 2014. **https://www.fda.gov/media/85473/download**. Accessed May 30, 2023.

41. Melendez I. Latex allergy management guidelines. AANA Board of Directors 2018. **https://issuu.com/aanapublishing/docs/5_-_latex_allergy_management?fr=sZWU1NTU2NDAxMjU**. Accessed August 25, 2023.

42. Association of Surgical Technologists. Guidelines for best practices for the natural rubber latex allergic and metal allergic patient. **https://www.ast.org/uploadedFiles/Main_Site/Content/About_Us/Guideline_Latex_Allergy.pdf**. Revised April 9, 2018. Accessed June 11, 2023,

43. Côté S. Stopper functionality – key considerations. West Pharma Blog. **https://www.westpharma.com/blog/2022/march/key-considerations-to-choose-rubber-stopper-for-vial-containment-system**. March 24, 2022. Accessed July 9, 2023.

44. Centers for Disease Control and Prevention. One & Only Campaign. **https://www.cdc.gov/injectionsafety/one-and-only.html**. Reviewed December 3, 2019. Accessed July 9, 2023.

SECTION 6: Quality Management

DOI 10.37573/9781585286492

DOCUMENTATION OF COMPOUNDED STERILE PREPARATIONS

30

David A. South

INTRODUCTION

Documentation is a record of activities. In the case of compounded sterile preparations (CSPs), appropriate documentation describes how a CSP was made, what quality tests it underwent, and what physical attributes it possesses. Robust documentation requirements help demonstrate that a system is in place that can consistently produce high quality, effective, and safe CSPs. Well-constructed documentation systems can even serve as a checklist for compounding procedures with built in quality assurance and quality control mechanisms. Documentation must be performed precisely, consistently, quickly, and in sufficient detail to permit another individual to investigate or replicate the exact compounding process (including the personnel, environment, raw materials, and process checks) that produced a CSP.

USES OF DOCUMENTATION

Outside Organizations

Many organizations, including state boards of pharmacy, the Centers for Medicare and Medicaid Services (CMS), third-party payers, The Joint Commission and other accrediting agencies, the Drug Enforcement Administration (DEA), and the U.S. Food and Drug Administration (FDA) may inspect the sterile compounding records. These organizations use documentation records when determining payments, granting licensure, and, possibly, justifying continued accreditation of certain programs. Standards of practice, including USP Chapter <797> Pharmaceutical Compounding—Sterile Preparations and USP Chapter <800> Hazardous Drugs—Handling in Healthcare Settings, provide requirements for documentation of environmental and equipment quality, personnel training and technique, compliance with compounding procedures, and safe handling of hazardous drugs.[1;2] The Federal Food, Drug and Cosmetic Act (FD&C Act) sections 503A and 503B also outline the documentation required for traditional compounders and outsourcing facilities respectively.[3] See Chapter 2 for more information on standards, guidelines and enforcement agencies for sterile compounding.

Legal Actions

If a patient pursues litigation related to a CSP, an attorney may subpoena the pharmacy's quality assurance records and other relevant documents. These records can also be reviewed by the organization's legal counsel and its malpractice insurance carrier. In this situation, the quality of documentation may prevent a costly lawsuit or judgment.

Process Deviation and Out-of-Specification Results Review

Whenever a process deviation occurs or a CSP is found to be out-of-specification, the documentation surrounding that preparation may be used for the facility's internal investigation and corrective action. Results from all investigations should be combined into corrective and preventive action (CAPA) plans (see Chapter 32). Data should be trended over time and incorporated into the facility's quality improvement processes (see Chapter 33). Root cause analyses (RCAs) and other investigative actions can use the process documentation to determine exactly where the deviation occurred and what to do to prevent the error in future compounding processes.

Workload Justification

Besides serving as a record of past actions, documentation of goods and services provided by the pharmacy can be used to develop workload statistics and productivity ratios. This information can subsequently support a formal request for adding staff, equipment, or workspace or for reallocating these same resources elsewhere.

Note: The author acknowledges Ryan A. Forrey and E. Clyde Buchanan who authored this chapter in previous editions.

DOI 10.37573/9781585286492.030

CAPTURING DOCUMENTATION AND RECORD RETENTION

Methods for Capturing Documentation

Documentation can be brief or extensive, as long as important facts are not omitted. Best practice includes capturing documentation where the work is completed and while it is in progress. Forms, worksheets, and computer software can prompt the user to document essential information. Computerized labels and auto-populated forms may save time by avoiding duplicate data entries (eg, patient names and locations). Many integrated electronic medical records and pharmacy information systems have the required compounding information (eg, lot numbers, expiration dates, beyond use dates [BUDs], and formulation records) within the electronic system, and they can be designed to capture this information at the point-of-care.

Newer information systems, often referred to as IV workflow automation systems, provide an integrated approach to directing workflow and capturing required documentation. Most of the available systems are built on a formulary database specific to the institution. They contain information about the appropriate drug, diluent, volume, and process checks required for a particular CSP. When set up properly, IV workflow automation systems allow for robust documentation of the compounding process and should be utilized to aid the facility in capturing required documentation. See Chapter 9 for more information on IV workflow automation systems and other sterile compounding technology that may be used for capturing documentation.

Record Retention

Each facility must develop a policy and procedure that describes what records are to be kept, how long each type of record must be kept, where these records are stored, and how to retrieve the records if needed. USP Chapter <797> specifies "all required documentation for a particular CSP (e.g., MFR, CR, and release inspection and testing results) must be readily retrievable for at least 2 years after preparation or as required by laws and regulations of the applicable regulatory jurisdiction or accrediting organization(s), whichever is longer."[1] Additionally, records must be stored in a manner that prevents any damage, deterioration, or loss. When paper or hard copy records are required or used, many facilities now use commercial record storage and retrieval companies for this purpose.

Because record retention requirements may vary based on given requirement or regulatory body oversight, many hospitals and home care organizations utilize electronic data files for long-term storage of records. Patient-specific records must be kept safe and secure to ensure their privacy. Pharmacists must refer to their state pharmacy laws and regulations to determine how long each type of record must be stored before its destruction. Compounding facilities should review each type of record generated and create a records retention policy or table to provide quick and explicit direction on the retention requirements for each type of document.

Handling Documentation Errors

Documentation errors must be handled carefully to avoid the appearance of a malfeasance or records tampering. As with any legal document or medical record, correction fluid should never be used on official records. Instead, a single line should be drawn through the mistake, and the word "error" and the person's initials should be written by it. Missed documentation that should have occurred at some regular interval (eg, daily temperature monitoring) should never be recorded after the fact. For electronic record systems, there must be a clear audit trail for any changes or modifications made to a record. Care must be taken when implementing a system that proper restrictions are in place to prevent alteration of records without a complete audit trail. Additional requirements for documentation errors related to investigational drugs and research studies may exist. It is important that the compounder follow any additional requirements of the study sponsor or principal investigator. USP Chapter <1168> Compounding for Phase 1 Investigational Studies provides some guidance on documentation for Phase 1 investigational study compounding.[4]

REQUIRED ELEMENTS OF DOCUMENTATION

USP Chapter <797> details multiple elements of required documentation.[1] The following section attempts to describe the required elements of documentation without redundantly describing overall requirements of the chapter.

Personnel Training, Competency Assessments, and Qualification Records

Training and evaluation of pharmacists and pharmacy technicians who compound sterile preparations must be documented prior to them performing their duties independently. It is not adequate to state that an employee passed an initial evaluation period. Specific training about aseptic technique, working in an ISO Class 5 environment, appropriate garb and personal hygiene, cleaning, disinfection practices, and storage and handling of drugs and supplies should be documented in facility standard operating procedures (SOPs). These elements should be in accordance with the facility's written training program.

Employees should also be trained in the setup, calibration, and use of all compounding devices and equipment. Training should be recorded for each type of equipment used. Any personnel who transport, compound, or administer hazardous drugs must be trained and have appropriate documentation of training.[2] The verification of acceptable practices must be documented before employees are allowed to compound sterile preparations for patients. Personnel records should also include documentation of employee health records (eg, annual physical, acknowledgment and medical surveillance documentation for those who handle hazardous drugs, hazardous drug exposures, tuberculin skin tests, and vaccinations against contagious diseases) and offers to provide vaccinations against diseases (eg, hepatitis B, influenza).[5]

Employee competencies must be re-evaluated and documented at the required interval according to their job function and the category of sterile compounds they produce. Documentation of retesting must include the following[1]:

- Evaluation of aseptic technique with media fills followed by immediate feedback
- Media fill and fingertip sterility testing: Sampling data must be collected and reviewed on a routine basis as a means of evaluating personnel aseptic technique and the overall control of the compounding environment.
- Observation of hand cleansing and garbing, aseptic technique and related practices, and cleaning and disinfection procedures

When documenting media fill and sterility testing, USP Chapter <797> requires the following information at a minimum:[1]

- Name of the person evaluated
- Evaluation date and time
- Media and components used, including their manufacturer or supplier
- Expiration dates and lot numbers
- Starting temperature for each interval of incubation
- Dates of incubation
- The results
- The names or other identification of the observer and the person who reads and documents the results

In addition to testing for appropriate hand hygiene, garbing (including gloved fingertip and thumb testing), and aseptic manipulation (including media fill and gloved fingertip testing), compounding personnel must complete training and demonstrate knowledge of compounding principles at least every 12 months according to the facility's written training program. Such exams should include a prespecified passing grade, and exam scores should be documented as part of the annual examination process. Records of these evaluations must be maintained to provide a record of ongoing assessment of personnel competency.

Certification Reports

The quality of ISO classified environments must be certified prior to initial use, following any changes to the area (redesign, construction, replacement or relocation of a primary engineering control [PEC] or other changes that can alter airflow and effectiveness of PECs or secondary engineering controls [SECs]) and at least every 6 months thereafter. The following elements of certification that must be performed and documented for all classified areas include[1]:

- Airflow testing, including air changes per hour (ACPH) and pressure differentials
- HEPA filter integrity testing
- Total particle count
- Dynamic airflow smoke pattern test
- The number of personnel present in each PEC or SEC during testing of total particle count and dynamic airflow smoke pattern

All certification records must be maintained and reviewed by supervising personnel or other designated employees to ensure that the controlled environments comply with the proper air cleanliness, room pressures, and ACPH. It is recommended that this review be formally documented, though not required by USP Chapter <797>. A corrective action plan must also be formulated and documented in response to any out-of-range results (see Chapter 32).

Environmental Monitoring and Facility Control

Monitoring the effectiveness, cleanliness, and overall appropriateness of the compounding environment is a core function of an effective compounding program. Not only should the environment be monitored, results of monitoring must be documented. It is easiest to think of the required elements of environmental monitoring and documentation in terms of daily, monthly, and every 6 months requirements.

Daily Facility Monitoring

The following elements related to the compounding environment, including component storage areas, must be monitored and documented on a daily basis. Results of certain elements may be recorded via a continuous recording device as long as the results are retrievable. Results should be reviewed as described in facility SOPs and the review documented.

- Temperature
- Relative humidity
- Pressure differentials (if applicable)

Monthly Environmental Monitoring

In addition to daily facility monitoring requirements, surfaces should be monitored for bacterial contamination on at least a monthly basis (see Chapter 31). These results must be documented. Results of a given sample should be recorded along with the given action level for the sample. If the action level is exceeded, a root cause analysis must be conducted, and corrective action must be taken (see Chapter 32). The results of the corrective action must be documented. In addition to the documentation of the results themselves, the incubator temperature must be monitored during incubation, either manually or by a continuous recording device, and the results must be reviewed and documented as described in the facility's SOPs.[1]

When conducting environmental monitoring, it is important to evaluate specific results and trend data over time. By monitoring trends over time, one may be able to see a particular area proceeding toward an out-of-control state even before an action level is exceeded.

A comprehensive cleaning strategy is one of the most important facets of an effective compounding program. The cleaning strategy must be described in facility SOPs and documented accordingly. Maintaining a checklist of required daily and monthly cleaning tasks can be a simple and reliable method for ensuring documentation is collected appropriately. Alternatively, many of the IV workflow automation systems available on the market today also offer the ability to capture daily, weekly, and monthly cleaning tasks.

Equipment Records

Personnel must maintain records of equipment calibration, verification, and maintenance in accordance with the requirements in USP Chapter <797>.[1] Examples of equipment utilized frequently during compounding include PECs, scales, and automated compounding devices. For automated compounding devices, the accuracy of the device must be documented each day the device is used. If a restricted-access barrier system (RABS) is used as the PEC, the recovery time after opening the transfer chamber to achieve ISO Class 5 must be documented (determined/stated by the manufacturer). Temperature and humidity measuring devices must be calibrated at least every 12 months or more frequently per manufacturer requirements. Any process evaluations to assess for containment of airborne chemical particles required for weighing, measuring, or manipulation must be documented in accordance with facility SOPs. Additionally, for facilities conducting their own environmental monitoring, the equipment used in those processes require routine inspection, calibration, and associated documentation.

Receipt of Components

In addition to the usual purchasing and inventory records for pharmaceuticals, the use of bulk chemicals (active pharmaceutical ingredients [APIs]) to compound high-risk CSPs must be documented accordingly. Whenever APIs are used, they must have a Certificate of Analysis (COA) that includes the specifications, test results, and proof that the API meets the specifications.[1] These COAs should be filed for future reference. When bulk chemicals are opened, the date of opening should be recorded on the container. When quantitative testing is done to verify the quality and purity of bulk ingredients, records of these tests should be kept. Each lot of commercially available sterile, depyrogenated containers and container closure systems must be accompanied by a COA or other documentation showing conformance with established specifications (ie, sterility and depyrogenation requirements). If sterilization and depyrogenation of supplies or container closure systems are performed on site, the efficacy of each process must be established and documented.[1]

Standard Operating Procedures, Master Formulation Records, and Compounding Records

Facility SOPs detail the procedures to be followed for every aspect of sterile compounding. They are essential components of facility documentation. SOPs must be reviewed initially and at least every 12 months by designated people to ensure that they reflect current practices, and the review must be documented. Any changes or alterations to an SOP can only be made by designated people, and changes must be documented. Revisions to SOPs must be communicated to all personnel involved in these processes and procedures, and personnel should document acknowledgment of the communication.[1]

The process of preparing each individual CSP must be documented via a compounding record (CR). Master formulation records (MFRs) are often used to dictate the compounding process and are required for certain types of CSPs. In many cases, the MFR can serve as the basis for creating a CR.

A compounding record is typically created during the compounding process or as soon as possible thereafter. It is intended to document the exact steps and components that were used in the preparation of a CSP. USP Chapter <797> specifies the exact information that must be recorded for each CSP.[1] The required elements include the following:

- Name, strength or activity, and dosage form of the CSP
- Date and time of preparation of the CSP
- Assigned internal identification number (eg, prescription, order, or lot number)
- A method to identify the individuals involved in the compounding process and individuals verifying the final CSP
- Name of each component
- Vendor, lot number, and expiration date for each component for CSPs prepared for more than one patient and for CSPs prepared from nonsterile ingredients(s)
- Weight or volume of each component
- Strength of activity of each component
- Total quantity compounded
- Final yield (eg, quantity, containers, number of units)
- Assigned BUD and storage requirements

- Results of quality control (QC) procedures (eg, visual inspection, filter integrity testing, pH testing)
- Master Formulation Record reference (if applicable)
- Calculations made to determine and verify quantities and/or concentrations of components (if applicable)

Whereas the compounding process for all prepared CSPs should be documented on the CR as described above, certain CSPs must also be prepared according to an MFR. The MFR is required when preparing CSPs for more than one patient and when preparing CSPs from nonsterile ingredients. While compounding records are essentially created during the process of compounding, an MFR is prepared in advance of the compounding process and can be thought of as a recipe that can be easily reproduced each time a particular CSP is needed. As such, changes to the MFR should be made cautiously, and they must be approved and documented according to a facility's SOP. As with compounding records, USP Chapter <797> specifies the exact information that must be contained within each MFR. These elements include the following[1]:

- Name, strength or activity, and dosage form of the CSP
- Identities, amounts of all ingredients, and if applicable, relevant characteristics of components (eg, particle size, salt form, purity grade, solubility)
- Type and size of container closure system(s)
- Complete instructions for preparing the CSP, including equipment, supplies, a description of the compounding steps, and any special precautions
- Physical description of the final CSP
- BUD and storage requirements
- Reference source to support the stability of the CSP
- QC procedures (eg, pH testing, filter integrity testing)
- Other information needed to describe the compounding process and ensure repeatability (eg, adjusting pH and tonicity or sterilization method, such as steam, dry heat, irradiation, or filter)

Ensuring that all required information is captured for both MFRs and CRs is paramount to an effective compounding program. However, actually collecting all required information need not be more time intensive than necessary. It is both feasible and recommended to design MFR template documents with all the required information for a given CSP that can be stored electronically prior to use. When a particular CSP is needed, the MFR document can be used to guide the compounding process and document the required information for the particular CSP, thus creating a CR in the process.

Additionally, some facilities have found it useful to print an additional production label for each patient-specific CSP being prepared. Not only can the pharmacy information system prepopulate most of the required elements of the CR, it can also serve as a useful guide for preparing the CSP and collecting the remaining required elements. These production labels can then be kept per the facilities SOP to serve as the CR for that particular CSP. As mentioned above, IV workflow technologies are changing the landscape in automating both the preparation and documentation of CSPs. When effectively designed, these technologies assist with the capture of all required elements of both MFRs and CRs, allowing all documentation to be captured and stored electronically.

Release Inspection and Testing Records

All release testing procedures must be included in the facilities documentation (namely MFRs and SOPs). The MFR and/or SOP should describe the documentation required following appropriate testing and before release can occur. Additionally, any documentation produced in conjunction with an out-of-specification result investigation and corrective action plan must be maintained as part of the quality assurance and QC program (see Chapters 31, 32).

Information Related to Complaints and Adverse Events, Including Corrective Actions Taken

Any complaints received or notification of adverse events resulting from the administration of a compounded product must be documented. A readily retrievable written or electronic record of each complaint must be kept by the facility, regardless of the source of the complaint (eg, email, telephone, or mail). The record must contain the name of the complainant or other unique identifier, the date the complaint was received, the nature of the complaint, and the response to the complaint. Additionally, if available, the name, strength, and assigned internal identification number should be recorded. The record must also include the findings of any investigation and any follow up. Records of complaints must be easily retrievable for review and evaluation for possible trends, and they must be retained for at least 2 years or longer if required by law.[1]

Results of Investigations and Corrective Actions

The assurance of CSP quality and packaging integrity is highly dependent on the proper adherence of all personnel to the pertinent SOPs.[1] For each compounding facility, a designated person must design, implement, and maintain a formal education, training, and quality assurance program that encompasses all the functions and tasks addressed in this chapter. The program should also include a record of all the personnel who are assigned these tasks, including nonpharmacy personnel (eg, home care nurses, employees of common carriers, and patients at home). Additionally, this program includes the assessment and documentation of procedural breaches, administration errors, side effects, allergic reactions, and complications associated with dosage or administration, such as extravasation. The quality assurance program should be coordinated with the institution's adverse events and incident reporting programs.[1]

Examples of the activities that may result in investigations and corrective action plans include aseptic technique simulation and gloved fingertip sampling, environmental monitoring (eg, surface sampling or viable airborne particle sampling), sterility and other release testing failures, and complaint and/or adverse event reports.

Compounding Allergenic Extracts

Allergenic extract prescription sets must follow standards as specified in the applicable section of USP Chapter <797>. Additional detail regarding considerations for allergenic extract compounding can be found in Chapter 24. Required elements of documentation include the following[1]:

- SOPs describing all aspects of the compounding process
- Personnel training records, competency assessments, and qualification records including corrective actions for any failures
- Certification reports of the PEC, if used, including corrective actions for any failures
- Temperature logs for refrigerator(s)
- Compounding records for individual allergenic extract prescription sets
- Information related to the complaints and adverse events including corrective actions taken
- Investigations and corrective actions

SUMMARY

Documentation is an important and essential part of any sterile compounding program. Best practices include capturing documentation where the work is completed and while it is in progress. Such documentation may be used to validate current processes, justify third-party payments, prevent or provide a basis for legal action, justify workloads, discover errors in practice and procedure, and quality improvement.

REFERENCES

1. USP <797> Pharmaceutical compounding—sterile preparations. In: *2023: USP Compounding Compendium*. Rockville, MD: The United States Pharmacopeial Convention. doi:10.31003/USPNF_M99925_07_01.
2. USP <800> Hazardous drugs—handling in healthcare settings. In: *2023: USP Compounding Compendium*. Rockville, MD: The United States Pharmacopeial Convention. doi:10.31003/USPNF_M7808_07_01.
3. Compounding Laws and Policies. U.S. Food and Drug Administration. **https://www.fda.gov/drugs/human-drug-compounding/compounding-laws-and-policies**. Accessed August 18, 2023.
4. USP <1168> Compounding for phase I investigational studies. In: *2023 USP Compounding Compendium*. Rockville, MD: The United States Pharmacopeial Convention. doi:10.31003/USPNF_M7807_04_01.
5. Uselton JP, Kienle P, Murdaugh LB. Human resource standards checklist. In: *Meeting accreditation standards: a pharmacy preparation guide*. 9th ed. Bethesda, MD: American Society of Health-System Pharmacists; 2019:297–312.

ENVIRONMENTAL QUALITY AND CONTROL

31

Patricia C. Kienle

INTRODUCTION AND REQUIREMENTS

A high-quality management program seeks to identify problems before they occur. Although there are several critical elements to consider when working in or managing a sterile compounding operation, environmental sampling has historically received minimal consideration in pharmacy practice. In other industries, great attention is placed on the influence and impact that the operating environment has on the quality of the product.[1] It is widely accepted in the pharmaceutical industry that production facility design, environment, and personnel have a direct effect on the integrity of aseptically prepared products.[2]

It is essential to ensure that quality be built into compounding sterile preparations before they are distributed. This system is known as quality by design. The characteristics of a quality-by-design system include the following:

- The preparation is designed to meet patient requirements.
- The process is designed to consistently meet preparation critical quality attributes.
- The impact of formulation components and process parameters on preparation quality is understood.
- Critical sources of process variability are identified and controlled.

The process must be continually monitored and updated to ensure consistent quality over time.[3] Proper sterile compounding requires "a strict design regime, not only on the process area, but on the interactions with surrounding areas and the movement of people, materials and equipment so as not to compromise the aseptic conditions."[4] The environment where sterile preparations are compounded must be suitable for its intended purposes.[5] One intended purpose of a properly designed, constructed, and operated compounding environment is to minimize the impact of human and process generated contamination that can affect sterility or stability. There are several interconnected and dynamic variables that form the foundation of a solid environmental monitoring program (see **Figure 31-1**). Failing to understand, maintain, and monitor the compounding environment and the personnel working in these areas has resulted in significant patient injury and death.[6-15] Primary and secondary engineering controls (PECs and SECs) are used to prevent, reduce, and control potential contaminants from being introduced into CSPs and to support environmental control programs (see Chapters 6 and 7 for details). They can, however, be thwarted by inappropriate personnel work practices.

An equally important variable is the contribution and influence of the employee's hand hygiene and garbing practices on the sterility of compounded sterile preparations (CSPs). In 1982, a study was published that demonstrated that there is a high correlation between the bacterial contamination on hands and on contaminated vials.[16] Several other studies have confirmed the significant contribution of employee technique and touch contamination to contaminated vials.[17-19]

USP Chapter <797> Pharmaceutical Compounding—Sterile Preparations requires each organization to have a written environmental quality and control plan. Common problem areas for compounding locations that received U.S. Food and Drug Administration (FDA) warnings for violating good practices include the following[20]:

- Lack of or not following standard operating procedures (SOPs)
- Visible microbial growth in the International Organization for Standardization (ISO) Class 5 area or surroundings

Note: The author acknowledges Eric S. Kastango who authored this chapter in the previous edition.

DOI 10.37573/9781585286492.031

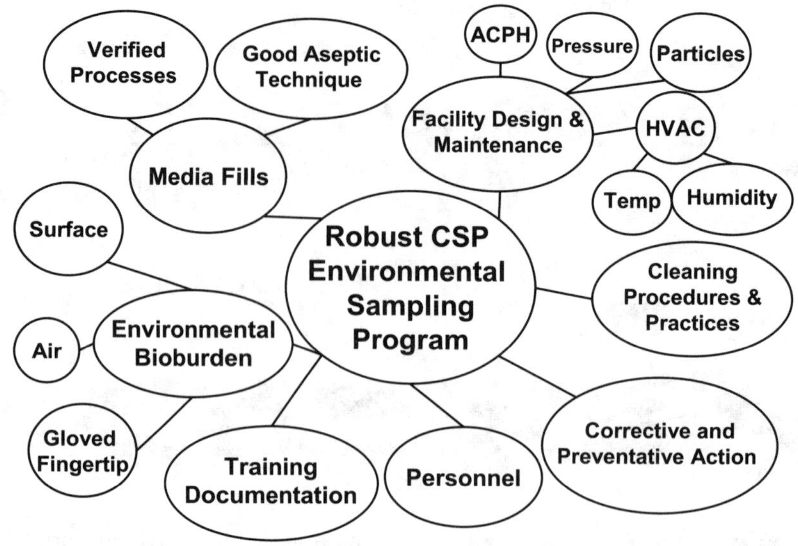

FIGURE 31-1. Elements of a robust environmental monitoring quality program

ACPH = air changes per hour; CSP = compounded sterile preparation; HVAC = heating, venting, and air conditioning; Temp = temperature.
Source: Reprinted with permission of CriticalPoint.

- Sources of nonmicrobial contamination in the ISO Class 5 area (eg, rust)
- Performing aseptic manipulations outside of an ISO Class 5 (or higher) area
- Personnel practices that are a contamination hazard to an exposed sterile product, component, or preparation
- Exposing sterile products or materials to lower than ISO 5 conditions for any length of time
- Cleanrooms with unsealed or loose ceiling tiles
- Poor technique, including inappropriate movement of materials in the cleanroom
- Using a filter for product sterilization that is not certified as pharmaceutical-grade and sterilizing-grade
- Using parameters for sterilization that are not lethal to resistant microorganisms

In recent years, most healthcare providers have been affected by drug shortages and the discontinuation of drug products. Some of these shortages and discontinuations have been caused by plant closures resulting from the FDA citations involving environmental control and monitoring programs. A comprehensive quality management program should include these elements:

- Staff education (both initially and ongoing)
- Aseptic technique media fill verification testing
- Gloved fingertip testing
- Certification of primary and secondary engineering controls
- Finished preparation release checks and tests
- Cleaning and disinfection controls
- Environmental quality and controls

This chapter focuses on environmental sampling requirements and controls to assist in the development and implementation of a robust compounding quality assurance program. USP Chapter <797> separated the viable environmental sampling requirements into facility-related sampling, including air sampling via volumetric impaction collection and surface sampling.

Viable air sampling is required at least every 6 months. Surface sampling is required for all classified areas and pass-through chambers opening into classified areas. Facilities compounding Category 1 and 2 CSPs must perform this at least monthly. Facilities compounding Category 3 CSPs must perform this at least weekly and at the end of each batch of Category 3 CSPs within the PEC. See USP Chapter <797> for a full explanation.

Environmentally controlled work areas (ie, ISO Class 5, 7, and 8) must operate within exact specifications and be adequate for the functions being performed in them. These controls must be monitored through the following[21]:

- Limiting access to environmentally controlled areas
- Proper design of compounding facilities
- Quality and quantity of high-efficiency particulate air (HEPA)–filtered supply air
- Maintenance and monitoring of continuous positive or negative pressure differentials between environmentally controlled and uncontrolled areas

- Maintaining air cleanliness limits based on critical activities in each respective engineering control (ie, ISO Class 5, 7, or 8)
- Routine monitoring of operating temperatures and humidity
- Routine environmental airborne particulates and microbial sampling
- ISO classified work area testing and certification
- Routine cleaning of work areas

CRITICAL SITES

Sterile components are manipulated in the direct compounding area (DCA). USP Chapter <797> requires that the DCA where critical sites are exposed be within an ISO Class 5 environment or better. Air particle counts for ISO Class 5 conditions call for no more than 3,520 particles (0.5 µm or larger) per cubic meter.

The key operating condition when working within a PEC, including laminar airflow workbenches (LAFWs), biological safety cabinet (BSCs), compounding aseptic isolators (CAIs), or compounding aseptic containment isolators (CACIs), is the unidirectional HEPA-filtered air (ie, first-air), which must move at a velocity sufficient to remove or sweep any particulate matter that may get introduced by personnel, components, containers, and equipment out of the PEC and downstream of the critical sites in the DCA. The recommended airflow velocity across the entire work surface should be maintained at 90 feet per minute (±20%) for LAFWs, but velocity is lower for BSCs and compounding isolators (see Chapter 6). This operating condition is pre-engineered into the equipment being used but needs to be routinely monitored to ensure that airflow velocity is being maintained. Any PEC used for sterile compounding must be operated continuously. All work surfaces must be disinfected with sterile 70% isopropyl alcohol (sIPA) prior to starting aseptic compounding. All engineering controls should run continuously so that the air cleanliness of the various controlled compounding environments is maintained. During the handling of packages of syringes and needles along with other materials, it is critical to work downstream of the DCA (see **Figure 31-2**) to prevent nonviable or viable contamination.

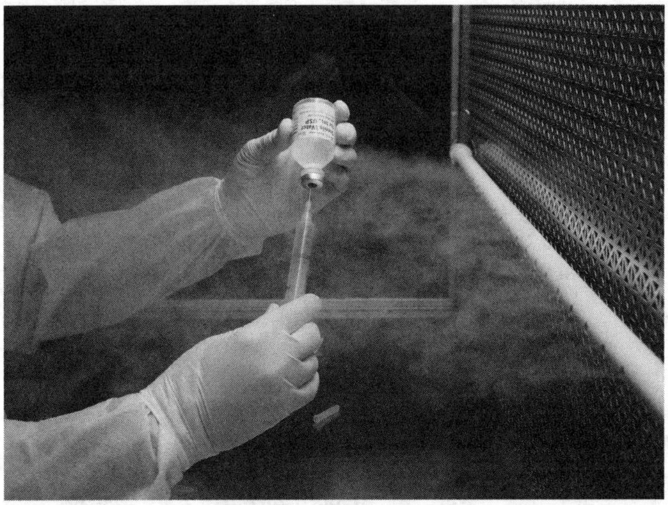

FIGURE 31-2. Working within the direct compounding area (DCA)

Source: Reprinted with permission of CriticalPoint.

PHYSICAL PLANT DESCRIPTIONS

USP Chapter <797> requires that the environments where pharmacy activities occur (eg, warehousing and storage, preparation and staging, and aseptic processing) be designed to provide the best level of cleanliness possible.[21] This is achieved through tiered zones of cleanliness where the closer things are to the DCA, the cleaner the environment (air and surfaces) should be. This level of cleanliness is achieved through various human and engineered methods. They include handwashing, gowning, masking, gloving, material transfer, and process and preparation workflows. The engineering controls include HEPA-filtered air, laminar airflow, isolation, room air exchanges, and positive or negative air pressure differentials between the various zones of cleanliness. It is important to define the physical plant areas (zones of cleanliness) in the pharmacy that will meet USP Chapter <797> standards. Rooms and areas in which CSPs are mixed are SECs, which include the anteroom, buffer room, segregated compounding area (SCA), and containment segregated compounding area (C-SCA).

Anteroom

An anteroom is an ISO class 8 or better room where personnel hand hygiene and garbing procedures and staging of components occurs. It is also a transition area that (1) ensures pressure relationships are constantly maintained so that air flows from clean to dirty areas, and (2) reduces the need for a heating, ventilating, and air conditioning (HVAC) control system to respond to large disturbances.[21] This room is considered clean and supports hand hygiene and garbing procedures. It should not be used for high particulate-generating activities that can be performed outside the ISO classified area. Temperature should be 68°F (20°C) or cooler. The relative humidity of this area should be no more than 60% to control mold and mildew. If an anteroom supports a hazardous buffer room, the air cleanliness classification of the anteroom must be at least ISO Class 7 and have at least 30 air changes per hour (ACPH).[21; 22] If the anteroom only supports a nonhazardous buffer area, it must be at least ISO Class 8 and have at least 20 ACPH.[21]

Buffer Room

A buffer room is the portion of the cleanroom in which the PEC is physically located. Activities that occur in this area include the preparation and staging of components and supplies used when compounding CSPs.[21] This space is designated for compounding sterile preparations. A buffer room has a controlled number of airborne particles and is constructed to minimize the introduction, generation, and retention of particles inside the room. The room also ensures that other critical operating factors, like temperature, humidity, and air pressure, are controlled as required by the facility design and type of compounding activities being performed. Temperature should be no higher than 68°F (20°C), and relative humidity should be no more than 60%. The minimum number of ACPH required in the buffer room is 30. PECs that are exhausted into the buffer area can contribute up to 15 ACPH.[21]

Segregated Compounding Area

SCAs are designated spaces with either a demarcated area or room that is restricted to preparing nonhazardous CSPs. Beyond-use dates (BUDs) assigned to CSPs compounded in a SCA cannot exceed 12 hours at room temperature or 24 hours if refrigerated. Such areas must contain a PEC that provides unidirectional airflow of ISO Class 5 air quality for preparation of CSPs, and they must not use activities and materials that are extraneous to sterile compounding.[21] The area does not need to be ISO classified.

Containment Segregated Compounding Area

A special type of SCA may be used for preparation of hazardous drugs (HDs). This C-SCA must be a room with fixed walls, a negative pressure of 0.010 to 0.030 inches water column (WC) negative to surrounding nonhazardous rooms, be vented to the outside, and have at least 12 ACPH.[22] The room does not need to be ISO classified. Like an SCA for non-HDs, BUDs assigned to CSPs compounded in a C-SCA cannot exceed 12 hours room temperature or 24 hours if refrigerated.

General Pharmacy Area

In the general pharmacy area, temperature should be controlled in the range between 15°C to 25°C (59°F to 77°F) and have a limited number of extreme temperature excursions. The mean kinetic temperature of this environment should not exceed 25°C (77°F).[23] To control mold, mildew, and electrostatic charges, the relative humidity of this area should be between 30% and 65%. This area does not need to be ISO classified with respect to air cleanliness.

PLACEMENT OF PRIMARY ENGINEERING CONTROLS

The PEC must be located in the SEC (ie, buffer area, SCA, or C-SCA) as stipulated by USP Chapter <797> and USP Chapter <800> Hazardous Drugs—Handling in Healthcare Settings.[21;22] PECs (including CAIs and CACIs) must be in a cleanroom suite in order to assign the full BUDs allowed in USP Chapter <797>.[21]

NONVIABLE ENVIRONMENTAL AIR SAMPLING

USP Chapter <797> specifies that the environmental sampling and testing program must demonstrate an environment in the compounding area that consistently ensures acceptably low viable and nonviable particle levels. The compounding areas include the ISO Class 5 PEC, buffer rooms, anterooms, SCAs, and C-SCAs.[21;22]

Certification must occur as part of a comprehensive quality management program (see Chapter 33). They must occur minimally under any of the following conditions[21]:

- As part of the commissioning and certification of new facilities and equipment
- At least every 6 months
- Following any servicing of facilities and equipment
- After any changes to the area (eg, redesign, construction, replacement or relocation of any PEC)
- Alteration to the room that could affect airflow or air quality

Certification must include airflow testing, HEPA filter integrity testing, total particulate counts, and dynamic airflow smoke pattern tests. A corrective action plan must be implemented and documented for any occurrences that are out of range. Confirmation that the action taken was effective must be documented. The environmental sampling program (see **Table 31-1**), which is required in all facilities that prepare, store, or transport CSPs, is designed to provide important information to staff and leadership. This program allows them to demonstrate that the compounding area is maintaining an environment that consistently ensures acceptably low viable and nonviable particle levels.

Environmental Nonviable Airborne Particle Testing Program

A program to monitor nonviable airborne particles differs from a viable particle monitoring program in that it is intended to directly measure the performance of the engineering controls used to create the various levels of air cleanliness (eg, ISO Class 5, 7, or 8).

Engineering Control Performance Verification

PECs and SECs are essential components of the overall contamination control strategy for aseptic compounding. It is imperative that they perform as designed and the resulting levels of contamination be within acceptable limits. Certification procedures, such as those outlined in the Controlled Environmental Testing Association *Certification Guide for Sterile Compounding Facilities* revised in 2022, must be performed by a qualified individual no less than every 6 months and whenever the device or room is relocated, altered, or major service to the facility is performed.[24]

TABLE 31-1. Required and Recommended Quality Program Elements

Element	Minimum Frequency
Temperature	Daily
Humidity	Daily
Pressure differential	Daily
Airflow testing	Every 6 months
HEPA filter integrity test	Every 6 months
Total particle count testing	Every 6 months
Dynamic airflow smoke pattern test of PEC	Every 6 months
Dynamic airflow smoke pattern test of SEC	Once, if air wall returns/exhausts are not close enough to the floor to establish the ability to control airflow in the room
Environmental electronic air by impaction of all ISO classified area	Every 6 months
Surface sampling of all ISO classified areas and pass-through chambers opening into ISO classified areas	Monthly

ISO = International Organization for Standardization; PEC = primary engineering control; SEC = secondary engineering control.

Source: Adapted with permission of USP <797> Pharmaceutical compounding—sterile preparations. In: *2023: USP Compounding Compendium.* Rockville, MD: United States Pharmacopeial Convention; 2023.

Total Particle Counts

Certification that each ISO classified room is within established guidelines must be performed no less than every 6 months and whenever the PEC is relocated or the physical structure of the buffer room or anteroom is altered. Testing must be performed by qualified operators using current, state-of-the-art electronic equipment and produce the following results:

- No more than 3,520 particles (0.5 µm and larger) per cubic meter of air (ISO Class 5) for any PEC
- No more than 352,000 particles (0.5 µm and larger) per cubic meter of air (ISO Class 7) for any buffer room or an anteroom leading to a negative pressure HD compounding buffer room
- No more than 3,520,000 particles (0.5 µm and larger) per cubic meter of air (ISO Class 8) for an anteroom leading only to a non-HD compounding area

A designated person must maintain and review all certification records to ensure that the controlled environments comply with the proper air cleanliness, room pressures, and ACPH.

PRESSURE DIFFERENTIAL MONITORING

To avoid particulates and contaminants from entering the sterile compounding area, positive air pressure must be maintained relative to adjacent support areas for non-HD compounding. The minimum industry standard of practice for air pressure differential for buffer rooms is at least 0.020 inches WC positive to adjacent spaces (WC is the unit of measurement commonly used to measure the difference between high and low pressures in controlled compounding environments). This prevents dirtier air that has more particulate matter from entering a cleaner area (see **Figure 31-3**).

For compounding HDs, a containment primary engineering control (C-PEC) must be located in a containment secondary engineering control (C-SEC), which can be an externally vented ISO Class 7 buffer room with an ISO Class 7 anteroom or an externally vented C-SCA. The ISO Class 7 buffer room must have a negative pressure between 0.010 and 0.030 inches WC relative to adjacent areas and a minimum of 30 ACPH. If the C-PEC is placed in an unclassified C-SCA, a negative pressure between 0.010 and 0.030 inches WC relative to the surrounding nonhazardous rooms and a minimum of 12 ACPH must be maintained.[22]

A pressure gauge must be installed to monitor the pressure differential and airflow between the buffer room and anteroom, the anteroom and the general environment outside the compounding area, and the C-SCA and the surrounding nonhazardous room. The results must be reviewed and documented in a log on a daily basis or by a recording device.

USP Chapter <797> created a quality schema for personnel-related environmental sampling that is an important quality assurance procedure required of all compounders (eg, pharmacists, technicians, nurses, physicians, etc.). These personnel-related environmental monitoring processes are tied to activities that pose the greatest risk of contamination to the CSP, such as hand hygiene, garbing and gloving, cleaning, and aseptic compounding procedures. By associating glove fingertip sampling to specific personnel-related activities, microbial bioburden can be tied directly to an individual.

The risk of contaminating a CSP is highly dependent on proper hand hygiene and garbing practices, compounding aseptic technique, and the presence of surface contamination. A sampling program in conjunction with an observational audit must be designed to evaluate the competency of compounding personnel work practices, allowing for the implementation of corrective actions on an ongoing basis. CSPs mixed with starting nonsterile components pose the greatest threat to patients because compounders are

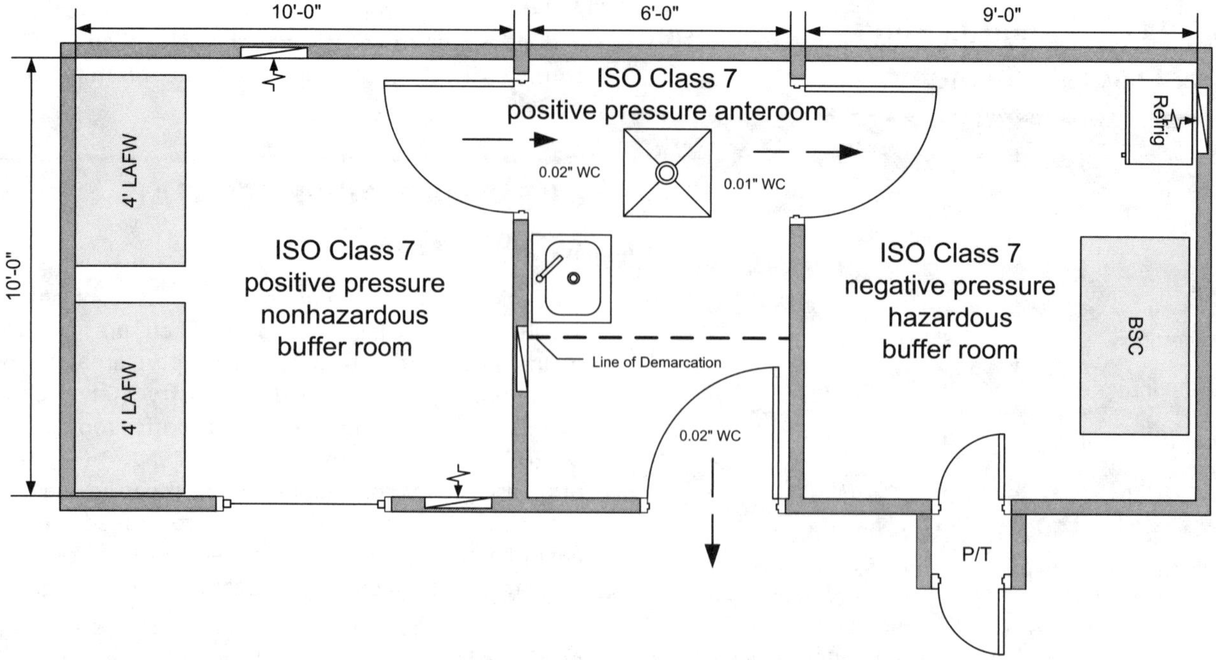

FIGURE 31-3. Sample floor plan for sterile compounding area and respective ISO classifications and pressure relationships

BSC = biological safety cabinet; HD = hazardous drug; ISO = International Organization for Standardization; LAFW = laminar airflow workbench; P/T = pass-through; Refrig = refrigerator; WC = water column.

Source: Reprinted with permission of CriticalPoint.

required to process nonsterile components and devices to achieve sterility.

Sampling Plan

An environmental sampling plan must be developed for airborne viable particles based on an assessment of compounding activities. USP Chapter <797> uses the term viable monitoring to differentiate monitoring for microbial contamination from nonviable (particle) monitoring. Selected sampling sites must include locations within each ISO Class 5 environment and in the ISO Class 7 and 8 rooms or the SCA and C-SCA at greatest risk of contamination. The plan must include sample locations, methods of collection, frequency of sampling, volumes of air sampled, and times of day related to each activity in the compounding area and action levels.

Review of the data generated during a sampling event may detect elevated amounts of airborne microbial bioburden. Such changes may indicate adverse changes within the environment. Compounding personnel should refer to USP Chapter <1116> Microbiological Control and Monitoring of Aseptic Processing Environments for more.[25]

Growth Medium

A general microbiological growth medium, such as soybean casein digest medium (eg, trypticase soy broth [TSB] and trypticase soy agar [TSA]), must be used to support the growth of bacteria. Malt extract agar (MEA) or similar media may be used to detect fungus. Media used for surface sampling must be supplemented with additives to neutralize the effects of disinfecting agents (eg, TSA with lecithin and polysorbate 80).

Air Sampling

Evaluation of airborne microorganisms in the controlled air environments (ISO Class 5, 7 and 8 rooms) must be performed by properly trained individuals for all compounding risk levels. The sampling devices must be properly calibrated and documented for appropriate use. Many organizations outsource this function, often to the company that performs their semiannual facility certification. Those certifiers contract with a laboratory specializing in environmental samples to perform the incubation and reading of the samples.[26]

Impaction is the required method of volumetric air sampling. Settling plates are not suitable for monitoring. The settling of airborne particles by gravity onto culture plates depends on the particle size and may be influenced by air movement. Consequently, the number of microbial colony forming units (CFUs) on a settling plate may not relate to the concentrations of viable particles in the sampled air.[27;28]

Air sampling must be performed for all risk levels of compounding at locations that are prone to contamination during compounding activities and during other activities, such as staging, labeling, gowning, and cleaning. Locations must include zones of air backwash turbulence within the LAWF and other areas where air backwash turbulence may enter the buffer and anterooms (eg, doorways, pass-through chambers, in and around ISO Class 5 engineering controls and environments). Consideration should be given to the overall effect the chosen sampling method will have on the unidirectional airflow within a compounding environment.

Air Sampling Devices

There are several manufacturers of electric air sampling equipment. Compounding personnel should refer to the manufacturer's recommended procedures when using the equipment to perform volumetric air sampling procedures. The instructions in the manufacturer's user manual for verification and use of electric air samplers must be followed. A sufficient volume of air (eg, 1,000 L) must be tested at each location to optimize sensitivity. The volumetric air sampling devices need to be serviced and calibrated as recommended by the manufacturer. Compounding personnel should also refer to USP Chapter <1116> for additional information on techniques that should be used to detect environmental bioburden excursions.[25]

Incubation Period

At the end of the designated sampling or exposure period for all environmental sampling activities (air, surface, or personnel), the plates must be retrieved, covers secured (eg, taped), inverted and incubated at a temperature and for a time period conducive to multiplication of microorganisms. See <797> for incubation times and temperatures based on the media used.[21]

The number of discrete colonies of micro-organisms must be counted and reported as CFUs and documented on an environmental monitoring form. Counts from air monitoring need to be transformed into CFU per cubic meter of air and evaluated for adverse trends (Chapter 11).

Action Levels, Documentation, and Data Evaluation

The greatest value of air microbial sampling within the compounding environment is realized when normal baseline CFU counts are evaluated over a period of time. Environmental sampling data that are collected and trended are a means of evaluating the overall control of the compounding environment. If an area consistently shows elevated levels of microbial growth, competent microbiology personnel must be consulted.

Table 31-2 lists the action levels required by USP Chapter <797>. Determining the baseline CFU counts permits identification of an increasing trend of microbial CFUs. An increasing trend in CFU counts should prompt re-evaluation of the adequacy of cleaning procedures, operational procedures, personnel work practices, and air filtration efficiency within the aseptic compounding location.

When action levels are exceeded, an investigation into the source of the contamination must be conducted. Sources may include HVAC systems, damaged HEPA filters, and changes in personnel garbing or working practices. It is important to eliminate the source of the problem, clean the affected area, and then resample.

TABLE 31-2. Microbial Sample Action Levels Required by USP Chapter <797>

Classification	Air	Gloved Fingertip	Surface
	CFU per 1,000 Liters of Air per Plate	CFUs per Set of Two Plates	CFU per Plate
ISO 5	>1	>3	>3
ISO 7	>10	NA	>5
ISO 8	>100	NA	>50

CFU = colony forming unit; ISO = International Organization for Standardization.

Source: Adapted with permission of USP <797> Pharmaceutical compounding—sterile preparations. In: *2023: USP Compounding Compendium*. Rockville, MD: United States Pharmacopeial Convention; 2023.

When gloved fingertip sample results exceeds action levels after proper incubation, a review of hand hygiene, garbing procedures, glove and surface disinfection procedures, and work practices must be performed and documented. Employee training may be required to correct the source of the problem.

ENVIRONMENTAL MONITORING FOR HAZARDOUS DRUG CONTAMINATION

When HDs are handled, monitoring for HD contamination should be performed to ensure a safe area for patient treatment and a safe workplace for personnel. USP Chapter <800> recommends baseline and periodic environmental monitoring by use of surface wipe samples for areas most likely to be contaminated.[22] These areas include surfaces within the C-PEC and any equipment contained in it, surfaces on counters and carts near the C-PEC, pass-through chambers between the anteroom or buffer room and the adjacent areas, floors immediately surrounding the C-PEC and in the anteroom, and patient treatment areas. Results of the surface wipe samples can be used to confirm lack of contamination or to improve processes to ensure mitigation of risk.

SUMMARY

Ensuring the quality of CSPs requires two critical factors:

1. A properly designed environment that can maintain a state of control by meeting specific air cleanliness requirements and other design and performance criteria.
2. An educated, trained, skilled, motivated, and vigilant workforce utilizing meticulous aseptic technique in properly functioning primary and secondary engineering controls.

Assuming that a properly designed and maintained anteroom and buffer room is built and maintained through routine cleaning and disinfecting practices, the greatest risk affecting the sterility of CSPs is the behavior of compounding personnel. These two factors need to be verified routinely through an effective environmental bioburden testing program that provides quantitative information on nonviable and viable bioburden. These data will serve to identify the source of the deviation and allow for proper remediation.

REFERENCES

1. Cebular VJ, Collins JS, AIA, et al. *Baseline Guide Volume 3: Sterile Product Manufacturing Facilities*. 3rd ed. Bethesda, MD: International Society for Pharmaceutical Engineering; 1999.
2. U.S. Food and Drug Administration. *Guidance for Industry: Sterile Drug Products Produced by Aseptic Processing—Current Good Manufacturing Practice*. Rockville, MD: U.S. Food and Drug Administration; September 2004. **www.fda.gov/downloads/Drugs/GuidanceComplianceRegulatoryInformation/Guidances/UCM070342.pdf**. Accessed August 18, 2023.
3. International Society for Pharmaceutical Engineering (ISPE). *Baseline pharmaceutical engineering guide for sterile manufacturing facilities*. Bethesda, MD: ISPE; 1999.
4. Chen C, Moore C. Roles of statistics in pharmaceutical development using quality-by-design approach—an FDA perspective [slideshow]. **https://slidetodoc.com/role-of-statistics-in-pharmaceutical-development-using-qualitybydesign/**. Presented September 27-29, 2006. Accessed August 18, 2023.
5. Kastango ES, Trissel LA, Bradshaw B. An ounce of prevention: controlling hazards in extemporaneous compounding practices. *Int J Pharm Compd*. 2003;5:401–416.
6. Hallissy E, Russell S. Chronic investigation/ Who's mixing your drugs?/ Bad medicine: pharmacy mix-ups a recipe for misery/ some drugstores operate with very little oversight. *San Francisco Chronicle*. June 23, 2002.
7. Centers for Disease Control and Prevention. Exophiala infection from contaminated injectable steroids prepared by a compounding pharmacy—United States, July–November 2002. *MMWR Weekly*. December 13, 2002;51(49):1109–1112.**www.cdc.gov/mmwr/preview/mmwrhtml/mm5149a1.htm**. Accessed August 18, 2023.
8. Selenic D, Dodson DR, Jensen B, et al. *Enterobacter cloacae* bloodstream infections in pediatric patients traced to a hospital pharmacy. *Am J Health Syst Pharm*. 2003;60(14):1440–1446. doi:10.1093/ajhp/60.14.1440.
9. Centers for Disease Control and Prevention. *Pseudomonas* bloodstream infections associated with a heparin/saline flush, Missouri, New York, Texas, and Michigan, 2004–2005. *MMWR Weekly*. March 25, 2005;54(11):269–272. **https://www.cdc.gov/Mmwr/Preview/Mmwrhtml/Mm5411a1.Htm**. Accessed August 18, 2023.
10. American Society of Health-System Pharmacists (ASHP). *Compounded IV solution linked to sepsis cases*. Bethesda, MD: ASHP; 2005.
11. American Society of Health-System Pharmacists (ASHP). *Pharmacy linked to multiple-state outbreak of serratia infections*. Bethesda, MD: ASHP; 2005.
12. Tresoldi AT, Padoveze MC, Trabasso P, et al. *Enterobacter cloacae* sepsis outbreak in a newborn unit caused by contaminated total parenteral nutrition solution. *Am J Infect Control*. 2000;28(3):258–261. doi:10.1067/mic.2000.105286.
13. Kainer MA, Reagan DR, Nguyen DB, et al. Fungal infections associated with contaminated methylprednisolone in Tennessee. *N Engl J Med*. 2012;367(23):2194–2203. doi:10.1056/NEJMoa1212972.
14. Moehring RW, Lewis SS, Isaacs PJ, et al. Outbreak of bacteremia due to *Burkholderia contaminans* linked to intravenous fentanyl from an institutional compounding pharmacy. *JAMA Intern Med*. 2014;174(4):606–612. doi:10.1001/jamainternmed.2013.13768.
15. Centers for Disease Control and Prevention. Multistate outbreak of fungal meningitis and other infections. **www.cdc.gov/HAI/outbreaks/meningitis.html**. Reviewed October 30, 2015. Accessed August 18, 2023.
16. Whyte W, Bailey PV, Tinkler J, et al. An evaluation of the routes of bacterial contamination occurring during aseptic pharmaceutical manufacturing. *J Parenter Sci Technol*. 1982;36(3):102–107. **https://pubmed.ncbi.nlm.nih.gov/7097451/**.
17. van Grafhorst JP, Foudraine NA, Nooteboom F, et al. Unexpected high risk of contamination with staphylococci species attributable to standard preparation of syringes for continuous intravenous drug administration in a simulation model in intensive care units. *Crit Care Med*. 2002;30(4):833–836. doi:10.1097/00003246-200204000-00019.
18. van Doorne H, Bakker JH, Meevis RF, et al. Influence of background air on microbial contamination during simulated i.v.-admixture preparation. *J Clin Pharm Ther*. 1994;19(3):181–187. doi:10.1111/j.1365-2710.1994.tb00670.x.

19. Trissel LA, Gentempo JA, Saenz LM, et al. Effect of two work practice changes on the microbial contamination rates of pharmacy-compounded sterile preparations. *Am J Health Syst Pharm*. 2007;64(8):837–841. doi:10.2146/060199.

20. U.S. Food and Drug Administration. *Insanitary Conditions at Compounding Facilities: Guidance for Industry*. Silver Spring, MD: U.S. Food and Drug Administration; November 2020. **https://www.fda.gov/regulatory-information/search-fda-guidance-documents/insanitary-conditions-compounding-facilities-guidance-industry**. Accessed August 18, 2023.

21. USP <797> Pharmaceutical compounding—sterile preparations. In: *2023: USP Compounding Compendium*. Rockville, MD: United States Pharmacopeial Convention; 2023.

22. USP <800> Hazardous drugs—handling in healthcare settings. In: *2023: USP Compounding Compendium*. Rockville, MD: United States Pharmacopeial Convention; 2023.

23. USP <659> Packaging and storage requirements. In: *2023: USP Compounding Compendium*. Rockville, MD: United States Pharmacopeial Convention; 2023.

24. Controlled Environment Testing Association. CAG-003–CETA certification guide for sterile compounding facilities for USP compliance (Revised 2022). **www.cetainternational.org/ceta-application-guides-for-nonmembers-**. Accessed August 18, 2023.

25. USP <1116> Microbiological control and monitoring of aseptic processing environments. In: *2023: USP Compounding Compendium*. Rockville, MD: United States Pharmacopeial Convention; 2023.

26. McAteer F. Environmental monitoring and control in the pharmacy. *Pharm Purch Prod*. 2015; 12:8,10,12.

27. Macher J. *Bioaerosols: assessment and control*. Cincinnati, OH: American Conference of Governmental Industrial Hygienists; 1999.

28. Hurst CJ. *Manual of environmental microbiology*. 3rd ed. Washington, DC: ASM Press; 2007.

32

CORRECTIVE AND PREVENTATIVE ACTION (CAPA) PLANS

Varsha Gaitonde and David Short

INTRODUCTION

The U.S. Food and Drug Administration (FDA) defines *corrective and preventive action* as a systematic approach that includes actions needed to correct (correction), prevent recurrence (corrective action), and eliminate the cause of potential nonconforming products and other quality problems (preventive action).[1] While corrective action is reactive, preventative action is a proactive approach to prevent further occurrences. The purpose of this chapter is to explain and establish the process for implementing and maintaining a corrective and preventive action (CAPA) system as it applies to compounding operations.

BACKGROUND

The 2006 FDA guidance *Quality Systems Approach to Pharmaceutical Current Good Manufacturing Practice Regulations*, states that a CAPA should focus on investigating, understanding, and correcting discrepancies while attempting to prevent their recurrence.[2] Procedures must be developed and documented to ensure that the need for action is evaluated with respect to the possible consequences, the root cause of the problem is investigated, possible actions are determined, a selected action is taken within a defined time frame, and the effectiveness of the action taken is evaluated. This involves analyzing processes, records, complaints, returned goods, and all such available data to identify existing as well as potential causes for a product defect. The investigation must be expanded to include any other batches that may have been associated with the specific result or discrepancy. Additionally, it is important that there are controls to prevent dispensing of affected product and, if needed, for tracking any product that is still in use.

The International Organization for Standardization (ISO) and the International Conference on Harmonization (ICH) have similar requirements to the FDA.[3;4] The Joint Commission includes a discussion of a root cause analysis as a response to a sentinel event, and they provide a framework for root cause analysis (RCA) and corrective actions to assist with conducting a comprehensive analysis in healthcare situations.[5]

TYPES OF ERRORS IN HOSPITALS

The Institution for Safe Medication Practices (ISMP) has identified typical types of errors that occur in hospitals through its voluntary reporting program. Reports from the past few years have identified incorrect route, incorrect preparation, smart pump programming errors, incorrect administration of drugs including insulin, inadvertent administration of drugs due to residual drug in line, and alert fatigue leading to overriding of alerts causing errors. The 2019 ISMP top ten medication error summary, which was the most recent report prior to the COVID-19 pandemic, identified several errors that may be prevalent in sterile compounding.[6]

- Selecting the wrong drug after entering a few letters of the drug name
- Look-alike labeling of manufacturers' products
- Misheard verbal orders
- Incorrect routes of administration
- Unsafe labeling of syringes and infusions by 503B compounders
- 1000-fold overdoses with components in parenteral nutrition

The American Society of Health-System Pharmacists (ASHP) guidelines on compounding sterile preparations identifies common errors more specific to sterile compounding. These

DOI 10.37573/9781585286492.032

errors made during the preparation of a compounded sterile preparation (CSP) include the following[7]:

- Wrong concentration
- Wrong drug
- Wrong dose
- Wrong base solution and/or diluent
- Wrong volume
- Wrong patient
- Wrong route

THE CAPA PROCESS

The CAPA applies to the corrective and preventative actions resulting from process errors, department investigations, complaints, agency inspections, internal and external audits, change controls, and supplier issues. The CAPA process provides two paths for completing a CAPA. The first is a standalone CAPA where root cause of the event has already been identified. An example of this is when a cleanroom goes down due to an unanticipated power outage from the local utility. The root cause is known, so the actions flow from the root cause. The second path is when a cause of the event is not evident and a root cause analysis method (RCA) is needed to identify appropriate CAPAs. An example of this is when a clean room environmental monitoring sample shows colony forming units outside of the specified limits. The cause of the colony forming units is not known and an investigation is needed to determine root cause to be able to identify appropriate CAPAs. When a CAPA is found not to be effective, then a new RCA must be initiated to identify more appropriate and effective CAPA. An overview of the CAPA process is shown in **Figure 32-1**.

DEFINE THE PROBLEM: IDENTIFICATION OF A PROCESS ERROR

Process errors may be identified by internal or external sources. These may result from an inappropriate dosage administered, different medication administered or an unapproved route of administration. Many are identified due to an adverse effect or lack of effect of a medication on a patient. Some process errors may also arise due to incorrect storage, incorrect restocking in medication cabinets, or incorrect/incomplete labeling.

Compounding error is a type of process error that can arise from various root causes; for example, using a different component vial that has a different concentration, calculation errors, measurement errors, look-alike containers of medications and diluents, and human factors. ISMP has identified some of the root causes for these errors as the following:

- Depreciating importance of compounding and dispensing in pharmacy practice
- Lack of knowledge and standardization of best practices
- Training gaps and learned tolerance of deviation and risks in practice[8]

In addition, it is important to learn from process errors that have occurred at other organizations. This information can help identify potential risk points to prevent similar errors. ISMP has determined that a medication error reported in one organization is also likely to occur in another.[9] Therefore, seeking out information about errors at other institutions and implementing preventative actions is imperative.

PERFORM CONTAINMENT

In some events, the containment of a problem cannot wait for a formal CAPA process. For example, a compounding error leads to the entire batch being ineligible for patient administration or a supplier safety recall of the starting component used in a batch. These errors may require immediate action to be taken and quarantine of the batch and/or removal from patient care areas or distribution. For these events, the department must complete and document the immediate corrective actions that were taken to prevent continuation of the problem and/or expansion of the impact. The CAPA owner includes the initial actions taken as corrective actions in the CAPA.

Part of these initial immediate steps include a completion of a health hazard assessment, also called a health risk assessment. A health hazard assessment is a tool for predicting possible harm that can come from a defective or malfunctioning product. The assessment helps the FDA and the firm determine if any actions are necessary, such as recalling the

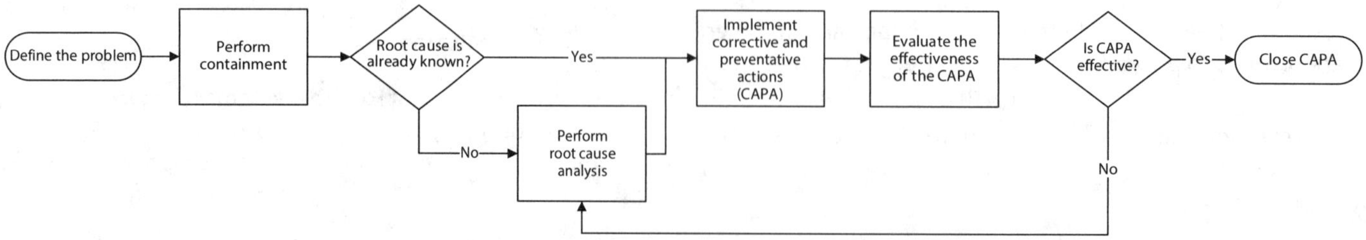

FIGURE 32-1. The CAPA process map

product or notifying the public about the risk. A health hazard assessment must be conducted and appropriate actions up to and including recall of the stated product may be necessary.

In a hospital, the investigation must include medical record review of any patients who received the impacted product to evaluate for adverse events. At an outsourcing facility or an infusion center, an error resulting in failure of the compounded product that has been shipped to the hospital must include analysis of impact to the patient performed by the outsourcing facility and the hospital.

INVESTIGATION OF AN ERROR

The investigation must be conducted in an unbiased fashion and must include a root cause analysis. A root cause analysis helps determine the actions to be conducted. The scope, severity, and cause of the error will determine appropriate corrective actions and preventative actions.

ROOT CAUSE ANALYSIS

For CAPAs where root cause has not previously been identified, the CAPA owner assigns an investigation owner to conduct an RCA investigation. The investigation includes the following:

- The scope of impact, including dates, times, people, product/component, process, etc. as appropriate to provide full traceability
- Documentation in chronological order details of the investigation (who, what, where, when, why and how)
- Descriptions (and references to data) of investigation activities undertaken that did not ultimately determine root (or most probable) cause, as appropriate
- Completed references and discussion of product codes, work orders, equipment numbers, etc. to provide full traceability to investigation activities, as appropriate
- Completed references to data (attachments) required to support the findings of the investigation
- Keep any collected items relevant to the investigation for review, as all evidence should be held until the investigation is complete

The RCA is performed by a team consisting of stakeholders and subject matter experts who can analyze the data collected and perform the analysis. The type of error determines the team involved. In the case of an unexpected patient response to a compounded product, in addition to direct care providers and pharmacy compounding staff, there may be a need to include biomedical engineering if a pump was involved and is suspected to be malfunctioning. If a look-alike vial or diluent is implicated in the error, supply chain pharmacists should be included. The investigation owner brainstorms possible root causes with the team. They may use various cause and effect tools to organize ideas from the brainstorming activities, such as failure mode and effects analysis (FMEA) and a frequency/severity matrix.

The investigation owner determines probable causes based on the above data, and then justifies this conclusion briefly and completely, summarizing the factual elements contained in the body of the investigation that support the claim being made. In addition to probable root causes, any other contributing causes should also be stated and justified if present.

COMMON AND SPECIAL CAUSE PROCESS ERRORS

Common cause process errors are variations inherent in a process. For example, the possibility of errors in a compounded medication depends on the number of steps involved in compounding the medication. A process that varies only because of a common cause is determined to be stable. Performance of a stable process can be changed by redesigning the process. An example would be providing automation for complicated compounded products such as total parenteral nutrition (TPN). Common cause variation is endogenous, meaning it is part of the process as designed, so correcting this prevents the same common cause from recurring.

Special cause process errors are variations due to unusual and unanticipated events. These are usually external, such as natural disasters or mechanical malfunctions. In addition, drug and supply shortages can contribute to medication selection errors, administration errors, and errors in compounding. Correcting one special cause does not prevent the next one from occurring.

RISK ASSESSMENT

Once a FMEA is conducted or a root cause is determined, it is important to assess the risk of the failure or potential causes of the error occurring in the future. Quantification of this risk is the first step in determining the impact and prioritizing the important corrective actions to be implemented. This quantification can be done by assigning a risk priority number (RPN) to the investigation based on the impact to the process and patient.[10] The RPN is calculated by multiplying three avenues for risk (severity, occurrence, and detection).

RPN = Severity × Occurrence × Detection

CAPA

Prevention of further errors is dependent on risk assessment, identification of specific risks associated with the process, and development of controls to mitigate this risk. This may be accomplished through enhanced monitoring and process controls, process improvements, or training and education, any of which must be documented in the CAPA.

ROLES AND RESPONSIBILITIES

In a hospital or healthcare system, a pharmacist in charge (PIC) has the overall responsibility of ensuring appropriate CAPA are implemented for medication related errors. This responsibility may be delegated to a compliance pharmacist or similar role. In an outsourcing facility, the responsibility to investigate discrepancies, failures, and oversight of CAPA falls to the quality assurance unit.

It is important that each CAPA be assigned to a CAPA owner who understands the scope of the CAPA, is experienced in documentation, and can liaise with all departments and functions to execute the CAPA to completion.

The CAPA owner manages the following:

- Prioritization: The owner works with departments to define an appropriate timeline for the CAPA that establishes priority with respect to other projects.
- Initiation: The owner ensures that the project is launched with a defined CAPA plan that provides roles and responsibilities including actions with appropriate timelines.
- Documentation: The owner ensures the CAPA has adequate information, allowing it to be independent of other systems.
- Performance: The owner ensures the roles and responsibilities are being completed within the defined timelines. Concerns are escalated to leadership if necessary.
- Completion: The owner ensures there is evidence of completion, including the effectiveness check.
- Effectiveness: The owner performs the CAPA effectiveness check.

The CAPA investigation owner is responsible for the following:

- Collecting the data: All relevant data as to who, what, and when should be collected (include voice of customer as needed) for CAPAs pursuant to a regulatory change. The change should be documented.
- Assembling a RCA team: The team should contain stakeholders and subject matter experts who can analyze the data collected and perform the analysis.
- Root Cause Analysis: Assign possible and probable root causes.

The PIC, medication safety pharmacist, or the compounding pharmacist manager should have oversight of the CAPA, and they must perform specific functions. In a 503A or 503B compounding facility, the following functions may be performed by the quality assurance unit:

- Initial review: They should review the CAPA details and decide whether the CAPA owner can proceed with the CAPA action plan or if the CAPA needs to be reviewed/revised or cancelled. Due diligence must be employed to assure that the CAPA under consideration does not already exist in the CAPA system.
- Approving RCA: They should ensure that the RCA is appropriate and that the action plan addresses the root cause and its rectification.
- Approving timeline extensions: They should ensure that rationale for extensions are adequate.
- Final review: CAPAs must be reviewed and approved to ensure adherence to the CAPA process.
- Effectiveness check: Reviewing and approving the CAPA effectiveness is essential. If a CAPA is deemed to be ineffective, they must approve next steps, which includes a new CAPA.

The pharmacy manager should also provide performance metrics to other departments and leadership at a defined frequency, usually monthly.

CAPA PLAN

The CAPA owner collaborates with stakeholders and subject matter experts to create a CAPA action plan based on the RCA outcome. The PIC and/or quality unit then accept the CAPA action plan if it is appropriate for the identified root cause or probable cause by reviewing supporting documentation that led to the creation of the corrective action. The action plan must outline all necessary activities, resources, and timelines to complete the CAPA, which includes but is not limited to the following:

- Tasks that must be completed
- Persons responsible for each task
- Completion date for each task
- Verification activities, responsibility, and timing

If document changes are required, such as policies and procedures, a list of all affected documents that need revision should be included in the CAPA form with a general description of what the modifications entail. Employee training is an essential part of any change that is made. Training should be a part of the action plan, and training documentation should be attached to the CAPA. If multiple CAPAs are required to eliminate, reduce, or remediate a single root cause, actions may be managed separately or collectively.

CAPA ACTION ITEMS

CAPA action items are assigned by the CAPA owner as needed to complete the CAPA action plan. The assignee must ensure action items are completed as assigned and within the given timeline. Upon completion of the action items, the CAPA owner provides a summary of all tasks completed and attaches appropriate supporting documentation to the CAPA.

CAPA REVIEW

Upon completion of the investigation, the PIC and/or quality assurance unit reviews the investigation for the following:

- Ensure that the entire investigation package is complete and correct.
- Ensure that the action plan is accurate and complete.
- Ensure that the investigation addresses the problem and identifies the correct root cause, as supported by documentation.
- Ensure that the action plan is in place to mitigate or eliminate the root cause with appropriate supporting documentation.
- Ensure that interim controls agreed upon by the CAPA owner and PIC/quality for the safety of the compounded product are in place until long term actions are completed to mitigate the root cause.
- If unacceptable, they reject the CAPA and provide comments as to why it was rejected.

A rejected CAPA is re-evaluated by the CAPA owner, who can then revise the action plan, add additional action items, or attach additional documentation as needed to address the comments. If there is a change in the action plan, the revised plan must be reviewed and approved prior to assignment of additional action items.

CAPA EFFECTIVENESS CHECKS

Once all action items have been completed and documented with appropriate supporting evidence, the CAPA owner reviews the effectiveness of the action. The CAPA owner should work with the PIC and/or quality assurance unit to determine an appropriate time period for the effectiveness check and list it in the effectiveness plan, which must provide details on how effectiveness will be measured. The time period is based on various factors and can be fluid. Ample time for confirming effectiveness should be allowed. Effectiveness check verification must be documented in the CAPA with supporting evidence, and it must be approved by the PIC and/or quality assurance unit. If the CAPA is determined not to be effective, then the CAPA owner initiates a new RCA that establishes new CAPA(s).

CAPA DUE DATES

Due dates for assigned CAPAs must be

- Realistic to allow the owner of the action adequate time in order to prevent short cuts being taken resulting in a failed CAPA effectiveness check
- Aggressive to create department prioritization for completion and address expectations following the health hazard assessment
- Suitable to allow collaboration between department leadership and PIC/Quality

Any corrective action (CA) or preventive action (PA) not completed by its assigned due date must be reviewed to determine if the due date should be extended.

CAPA AND EFFECTIVENESS CHECK EXTENSIONS

If completion of a CA or PA extends beyond the stated due date, the CAPA owner may request an extension. The extension request must contain written justification, including the status of the actions taken and a new target completion date. All extension requests must be reviewed and approved by the PIC and/or quality assurance unit.

A CAPA or effectiveness check extension must include the following information at minimum:

- Previous implementation due date
- New due date
- Reason and justification for extension
- Description of completed tasks and dates
- Description of remaining tasks (including action plan and timeline for tasks completion)
- Risk assessment/impact of not completing action by the original due date

CAPA CLOSURE

Once the CAPA is deemed to be effective, the CAPA may be closed with approval from the PIC and/or quality assurance unit. If the CAPA is not effective, an extension to assess the effectiveness may be requested. Alternately, the CAPA may be closed as being ineffective, while a new CAPA can be launched to address the problem.

SUMMARY

Compounding errors in hospitals must be thoroughly investigated, and corrective and preventative actions must be implemented to mitigate patient risk.[11] It is imperative to patient safety that measures are effective and in place to systematically investigate medication errors, perform interventions to prevent recurrence of errors, provide adequate documentation of actions taken, and complete training to educate staff in preventing recurrence.

REFERENCES

1. Code of Federal Regulations. 21 CFR § 820.100, last amended June 22, 2023. **https://www.ecfr.gov/current/title-21/chapter-I/subchapter-H/part-820/subpart-J/section-820.100**. Accessed August 18, 2023.
2. U.S. Food and Drug Administration. Guidance document: quality systems approach to pharmaceutical current good manufacturing practice regulations. **https://www.fda.gov/regulatory-information/search-fda-guidance-documents/quality-systems-approach-pharmaceutical-current-good-manufacturing-practice-regulations**. Published October 2006. Accessed August 18, 2023.
3. International Organization for Standardization. ISO 13485:2016. Medical devices — quality management systems — requirements for regulatory purposes. 3rd ed. Geneva, Switzerland: International Organization for Standardization; 2016.
4. European Medicines Agency. ICH guideline Q9 on quality risk management: step 5. **https://www.ema.europa.eu/en/documents/scientific-guideline/international-conference-harmonisation-technical-requirements-registration-pharmaceuticals-human-use_en-3.pdf**. Published September 2015. Accessed August 18, 2023.
5. The Joint Commission. Framework for root cause analysis and corrective actions. **https://www.jointcommission.org/resources/sentinel-event/**. Published 2017. Accessed August 18, 2023.
6. Institute for Safe Medication Practices. Start the new year off right by preventing these top 10 medication errors and hazards. *ISMP Medication Safety Alert!* 2020;25(17):1-4. Available at: **https://www.ismp.org/resources/start-new-year-right-preventing-these-top-10-medication-errors-and-hazards**. Accessed August 18, 2023.
7. American Society of Health-System Pharmacists. ASHP guidelines on compounding sterile preparations. *Am J Health Syst Pharm*. 2014;71(2):145–166.
8. Institute for Safe Medication Practices. Technology and error-prevention strategies: why are we still overlooking the IV room? *ISMP Medication Safety Alert!* 2015;20(1):1-4. Available at: **https://www.ismp.org/resources/technology-and-error-prevention-strategies-why-are-we-still-overlooking-iv-room**. Accessed August 18, 2023.
9. Institute for Safe Medication Practices. A lot happens when you report a hazard or error to ISMP—there's no "black hole" here! *ISMP Medication Safety Alert!* 2019;24(22):1-4. Available at: **https://www.ismp.org/resources/lot-happens-when-you-report-hazard-or-error-ismp-theres-no-black-hole-here**. Accessed August 18, 2023.
10. Feemster AA, Augustino M, Duncan R, et al. Use of failure modes and effects analysis to mitigate potential risks prior to implementation of an intravenous compounding technology. *Am J Health Syst Pharm*. 2021;78(14):1323–1329 10.1093/ajhp/zxab179.
11. Liu H-C. FMEA for proactive healthcare risk analysis: A systematic literature review. In: *Improved FMEA Methods for Proactive Healthcare Risk Analysis*. Singapore, Singapore: Springer; 2019:15–45., 10.1007/978-981-13-6366-5_2.

33

POLICIES, PROCEDURES, AND QUALITY ASSURANCE PROGRAMS

Patricia C. Kienle

INTRODUCTION

The American Society of Health-System Pharmacists' guideline for pharmacies in hospitals states, "The pharmacy shall be responsible for the procurement, distribution, and control of all drug products used in the hospital for inpatient and ambulatory patients. Policies and procedures governing these functions shall be developed by the pharmacy with input from other appropriate hospital staff and committees."[1]

WRITING POLICIES AND PROCEDURES

Tomich and Dydek defined policies and procedures as the following:

> Policies are written statements that provide guidance on the position and values of an organization. They are often considered broad operational guidelines, but they should clearly define the direction and activities of an organization or department. Procedures are written instructions that describe the recommended methods of sequential steps to follow to perform a task or activity. In short, procedures help define the process for completing a task.[2]

In compounding most sterile preparations, final sterility and accuracy testing is not possible. Thus, having robust policies and procedures and consistent work practices is mandatory. Compounders must use these policies and procedures correctly each time for uniformity of compounded sterile preparations (CSPs).

Policies and procedures should be organized (eg, numbered under headings) so that they are easy for employees to find. They should be available either in written form or electronically stored printable documentation. Policies and procedures have numerous benefits[2]:

- Inter- and intradepartmental communication
- Creation of standards of care
- Mechanism to document standards of care and other important activities
- Enhancement of staff orientation and training
- Ability to systematically, objectively, and efficiently measure staff and departmental performance
- Promotion of patient safety practices
- Consistency with state regulations
- Quality improvement processes
- Cost-effective use of resources
- Effective administrative tool for planning, developing, and improving pharmacy services and patient care
- Comprehensive source of information about departmental operations

Policies and procedures, also known as standard operating procedures (SOPs), should be available to all personnel involved in the process of creating and distributing CSPs. USP Chapter <797> specifies many SOPs and important statements that must be included in policies. SOPs should be drafted by or in cooperation with personnel that perform compounding processes. SOPs must be updated at least annually by a sterile compounding designated person to reflect current standards of practice. Revisions of policies and procedures should be communicated to affected personnel.

Tomich and Dydek describe the format and style for writing policies and procedures. Although many policy and

Note: The author acknowledges E. Clyde Buchanan who authored this chapter in a previous edition.

DOI 10.37573/9781585286492.033

procedure formats have been described, most policy and procedure manuals document the following information[2-4]:

- Policy title
- Policy number
- Policy statement
- Purpose of the policy
- References for the policy
- Applicability to work areas or personnel types
- Use of definitions, terms, acronyms, words, or abbreviations
- Responsibilities of personnel involved with the procedure
- Procedures

Appendix 33-A shows an example of a typical policy and procedure for format, style, and content reference.

All significant procedures performed in the compounding areas must be covered by SOPs and must have records or documentation. Procedures should be developed for the facility, equipment, personnel, preparation, labeling, packaging, and storage of compounded preparations to ensure accountability, accuracy, quality, safety, and uniformity in compounding practices. Documentation should enable a compounding supervisor to systematically trace, evaluate, and replicate the steps included throughout the process of compounding a sterile preparation.

Job Descriptions

Complete job descriptions for personnel compounding sterile preparations are essential for hiring and orientation. These descriptions are often included in policy and procedure manuals. Job descriptions should include the following:

- Basic qualifications (eg, education level, certification, registration, and length and type of experience)
- Physical requirements (eg, ability to lift moderately heavy weights, push carts, and perform rapid, repetitive, and accurate manipulations)
- Working conditions (eg, shifts, environment, hazards [including hazardous drugs and hazardous materials], and attire)
- Responsibilities and competencies (eg, ability to compound a pharmaceutical preparation that is free of errors in content and free of microbial, particulate, and pyrogenic contaminants)

Additionally, the job description of designated persons should include the following tasks:

- Develop and approve standard operating procedures and review them at least annually
- Oversee the training of personnel
- Oversee personnel monitoring and testing
- Ensure that all personnel who enter the compounding areas maintain the quality of the environment
- Evaluate if individuals should be excused from working in the compounding area due to health issues
- Ensure International Organization for Standardization (ISO) classified devices and areas are monitored and certified
- Select acceptable sources of drugs and other components
- Develop and monitor quality standards
- Review complaints

RESPONSIBILITY OF COMPOUNDING PERSONNEL

This chapter identifies topics pertinent to compounding sterile preparations that should be covered in a policy and procedure manual. The same topics are presented in detail throughout this book. According to the *United States Pharmacopeia–National Formulary* (*USP–NF* or USP) Chapter <797> Pharmaceutical Compounding—Sterile Preparations and USP Chapter <800> Hazardous Drugs—Handling in Healthcare Settings, all compounding personnel are responsible for understanding fundamental practices and precautions, developing and implementing appropriate procedures, and continuously evaluating these procedures and the quality of final CSPs to prevent harm to patients and personnel.[5;6] Each pharmacy that compounds sterile preparations or handles hazardous drugs must appoint a designated person to oversee these activities.

TOPICS COVERED BY POLICIES AND PROCEDURES

USP Chapter <797> is divided into sections that should be covered in departmental policies and procedures[5]:

- Scope of sterile compounding
- Personnel training and evaluation
- Personal hygiene and garbing
- Facilities and engineering controls
- Certification and recertification
- Microbiological air and surface monitoring
- Cleaning, disinfecting, and applying sporicidal disinfectants and sterile 70% isopropyl alcohol
- Introducing items into the secondary and primary engineering controls
- Equipment, supplies, and components

- Sterilization and depyrogenation
- Master formulation and compounding records
- Release inspection and testing
- Labeling
- Establishing beyond-use dates (BUDs)
- Use of conventionally manufactured products as components
- Use of CSPs as components
- SOPs
- Quality assurance and quality control
- CSP handling, storage, packaging, shipping, and transport
- Documentation

Special types of CSPs, such as allergenic extracts or radiopharmaceuticals, have additional specific requirements that must be delineated in SOPs related to these practices.[7]

USP has several other general chapters that can be used to guide pharmacists in developing SOPs. The *USP Compounding Compendium* is an electronic publication that extracts compounding-related USP chapters in a dedicated reference. The 2023 edition of the *USP Compounding Compendium*[8] contains general chapters on compounding, compounding support information, and over 200 compounding monographs. General chapters include good compounding practices; nonsterile and sterile compounding; pharmaceutical calculations in compounding; weighing and measuring; containers, packaging, and storage; labeling; dosage forms; sterility and endotoxin testing; analytical tests and procedures; and many other topics.

Professional organizations have guidance documents that may also assist in developing SOPs that reflect best practices. *ASHP Guidelines on Compounding Sterile Preparations*, *ASHP Guidelines on Outsourcing Sterile Compounding Services*, ASHP's vendor assessment tool, and the Institute for Safe Medication Practices' *Guidelines for Sterile Compounding and the Sage Use of Sterile Compounding Technology* provide additional advice when developing and revising sterile compounding policies and procedures.[9 12]

Personnel Training and Evaluation

All training activities must be covered by appropriate SOPs and documentation. A designated person or other designated skilled compounder must demonstrate procedures to each compounder. They must also observe and guide each compounder through the procedures. The compounder should repeat the procedure without any assistance, but they should do so under the observation of the designated person. When the compounder has demonstrated a verbal and functional knowledge of the procedure, only then may the compounder independently prepare CSPs. Documentation, including successful completion of tests (based on established passing test scores) and hands-on observation, must be completed and retained. The designated person should continue to monitor the work of the compounder and answer any questions the compounder may have concerning the SOPs.

Suggested Standard Operating Procedures

USP Chapter <797> requires the compounding facility to have written, properly approved SOPs designed to ensure the quality of the environment in which a CSP is prepared. The SOPs must be reviewed at least every 12 months. **Table 33-1** lists required and recommended SOPs from USP Chapter <797>. **Table 33-2** lists additional required and recommended SOPs from USP Chapter <800>.[13,14]

Other Sources of Policies and Procedures

Compounding personnel can write policies and procedures more completely and efficiently by starting with SOPs for compounding sterile preparations that are already available. Practitioners often post pharmacy policies and procedures on ASHP's Practice Management Resource Center and on ASHP Connect.[15] ASHP's best practices and guidelines also provide ample amounts of guidance for writing SOPs. SOPs must be modified to match actual practices, otherwise a generic SOP may be used by an inspector or surveyor to point out differences and deficiencies between practice and written policy.

COMPOUNDING RECORDS AND DOCUMENTS

All compounders must comply with record keeping and retention requirements designated by individual states. The objective of documentation is to allow another compounder to reproduce the identical order or prescription at a future date. Policies and procedures should specify pharmacist verification of ingredients and their amounts, the order of compounding additives, and the compounding process for both manual and automated additives.[16]

Master Formulation Records

A master formulation record (MFR) must be created for a CSP that is mixed for more than one patient or for any CSP containing a nonsterile starting component. The MFR must delineate the following[5]:

- Name, strength or activity, and dosage form of the CSP
- Identities and amounts of all ingredients
- Type and size of container closure system

TABLE 33-1. Policies Required and Recommended in USP Chapter <797>

General

- Standard operating procedures (SOPs) must be written and available to all compounding personnel.
- SOPs must include the types of compounded sterile preparations (CSPs) prepared (eg, Category 1, Category 2, Category 3).
- When compounding activities require the manipulation of a patient's blood-derived or other biological material (eg, autologous serum), the manipulations must be clearly separated from other compounding activities and equipment used in CSP preparation activities, and they must be controlled by specific standard operating procedures (SOPs) to avoid any cross-contamination. Handling of blood components and other biological materials must also comply with laws and regulations of the applicable regulatory jurisdiction.
- A designated person must ensure that SOPs are appropriate and are implemented, which includes ensuring that personnel demonstrate competency in performing every procedure that relates to their job function.
- A designated person must follow up to ensure that corrective actions are taken if problems, deviations, failures, or errors are identified. The corrective action must be documented.
- A designated person is responsible for addressing other areas of risk in the facility's SOPs.
- All personnel who perform or oversee compounding or support activities must be trained in SOPs and the following:
    - Recognize potential problems, deviations, failures, and errors associated with preparing a CSP (eg, those related to equipment, facilities, materials, personnel, the compounding process, or testing) that could potentially result in contamination or other adverse impact on CSP quality.
    - Report any problems, deviations, failures, or errors to the designated person.
- SOPs must be reviewed initially and at least every 12 months by a designated person to ensure that they reflect current practices. The review must be documented.
- Any changes or alterations to an SOP must only be made by a designated person, and it must be documented.
- Revisions to SOPs must be communicated to all personnel involved in these processes and procedures. Personnel should document acknowledgment of the communication.

Documentation

- All facilities where CSPs are prepared must have and maintain written or electronic documentation to demonstrate compliance with the requirements outlined in this chapter. This documentation must include but is not limited to the following:
    - Personnel training, competency assessments, and qualification records, including corrective actions for any failures
    - Certification reports, including corrective actions for any failures
    - Environmental air and surface monitoring procedures and results
    - Equipment records (eg, calibration, verification, and maintenance reports)
    - Receipt of components
    - SOPs
    - Master formulation records (MFRs)
    - Compounding records (CRs)
    - All required CRs for a particular CSP (eg, MFR, CR, and release inspection and testing results) must be readily retrievable for at least 2 years after preparation or as required by laws and regulations of applicable regulatory jurisdiction or accrediting organizations (whichever is longer)
    - Release inspection and testing records
    - Information related to complaints and adverse events, including corrective actions taken
    - Results of investigations and corrective actions
    - Documentation must comply with all laws and regulations of the applicable regulatory jurisdiction.
    - Records must be legible and stored in a manner that prevents their deterioration and loss.

Personnel Training

- All training must be documented.
- Personnel compounding only immediate-use CSPs must complete training as required by the facility's SOPs. Immediate use SOPs must include aseptic techniques, processes, and procedures to be followed in order to minimize the potential for contact with nonsterile surfaces, introduction of particulate matter or biological fluids, and mix-ups with other conventionally manufactured products or CSPs.

TABLE 33-1. (Continued)

Personnel Training (Cont.)

- Personnel who only perform restocking or cleaning and disinfecting duties outside of the primary engineering control (PEC) must complete ongoing training as required by the facility's SOPs.
- Processes and techniques for handling, storing, packaging, and transporting CSPs must be outlined in the facility's SOPs. Personnel who handle, store, package, and transport CSPs within the facility must be trained in accordance with the relevant SOPs. The training must be documented.
- A written training program must describe required training, the frequency of training, and the process for evaluating the performance of individuals who compound, have direct oversight of compounding personnel, perform in-process checks and final verifications, and dispense CSPs. This program must equip personnel with appropriate knowledge and train them in the required skills necessary to perform their assigned tasks, which are specified in SOPs.
- Initial training for compounders, designated persons, and personnel with direct oversight of compounding must include the following:
    - Training and competency in maintaining the quality of the sterile compounding environment
    - Training and competency in sterile compounding principles and practices
    - Garbing competency (including gloved fingertip testing [GFT])
    - Media fill with post GFT and surface sampling
- Initial training must be defined for the following facility personnel:
    - Personnel who do not compound but restock or clean and disinfect the sterile compounding areas
    - Personnel who perform in-process checks or final verification of CSPs
    - Personnel who only compound immediate-use CSPs
    - Others, such as maintenance personnel, certifiers, contractors, inspectors, surveyors, etc.
- Ongoing training and competency for compounders must occur
    - At least every 12 months
        - Training and competency in sterile compounding principles and practices
    - At least every 6 months for those who compound Category 1 and Category 2 CSPs
        - Garbing competency (including GFT)
        - Media fill with post GFT and surface sampling
    - At least every 3 months for those who compound Category 3 CSPs
        - Garbing competency (including GFT)
        - Media fill with post GFT and surface sampling
- For designated persons and personnel with direct oversight of compounding who do not compound, ongoing training and competency must be completed at least every 12 months and must include the following:
    - Training and competency in sterile compounding principles and practices
    - Garbing competency (including GFT)
    - Media fill with post GFT and surface sampling
- Ongoing training must be defined by facility personnel for
    - Personnel who do not compound but restock or clean and disinfect the sterile compounding areas
    - Personnel who perform in-process checks or final verification of CSPs
    - Personnel who only compound immediate-use CSPs
    - Others, such as maintenance personnel, certifiers, contractors, inspectors, surveyors, etc.

Garbing

- The required garb, manner of storage, and order of garbing must be determined by the facility and documented in the facility's SOPs.
- The facility's SOPs must describe disinfection procedures for reusing goggles, respirators, and other reusable equipment.

RABS Sleeves and Gloves

- The RABS sleeves and gloves and pharmaceutical isolator sleeves and gloves should be changed per the manufacturer's recommendations and as defined in the facility's SOPs.

TABLE 33-1. (Continued)

Components
• Compounding personnel must follow the facility's SOPs, which must address the selection, receipt, evaluation, handling, storage, and documentation of all CSP components, including all ingredients and container closure. • Weighing, measuring, or other component manipulation activities that could generate airborne chemical particles (eg, active pharmaceutical ingredients [APIs], added substances, conventionally manufactured products) must be evaluated to determine if they should be performed in a PEC or other closed system processing device (eg, single use containment glove bag) to reduce potential exposure to personnel and contamination of the facility or CSPs. The process evaluation must be carried out in accordance with the facility's SOPs. The assessment must be documented.
Equipment
• Compounding personnel must follow established SOPs for calibration, maintenance, cleaning, and use of equipment based on the manufacturer's recommendations.
Incubation Temperature
• Incubator temperatures must be monitored during incubation, either manually or by a continuous recording device, and the results must be reviewed and documented as described in the facility's SOPs. • The order of the incubation temperatures for media fill must be described in the facility's SOPs.
MFRs
• Any changes or alterations to the MFR must be approved and documented according to the facility's SOPs.
Terminal Sterilization
• A description of the terminal sterilization and depyrogenation process, including the temperature, pressure, duration, permissible load conditions for each cycle, and the use of biological indicators and endotoxin challenge vials (ECVs), must be included in the facility's SOPs. SOPs must include training and competency of personnel on all sterilization methods and equipment used by the facility. In addition, the SOPs must include a schedule and method for establishing and verifying the effectiveness of the terminal sterilization and depyrogenation methods selected and the methods for maintaining and cleaning the sterilizing and depyrogenation equipment. • The effectiveness of the depyrogenation cycle must be re-established if there are changes to the depyrogenation cycle described in the SOPs (eg, changes in load conditions, duration, or temperature). This verification must be documented.
Labeling
• Labeling procedures must be followed as described in the facility's SOPs to prevent labeling errors and CSP mix-ups. • The label of the CSP must be verified to ensure that it conforms with the prescription or medication order, MFR, and CR.
Nonviable Monitoring
• The temperature and humidity readings must be reviewed as described in the facility's SOPs. • All total airborne sampling sites and procedures must be described in the facility's SOPs. • The results of the temperature readings must be documented in a temperature log per facility SOPs or stored in and retrievable from a continuous temperature recording device. • Temperature monitoring devices must be verified for accuracy at least every 12 months or as required by the manufacturer.
Viable Monitoring
• Sterile compounding facilities must develop and implement written procedures for microbiological air and surface monitoring. • The microbiological air and surface monitoring program must be clearly described in the facility's SOPs, which must include a diagram of the sampling locations, procedures for collecting samples, frequency of sampling, size of samples (eg, surface area, volume of air), time of day of sampling in relation to activities in the compounding area, and action levels that trigger corrective action. • All sampling sites and procedures must be described in the facility's SOPs.

TABLE 33-1. (Continued)

Cleaning

- All cleaning and disinfecting activities must be performed by trained and appropriately garbed personnel using facility-approved agents and procedures, which must be described in written SOPs.
- The frequency, methods, and locations of cleaning, disinfecting, and applying sporicidal disinfectants must be established in written SOPs in accordance with the manufacturer's instructions. They must be followed by all cleaning personnel. The manufacturer's directions or published data for minimum contact time must be followed for each of the cleaning, disinfecting, and sporicidal disinfectants used.
- When sterile 70% IPA is used, it must be allowed to dry. All cleaning, disinfecting, and application of sporicidal disinfectants must be documented according to the facility's SOP.
- Once opened, sterile cleaning and disinfecting agents and supplies (eg, closed containers of sterile wipers) and sterile 70% IPA may be reused for a time period specified by the manufacturer and/or described in the facility written SOP.

Release Testing

- All release testing procedures (eg, visual inspections and testing) must be included in the facility's documentation for MFRs and CRs.
- Visual inspection defects that indicate sterility or stability problems must be investigated to determine the cause according to the facility's SOPs.

Quality Assurance (QA) and Quality Control Program (QC)

- A facility's QA and QC programs must be formally established and documented in the facility's SOPs. They should be used to ensure that all aspects of the preparation of CSPs are conducted in accordance with the requirements in USP Chapter <797> and laws and regulations of applicable regulatory jurisdictions.
- The facility's SOPs must describe the roles, duties, and training of the personnel responsible for each aspect of the QA program. Designated persons responsible for the QA program must have the training, experience, responsibility, and authority to perform these duties. The overall QA and QC program must be reviewed at least once every 12 months by the designated person. The results of the review must be documented, and appropriate action must be taken if needed.
- An SOP for recall of out-of-specification dispensed CSPs must contain the following:
  - Procedures to determine the severity of the problem and the urgency for implementation and completion of the recall.
  - Procedures to determine the distribution of any affected CSP, including the date and quantity of distribution.
  - Procedures to identify patients who have received the CSP.
  - Procedures for disposal and documentation of the recalled CSP.
  - Procedures to investigate and document the reason for failure.
- The sterile compounding facility must document the implementation of recall procedures. The recall must be reported to appropriate regulatory bodies as required by laws and regulations of the applicable regulatory jurisdiction.
- Compounding facilities must develop and implement SOPs for handling complaints.
- Adverse events potentially associated with the quality of CSPs must be reported in accordance with the facility's SOPs and all laws and regulations of the applicable regulatory jurisdiction.

Source: Reprinted with permission of *The Chapter <797> Answer Book*. 2nd ed. Bethesda, MD: American Society of Health-System Pharmacists; 2023.

- Complete instructions for preparing the CSP
- Physical description of the final CSP
- BUD and storage requirements
- Reference source to support the stability of the CSP
- Quality control procedures
- Other information needed to ensure repeatability

Compounding Record

A compounding record (CR) must be created for all Category 1, Category 2, and Category 3 CSPs and for immediate use CSPs mixed for more than one patient. The CR must delineate the following[5]:

- Name, strength or activity, and dosage form of the CSP
- Date and time of preparation
- Assigned internal identification number
- A method to identify the individuals involved in the compounding process and verifying the final CSP
- Name of each component

TABLE 33-2. Written Standard Operating Procedures Cited in USP Chapter <800>

Occupational Safety Plan • The pharmacy's written plan must be consistent with OSHA requirements and include a list of hazardous drugs and dosage forms handled; the facility and engineering controls employed; competency of personnel, safe work practices, personal protective equipment used; and policies for waste segregation and disposal.
Medical Surveillance • The health-system's medical surveillance plan must be used to protect workers from hazards.
Assessment of Risk • If performed, it must include the type of hazardous drug, dosage form of the specific hazardous drug, risk of exposure to personnel, manipulation used, and required packaging.
Designated Person • This is a specific person responsible for development and implementation of policies and procedures; oversight of compliance with standards, laws, and regulations; ensuring competency of personnel; ensuring environmental controls of storage and compounding facilities (including maintenance of reports and testing and acting on the results).
Consideration for Hazardous Drug Movement Within the Organizations • This includes the recognition of risk and mitigation of hazards related to receiving, unpacking, storing, compounding, transporting, labeling administration, and waste control of hazardous drugs.
Personal Protective Equipment • Proper use of gloves, gowns, hair covers, shoe covers, eye and face protection, and respiratory protection designed to minimize occupational exposure to hazardous drugs must be defined.
Use of Closed System Drug-Transfer Devices • The use of a closed system drug-transfer device for the administration of hazardous drugs and integration with CSPs compounded by the pharmacy must be defined.
Deactivation and Decontamination of Hazardous Drug Areas • Use of appropriate oxidizers, germicidal detergents, and disinfectants to clean hazardous drug areas must be defined.
Environmental Monitoring • Detection of hazardous drug residue in storage, compounding, and administration areas must be defined.
Spill Management Plan • Proactive process to handle spills throughout the organization must be defined.

CSPs = compounded sterile preparations; OSHA = Occupational Safety and Health Administration.

Source: Adapted with permission of USP <800> Hazardous drugs—handling in healthcare settings. In: *2023: USP Compounding Compendium*. Rockville, MD: United States Pharmacopeial Convention; 2023 and Kienle PC. *The Chapter <800> Answer Book*. Bethesda, MD: American Society of Health-System Pharmacists; 2017.

- If mixed for more than one patient or for any CSP containing a nonsterile component: vendor, lot number, and expiration date for each component
- Weight or volume of each component
- Strength or activity of each component
- Total quantity compounded
- Final yield
- Assigned BUD and storage requirements
- Results of quality control procedures

If applicable, the compounding record must also include the following:

- Master formulation record reference for the CSP
- Calculations made to determine and verify quantities and/or concentrations of components

Compounding procedures that are routinely performed must be completed and verified according to SOPs. State regulations may detail processes for compounding single items or when CSPs are mixed according to FDA-approved labeling for a specific dosage form. Specific documentation may be required when mixtures are compounded outside of the FDA-approved labeling.

Other Documentation Records

Policies and procedures concerning documentation records should specify the location of stored records and the required storage time. Records must be legible and stored in a manner that prevents their deterioration and loss. All required CRs for a particular CSP (eg, MFR, CR, and release inspection and testing results) must be readily retrievable for at least 2 years after preparation or as required by laws and regulations of the applicable regulatory jurisdiction or accrediting organizations (whichever is longer). The following records should be kept (storage periods vary according to laws, regulations, and professional standards):

- Training records and competence tests for each employee (eg, test scores, technique observation, hand hygiene and garbing observation, media fills, and gloved fingertip tests)
- Refrigerator, freezer, warmer, and incubator temperature logs or charts
- Initial and preventive maintenance calibration of balances, automated compounding devices, repeater pumps, and other devices
- Certification of primary engineering controls
- Certification of cleanroom suites and segregated compounding areas
- Master formulation records
- Compounding records
- Environmental sampling test results (including surface samples and electronic air samples for microbial detection)
- Process validation
- Drug recalls
- Product problem reports to manufacturers and USP
- Adverse drug reaction reports to manufacturers and the FDA
- Patient complaints, problem handling, and outcome
- Agreements and reports from outsourcing facilities and external compounding pharmacies
- Quality reports

Labeling

Policies and procedures for labeling should outline required information for the following:

- Preparations compounded in batches in anticipation of routine orders
- Preparations dispensed for administration within the institution

SOPs should indicate where labels are obtained and stored in the pharmacy. They should also require sequestration of batch labels with their preparation batch.

STORAGE AND BEYOND-USE DATING

Policies and procedures concerning storage should be based on USP or manufacturer-specified conditions. Written procedures are needed for temperature monitoring of refrigerators, freezers, warmers, and incubators; light, ventilation, and humidity standards; stock rotation and inspection; and locations of quarantined preparations (ingredients and end preparations).

SOPs for handling expired drugs and supplies should encompass their removal, quarantine, and their return or disposal. Preparation recall procedures should detail notification of recalls, removal from stock and nursing areas, and retrieval from patients.

MAINTAINING QUALITY OF COMPOUNDED PREPARATIONS

SOPs should cover packing for transport, in-transit temperatures, precautions for toxic preparation transport, commercial carrier expectations, evaluations of shipper performance, and in-home conditions. For CSPs to be used in a patient's home, procedures should include the following:

- Assurance of proper storage capability
- Written instructions for storage, use (eg, handwashing, aseptic technique, site care, etc.), and suitability for use
- Home visitation and inspection

Patient or Caregiver Training

Policies and procedures for patient or caregiver training should be formalized and include the following:

- Understanding of the therapy provided
- Handling and storage of the sterile preparation
- Appropriate administration techniques
- Use and maintenance of any infusion device used
- Use of printed material
- Appropriate post training verbal counseling

Patient Monitoring and Complaint System

SOPs for shipping CSPs to patients and customers should also define the action to be taken in the event that a patient reports a deviation from required storage conditions, including any environmentally sensitive CSPs, prior to the point of receipt.[17]

QUALITY ASSURANCE PROGRAM

The pharmacy should have written policies and procedures for monitoring, evaluating, correcting, and improving sterile preparation activities and processes. These policies and procedures (ie, the quality assurance [QA] program) should be applied to training and education, competency evaluation, preparation compounding, sterilization methods, media fill testing, and end-preparation evaluation. The program must delineate individual responsibilities for each aspect of the program. Specific responsibilities should include the following[18]:

- Formalization in writing
- Compliance with Centers for Medicare & Medicaid Services (CMS) requirements and accreditation standards
- Consideration of all aspects of the preparation and dispensing of products as described in USP Chapter <797> and USP Chapter <800>
- Description of specific monitoring and evaluation activities
- Specification of how results are reported and evaluated
- Identification of appropriate follow-up mechanisms when action levels are exceeded
- Delineation of the individuals responsible for each aspect of the QA program

There can be some confusion regarding terms quality control, QA, quality management, and quality improvement. Quality control is about testing (eg, testing of a finished CSP for accuracy, purity, sterility, nonpyrogenicity, pH, osmolality). A QA program is a system of steps and actions taken to ensure the maintenance of proper standards in compounded preparations.[19] QA is the system that ensures that SOPs are followed and documented consistently and uniformly and that results of testing outside acceptable limits are followed up with corrective actions. QA does not necessarily change the processes or procedures themselves, which is where quality management or performance improvement is evident.

CMS, The Joint Commission (TJC), Det Norske Veritas Healthcare (DNV) Healthcare, the Accreditation Commission for Health Care (ACHC), the Center for Healthcare Facilities Accreditation Program (HFAP), the Center for Improvement in Healthcare Quality (CIHQ), and many ambulatory accreditation organizations require hospitals and health systems to improve their performance on a continuing basis. For example, TJC performance improvement (PI) standards may be described in a separate organizational plan or within other planning documents. Departments in all TJC accredited organizations must participate in performance improvement. TJC does not specify what the organization calls their program (it can be quality improvement, quality management, continuous quality improvement, etc.). They also don't require that organizations follow a specific approach to performance improvement. Their PI standards applied to pharmacy require the following[20]:

- Collect data to measure the performance of medication management and other high-risk processes.
- Systematically aggregate and analyze data at an appropriate frequency using statistical tools and techniques.
- Analyze undesirable patterns and trends relating to serious adverse drug events and significant medication errors.
- Compare data internally and with external information sources to determine if the data vary excessively or performance is at an unacceptable level.
- Identify and manage sentinel events.
- Use information from data analysis to make changes that improve performance and patient safety and reduce the risk of sentinel events.
- Have an ongoing, proactive program for identifying and reducing unanticipated adverse events and safety risks to patients.
- Include the use of failure mode and effects analysis in its proactive activities.

The intent of a QA program is to ensure that adequate controls exist throughout the life cycle of CSPs. Many of the elements of USP Chapter <797> focus on controls through formalized SOPs, defined processes, and established best practices and procedures. Documentation serves as proof that SOPs are being followed and that quality is being maintained by compounding staff. Documentation links personnel with operational responsibility. It is important that data be collected, documented, and reviewed for operational compliance, process excursions, and procedural deviations.[21]

The following is a list of documents to include in a pharmacy's sterile compounding QA program:

- Leadership documentation
    - Review and approval of the use of any outsourced clinical services (eg, outsourcing facilities, compounding pharmacies, or nuclear pharmacies that may provide CSPs to the hospital)
    - Development and monitoring of expectation standards for these providers
- Personnel records
    - Orientation check list
    - Didactic training test results
    - Form for assessing hand hygiene and garbing related practices
    - Form for assessing aseptic technique and related practices
    - Form for assessing cleaning and disinfection procedures
    - Media fill results
    - Gloved fingertip testing results
    - Hazardous drug handling training
- Refrigerator, freezer, warmer, and incubator temperature logs

- Compounding area and drug storage room temperature logs
- Air pressure differentials, air velocities, and air changes per hour
- Cleaning logs for primary engineering controls, compounding areas (compounding suites and segregated compounding areas), and compounding equipment
- Equipment calibration logs
- Surface microbial testing logs
- Hazardous drug surface contamination logs
- Master formulation records and compounding records
- CSP orders or prescriptions and corresponding release checks (eg, accuracy, particulates, closures) and tests (eg, sterility, nonpyrogenicity)
- Primary and secondary engineering control certification reports
- Patient incident, adverse drug reaction, and complaint logs
- Annual policy and procedure review statement
- Annual review of effectiveness of QA program

Well-kept documents provide a means of tracing or recreating a set of events that can be investigated and acted on. Many of the newer automated compounding devices automatically generate documents that capture and record each of the critical elements when compounding a sterile preparation.

Preparation traceability is an essential element of any sterile preparation compounding program. Proper documentation follows the final preparation back to the source providing the necessary assurance for the configuration, characteristics, and integrity of the preparation. Preparation traceability through distribution channels is an essential element of an effective and targeted preparation withdrawal and recall.

Gap Analysis

Performing a gap analysis of the operation every year or whenever changes occur in facilities, supervision, federal or state regulations, standards, or health-system policies provides a fresh perspective for potential issues. Several sources provide gap analysis tools.[22;23]

Data Collection

Data should be collected in formats that help pharmacists assess processes, set priorities, and determine patterns and trends. Tools, such as flow charts, check sheets, cause-and-effect diagrams, Pareto diagrams, scatter plots, histograms, run charts, and control charts, help organize data in a way that visibly reflects trends.

Data Analysis

Action levels can be set for some types of data. If a trend becomes negative to the point of passing a predetermined threshold, corrective action is required. Types of data for which action levels can be set include but are not limited to air particulate counts, microbial testing results, temperature and humidity, air pressure, velocity, and air changes per hour.

CORRECTIVE ACTIONS

USP Chapter <797> includes action level tables. When results exceed the action level, steps must be taken to remediate the issue. Many organizations also develop alert levels, which are lower than action levels but still trigger steps outlined in SOPs.

Action levels for glove fingertip sampling for personnel are detection of any colony forming units (CFUs) when sampled after initial garbing processes. The action level for glove fingertip testing following media fill is greater than 3 CFUs from both hands. Action levels for microbial sampling are summarized in **Tables 33-3** and **33-4**. **Table 33-5**

TABLE 33-3. USP Chapter <797> Action Levels for Microbial Contamination

Air Microbial Sampling Action Levels	
Classification	Air Sample Test Result (CFUs/m^3 air)
ISO Class 5	>1
ISO Class 7	>10
ISO Class 8	>100

CFUs = colony-forming units; ISO = International Organization for Standardization.

Source: Reprinted with permission of USP <797> Pharmaceutical compounding—sterile preparations. In: *2023: USP Compounding Compendium*. Rockville, MD: United States Pharmacopeial Convention; 2023.

TABLE 33-4. USP Chapter <797> Action Levels for Microbial Contamination

Surface Sampling Action Levels	
Classification	Surface Sample Test Result (CFU per device or swab)
ISO Class 5	>3
ISO Class 7	>5
ISO Class 8	>50

CFUs = colony-forming units; ISO = International Organization for Standardization.

Source: Reprinted with permission of USP <797> Pharmaceutical compounding—sterile preparations. In: *2023: USP Compounding Compendium*. Rockville, MD: United States Pharmacopeial Convention; 2023.

TABLE 33-5. Quality Assurance Indicators

Quality Indicator	Purpose	Action Level Guidelines	Types of Corrective Action
Media fill tests	To trend failures in media fill evaluations	Any growth or discoloration	Review trend for sources of contamination; identify microbe at genus level for pathogenic potential
Initial gloved fingertip tests Ongoing gloved fingertip tests	To trend failures in fingertip media tests To trend failures in fingertip media tests	>0 CFU >3 CFU based on CFU on both gloves (not per glove)	Review to detect problems with garbing procedures Review trend to detect problems with hand hygiene and garbing procedures, surface disinfection procedures, and work practices
Refrigerator log	To ensure that drugs are stored at required temperatures	Below 2°C or over 8°C	Transient excursions between 0°C and 15°C may be permitted; otherwise have refrigerator serviced
Freezer log	To ensure that drugs are stored at required temperatures	Below –25°C or above –10°C	Transient excursions above –10°C may be permitted; otherwise have freezer serviced
Warmer log	To ensure that drugs are stored at required temperatures	Within range defined	Transient excursions may be permitted; otherwise have warmer serviced
Incubator log	To ensure proper incubation of samples	Within range defined	Evaluate need to retest; have incubator serviced
Room temperature log	To ensure comfort of compounding personnel	Above 20°C	Transient excursions outside comfort range may be permitted; otherwise have HVAC serviced
Room humidity log	To ensure that compounding personnel are comfortable and ensure that conditions do not favor mold growth	Above 60% relative humidity	Transient excursions outside moderate humidity may be permitted; otherwise have HVAC serviced
Air pressure differential log	To ensure that air currents do not push contaminated air into a cleaner area	0.020 inches WC for positive pressure; 0.010 to 0.030 inches WC for negative pressure	Investigate excursions; if measurements remain outside parameters, have HVAC serviced
ACPH log	To ensure that air currents do not push contaminated air into a cleaner area	30 ACPH or more in ISO 7 areas; 20 ACPH or more in ISO 8 areas; 12 ACPH or more in containment segregated compounding areas and hazardous drug storage area	Transient excursions may be permitted; otherwise have HVAC serviced
Automated compounding or repeater pump device calibration log	To ensure that automated compounding devices maintain precision (ie, cumulative errors over time)	Excursions of >5% from accurate measure	Have ACD or repeater pump serviced
Surface test log	To determine the effectiveness of cleaning and disinfecting procedures	>3 CFU for ISO Class 5 >5 CFU for ISO Class 7 > 50 for ISO Class 8	Retrain personnel and redo test; identify microbes for pathogenic potential

TABLE 33-5. (Continued)

Quality Indicator	Purpose	Action Level Guidelines	Types of Corrective Action
Hazardous drug wipe sampling records	To determine whether hazardous drug cleanup in PEC is effective and whether hazardous drug has escaped containment into environment	As designated by results	Retrain personnel and redo surface test; clean thoroughly and change cleaning process; improve BSC or CACI function or use CSTDs
Primary engineering control air particulate tests	To determine whether PEC provides ISO Class 5 compounding environment	>3,520 particles ≥0.5 μm/m^3 air	Have service company test HEPA filter for leaks and fan for effectiveness
Buffer area air particulate tests	To determine whether buffer area provides ISO Class 7 protection around the PEC	>352,000 particles ≥0.5 μm/m^3 air	Have service company test HEPA filter for leaks and fan for effectiveness
Anteroom air particulate count log	To determine whether anteroom provides ISO Class 8 protection for the buffer area	>3,520,000 particles ≥0.5 μm/m^3 air	Have service company test HEPA filter for leaks and fan for effectiveness
Primary and secondary engineering controls air microbial counts trended over time	To evaluate overall control inside the PEC compounding environment	>1 CFU/m^3 air within PECs; >10 CFUs/m^3 within buffer areas; >50 CFUs/m^3 within anteroom and segregated compounding areas Highly pathogenic microbes must be immediately remedied regardless of CFU count	Consistent elevated levels of microbial growth require consultation with competent microbiology personnel; evaluate and eliminate source of contamination; re-evaluate work practices, cleaning procedures, operational procedures, and air filtration efficiency; resample area

ACPH = air changes per hour; BSC = biological safety cabinet; CACI = compounding aseptic containment isolator; CFU = colony-forming units; CSTDs = closed-system drug transfer devices; HEPA = high-efficiency particulate air; HVAC = heating, venting, and air conditioning; ISO = International Organization for Standardization; PEC = primary engineering controls; WC = inches of water column.

summarizes quality indicator data, purpose, action levels if specified, and types of action that might be used to correct negative trends.

SUMMARY

Establishing policies and procedures is a critical step in any sterile drug preparation program. A thorough policy and procedure manual must be available to all involved personnel. These employees must show an understanding of each policy and procedure before being allowed to compound sterile preparations. Moreover, their competency in performing these procedures and interpreting each policy must be assessed periodically. Excellent policies and procedures form the foundation for a QA program, which is a mechanism for monitoring, evaluating, correcting, and improving the activities and processes related to compounding sterile preparations. The QA program delineates individuals responsible for each act of the program. QA plans focus on objective, measurable indicators that reflect standards set by USP Chapter <797>.

REFERENCES

1. American Society of Health-System Pharmacists. ASHP guidelines: minimum standard for pharmacies in hospitals. *Am J Health Syst Pharm*. 2013;70(18): 1619–1630. doi:10.2146/sp130001.
2. Tomich DJ, Dydek GJ. The policy and procedure manual. In: Brown TR, ed. *Handbook of institutional pharmacy practice*. 4th ed. Bethesda, MD: American Society of Health-System Pharmacists; 2005:297–312.
3. Page SB, ed. *Establishing a system of policies and procedures*. Westerville, OH: Process Improvement Publishing; 2002.
4. Page SB, ed. *7 steps to better policies and procedures*. Westerville, OH: Process Improvement Publishing; 2004.
5. USP <797> Pharmaceutical compounding—sterile preparations. In: *2023: USP Compounding Compendium*. Rockville, MD: United States Pharmacopeial Convention; 2023.

6. USP <800> Hazardous drugs—handling in healthcare settings. In: *2023: USP Compounding Compendium*. Rockville, MD: United States Pharmacopeial Convention; 2023.
7. USP <825> Radiopharmaceuticals—preparation, compounding, dispensing, and repackaging. In: *2023: USP Compounding Compendium*. Rockville, MD: United States Pharmacopeial Convention; 2023.
8. U.S. Pharmacopeial Convention. *2023 USP Compounding Compendium*. Rockville, MD: United States Pharmacopeial Convention; 2023.
9. American Society of Health-System Pharmacists (ASHP). ASHP guidelines on compounding sterile preparations. *Am J Health Syst Pharm*. 2014;71(2): 145–166. doi:10.2146/sp140001.
10. American Society of Health-System Pharmacists (ASHP). ASHP guidelines on outsourcing sterile compounding services. *Am J Health Syst Pharm*. 2015;72(19):1664–1675. doi:10.2146/sp150024.
11. American Society of Health-System Pharmacists (ASHP). Outsourcing sterile products preparation: vendor assessment tool. ASHP Website. **https://outsourcing.ashp.org/**. Accessed August 18, 2023.
12. Institute for Safe Medication Practices (ISMP). Guidelines for sterile compounding and the safe use of sterile compounding technology. **https://www.ismp.org/resources/guidelines-sterile-compounding-and-safe-use-sterile-compounding-technology**. Published May 4, 2022. Accessed August 18, 2023.
13. Kienle PC. *The Chapter <797> Answer Book*. 2nd ed. Bethesda, MD: American Society of Health-System Pharmacists; 2023.
14. Kienle PC. *The Chapter <800> Answer Book*. 2nd ed. Bethesda, MD: American Society of Health-System Pharmacists; 2023.
15. American Society of Health-System Pharmacists. Practice management. **https://www.ashp.org/Pharmacy-Practice/Resource-Centers/Practice-Management**. Accessed August 18, 2023.
16. Ashworth LD. Quality-control standard operating procedures—an essential tool for developing quality preparations. *Int J Pharm Compd*. 2007;11(3):226–228. **https://pubmed.ncbi.nlm.nih.gov/23996025/**.
17. USP <1079> Risks and mitigation strategies for the storage and transportation of finished drug products. In: *2023: USP Compounding Compendium*. Rockville, MD: United States Pharmacopeial Convention; 2023.
18. McAteer F. Establishing a quality unit: a formal quality unit not only helps assess overall performance but also provides continuous improvement to patient care. *Cleanrooms*. 2007;24:47–48.
19. USP <1163> quality assurance in pharmaceutical compounding. In: *2023: USP Compounding Compendium*. Rockville, MD: United States Pharmacopeial Convention; 2023.
20. Uselton JP, Kienle PC, Murdaugh LB. Performance improvement activities. In: *Preparing to Meeting Accreditation Standards: A Pharmacy Preparation Guide*. Bethesda, MD: American Society of Health-System Pharmacists; 2019.
21. Kastango ES. Blueprint for implementing USP chapter 797 for compounding sterile preparations. *Am J Health Syst Pharm*. 2005;62(12):1271–1288. doi:10.1093/ajhp/62.12.1271.
22. American Society of Health-System Pharmacists (ASHP). Compounding competency assessment center. **https://elearning.ashp.org/subscriptions/1001/ashp-sterile-compounding-competency-library**. Accessed August 18, 2023.
23. Gap analysis. International Journal of Pharmaceutical Compounding Website. **www.compoundingtoday.com/Compliance/USPGAP.cfm**. Accessed August 18, 2023.

APPENDIX 33-A. CLEANING AND DISINFECTING THE BUFFER ROOM AND ANTEROOM

Cleaning and Disinfecting Positive Pressure Buffer Room and Anteroom

Organization: ______________________ Department: Pharmacy

Department Director: ______________________ Phone Number: ____________

Responsible Supervisor: ______________________ Phone Number: ____________

Policy 10-4 Effective Date: June 1, 2023

I. **POLICY:** It is the intent of this organization to protect the health and safety of our patients, visitors, and employees and to abide by applicable laws, regulations, and professional standards. Therefore, cleaning and disinfecting the buffer room and anteroom according to the procedures below must occur on a regular basis at delineated intervals, when spills occur, when surfaces are visibly soiled, and when microbial contamination is suspected of having been introduced into the compounding work areas. Note that no hazardous drug compounding is conducted in the positive pressure buffer room or anteroom (see separate policy Decontaminating, Cleaning, and Disinfecting Negative Pressure Buffer Room for compounding hazardous drugs).

II. **PURPOSE:** Scrupulous attention to cleaning and disinfecting the sterile compounding areas is paid to minimize environmental microbial growth as a source of contamination of compounded sterile preparations.

III. **REFERENCES:**

a. USP Chapter <797> Pharmaceutical Compounding—Sterile Preparations

b. Institutional policies and procedures on selection of detergents, disinfectants, and cleaning agents

IV. **APPLICABILITY:** This standard operating procedure (SOP) applies only to sterile compounding areas (pharmacy positive pressure buffer room and anteroom). Related SOPs, such as the use and care of laminar air flow workbenches (LAFWs) and environmental monitoring, also apply to the compounding areas.

V. **RESPONSIBILITIES:** The supervisor of sterile compounding who serves as the designated person is responsible for enforcing this SOP and for its annual review and revision. Compounding personnel and environmental services personnel are responsible for carrying out the procedures outlined below. Trained compounding personnel clean and disinfect storage shelving, counters, carts, and other equipment. Trained environmental services personnel clean and disinfect floors, walls, and ceilings.

VI. **DEFINITIONS:**

a. **Anteroom:** The ISO Class 8 area where compounding personnel garb and wash hands, stage and clean components, label compounded sterile preparations, and perform other defined CSP-related activities.

b. **Buffer room:** The ISO Class 7 area where LAWFs are located and in which sterile compounding occurs.

c. **Detergent:** A cleansing agent including a surfactant that acts to remove impurities. The detergent used must be approved by the Infection Control Committee.

d. **Disinfectant:** A chemical or physical agent used on inanimate surfaces and objects to destroy fungi, viruses, and bacteria. Sporicidal disinfectants are considered a special class of disinfectants that also are effective against bacterial and fungal spores.

VII. **PROCEDURES:**

a. **Access:** Access to the sterile compounding suite is limited to authorized personnel.

b. **Traffic:** Only properly trained, garbed, and hand-washed personnel may clean and disinfect the buffer room and anteroom.

c. **Surfaces:** Environmental services cleaning and disinfecting of floors, walls, and ceiling in the buffer room and anteroom is performed after sterile compounding ceases on the night shift.

i. **Floors:** The buffer room floor is mopped, beginning in the cleanest section around and under the LAFWs and proceeding to the exit to the anteroom, with the appropriately diluted detergent solution and disposable mop head. The mop should be damp, not dripping wet, and should be rinsed frequently during the cleaning process. The mop is moved left and right in parallel lines so as not to contaminate previously mopped space. Circular motions with mops are avoided to prevent recontamination. With the same mop, the anteroom is mopped next, proceeding from the exit from the buffer room to the exit from the anteroom to the main pharmacy. Then the mop head is discarded.

ii. **Ceilings:** The buffer room ceiling is wiped from the cleanest areas around the HEPA air inputs toward the door exiting to the anteroom with the appropriately diluted detergent solution and disposable wipers. The wiper is moved left and right in parallel lines so as not to contaminate previously wiped space. Circular motions with wipers are avoided to prevent recontamination. The anteroom ceiling is wiped from the exit from the buffer room to the exit from the anteroom to the main pharmacy. Then the wipers are discarded. After ceilings are cleaned, proceed to clean walls.

iii. **Walls:** After the ceilings have been wiped, the buffer room walls are wiped from the top of the cleanest wall behind the LAFWs to the bottom of that wall with the appropriately diluted detergent solution and disposable wipers. Then the two side walls are wiped from top to bottom. The wiper is moved left and right in parallel lines so as not to contaminate previously wiped space. Circular motions with wipers are avoided to prevent recontamination. Then the two side walls of the anteroom are wiped top to bottom. Finally, the back wall with the exit to the main pharmacy is wiped from top to bottom. Then the wipers are discarded. After walls are cleaned, proceed to clean floors.

iv. **Counters:** Wipers are wetted with the appropriately diluted detergent. Counters and cart shelves are wiped from cleanest side to dirtiest side. The wiper is moved left and right in parallel lines so as not to contaminate previously wiped space. Circular motions with wipers are avoided to prevent recontamination. After the counters are dry, sterile IPA is used to disinfect the surface. The IPA is allowed to dry before compounding activity is resumed.

v. **Pass-through chambers:** Wipers are wetted with the appropriately diluted detergent. One door of the pass-through chamber is opened (do not open both doors at the same time). All surfaces inside the pass-through chambers are cleaned in the following order, top (ceiling of the chamber), walls, and deck. The wiper is moved left and right in parallel lines so as not to contaminate previously wiped space. Circular motions with wipers are avoided to prevent recontamination. After the pass-through chamber surfaces are dry, sterile IPA is used to disinfect the surface. The IPA is allowed to dry before compounding activity is resumed.

vi. **Storage shelving:** Wipers are wetted with the appropriately diluted detergent. Storage shelves are wiped from cleanest side to dirtiest side. The wiper is moved left and right in parallel lines so as not to contaminate previously wiped space. Circular motions with wipers are avoided to prevent recontamination. After the shelving is dry, sterile IPA is used to disinfect the surface. The IPA is allowed to dry before compounding activity is resumed.

vii. **Supplies:** No corrugated cardboard, shipping, or other external cartons may be taken into the anteroom or buffer room. When removed from shipping cartons, supplies and components are wiped with sterile 70% IPA. The IPA is allowed to dry before supplies and components are transferred to the cleanroom storage area. When sterile supplies are packaged in sealed pouches designed to keep them sterile until opening, the sterile supplies are removed just as the supplies are introduced into the LAFWs as part of the active compounding process.

viii. **Equipment:** When removed from shipping cartons, equipment is wiped with sterile 70% IPA if IPA is compatible with the surface of the equipment. The IPA is allowed to dry before equipment is transferred from the anteroom to the buffer room. The external surfaces of the LAFWs and trash receptacles are cleaned and disinfected on a monthly basis.

d. **Methods and materials:** All cleaning materials, such as wipers and mop heads, must be low-linting (ie, made of synthetic microfibers) and dedicated to the buffer room and anteroom. Once taken into the buffer room and anteroom, cleaning materials are not removed except for disposal.

i. **Wiping:** Approved sterile wipers packaged in pouches are stored in the anteroom and may be used in the buffer room or anteroom, but only in that order. Single-use, disposable, low-lint wipers are used.

ii. **Mopping:** Approved, clean floor mop handles and mop heads are stored in the anteroom and may be used in the buffer room or anteroom, but only in that order. Single-use, disposable mop heads are used. After mopping, mop buckets are removed from the anteroom and cleaned and disinfected outside of the sterile compounding suite.

e. **Schedule:** Example of a schedule for minimum frequency of cleaning and disinfecting the buffer room and anteroom is as follows:

Site	Minimum Frequency
Counters and easily cleanable work surfaces (eg, clean transfer cart shelves)	Daily or when spills or visible or suspected soiling occurs
Floors	Daily or when spills or suspected soiling occurs
Walls	First Wednesday of each month
Ceiling	First Wednesday of each month
Storage shelves	First Wednesday of each month or when spills or visible or suspected soiling occurs; all supplies must be removed before storage shelves are cleaned and disinfected
External surfaces of LAFWs and trash receptacles	First Wednesday of each month or when spills or visible or suspected soiling occurs

f. **Detergents and disinfectants:** Cleaning and disinfecting agents are approved by the Infection Control Committee with careful consideration of compatibilities, effectiveness, ambient microbial flora, and inappropriate or toxic residues.

i. **Protection:** Personnel involved with cleaning and disinfection must wear appropriate personal protective equipment (ie, shoe covers, hair covers, face mask or shield, gowns, and sterile gloves).

ii. **Selection:** Approved cleaning and disinfecting agents include the following:

Agent Type	Product and Source Approved by Infection Control Committee
Sterile 70% IPA for counters, shelves, carts, and other equipment	
Detergent for ceilings, walls, and floors	
Germicidal for ceilings, walls, and floors	
Purified water, USP	

iii. **Preparation:** Ready-to-use solutions are preferred. If dilution of concentrated disinfectant and sodium hypochlorite solutions is required, it is performed by the sterile compounding designated person or designee.

iv. **Storage:** Cleaning and disinfecting agents dedicated to the sterile compounding areas are stored in designated locations in the anteroom. No food or drug products or preparations may be stored in the locations designated for cleaning and disinfecting agents.

g. **Personnel training:** Personnel who clean and disinfect the buffer room and anteroom must be properly trained before being given the above cleaning and disinfecting responsibilities. Effectiveness of personnel training must be demonstrated to and documented by the designated person. Every six months, the designated person evaluates the performance of all personnel involved with cleaning and disinfecting the buffer room and anteroom as to proper hand hygiene, garbing, and all applicable cleaning and disinfecting procedures.

h. **Documentation:** Compounding personnel maintain a log of cleaning and disinfecting activities described in this policy and procedure. The designated person documents the training and competency of personnel that clean and disinfect the buffer room and anteroom. Records are stored in designated locations for approved periods of time.

CSP = compounded sterile preparation; ISO = International Organization of Standardization; HEPA = high-efficiency particulate air; IPA = isopropyl alcohol.

34

OUTSOURCING THE COMPOUNDING OF STERILE PREPARATIONS

Angela T. Cassano

INTRODUCTION

Laws, regulations, drug shortages, and professional guidelines make compounding sterile preparations very complex (see Chapter 2 for details). Faced with these challenges, pharmacists may elect to outsource sterile compounding operations to pharmacies and outsourcing facilities that have a proven track record of having trained staff, appropriate facilities, and a supply of ingredients to make the compounded sterile preparations (CSPs) needed for their patients.

NATIONAL TRENDS

According to a 2012 survey of 298 hospitals by the U.S. Office of Inspector General (OIG), ensuring an adequate supply of CSPs was very important to hospitals when determining whether to outsource them. Many hospitals cited shortages of commercial products (68%), the availability of CSPs with extended shelf lives (62%), and CSP stability (69%) as very important factors in their decision to outsource. Historically, hospitals took limited steps to ensure the quality of outsourced CSPs but had few problems (that they knew about) with the quality of products from outside pharmacies.[1]

Pedersen et al. reported in 2020 that 79% of hospitals outsourced some of their sterile preparation activities, including patient-specific (503A) and nonpatient-specific (503B) preparations.[2] The 2002 national survey, which was conducted prior to *United States Pharmacopeia* (USP) Chapter <797> setting the minimum standard for compounding sterile preparations, reported only 21% of hospitals outsourced some sterile preparation activities. Survey results increased to 41.8% in 2008, which was the first time the survey was conducted after USP Chapter <797> was fully enforceable.[3;4] A sharp increase in outsourcing CSPs was documented in 2011 (70.9%) and remains at or above that level today.[2;5] Of the hospitals that outsourced some preparation activities in the 2017 survey, 76.7% outsourced patient-controlled analgesia (PCA) and epidurals, 62.3% outsourced syringe-based anesthesia medications, 60.5% outsourced oxytocin preparations, 33.6% outsourced routine intravenous (IV) admixtures and piggybacks, and 32.4% outsourced total parenteral nutrition (TPN).[6] Less than 25% of hospitals outsourced high-risk products made from nonsterile components or cardioplegia.[6]

Why do so many hospitals choose an outside pharmacy or outsourcing facility to provide CSPs for their patients? In addition to the reasons in the OIG survey, other reasons include but are not limited to the following[2]:

- Extended beyond-use dates
- Purchasing repackaged or compounded drugs for procedures
- Staffing shortages
- Purchasing drugs on the U.S. Food and Drug Administration (FDA) drug shortages list
- Complex formulations (eg, TPNs)
- Preparation of large batches for anticipatory use
- Nonsterile to sterile compounding

Furthermore, pharmacists and technicians are often not adequately trained to compound all types of sterile preparations, especially those that are made from nonsterile components.[7] This gap is widened with the introduction of new technologies and pharmacologic advances, such as specialty pharmaceuticals, cell and gene therapies, and individualized dosing based on pharmacogenomics, which are creating an increased need for trained compounding pharmacists and technicians. Outsourcing of CSPs may be an answer for some of the issues hospital pharmacies are facing.

Note: The author acknowledges E. Clyde Buchanan who authored this chapter in the previous edition.

DOI 10.37573/9781585286492.034

Syringes for CSP Storage

In July 2015, the Institute for Safe Medication Practices published a special alert on the loss of drug potency when stored in 3-mL or 5-mL syringes manufactured by Becton, Dickinson and Company (BD).[8] The manufacturer recommended preparing medication syringes as close to the time of administration as possible. By August 2015, the FDA published a MedWatch Safety Alert suggesting that drugs stored in these syringes may lose potency over time due to a possible interaction with the rubber stopper in the syringe. In the same alert, BD asked their customers not to use their 10-mL, 20-mL, and 30-mL syringes for drug storage as well.[9] All of these syringes had been cleared as medical devices for general purpose fluid aspiration and injection only, not for use as a closed-container storage system for drug products. The FDA also stated that this issue likely extends to other manufacturer general use syringes that were not cleared for the purpose of closed container storage. In 2018, BD alerted the FDA that the stoppers in question had been changed out and should not cause loss of potency. The FDA alerted clinicians of this change, but they did not make a formal comment as to how this should be interpreted in practice.[9]

The issue of use of a syringe for closed container storage is a particularly important consideration for outsourcing of CSPs. As reported previously, 62.3% of hospitals outsourced syringe-based anesthesia medications.[6] Therefore, 503A and 503B compounding pharmacies must test potency and stability of each drug, drug concentration, and syringe size or present published stability studies to back up the quality of their products.

Laws, Regulations, and Standards

A licensed pharmacy director or pharmacist-in-charge must take responsibility for patient outcomes from all medication-related activities performed at or for the organization's work sites whether they are carried out by the organization's staff, in-house contracted pharmacy staff, or by an outside pharmacy. Pharmacy leadership should arrange a legal contract with outside compounding pharmacies to support purchases of CSPs whether the CSP is for a patient-specific order or a nonpatient-specific lot. For the purposes of this discussion, the outside pharmacy may be either a 503A traditional compounding pharmacy or a 503B outsourcing facility.

Compounding Quality Act

In September 2012, a sole case report sparked an investigation into a nationwide outbreak of fungal meningitis due to contaminated injectable drugs. The compounder of contaminated preparations, New England Compounding Center (NECC), was in violation of several state and federal laws. The regulation of compounding pharmacies has historically been left to the states, but sterile pharmaceutical manufacturing fell under the jurisdiction of FDA. However, as more compounders took part in large-scale interstate distribution of CSPs, the state-based regulatory system was not equipped to provide oversight.[10]

The U.S. Congress passed H.R. 3204 to build safeguards for large-scale compounding by increasing inspections, adopting stricter licensing requirements under the Compounding Quality Act (CQA) subsection of the Drug Quality and Security Act (DQSA) of 2013.[11]

503A Compounding Pharmacies

Section 503A of the Food, Drug, and Cosmetic (FD&C) Act was originally added in 1997 as part of the Food and Drug Administration Modernization Act (FDAMA), which described "[c]onditions that must be satisfied for drug products compounded by a licensed pharmacist or licensed physician to be exempt from the following three sections of the FD&C Act: (1) section 501(a)(2)(B) (concerning current good manufacturing practice); (2) section 502(f)(1) (concerning the labeling of drugs with adequate directions for use); and (3) section 505 (concerning the approval of drugs under new drug applications (NDAs) or abbreviated new drug applications [ANDAs])."[12]

Section 503A also included advertising and promotional restrictions on pharmacy compounding of any drugs. This advertising portion of the law was challenged by compounding pharmacies and was subsequently found to be unconstitutional by the U.S. Supreme Court, resulting in confusion over which agencies were responsible for oversight of drug compounding, nonmanufacturing operations. The 2013 DQSA amended section 503A of the FD&C Act, outlining what constitutes traditional compounding, which standards are to be followed, and which agencies are responsible for oversight. In short, 503A compounding includes traditional pharmacy compounding, must comply with USP Chapter <797> and other applicable USP chapters, and is most often subject to inspections by state boards of pharmacy (see **Table 34-1** for an overview of compounding pharmacies and outsourcing facilities).[13] Under DQSA, compounding performed by health-system pharmacies continues to be governed by section 503A in most situations.

503B Outsourcing Facilities

Additionally, H.R. 3204 created a new section, 503B of the FD&C Act, which describes outsourcing facilities (OFs).[11] Section 503B allows outsourcing facilities to voluntarily register with FDA and submit to inspections on a risk-based schedule set by the Secretary of Health and Human Services (HHS). As of 2017, 89% of the over 400 Medicare-participating, acute-care hospitals that responded to an OIG survey reported they only purchased CSPs from FDA-registered OFs.[14] While registration is technically voluntary, market forces have dictated mandatory registration with the FDA for an outsourcing facility to remain competitive. As of February 2023, over 70 outsourcing facilities are registered with FDA, which represents only a modest increase over the prior version of this text that reported 55.[15;16]

An *outsourcing facility* is defined as a facility at one geographic location that performs the following[11]:

- Compounds sterile drugs
- Has registered as an outsourcing facility with FDA

TABLE 34-1. Differences Between Compounding Pharmacies and Outsourcing Facilities

Variable	Section 503A Compounding Pharmacies	Section 503B Registered Outsourcing Facilities
Regulatory authority	State boards of pharmacy	FDA and according to guidelines established by federal legislation States may add requirements
Applicable standards	USP compounding standards FDA Compliance Policy Guide on Pharmacy Compounding of Human Drug Products under Section 503A of the Federal Food, Drug, and Cosmetic Act	Applicable section 503B-specific FDA current good manufacturing practice Subject to additional state requirements
FDA inspection	Subject to FDA inspection under authority to enforce section 503A	Subject to risk-based FDA inspection and enforcement procedures
State inspection	Subject to state board of pharmacy inspection	May be subject to state inspection if state law imposes additional requirements
Limitations on services	May only dispense pursuant to an individual prescription or medication order for an identified patient Anticipatory compounding of limited quantities is permitted, but a prescription or medication order is required before dispensing FDA limitation on interstate distribution, either 5% or 50%, depending on whether the state has entered into an MOU with FDA May not compound: • Drugs that present demonstrable difficulties for compounding • Copies of FDA-approved products • Drugs using certain prohibited bulk substances	Not required to be a licensed pharmacy or obtain prescriptions for specific patients May compound and maintain inventory of compounded products in anticipation of customer orders No federal limit on interstate commerce (some state regulations may apply) Compounding from bulk APIs only allowed for drugs on FDA-approved bulk list May compound copies of FDA-approved products from bulk substances if on FDA shortage list
Office-use compounding	Not yet addressed in FDA guidance	Permitted (resale prohibited but resale does not include administration or dispensing by the purchaser)
Labeling requirements	As mandated by state law and regulation	Must include "Office use", "This is a compounded drug," and "Not for resale"

FDA = U.S. Food and Drug Administration; USP = *United States Pharmacopeia.*

Source: Adapted with permission of the American Society of Health-System Pharmacists (ASHP). Guidelines on Outsourcing Sterile Compounding Services. *Am J Health-Syst Pharm.* 2015; 72:1664-1675.

- Complies with 503B requirements established in H.R. 3204

Although an outsourcing facility is not a pharmaceutical manufacturer, it is not required to be a licensed pharmacy and may or may not obtain patient-specific prescriptions. If an outsourcing facility chooses to have patient-specific prescriptions filled under 503A provisions (ie, not subject to current good manufacturing practices [CGMPs]), the compounding of such CSPs must occur in a completely segregated area from any 503B operations in the same building.[17] The FDA published guidance on what typically indicates complete segregation but noted that it is handled on a case-by-case basis. Examples of outsourcing facilities and 503A establishments being completely segregated include the following[17]:

- No shared rooms
- No shared fixed equipment or compounding supplies
- The 503A and 503B areas must have separate entrances and exits, not share pass-throughs, and are separated by permanent fixed barriers (ie, walls)

An outsourcing facility must submit a list of compounded drugs made by the facility every 6 months to the FDA.[18] As a reference point on the volume of outsourcing, a 2017 report by the FDA Center for Drug Evaluation and Research (CDER) highlighted 59 outsourcing facilities that reported preparing 12,305,873 units of drugs in the preceding 6-month period.[18] The following information must be identified for each compounded drug submitted to FDA:

- The active ingredient, its source, and its strength per unit
- The National Drug Code (NDC) number of the source drug or bulk active ingredient
- The dosage form and route of administration
- The package description
- The number of individual units produced
- The NDC number of the final product

Outsourcing facilities are exempt from FDA requirements for safety and effectiveness and labeling for directions for patient use, but they must submit adverse event reports to FDA.[11]

Compounding with a bulk drug substance is allowed as long as that substance is on the FDA's drug shortage list or can be found on an FDA-issued list for which there is a clinical need. Bulk drug substances must be accompanied by a valid certificate of analysis and must have been manufactured by an establishment registered with the FDA under section 510 of the FD&C Act. Additionally, if an applicable USP or National Formulary (NF) monograph exists, bulk drug substances must comply with the monograph. Extensive guidance is provided by the FDA in the form of guidance documents relating to bulk substances and the lists mentioned above.[19] The drug shortages list changes frequently, requiring 503B outsourcing facilities to routinely monitor this list or risk being noncompliant. Physicians, pharmacists, and advocacy groups that want patients to use substances not on the FDA's bulk drug substances list can submit treatment investigational new drug applications.[20]

Once registered, outsourcing facilities have no limits on the amount of CSPs they can compound from the FDA-approved list, but they cannot make false or misleading statements in advertisements or promotions. Each outsourcing facility (individual location) must pay an annual establishment fee equal to $15,000 multiplied by the inflation adjustment factor, plus the small business adjustment factor. In the 2023 fiscal year, the annual reinspection fee was $17,823.[21]

Current Good Manufacturing Practices

In contrast to state-licensed 503A compounding pharmacies, which must comply with applicable USP standards, FDA-registered outsourcing facilities are subject to more rigorous quality and safety standards modeled on CGMPs that apply to pharmaceutical manufacturers. CGMPs are not best practice standards. They are minimum rules for practice in the manufacture, processing, packaging, and storing of drug products to be administered to humans. The purpose of CGMPs is to ensure that all pharmaceutical products are produced with consistent quality and integrity.[22]

Based in part on findings during FDA inspections of outsourcing facilities, the FDA did release draft guidance for outsourcing facilities in July of 2014 with revisions published in 2020.[22] These standards are closer to CGMP regulations for pharmaceutical manufacturing than they are to USP Chapter <797>. As of the time of this writing, the FDA has not published a final guidance for CGMPs for 503B outsourcing facilities, so there is still some uncertainty regarding requirements during inspection. A review of inspection reports of 503B outsourcing facilities by the FDA may provide additional insight into expectations of CGMPs for such facilities.

INSPECTIONS AND ENFORCEMENT

As outlined in Table 34-1, 503A compounding pharmacies typically fall under the purview of state boards of pharmacy and 503B outsourcing facilities are subject to routine, risk-based inspections by the FDA. However, the FDA is not limited to only inspecting 503B outsourcing facilities, as it is within its jurisdiction to conduct proactive and for-cause inspections of any compounding pharmacy, producers of sterile drug products, and laboratories that perform sterility and stability testing as appropriate to protect public health. Any findings by the FDA during an inspection of a 503A compounding pharmacy are shared with the corresponding state board of pharmacy.

FDA Form 483

An FDA Form 483 (Inspectional Observations) is issued at most inspections. FDA inspections are conducted by comparing compounding organizations against CGMPs regardless of 503A or 503B status. Even though 503A compounders are not subject to CGMPs during inspection, they are not exempt from the prohibition on insanitary conditions and may be cited for violations under this provision or if they are found to be compounding drugs that do not qualify for the 503A exemption.[23] As the forms reflect, FDA inspectors have observed serious quality problems, including contaminated products and sterile practices, that create risks of contamination.[24] Numerous recalls of CSPs have resulted, and several pharmacies chose to halt sterile compounding after the FDA identified problems with their sterile compounding processes. New problems continue to be identified at compounding pharmacies and outsourcing facilities across the country. **Table 34-2** shows the types of compounding issues identified by FDA inspectors.

State Boards of Pharmacy

According to the DQSA, in consultation with the National Association of the Boards of Pharmacy (NABP), the HHS secretary is required to receive information from state boards of

TABLE 34-2. Top Ten FDA Form 483 Observations at 503A and 503B Organizations (2012-2022)

FDA Form 483 Issue	Occurrences*	Frequency†
Aseptic processing areas are deficient regarding the system for monitoring environmental conditions.	380	42%
Aseptic processing areas are deficient regarding the system for cleaning and disinfecting the room and equipment to produce aseptic conditions.	365	40.4%
Procedures designed to prevent microbiological contamination of drug products purporting to be sterile are not established, written, or followed.	298	33.0%
Clothing of personnel engaged in the manufacturing, processing, packing, and holding of drug products is not appropriate for the duties they perform.	271	30%
There is a failure to thoroughly review any unexplained discrepancy and the failure of a batch or any of its components to meet any of its specifications whether or not the batch has already been distributed.	216	23.9%
Procedures designed to prevent microbiological contamination of drug products purporting to be sterile do not include adequate validation of the sterilization process.	216	23.9%
Testing and release of drug product for distribution does not include appropriate laboratory determination of satisfactory conformance to the final specifications and identity and strength of each active ingredient prior to release.	210	23.2%
There is no written testing program designed to assess the stability characteristics of drug products.	178	19.7%
Each batch of drug product purporting to be sterile and pyrogen-free is not laboratory tested to determine conformance to such requirements.	160	17.7%
Production personnel were not practicing good sanitation and health habits.	143	15.8%

FDA = U.S. Food and Drug Administration; HVAC = heating, ventilation, and air conditioning; SOP = standard operating procedure; USP = *United States Pharmacopeia*.

* This report represents findings from 904 inspections of 540 total facilities across 46 states.

† Frequency indicates the percentage of pharmacy 483 reports that reference this issue. Interpretation of the 483 findings and assignment to a particular category were performed by LDT Health Solutions.

Source: Adapted with permission of LDT Health Solutions, Inc. (Dave Thomas, RPh, MBA, e-mail communication, February 27, 2023).

pharmacy about 503A compounding pharmacies and 503B outsourcing facilities.[11] This information includes descriptions of actions they have taken against these entities for compounding violations (eg, imposing sanctions or penalties), suspending or revoking a pharmacy license or registration, or the recall of a compounded drug. A state board of pharmacy can also submit to HHS any concerns that a compounding pharmacy could be exceeding the scope of Section 503A activity (eg, conducting large-scale compounding, participating in interstate commerce). The HHS secretary is required to notify all state boards of pharmacy when information is received from one of the state boards regarding actions taken against a compounding pharmacy or when the secretary determines a pharmacy is acting contrary to Section 503A.[11]

Section 503A (b)(3) directs the FDA to develop a memorandum of understanding (MOU) between the FDA and boards of pharmacy.[11] The FDA finalized the MOU in October 2020 with an implementation date set for 2022. Subsequently, several compounding pharmacies filed lawsuits against the FDA, which resulted in a remanding of the MOU to the FDA to either certify it will not have a significant economic impact on small businesses or the FDA must prepare a regulatory flexibility analysis.[25] As of August 2023, the MOU was not implemented and the required analysis was not complete. The MOU in question outlines the following [25]:

- Interstate distribution of inordinate amounts of compounded drug products by traditional compounding pharmacies (ie, 503A pharmacies)
- Appropriate investigation by a state agency of complaints relating to compounded drug products distributed outside the state
- Under Section 503A (b)(3), a pharmacist, pharmacy, or physician in a state board MOU state has

distributed an inordinate amount of compounded human drug products interstate if the number of units of compounded human drug products distributed interstate during any calendar month is greater than 50% of the number of units of compounded and noncompounded drug products distributed or dispensed intrastate and interstate by such pharmacist, pharmacy, or physician during that month

- Under Section 503A (b)(3)(B)(ii), in a state that does not enter into an MOU with the FDA, the licensed pharmacist, licensed pharmacy, or licensed physician may distribute (or cause to be distributed) compounded human drug products out of the state in which they are compounded only in quantities that do not exceed 5% of the total prescription orders dispensed or distributed by such pharmacy or physician

The NABP Survey of Pharmacy Law provides an illustration of variability among states in regulation of outsourcing facilities.[26] Some states require separate licenses for organizations registered as outsourcing facilities with the FDA. Some states also indicate that licensure or registration is in the form of a wholesaler or manufacturer designation. Some states require outsourcing facilities to register with an entity other than the state board of pharmacy.

Enforcement and oversight of out of state compounding pharmacies also varies widely and was highlighted in the 2018 report by Pew Charitable Trusts.[27] Few states reported sending inspectors to outsourcing facilities in other states. Many states rely on the inspections of the state in which the facility resides. Since there is some minor variation in state laws on sterile compounding, many states require that the outsourcing facility must comply with the laws of the state receiving shipments of the outsourced drugs.

Accrediting Organizations

Hospitals and other healthcare organizations strive to achieve and maintain accreditation to be a deemed provider by the Centers for Medicare & Medicaid Services (CMS) and to be recognized for quality in their communities.[28] Different professional bodies may accredit outside pharmacies (503A and 503B) on a voluntary basis, but this is not associated with hospital accrediting organizations. Two compounding pharmacy accreditation agencies are the Accreditation Commission for Health Care (ACHC) and The Joint Commission (TJC).

Few U.S. hospitals can afford not to be CMS-accredited because of the substantial number of Medicare and Medicaid patients. Outside compounding pharmacies do not have to be accredited to serve patients who choose to use their services. Nevertheless, CMS may amend its interpretative guidelines to address hospital contracts with outside pharmacies that supply CSPs to respective hospitals.

Working for CMS in 2015, the federal OIG for Health and Human Services found that only one of the four accrediting organizations always reviews hospital contracts with outside pharmacies (503A and 503B). Accrediting organization surveyors receive limited training specific to compounding, and only three accrediting organizations determine whether an outside pharmacy has voluntarily registered with the FDA as a 503B outsourcing facility. Consequently, OIG recommended that accrediting organizations (1) ensure that hospital surveyors receive training on standards from nationally recognized organizations related to safe compounding practices and (2) amend their interpretive guidelines to address hospital contracts with outside compounding pharmacies. CMS concurred with both recommendations.[29]

What do hospital accrediting organizations require when hospitals purchase drugs from an outside compounding pharmacy? When pharmacy services are outsourced or provided through a contract, the contract should address responsibility for meeting medication management standards. TJC-accredited hospitals must ensure that outsourced contracted pharmacy services comply with other TJC standards.

Health Insurance Portability and Accountability Act

An outside pharmacy is a business associate to the organization in terms of the Health Insurance Portability and Accountability Act (HIPAA) of 1996.[30] For patient-specific compounding, this means that the organization pharmacy must disclose protected healthcare information (PHI) to the outside pharmacy (eg, patient names, identifying numbers, medical information). To make these disclosures, the outside pharmacy must sign a business associate agreement that gives the outside pharmacy legal access to the information needed to prepare and label a sterile prescription, and it requires the outside pharmacy to follow rules to protect patient PHI. Only medical information that is needed to perform the compounding service can be sent to the outside pharmacy. Patients must sign a general consent on hospital admission that their PHI may be used by a third party to provide treatments. Data transmitted in either direction between the organizational pharmacy and the outside pharmacy must be secured by authentication, encryption, or alarms.

Drug Enforcement Administration

The Drug Enforcement Administration (DEA) requires the use of DEA Form 222 for the transfer of Schedule II controlled drugs between pharmacies. This has implications for compounding opioids for PCA and epidural analgesia. The DEA requires record keeping and security for all schedules of controlled drugs that are purchased by one pharmacy from another pharmacy. Records of purchases, storage, distribution, and administration or destruction are required for any controlled drug.[31] DEA security measures also dictate that any transporter of controlled drugs must be licensed and bonded. Therefore, taxi cabs and most common carriers cannot be used to transport controlled drugs from an outside compounding pharmacy to the organization pharmacy.

Antitrust Laws

The Robinson-Patman Act requires that a hospital that purchases drugs at preferential prices (eg, through an acute care hospital group purchasing organization) limit the use of those drugs to their own use.[32] Outside compounding pharmacies are usually in a different class of trade from hospital pharmacies. For example, they may be classified as retail pharmacies, not acute care hospital pharmacies. This difference in class of trade means that the outside pharmacy may not be able to purchase drugs at the same discounted price. This becomes significant for sterile preparations, such as TPN and cardioplegia. Therefore, organization pharmacies sometimes find ways to have the outside pharmacy use the organization's pharmaceutical ingredients in compounding. This may require the outside pharmacy to have the organization pharmacy purchase the pharmaceutical ingredients for delivery to the outside pharmacy, which in turn must maintain a separate inventory for each organization that it serves. This practice often increases the inventory cost for the organization pharmacy, which must have two inventories of compounding ingredients, one for stat orders within the organization and one in the outside pharmacy for routine compounding.

ASHP

More than 2,000 pharmacy residency programs are accredited by ASHP.[33] To maintain their accreditation, pharmacies with residency programs must meet all ASHP guidelines and, by extension, any outside pharmacy should meet ASHP guidelines. Some of the ASHP guidelines that pertain to outsourcing the compounding of sterile preparations include the following:

- ASHP guidelines for selecting pharmaceutical manufacturers and suppliers[34]
- ASHP guidelines on outsourcing pharmaceutical services[35]
- ASHP guidelines on compounding sterile preparations[36]
- ASHP guidelines on outsourcing sterile compounding services[13]

The outsourcing guidelines describe services available from compounding pharmacies or outsourcing facilities, reasons for outsourcing and reasons for not outsourcing, the outsourcing process and outsourcing arrangements, and recommendations for evaluating a contractor's performance. The concepts presented in this document should be used for strategic planning with the organization's decision-makers, designing and evaluating requests for information and proposals from 503A compounding pharmacies or 503B outsourcing facilities, evaluative visits to compounding pharmacies and outsourcing facilities, assessing the quality of CSPs or products, drafting contract provisions, comparing prospective contractors, preparing for contract negotiations, and evaluating contractor performance.

Organizational Pharmacy Responsibilities in Outsourcing

The pharmacy director is responsible for the legality and quality of pharmaceuticals obtained from outside pharmacies, but they also have other fiduciary responsibilities to their organization.[35]

Evaluation of Outsourcing Facilities and Compounding Pharmacies

For departments that choose to outsource the preparation of parenteral medications, the following framework, originally developed for the ASHP Research and Education Foundation Outsourcing Sterile Products Preparation Vendor Assessment Tool, can be used to evaluate a response to a request for proposal during the selection of an outside compounding pharmacy (503A or 503B).[36] Assessment should evaluate each of the following areas:

- Regulatory compliance
- Quality and patient safety measures
- Medication administration safety features
- Service excellence

All outsourcing facilities and compounding pharmacies are not alike in their quality. The ASHP Vendor Assessment Tool recommends identifying suitable outsourcing facilities by reviewing the outstanding issues pertaining to each of the pharmacies being considered for purchasing (FDA Form 483 reports and related documents are available on the FDA website). It is important to pay particular attention to facilities that received warning letters because warning letters reflect the FDA district office's elevated level of concern (warning letters are available with the FDA list of 503B registrants).[37] Furthermore, what is the entity's response to the FDA Form 483? Just as FDA Form 483s should be evaluated by a prospective outsourcer, so should the responses to the FDA Form 483s. The FDA makes these response letters available on their website, but there is a lag time. Request responses and documentation of changes directly from prospective or current outsourcers. It is critical for organizations to evaluate whether they are comfortable with the responses of the outsourcer to the allegations in the FDA Form 483.[37]

Hospital Administration

All organizations have a culture. Some favor outsourcing, others do not. The pharmacy director should first assess the willingness of the chief executive officer to enter into an outsourcing contract. Outsourcing has implications for the organization's patient satisfaction, nursing and medical staff relations, and reputation within the community. Sometimes, the decision to outsource can be reversed only with great difficulty. The administrator or medical staff may not wish to lose control over decisions about pharmaceutical services.

Fiscal Responsibilities

The pharmacy director must make sure that the organization makes the best decisions to protect the organization's financial health. A full cost analysis and business plan is needed before any outsourcing pharmacy contracts are signed. All direct and indirect costs must be considered, including technical support for information systems (IS); computer hardware connections (eg, internet service provider) and interfaces; legal services and liability insurance; accounting and tax services; transportation charges, including licensing and bonding; pharmaceutical ingredient inventory at the outside contract pharmacy; and, of course, all product and support fees for the outside pharmacy. All these costs must be compared with performing the same sterile compounding services within the organization.

Information System Responsibilities

Prescription orders (eg, PHI) may need to be transmitted between pharmacies. The pharmacy director must involve the IS department early on to ascertain whether IS has the time and resources to support efficient, accurate, and secure information transfer.

Material Responsibilities

The pharmacy director must arrange for receiving CSPs from the outside contract pharmacy. Arrangements should be coordinated with the receiving department for hours of service, space, refrigeration, and security for deliveries.

Risk Management

Most organizations have risk management and accreditation departments. The pharmacy director must get support from the risk manager to use CSPs from an outside contract pharmacy. The pharmacy director may have to explain all the liabilities for clarity in the decision-making process. Performing due diligence on outsourcing facilities or compounding pharmacies doesn't end once the contract is signed. Hospitals must develop a way to conduct periodic reviews and or inspections of outsourcers utilizing similar questions to those used when evaluating requests for proposals.[13;37]

Recalls

One report describes how CSPs that are compounded by outsourcers can cause problems in a recall. Only 67% of the facilities were able to identify all the patients who received recalled outsourced products compared with 80% for in-house compounded prouducts.[38]

SUMMARY

Outsourcing CSP compounding to outside pharmacies is often considered because of market shortages, personnel shortages, costs of space and equipment, or a lack of expertise within the pharmacy to safely compound more complex sterile preparations. There are many obstacles for outsourcing, including the organization's responsibility to ensure the same (or better quality of) compounding as the organization is expected to provide, legalities and liabilities of outsourced compounding services, and the finances and logistics of outsourcing. Buying from an outside compounding pharmacy is not the same as buying from a pharmaceutical manufacturer. It should be handled like other services contracted from third parties. Choosing outside pharmacies to provide services to hospital patients is a big decision that is likely to draw attention from accrediting and licensing agencies.

REFERENCES

1. U.S Department of Health and Human Services Office of Inspector General. High-risk compounded sterile preparations and outsourcing by hospitals that use them. Report (OEI-01-13-00150). **https://oig.hhs.gov/oei/reports/oei-01-13-00150.asp**. Published April 10, 2013. Accessed March 4, 2023.
2. Pedersen CA, Schneider PJ, Ganio MC, Scheckelhoff DJ. ASHP national survey of pharmacy practice in hospital settings: Dispensing and administration-2020. *Am J Health Syst Pharm*. 2021;78(12):1074–1093. doi:10.1093/ajhp/zxab120.
3. Pedersen CA, Schneider PJ, Scheckelhoff DJ, Scheckelhoff DJ. ASHP national survey of pharmacy practice in hospital settings: dispensing and administration–2002. *Am J Health Syst Pharm*. 2003;60(1):52–68. doi:10.1093/ajhp/60.1.52.
4. Pedersen CA, Schneider PJ, Scheckelhoff DJ, Scheckelhoff DJ. ASHP national survey of pharmacy practice in hospital settings: dispensing and administration–2008. *Am J Health Syst Pharm*. 2009;66(10):926–946. doi:10.2146/ajhp080715.
5. Pedersen CA, Schneider PJ, Scheckelhoff DJ, Scheckelhoff DJ. ASHP national survey of pharmacy practice in hospital settings: dispensing and administration–2011. *Am J Health Syst Pharm*. 2012;69(9):768–785. doi:10.2146/ajhp110735.
6. Schneider PJ, Pedersen CA, Scheckelhoff DJ. ASHP national survey of pharmacy practice in hospital settings: Dispensing and administration-2017. *Am J Health Syst Pharm*. 2018;75(16):1203–1226. doi:10.2146/ajhp180151.
7. Hellums M, Alverson SP, Monk-Tutor MR. Instruction on compounded sterile preparations at U.S. schools of pharmacy. *Am J Health Syst Pharm*. 2007;64(21):2267–2274. doi:10.2146/ajhp060531.
8. Institute for Safe Medication Practices (ISMP). ISMP special alert—loss of drug potency. *ISMP Medication Safety Alert!* 2015;20(15).
9. U.S. Food and Drug Administration. FDA compounded or repackaged drugs stored in Becton-Dickinson (BD) 3 mL and 5 mL syringes: FDA alert—do not use unless there is no suitable alternative. In: FDA notifies health care professionals that Becton-Dickinson replaced problematic rubber stoppers in its syringes. **https://www.fda.gov/drugs/drug-safety-and-availability/fda-notifies-health-care-professionals-becton-dickinson-replaced-problematic-rubber-stoppers-its**. Updated January 12, 2018. Accessed February 27, 2023.

10. Teshome BF, Reveles KR, Lee GC, et al. How gaps in regulation of compounding pharmacy set the stage for a multistate fungal meningitis outbreak. *J Am Pharm Assoc (2003)*. 2014;54(4):441–445. doi:10.1331/JAPhA.2014.14011.

11. Drug Quality and Security Act of 2013. HR 3204, 113th Cong, 1st Session. 2013. **https://www.govinfo.gov/content/pkg/BILLS-113hr3204eh/pdf/BILLS-113hr3204eh.pdf**. Accessed March 5, 2023.

12. U.S. Food and Drug Administration. *Pharmacy Compounding of Human Drug Products Under Section 503A of the Federal Food, Drug, and Cosmetic Act: Guidance*. Silver Spring, MD: U.S. Food and Drug Administration; June 2016. **https://www.fda.gov/regulatory-information/search-fda-guidance-documents/pharmacy-compounding-human-drug-products-under-section-503a-federal-food-drug-and-cosmetic-act**. Accessed March 5, 2023.

13. American Society of Health-System Pharmacists (ASHP). ASHP guidelines on outsourcing sterile compounding services. *Am J Health Syst Pharm*. 2015;72(19):1664–1675. doi:10.2146/sp150024.

14. U.S. Department of Health and Human Services Office of Inspector General. *Most Hospitals Obtain Compounded Drugs From Outsourcing Facilities, Which Must Meet FDA Quality Standards*. U.S. Department of Health and Human Services; June 2019. **https://oig.hhs.gov/oei/reports/oei-01-17-00090.pdf**. Accessed April 1, 2023.

15. U.S. Food and Drug Administration. Registered outsourcing facilities. **https://www.fda.gov/drugs/human-drug-compounding/registered-outsourcing-facilities**. Updated February 22, 2023. Accessed February 27, 2023.

16. Buchanan EC, Schneider PJ, Forrey RA. *Compounding Sterile Preparations*. 4th ed. Bethesda, MD: ASHP; 2018:478.

17. U.S. Food and Drug Administration. *Facility Definition Under Section 503B of the Federal Food, Drug, and Cosmetic Act: Guidance for Industry*. Silver Spring, MD: U.S. Food and Drug Administration; May 2018. **https://www.fda.gov/regulatory-information/search-fda-guidance-documents/facility-definition-under-section-503b-federal-food-drug-and-cosmetic-act**. Accessed February 27, 2023.

18. U.S. Food & Drug Administration. Human Drug Compounding Registration and Product Reporting Procedures. **https://www.fda.gov/drugs/electronic-drug-registration-and-listing-system-edrls/human-drug-compounding-registration-and-product-reporting-procedures#:~:text=Each%20report%20must%20identify%20all,of%20active%20ingredient%20per%20unit**. Accessed August 7, 2023.

19. U.S. Food and Drug Administration. Bulk drug substances used in compounding under Section 503B of the FD&C Act. **https://www.fda.gov/drugs/human-drug-compounding/bulk-drug-substances-used-compounding-under-section-503b-fdc-act**. Updated February 20, 2020. Accessed February 27, 2023.

20. Thompson CA. Substances doubtful for bulk drug substances list could be INDs. *Am J Health Syst Pharm*. 2016;73(8):512–514. doi:10.2146/news160025.

21. U.S. Food and Drug Administration. Human drug compounding outsourcing facility fees. **https://www.fda.gov/industry/fda-user-fee-programs/human-drug-compounding-outsourcing-facility-fees**. Updated August 5, 2022. Accessed February 27, 2023.

22. U.S. Food and Drug Administration. *Current Good Manufacturing Practice—Guidance for Human Drug Compounding Outsourcing Facilities Under Section 503B of the FD&C Act: Guidance for Industry: Draft Guidance*. Silver Spring, MD: U.S. Food and Drug Administration; January 2020. **https://www.fda.gov/regulatory-information/search-fda-guidance-documents/current-good-manufacturing-practice-guidance-human-drug-compounding-outsourcing-facilities-under**. Accessed February 27, 2023.

23. Department of Health & Human Services. Notice. Silver Spring, MD: U.S. Food and Drug Administration. **https://www.fda.gov/media/98911/download**. Accessed February 27, 2023.

24. Statement from FDA Commissioner Scott Gottlieb M.D. and Deputy Commissioner Anna Abram on new 2019 efforts to improve the quality of compounded drugs [news release]. Rockville, MD: U.S. Food and Drug Administration; April 3, 2019. **https://www.fda.gov/news-events/press-announcements/statement-fda-commissioner-scott-gottlieb-md-and-deputy-commissioner-anna-abram-new-2019-efforts**. Accessed February 27, 2023.

25. U.S. Food and Drug Administration. Memorandum of understanding addressing certain distributions of compounded drugs. **https://www.fda.gov/drugs/human-drug-compounding/memorandum-understanding-addressing-certain-distributions-compounded-drugs**. Published October 20, 2022. Accessed February 27, 2023.

26. National Association of Boards of Pharmacy (NABP). *2021 Survey of Pharmacy Law*. Mount Prospect, IL: National Association of Boards of Pharmacy; 2020.

27. Urahn SK, Coukell A, Jungman E, et al. State oversight of drug compounding. Pew Charitable Trusts. February 2018. **https://www.pewtrusts.org/en/research-and-analysis/reports/2018/02/state-oversight-of-drug-compounding**. Accessed August 31, 2023.

28. Centers and Medicare and Medicaid Services (CMS). CMS-approved accrediting organizations contacts for prospective clients. **https://www.cms.gov/Medicare/Provider-Enrollment-and-Certification/SurveyCertificationGenInfo/Downloads/Accrediting-Organization-Contacts-for-Prospective-Clients-.pdf**. July 22, 2022. Accessed February 27, 2023.

29. Office of Inspector General. Medicare's oversight of compounded pharmaceuticals used in hospitals. Report (OEI-01-13-00400). **https://oig.hhs.gov/oei/reports/oei-01-13-00400.asp**. Published January 21, 2015. Accessed February 27, 2023.

30. Tribble DA. The Health Insurance Portability and Accountability Act: security and privacy requirements. *Am J Health Syst Pharm*. 2001;58(9):763–770. doi:10.1093/ajhp/58.9.763.

31. U.S Food and Drug Administration. Code of Federal Regulations (CFR) Title 21: Part 1308 Schedules of Controlled Substances. September 24, 1973.**https://www.accessdata.fda.gov/scripts/cdrh/cfdocs/cfcfr/CFRSearch.cfm?CFRPart=1308&showFR=1**. Accessed February 27, 2023.

32. Welch CW. Robinson-Patman Act and the own-use exemption in health systems. *Am J Health Syst Pharm*. 1999;56(10):990–994. doi:10.1093/ajhp/56.10.990.

33. ASHP reaches milestone with 2,000 residency programs [news release]. Bethesda, MD: American Society of Health-System Pharmacists; October 21, 2015. **https://www.ashp.org/news/2015/10/21/ashp_reaches_milestone_with_2_000_residency_programs**. Accessed February 27, 2023.

34. American Society of Health-System Pharmacists. ASHP guidelines for selecting pharmaceutical manufacturers and suppliers. *Am J Hosp Pharm*. 1991;48(3):523–524. **https://pubmed.ncbi.nlm.nih.gov/2029002/**.

35. American Society of Health-System Pharmacists. ASHP guidelines on outsourcing pharmaceutical services. *Am J Health Syst Pharm*. 1998;55(15):1611–1617. doi:10.1093/ajhp/55.15.1611.

36. American Society of Health-System Pharmacists. ASHP guidelines on compounding sterile preparations. *Am J Health Syst Pharm*. 2014;71(2):145–166. doi:10.2146/sp140001.

37. American Society of Health-System Pharmacists (ASHP). Outsourcing sterile products preparation: vendor assessment tool. **https://outsourcing.ashp.org**. Accessed February 27, 2023.

38. State of Pharmacy Compounding Survey: Recalls. *Pharm Purchasing & Products*. 2020;17(4): S54, S56.

Glossary

Accuracy—A measure of the volume or weight of an ingredient to determine that the correct quantities of nutrients, electrolytes, or other components are delivered.[1]

Action items—A list of items that need to be completed in a defined time and assigned to a specific owner.

Action limit—The minimum and maximum values of a quality assurance measurement that can be interpreted as representing acceptable performance with respect to the parameter being tested. An action limit that is exceeded should trigger appropriate investigation and corrective action based on the investigation.

Active pharmaceutical ingredient (API)—Any substance or mixture of substances intended to be used in the compounding of a drug preparation, thereby becoming the active ingredient in the preparation and furnishing of pharmacological activity or other direct effect in the diagnosis, cure, mitigation, treatment, or prevention of disease in humans and animals or affecting the structure and function of the body.[3]

Added substances—Suitable substances added to preparations intended for injection to increase stability or usefulness, unless proscribed in the individual *USP–NF* monograph, provided they are harmless in the amounts administered and do not interfere with the therapeutic efficacy or with the responses to the specified assays and tests.[4]

Agency—A generic term used to reference the Food and Drug Administration, the Drug Enforcement Agency, and State Boards of Pharmacy.

Air changes—The frequency per unit of time (eg, minutes, hours, etc.) that the air within a controlled environment is replaced. The air can be recirculated partially or totally replaced.[5]

Air sampler—Device or equipment used to sample a measured amount of air in a specified time to quantitate the particulate or microbiological status of air in the controlled environment.[5]

Airborne particulate count (also referred to as total particulate count)—The total number of particles of a given size per unit volume of air.[5]

Airborne viable particulate count (also referred to as total airborne aerobic microbial count)—The recovered number of colony-forming units (CFUs) per unit volume of air.[5]

Alert level—An established microbial or airborne particulate count giving early warning of potential drift from normal operating conditions and triggering appropriate scrutiny and follow-up to address the potential problem. Alert levels are always lower than action levels.[6]

DOI 10.37573/9781585286492.035

Alternative duty—Performance of other tasks that do not include the direct handling of hazardous drugs.[3]

Ampul—Single-use container composed entirely of glass.

Ante-area—An ISO Class 8 or better area where personnel hand hygiene and garbing procedures, staging of components, order entry, labeling of compounded sterile preparations, and other high-particulate-generating activities are performed. It is also a transition area that (1) provides assurance that pressure relationships are constantly maintained so that air flows from clean to dirty areas, and (2) reduces the need for the heating, ventilation, and air conditioning (HVAC) control system to respond to large disturbances.[1]

Anteroom for HD handling—An ISO Class 7 or cleaner room where personnel hand hygiene, garbing procedures, and other activities that generate high particulate levels are performed. The anteroom is the transition room between the unclassified area of the facility and the buffer room.[3]

Antibody—Specific immunoglobulin produced by specialized blood cells (plasma cells) as a reaction to an antigen for the purpose of host defense. Antibodies are blood proteins that are produced in response to a foreign substance or antigen.

Antigen—Macromolecule that elicits an immune response in the body. The most common antigens are proteins (eg, natural rubber latex) and polysaccharides (eg, starch). Antigens may be either exogenous or endogenous to the body.

Antineoplastic drug—Chemotherapeutic agent that controls or kills cancer cells. Drugs used in the treatment of cancer are cytotoxic but are generally more damaging to dividing cells than to resting cells.[7]

Antiseptic (germicide)—Agents used to prevent infection and decay by inhibiting the growth of microorganisms. Because these products are used in or on living humans or animals, they are considered drugs and thus are approved and regulated by the FDA.

Audits—When a person or group of people review documentation and systems for accuracy, robustness, completeness, and compliance. This can be internal or external to the company.

Aseptic—Free of living pathogenic organisms or infected materials.[7]

Aseptic processing—Mode of processing pharmaceutical and medical products that involves the separate sterilization of the product and of the package (containers/closures or packaging material for medical devices) and the transfer of the product into the container and its closure under at least ISO Class 5 conditions.[1]

Aseptic technique—Methods used to manipulate sterile products so that they remain sterile.

Assessment of risk—Evaluation of risk to determine alternative containment strategies and/or work practices.[3]

Batch compounding—Compounding of multiple sterile preparation units, in a single discrete process, by the same individuals, carried out during one limited time period.

Beyond-use date (BUD)—The date, or hour and the date, after which a CSP must not be used, stored, or transported. The date is determined from the date and time the preparation is compounded.

Bioburden—Total number of microorganisms associated with a specific item prior to sterilization.[8]

Biohazard—Infectious agent or hazardous biological material that presents a risk to the health of humans or the environment. Biohazards include tissue, blood or body fluids, and materials such as needles or other equipment contaminated with these infectious agents or hazardous biological materials.[7]

Biological indicator (BI)—A population of microorganisms inoculated onto a suitable medium (eg, solution, container, or closure) and placed within appropriate sterilizer load locations to determine the sterilization cycle efficacy of a physical or chemical process. The challenge microorganism is selected based on its resistance to the given process. Incoming lot D-value and microbiological count define the quality of the BI.[2]

Biological safety cabinet (BSC)—A ventilated cabinet often used for preparation of hazardous drugs. These cabinets are divided into three general classes (Class I, Class II, and Class III). Class II BSCs are further divided into types (Type A1, Type A2, Type B1, and Type B2).[3] (See Chapter 6 for a detailed description of BSCs.)

Biomarker—Biological, biochemical, or structural change that serves as an indicator of potential damage to cellular components, whole cells, tissues, or organs.[7]

Bubble diagram—Schematic drawing of a floor plan that shows which functional areas need to be next to each other. For example, the buffer area must be adjacent to the ante-area. The "bubbles" can be rectangular or oblong shapes that indicate the relative size of the functional areas.

Buffer area—Area where the primary engineering control (PEC) is physically located. Activities that occur in this area include the preparation and staging of components and supplies used when compounding sterile preparations.[1]

Buffer room—As pertains to handling hazardous drugs, a type of containment secondary engineering control (C-SEC) under negative pressure that meets ISO Class 7 or better air quality where the containment primary engineering control (C-PEC) that generates and maintains an ISO Class 5 environment is physically located. Activities that occur in this area are limited to the preparation and staging of components and supplies used when compounding HDs.[3]

Calibration—The demonstration that a particular instrument or measuring device produces results within specified limits by comparison with those produced by a reference or traceable standard over an appropriate range of measurements.

CAPA—An acronym for Corrective Action/Preventive Action or Corrective Action and Preventive Action.

CAPA owner—The person responsible for ensuring execution of all CAPA activities.

CAPA investigation owner—The person responsible for collecting the data and the documentation of the investigation summary including root cause and corrective actions.

CAPA plan—A defined list of actions with assigned timelines and owners.

Cause—A situation or event that produces an effect or result.

Certificate of analysis (COA)—A document that reports the results of a test of a representative sample drawn from the batch of material that will be delivered.[9]

Certification—Process by which a nongovernmental agency or organization grants recognition to an individual who has met certain predetermined qualifications specified by that agency or organization. Certification is usually voluntary and usually involves passing a validated, standardized examination.

Change control—Controlled documentation defining and tracking specific changes (action items) to a critical system or document that requires review and approval.

Chelating agent—A chemical that bonds to trace amounts of metals to prevent the metals from catalyzing an oxidation process.

Chemical disinfectant—A chemical agent used on inanimate surfaces and objects to destroy infectious fungi, viruses, and bacteria, but not necessarily their spores. Sporicidal and antiviral agents may be considered a special class of disinfectants. Disinfectants are often categorized as high-level, intermediate-level, and low-level by medically oriented groups based on their efficacy against various microorganisms.[10]

Chemical stability—Extent to which a product retains, within specified limits and throughout its period of storage and use, the same properties and characteristics that it possessed at the time of preparation.

Chemotherapy drug—Chemical agent used to treat diseases. The term usually refers to a drug used to treat cancer.[7]

Chemotherapy glove—A medical glove that meets the ASTM Standard Practice for Assessment of Resistance of Medical Gloves to Permeation by Chemotherapy Drugs (D6978) or its successor.[3]

Chemotherapy waste—Discarded items such as gowns, gloves, masks, IV tubing, empty bags, empty drug vials, needles and syringes, and other items generated while preparing and administering antineoplastic agents.[7]

Classified space—An area that maintains an air cleanliness classification based on the International Organization for Standardization (ISO).[3]

Cleaning—The process of removing soil (eg, organic and inorganic material) from objects and surfaces, normally accomplished by manually or mechanically using water with detergents or enzymatic products.[3]

Cleanroom—Room in which the concentration of airborne particles is controlled to meet a specified airborne particulate cleanliness class. Microorganisms in the environment are monitored so that a microbial level for air, surface, and personnel gear are not exceeded for a specified cleanliness class.[1]

Closed-system drug transfer device (CSTD)—A drug-transfer device that mechanically prohibits the transfer of environmental contaminants into the system and the escape of hazardous drugs (HDs) or vapor concentrations outside the system.[3]

Closed system—A device that does not exchange unfiltered air or contaminants with the adjacent environment.[7]

Closure—Seal on a sterile container that prevents leakage, tampering, or entry of contaminants. A closure is part of a container.

Cold temperatures—Temperature not exceeding 8°C (46°F).[11]

Colony-forming unit (CFU)—A microbiological term that describes the formation of a single macroscopic colony after the introduction of one or more microorganisms to microbiological growth media. One colony-forming unit is expressed as 1 CFU.[6]

Commissioning of a controlled environment—Certification by engineering and quality control that an environment has been built according to the specifications of the desired cleanliness Class and that, under conditions likely to be encountered under normal operating conditions (or worst-case conditions), it is capable of delivering an aseptic process. Commissioning includes media fill runs and results of the environmental monitoring program.[5]

Component—Any ingredient used in the compounding of a drug preparation, including any active ingredient or added substance that is used in its preparation.[1]

Compounded preparation—A nonsterile or sterile drug or nutrient preparation that is compounded in a licensed pharmacy or other healthcare-related facility in response to or anticipation of a prescription or a medication order from a licensed prescriber.[3]

Compounding—The process of combining, admixing, diluting, pooling, reconstituting, repackaging, or otherwise altering a drug product or bulk drug substance to create a sterile preparation.

Compounding aseptic containment isolator (CACI)—A specific type of CAI that is designed for the compounding of sterile hazardous drugs (HDs). The CACI is designed to provide worker protection from exposure to undesirable levels of airborne drugs throughout the compounding and material transfer processes and to provide an aseptic environment with unidirectional airflow for compounding sterile preparations.[3]

Compounding aseptic isolator (CAI)—An isolator specifically designed for compounding sterile, nonhazardous pharmaceutical ingredients or preparations. The CAI is designed to maintain an aseptic compounding environment throughout the compounding and material transfer processes.[3]

Compounding personnel—Individuals who participate in the compounding process.[3]

Compounding record—A compounding record documents the compounding of each CSP. A compounding record must be created for all Category 1, Category 2, Category 3, and immediate-use CSPs prepared for more than one patient and for CSPs prepared from non-sterile ingredients.

Compounding supervisor—Individual(s) responsible for developing and implementing appropriate procedures; overseeing facility compliance with USP chapters and other applicable laws, regulations, and standards; ensuring the competency of personnel; and maintaining environmental control of the compounding areas.[3]

Container—That which holds the preparation and is or may be in direct contact with the preparation. The closure is part of the container.

Containment—An immediate corrective action that is implemented to prevent an event from continuing and to minimize impact before a formal corrective action plan can be developed.

Containment primary engineering control (C-PEC)—A ventilated device designed and operated to minimize worker environmental exposures to hazardous drugs by controlling emissions of airborne contaminants through the following:

- The full or partial enclosure of a potential contaminant source
- The use of airflow capture velocities to trap and remove airborne contaminants near their point of generation

- The use of air pressure relationships that define the direction of airflow into the cabinet
- The use of HEPA filtration on all potentially contaminated exhaust streams[3]

Containment secondary engineering control (C-SEC)—The room with fixed walls in which the containment primary engineering control (C-PEC) is placed. It incorporates specific design and operational parameters required to contain the potential hazard within the compounding room.[3]

Containment segregated compounding area (C-SCA)—A type of containment secondary engineering control (C-SEC) with nominal requirements for airflow and room pressurization as they pertain to hazardous drug compounding.[3]

Contamination—The undesired introduction of impurities of a chemical or microbiological nature or foreign matter into or onto a raw material, intermediate, or compounded preparation during production, sampling, packaging or repackaging, storage, or transport.[9]

Continuing education—Teaching and learning usually approved by an accrediting organization. Continuing education is designed to update the knowledge of a competent practitioner.

Controlled area—Space designated for compounding sterile preparations. This is referred to as the buffer area (eg, the cleanroom in which the laminar-airflow workbench is located).

Cool temperatures—Temperature between 8°C and 15°C (46°F and 59°F).[11]

Contributing cause—A factor or condition that facilitates a root (or most probable) cause acting to generate a deviation; a contributing cause cannot in and of itself generate a deviation.

Corrective action (CA)—Action taken to eliminate the cause(s) of a detected nonconformity, defect, negative trend, or other undesirable situation. Corrective actions are typically specific to lots of products or processes impacted by nonconformity or defect.

Critical area—An ISO Class 5 environment.[1]

Critical site—Location that includes any component or fluid pathway surface (eg, vial septa, injection ports, beakers) or openings (eg, opened ampuls, needle hubs) exposed and at risk of direct contact with air (eg, ambient room or HEPA-filtered), moisture (eg, oral and mucosal secretions), or touch contamination. Risk of microbial particulate contamination of the critical site increases with the size of the openings and exposure time.[1]

Cytotoxic—Pharmacologic compound that is detrimental or destructive to cells within the body.[3]

Deactivation—Treatment of a hazardous drug (HD) contaminant on surfaces with a chemical, heat, ultraviolet light, or another agent to transform the HD into a less hazardous agent.[3]

Decibel—A unit used to measure the intensity of a sound by comparing it with a standard level on a logarithmic scale, thereby indicating the degree of loudness. A scale is commonly used when measuring decibels, because it most closely represents what the human ear perceives in terms of loudness.[12]

Decontamination—Inactivation, neutralization, or removal of hazardous drug contaminants on surfaces, usually by chemical means.[3]

Demarcation line—The boundary of a specific area.

Direct compounding area (DCA)—Critical area within the ISO Class 5 primary engineering control (PEC) where critical sites are exposed to unidirectional HEPA-filtered air, also known as first air.[1]

Disinfectant—A chemical or physical agent that destroys or removes vegetative forms of harmful microorganisms when applied to a surface.[10]

Disinfection—The process of inhibiting or destroying microorganisms.[3]

Documentation—Record of how a drug was processed and what quality attributes it possesses.

Doff—To remove personal protective equipment (PPE).[3]

Don—To put on personal protective equipment (PPE).[3]

Dry natural rubber (DNR) process—A rubber manufacturing process using natural latex that has been acid coagulated into dry sheets or crumbled particles. The rubber undergoes prolonged treatment at high heat and is used to form *solid* rubber products by compression, molding, or extrusion.

Dynamic—Conditions relating to clean area classification under conditions of normal production.[6] For example, dynamic operating conditions for environmental monitoring means during normal levels of sterile compounding not worst case or simulated compounding conditions.

Effectiveness check (EC)—A documented process to establish if actions taken were effective and accomplished the intended objective.

Effectiveness check verification—A review of the effectiveness check. If the CAPA prevented recurrence then the effectiveness check (EC) can be closed if desired. If the CAPA did not prevent recurrence, then an additional root cause analysis may be performed.

Engineering controls—Devices designed to eliminate or reduce worker exposures to chemical, biological, radiological, ergonomic, or physical hazards. Examples include laboratory fume hoods, glove bags, retracting syringe needles, safety interlocks, and radiation shielding.[7]

Engineering control for handling hazardous drugs (HDs)—Primary, secondary, and supplemental devices designed to eliminate or reduce worker exposure to HDs.[3]

Environmental monitoring program—Documented program implemented via standard operating procedures that describes in detail the methods and acceptance criteria for monitoring particulates and microorganisms in controlled environments (air, surface, personnel gear). The program includes sampling sites, frequency of sampling, and investigative and corrective actions.[5]

EPA-registered disinfectant—Antimicrobial products registered with the Environmental Protection Agency (EPA) for healthcare use against pathogens specified in the product labeling.[3]

Ergonomic design—Arrangement of a workspace to accommodate each individual's capacities and limitations, allowing them to work safely and efficiently. This includes an optimum ambient environment and adjustable furniture.[12]

Expiration date—The time during which a product can be expected to meet the requirements of the *USP-NF* monograph, if one exists, or maintain expected quality provided it is kept under the specified storage conditions.

Externally vented—Exhausted to the outside.[3]

Failure mode and effects analysis (FMEA)—The process of reviewing components, procedures, and workflows to identify potential points of failure and their causes and effects.

First air—Air exiting the HEPA filter in a unidirectional air stream that is essentially particle free.[1]

Freezer—Cold place in which the temperature is maintained thermostatically between −20°C and −10°C (−4°F and −14°F).[11]

Gap analysis—Resource assessment tool enabling an organization to compare its actual performance with its expected performance. At its core are two questions: Where are we? Where do we want to be?

Genotoxic—Capable of damaging the DNA and leading to mutations.[7]

Globally Harmonized System of Classification and Labeling of Chemicals (GHS)—A system for standardizing and harmonizing the classification and labeling of chemicals.[3]

Goggles—Tight-fitting eye protection that completely covers the eyes, eye sockets, and facial area that immediately surrounds the eyes. Goggles provide protection from impact, dust, and splashes. Some goggles fit over corrective lenses.[3]

Hard stop—Command that is placed in automated compounding device software, which does not allow parenteral nutrition to be compounded when certain conditions are met or not met.

Hazard analysis and critical control points (HACCP)—Analyzing the compounding process and flow charting it to ensure that it reflects the actual procedure that is performed. Once the procedure has been clearly identified, the hazards within the procedures are identified.

Hazardous drug (HD)—Any drug identified by at least one of the following criteria:

- Carcinogenicity, teratogenicity, or developmental toxicity
- Reproductive toxicity in humans
- Organ toxicity at low dose in humans or animals
- Genotoxicity
- New drugs that mimic existing HDs in structure or toxicity[3]

Hazardous waste—Waste that is a Resource Conservation and Recovery Act (RCRA) Subtitle C (RCRA) listed as hazardous waste [40 CFR 261.30–33] or that meets a RCRA characteristic of ignitability, corrosivity, reactivity, or toxicity as defined in 40 CFR 261.21–24.[7]

Health Hazard Assessment (or Health Risk Assessment)—Tool for predicting possible harm that can come from a defective or malfunctioning device. The assessment helps the FDA and the firm determine if any actions are necessary such as recalling the devices or notifying the public about the risk.

Health Level-7, HL7—A set of international standards for transfer of clinical and administrative data between software applications used by various healthcare providers. These standards focus on the application layer, which is "layer 7" in the OSI model. The HL7 standards are produced by the Health Level Seven International, an international standards organization, and are adopted by other standards issuing bodies such as American National Standards Institute and International Organization for Standardization.[13]

High-efficiency particulate air (HEPA) filtration—An extended-medium, dry-type filter in a rigid frame, having a minimum particle collection efficiency of 99.97% for particles with a mass median diameter of 0.3 µm when tested at a rated airflow in accordance with MIL STD 282 using IEST Recommended Standard RP-CC001.5.[3]

Horizontal laminar flow workbench (HLF)—Device that protects the work product and the work area by supplying HEPA-filtered air to the rear of the cabinet and producing a horizontal flow across the work area and out toward the worker.[7]

Human factors—The scientific discipline concerned with interactions among humans and other elements of a system, and the profession that applies the theory, principles, data, and methods to design systems that optimize human well-being and overall system performance.[12]

Hydrolysis—Attack of labile bonds in dissolved drug molecules by water with resultant molecular changes.

Illumination level—The quantity of light energy reaching an area as measured (in lux or footcandles) by a photometer with an illuminance sensor; this indicates brightness. A lux is a unit of illuminance, measured in lumens per square meter. A foot-candle (fc) is lumens per square foot, and it is also commonly measured by light meters. The term candela replaced fc as the International System (SI) measure of luminous intensity and represents 1 lumen/steradian (lm/st).[12]

Immediate corrective action—Action to eliminate or control a detected nonconformity taken prior to root cause determination. Immediate corrective action is often required to establish containment of an event.

Incompatibility—Physical or chemical phenomenon that reduces the concentration of the active ingredient(s).

Infusion time (also hang time)—Allowable length of time for an infusion to be used before it must be taken down or exchanged. The time is determined from the date and time the infusion is spiked or accessed with administration set.

In-process testing—Method to verify that the compounding environment and the actual preparation meet established criteria.

In-use time—The maximum amount of time that can be allowed to elapse between penetration of a container-closure system containing a sterile drug product, or after a lyophilized drug product has been reconstituted, and before patient administration.

Instability—Chemical processes that result in degradation or change in the active ingredients, including hydrolysis, oxidation, reduction, and photo-degradation reactions.

Isolator—Device that is sealed or is supplied with air through a microbially retentive filtration system (HEPA minimum) and may be reproducibly decontaminated. When closed, an isolator uses only decontaminated interfaces or rapid transfer ports (RTPs) for materials transfer. When open, it allows for the ingress and/or egress of materials through defined openings that have been designed and validated to preclude the transfer of contaminants or unfiltered air to adjacent environments. An isolator can be used for aseptic processing, for containment of potent compounds, or for simultaneous asepsis and containment.[7]

Labeling—Term that designates all labels and other written, printed, or graphic matter on an immediate container of an article or preparation or on, or in, any package or wrapper in which it is enclosed, except any outer shipping container. The term label designates that part of the labeling on the immediate container.[1]

Laminar airflow workbenches (LAFWs)—A controlled environment created by a HEPA filter to retain airborne particles and microorganisms, and its use decreases the chance of contamination of compounded preparations.

Latex—Any polymer (natural or synthetic) in a water-based liquid or viscous state.

Latex allergy—An immune-mediated reaction to Hev b (*H. brasiliensis*) protein associated with clinical symptoms.

Latex sensitization—The presence of immunoglobulin antibodies to Hev b (*H. brasiliensis*) protein without clinical manifestations.

Licensure—Process by which a government agency or board grants permission to an individual to engage in a given occupation or professional practice. Licensure is contingent on an applicant's successful completion of certain specified minimal levels of competency necessary to ensure the public's health, safety, and welfare.

Manufacturing—The production, propagation, conversion, or processing of a drug or device, either directly or indirectly, by extraction of the drug from substances of natural origin or by means of chemical or biological synthesis. Manufacturing may also include any packaging or repackaging of the substance(s) or labeling or relabeling of containers for resale by pharmacies, practitioners, or other persons.[1]

Mass reconstitution—Reconstitution of parenteral drugs in bulk and then refrigerating or freezing them for later use.

Master facilities plan—Floor plan based on the strategic plan of the organization in terms of the facilities needed to accommodate all planned activities, along with a timeline to show when facility needs will occur. A department master facilities plan should be congruent with the master facilities plan for the parent organization.[14]

Master formulation record—A master formulation record (MFR) is a detailed record of procedures that describes how the CSP is to be prepared. An MFR must be created for Category 1, Category 2, Category 3, and immediate-use CSPs prepared for more than one patient and for CSPs prepared from non-sterile ingredient(s).

Media fill test—Test used to qualify aseptic technique of compounding personnel or processes and to ensure that the processes used are able to produce a sterile product without microbial contamination. During this test, a microbiological growth medium such as soybean–casein digest medium is substituted for the actual drug product to simulate admixture compounding.[1]

Multiple-dose container (or multidose container)—A *Container–closure system* that holds a sterile medication for parenteral administration (injection or infusion) that has met antimicrobial effectiveness testing requirements, or is excluded from such testing requirements by FDA regulation. A *Multiple-dose container* is intended to contain more than one dose of a drug product. The beyond-use date for an opened or entered (eg, needle-punctured) *Multiple-dose container* is 28 days unless otherwise specified by the manufacturer on the label.[11]

Mutagenic—Capable of increasing the spontaneous mutation rate by causing changes in the DNA.[7]

Natural latex—A milky fluid consisting of very small rubber particles obtained from plants (usually *H. brasiliensis*) and dispersed in an aqueous medium.

Natural rubber—Includes all materials made from or containing natural latex. Products containing natural rubber may be produced by the dry natural rubber (DNR) or the natural rubber latex (NRL) process.

Natural rubber latex (NRL) process—A manufacturing process using a concentrated colloidal suspension of natural latex that has been ammoniated to prevent bacterial growth. Products are formed by dipping, extruding, or coating.

Negative-pressure room—A room that is maintained at a lower pressure than the adjacent areas; therefore, the net flow of air is into the room.[3]

Occupational exposure limit (OEL)—Industry or other nongovernment exposure limit usually based on scientific calculations of airborne concentrations of a substance that are considered to be acceptable for healthy workers.[7]

Open reservoir mixing—Combining either sterile or nonsterile ingredients using an open-system transfer or an open reservoir before terminal sterilization or subdivision into units.

Orientation—On-the-job training necessary for an individual to understand the policies and procedures used at a specific practice site.

Outsourcing facility—Compounding pharmacy at one geographic location or address that (1) is engaged in the compounding of sterile drugs; (2) has elected to register with the FDA as an outsourcing facility; and (3) complies with all of the requirements of Section 503B. Major requirements include registration with FDA, reporting of adverse events and products compounded to FDA, and payment of fees to FDA. Outsourcing facilities are permitted to compound and distribute drugs without receiving individual patient prescriptions, but they are not exempt from current good manufacturing practices.[15]

Parenteral—General route of administration which is characterized by injection through the skin or other external boundary tissue or implantation within the body. Specific parenteral routes include intravenous, intraventricular, intra-arterial, intra-articular, subcutaneous, intramuscular, intrathecal, intracisternal, and intraocular.[16]

Particulates—Airborne particles found in the environment are pollen, dust, bacteria, miscellaneous living and dead organisms, skin flakes, hair, clothing lint, cosmetics, respiratory gases, and bacteria from perspiration.

Pass-through—An enclosure with interlocking doors that is positioned between two spaces for the purpose of reducing particulate transfer while moving materials from one space to another. A pass-through serving negative-pressure rooms needs to be equipped with sealed doors.[3]

Permissible exposure limit (PEL)—Time-weighted average concentration of a substance to which nearly all workers may be exposed for up to 8 hours per day, 40 hours per week for 30 years without adverse effects. A PEL may also include a skin designation.[7]

Personal protective equipment (PPE)—Items such as gloves, gowns, respirators, goggles, face shields that protect individual workers from hazardous physical or chemical exposures.[3]

Pharmacy bulk package—A container of a sterile preparation for parenteral use that contains many single doses. The contents are intended for use in a pharmacy admixture program and are restricted to the preparation of admixtures for infusion or, through a sterile transfer device, for the filling of empty sterile syringes. The closure shall be penetrated only one time after constitution with a suitable sterile transfer device or dispensing set, which allows measured dispensing of the contents. The pharmacy bulk package is to be used only in a suitable work area such as a laminar flow hood (or an equivalent clean air compounding area).[1]

Photodegradation—Catalysis of degradation reactions by light.

Photolysis—Catalysis of degradation reactions by light.

Physical incompatibility—Visible changes in a preparation, such as precipitation, cloudiness or haziness, color change, viscosity change, cracking, and effervescence. (See also *Visual Incompatibility*.)

PIC—Pharmacist-in-Charge.

Plenum—Space in a ventilation system or device that receives air for distribution.

Policy—General statement that provides a basis for decision-making. It addresses what must be done and, sometimes, why and when. Policies are written statements that provide guidance on the position and values of an organization. They are often considered broad operational guidelines, but they should clearly define the direction and activities of an organization or department.

Pooling—Combining sterile ingredients in a sterile closed system, by aseptic transfer, before subdivision into patient units.

Positive-pressure room—A room that is maintained at a higher pressure than the adjacent areas; therefore, the net flow of air is out of the room.[3]

Precision—A measure or trend of the day-to-day variations in performance of the accuracy measures.[1]

Preparation—An article of drug or nutrient compounded in a a licensed pharmacy or other healthcare-related facility pursuant to the order of a licensed prescriber; the article may or may not contain sterile products. If it is aseptically prepared with sterile products or terminally sterilized, it is a compounded sterile preparation (CSP).[1]

Preparation traceability—Essential element of any sterile preparation compounding program, that includes complete documentation for a compounded sterile preparation (CSP), such as drug name, manufacturer, lot number and expiration date, name or initials of pharmacist or technician who compounded the CSP and unique identifier (batch number or lot number) that allows the final preparation to be traced back to source providing the necessary assurance as to the formulation, characteristics, and integrity of the preparation.

Pressure differential—Measurement of air pressures between two adjoining areas where the air pressure in the more stringently classified area is higher than the pressure of the next classified area.

Preventive action (PA)—Action taken to eliminate the cause(s) of a potential nonconformity, defect, negative trend, or other undesirable situation in order to prevent recurrence. Preventive actions may extend to other product lines, processes, and systems.

Primary engineering control (PEC)—Device or room that provides an ISO Class 5 environment for the exposure of critical sites when compounding sterile preparations. Such devices include, but may not be limited to, laminar airflow workbenches (LAFWs), biological safety cabinets (BSCs), compounding aseptic isolators (CAIs), and compounding aseptic containment isolators (CACIs).[1]

Probability of a nonsterile unit (PNSU)—Probability of a compounded sterile preparation being nonsterile after it has been exposed to a validated sterilization process (eg, filtration, moist heat, ionizing radiation, ethylene oxide) or to aseptic compounding techniques.

Probable cause (PC)—A most likely root cause that cannot be established beyond doubt, but is, nonetheless, adequately and substantially supported by data gathered during the investigation using scientific and logical approaches. A most probable cause is only identified in an investigation report in cases wherein the level of certainty required establishing root cause could not be reasonably determined.

Procedure—A "how to" document that provides methods for carrying out a policy. Procedures outline the complete cycle of a task, step by step, and assign responsibility to specific personnel. Procedures are written instructions that describe the recommended methods of sequential steps to follow to perform a task or activity. Procedures define the process for completing a task. (See *Standard Operating Procedure*.)

Process validation—Test that mimics an actual and entire compounding procedure using a suitable growth medium such as tryptic soy broth (TSB) instead of using ingredients to prepare a finished compounded preparation. (See *Media Fill Test*.)

Product—Commercially manufactured sterile drug or nutrient that has been evaluated for safety and efficacy by the FDA. Products are accompanied by full prescribing information, which is commonly known as the FDA-approved manufacturer's labeling or product package insert.[1]

Product quality and characteristics—Product attributes like sterility, potency, identity, strength, quality, and purity associated with environmental quality, preparation activities, and checks and tests.[8]

Quality assurance (QA)—The total of the organized arrangements made to ensure that all compounded sterile preparations are of the quality required for their intended use and that quality systems are maintained.[9]

Quality control (QC)—Checking or testing that specifications are met.[9]

Quality Department—An independent group that has oversight of the CAPA system to ensure it is in a state of control and in compliance.

Quarantine—The status of materials isolated physically or by other effective means pending a decision about their subsequent approval or rejection.[9]

Radionuclide—Atom with an unstable nucleus, which is a nucleus characterized by excess energy that is available to be imparted either to a newly-created radiation particle within the nucleus, or else to an atomic electron. The radionuclide undergoes radioactive decay and emits gamma rays and/or subatomic particles. These particles constitute ionizing radiation. Radionuclides may occur naturally, but they can also be artificially produced.

Recommended exposure limit (REL)—Occupational exposure limit recommended by the National Institute of Occupational Safety and Health (NIOSH) as being protective of worker health and safety over a working lifetime. The REL is frequently expressed as a time-weighted average exposure to a substance for up to a 10-hour workday during a 40-hour work week.[7]

Refrigerator—Cold place in which the temperature is maintained thermostatically between 2°C and 8°C (36°F to 46°F).[11]

Registration—Process of including a person's name on a registry with a state agency or regulatory board. Registration is the lowest form of "regulating" a group of individuals. Registration enables the agency or board to track where those individuals are employed to practice.

Regulations—Rules promulgated by a state or federal agency as needed to apply the concepts encompassed in a law or statute.

Relative humidity (RH)—Ratio of the amount of water vapor present in the air relative to the greatest amount possible of water vapor at the same temperature.

Repackaging—The act of removing a product from its original primary container and placing it into another primary container, usually of smaller size.[3]

Repetitive motion injury—An injury that is temporary or permanent to muscles, nerves, ligaments, and tendons caused by doing the same motion over and over again. A common repetitive motion injury is carpal tunnel syndrome.[17] Also called *repetitive stress injury*.

Respirator—Type of personal protective equipment (PPE) that prevents harmful materials from entering the respiratory tract, usually by filtering hazardous agents from workplace air. A surgical mask does not offer respiratory protection.[7]

Risk assessment—Characterization of potentially adverse health effects from human exposure to environmental or occupational hazards. Risk assessment can be divided into five major steps: hazard identification, dose-response assessment, exposure assessment, risk characterization, and risk communication.[7]

Risk priority number (RPN)—A numerical assessment of the risk arising from a failure. It ranks the failure mode in terms of severity, probability of occurrence and likelihood of detection and computes the risks based on the three ranks.

Root cause (RC)—The central underlying reason for the deviation. It is confirmed by evidence of a known sequence of events, observations, and/or experimentations.

Root cause analysis (RCA)—The part of an investigation that is used to determine why and how an error or event has occurred.

Safety data sheet (SDS)—An informational document that provides written or printed material concerning a hazardous chemical. The SDS is prepared in accordance with the Health Communication Standard (previously known as a material safety data sheet [MSDS]).[3]

Sampling plan—A documented plan that describes the procedures and methods for sampling a controlled environment; identifies the sampling sites, the sampling frequency, and number of samples; and describes the method of analysis and how to interpret the results.[5]

Sampling sites—Documented geographical location, within a controlled environment, where sampling for microbiological evaluation is taken. In general, sampling sites are selected because of their potential for product/container closure contacts.[5]

Sanitizing agent—Agent for reducing, on inanimate surfaces, the number of all forms of microbial life including fungi, viruses, and bacteria.[10]

Secondary engineering control—Term that refers to cleanrooms, buffer areas, or ante-areas in which air quality meets cleanliness standards of the International Organization for Standardization (ISO) and which serve as a core for the location of the primary engineering control.[1]

Segregated compounding area—Designated space, either a demarcated area or room, that is restricted to preparing low-risk level compounded sterile preparations (CSPs) with 12-hour or less beyond-use dates. Such an area must contain a device that provides unidirectional airflow of ISO Class 5 air quality for preparation of CSPs and shall be void of activities and materials that are extraneous to sterile compounding.[1]

Shelf life—Longest time period during which 90 percent or more of the labeled active ingredient is available for delivery. (See also *Expiration Date*.)

Single-dose container (or single-use container)—Single-unit container for articles or preparations intended for parenteral administration only. It is intended for a single use. A single-dose container is labeled as such. Examples of single-dose containers include prefilled syringes, cartridges, fusion-sealed containers, and closure-sealed containers when so labeled.[1]

Sorption—Situation in which drug is lost (from the solution to be administered) by adsorption to the surface or absorption into the matrix of the container material, administration set, or filter.

Spill kit—A container of supplies, warning signage, and related materials used to contain the spill of a hazardous drug.[3]

Sporicidal agent—An agent that destroys bacterial and fungal spores when used in sufficient concentration for a specified contact time. It is expected to kill all vegetative microorganisms.[10]

Stability—Extent to which a preparation retains, within specified limits, and throughout its period of storage and use, the same properties and characteristics that it possessed at the time of compounding.

Standard operating procedure (SOP)—Written procedures describing operations, testing, sampling, interpretation results, and corrective actions that relate to the operations that are taking place.[3]

Standard precautions (formerly universal precautions)—Practice in healthcare of treating all patients as if they were infected with HIV or other similar diseases by using barriers to avoid known means of transmitting infectious agents (Centers for Disease Control; 1987, 1988). Barriers can include nonporous gloves, goggles, and face shields. Careful handling and disposal of sharps or the use of needleless systems are also important.[7]

Sterility assurance level (SAL)—A term used in microbiology to describe the probability of a single unit being nonsterile after it has been subjected to the sterilization process. SAL is also used to describe the killing efficacy of a sterilization process, where a very effective sterilization process has a very high SAL.

Sterilization—Validated process used to render a preparation free of viable organisms.

Sterilization by filtration—Passage of a fluid or solution through a sterilizing grade membrane to produce a sterile effluent.[1]

Sterilizing grade membranes—Membranes that are documented to retain 100% of a culture of 10^7 microorganisms of a strain of *Brevundimonas* (Pseudomonas) *diminuta* per square centimeter of membrane surface under a pressure of not less than 30 pounds per square inch (2.0 bar). Such filter membranes are nominally at 0.22 µm or 0.2 µm nominal pore size, depending on the manufacturer's practice.[1]

Subcutaneous allergy immunotherapy extracts—Vials or sets of vials of premixed licensed standardized and non-standardized allergenic extracts for subcutaneous immunotherapy diluted with an appropriate diluent prepared by a licensed physician for an individual patient according to instructions from a valid prescription.

Supplemental engineering control—An adjunct control (eg, closed-system drug transfer device [CSTD]) that may be used concurrently with primary and secondary engineering controls. Supplemental engineering controls offer additional levels of protection and may facilitate enhanced occupational protection, especially when handling hazardous drugs outside of primary and secondary engineering controls (eg, during administration).[3]

Supplier—The group that provides materials to be able to produce a product or service. The supplier can be external or internal to the company.

Swabs (for microbiological sampling)—Devices used to remove microorganisms from irregular or regular surfaces for cultivation to identify the microbial population of the surface. A swab is generally composed of a stick with an absorbent tip that is moistened before sampling and is rubbed across a specified area of the sample surface. The swab is then rinsed in a sterile solution to suspend the microorganisms, and the solution is transferred to growth medium for cultivation of the microbial population.[5]

Temperature—Degree of hotness or coldness measured on a definite scale. Units of measure are either in Fahrenheit (U.S.) or Celsius (metric).

Terminal sterilization—Application of a lethal process (eg, steam under pressure or autoclaving) to sealed containers for the purpose of achieving a predetermined sterility assurance level of usually less than 10^{-6} or a probability of less than one in one million of a nonsterile unit.[1]

Threshold limit values (TLVs)—Values are exposure limits of airborne concentrations of chemical substances and represent conditions under which it is believed that nearly all workers may be repeatedly exposed, day after day, over a working lifetime, without adverse health effects.[7]

Total nutrient admixture (TNA)—Dextrose, amino acids, and fat emulsions/lipids combined in one container.

Training—Process of making or becoming prepared to perform a skill.

Trend—A positive or negative pattern identified during analysis of time-dependent data.

Trend report—A report that presents an analysis of data over a specified period sufficient to identify any changes over time for the specific type of data analyzed.

Unclassified space—A space not required to meet any air cleanliness classification based on the International Organization for Standardization (ISO).[3]

Unidirectional flow—Airflow moving in a single direction in a robust and uniform manner and at sufficient speed to reproducibly sweep particles away from the critical processing or testing area.[1]

Validation—A documented program that provides a high degree of assurance that a specific process, method, or system will consistently produce a result meeting predetermined acceptance criteria.[9]

Ventilated cabinet—Type of engineering control designed for purposes of worker protection. These devices are designed to minimize worker exposures by controlling emissions of airborne contaminants through the following:

- Full or partial enclosure of a potential contaminant source
- Use of airflow capture velocities to capture and remove airborne contaminants near their point of generation
- Use of air pressure relationships that define the direction of airflow into the cabinet
- Examples of ventilated cabinets include biological safety cabinets, containment isolators, and laboratory fume hoods.[7]

Ventilated control—A device such as a biological safety cabinet or isolator that vents exhaust away from the critical area.

Verification—Authoritatively signed assurance and documentation that a process, procedure, or piece of equipment is functioning properly and producing the expected results. The act of verification of a compounding procedure involves checking to ensure the calculations, weighing and measuring, order of mixing, and compounding techniques and equipment were appropriate and accurately performed.[18]

Vial—A plastic or glass container with a rubber closure secured to its top by a metal ring.

Visual incompatibility—Visible changes in a preparation, such as precipitation, cloudiness or haziness, color change, viscosity change, cracking, and effervescence. (See also *Physical Incompatibility*.)

Workflow system—In the context of sterile compounding, a workflow system is software that accepts CSP orders from the pharmacy system, populates a workflow queue, generates a compounding label, allows verification via either barcode scan or gravimetric check, and captures images of relevant steps in the compounding process. When doses are ready to be verified, a pharmacist accesses the system reviewing each step the technician took to prepare the CSP and verifies the images associated with each dose for accuracy. The pharmacist is able to complete this verification process remotely from any workstation with access to the workflow system. As the pharmacist verifies a dose as correct, the workload system produces a single barcode label to be applied to that dose indicating the dose is ready for delivery. Verified doses then can be scanned during subsequent steps of the delivery process, which creates an audit trail and allows pharmacy staff to view status and/or location of the dose during the compounding and delivery processes.[19] (See details in Chapter 9.)

Workplace environmental exposure level (WEEL)—Occupational exposure limits developed by the American Industrial Hygiene Association as a chemical concentration to which nearly all workers may be repeatedly exposed for a working lifetime without adverse health effects.[7]

Worst-case scenarios—Situations that occur when compounding operations are at their greatest risk of introducing contamination into sterile preparations (eg, late in a work shift when personnel are tired, volume is high, and cleaning/disinfecting has yet to be done).

Zone of turbulence—Pattern of flow of air from the HEPA filter created behind an object placed within the laminar airflow workbench pulling or allowing contaminated room air into the aseptic environment.

REFERENCES

1. USP <797> Pharmaceutical compounding—sterile preparations. In: *2023: USP Compounding Compendium*. Rockville, MD: United States Pharmacopeial Convention; November 1, 2023. **https://doi.org/10.31003/USPNF_M99925_07_01**.
2. Food and Drug Administration (FDA). Current good manufacturing practice—guidance for human drug compounding outsourcing facilities under Section 503B of the FD&C Act: guidance for industry. Draft guidance, Revision 2. **https://www.fda.gov/media/88905/download**. Published January 2020.
3. USP <800> Hazardous drugs—handling in healthcare settings. In: *2020: USP Compounding Compendium*. Rockville, MD: United States Pharmacopeial Convention; July 1, 2020. **https://doi.org/10.31003/USPNF_M7808_07_01**.
4. USP <1> Injections and implanted drug products (parenterals)—product quality tests. In: *2020: USP Compounding Compendium*. Rockville, MD: United States Pharmacopeial Convention; December 1, 2020. **https://doi.org/10.31003/USPNF_M98730_03_01**.
5. USP <1116> Microbiological control and monitoring of aseptic processing environments. In: *USP Compounding Compendium*. Rockville, MD: United States Pharmacopeial Convention; 2013. doi:10.31003/USPNF_M99835_01_01.
6. Christensen J, Darius R, DelBoca J, et al. Glossary. In: *Global sterile manufacturing regulatory guidance comparison*. Bethesda, MD: Parenteral Drug Association; 2016.
7. National Institute for Occupational Safety and Health (NIOSH). *NIOSH Alert: Preventing Occupational Exposure to Antineoplastic and Other Hazardous Drugs in Health Care Settings*. Cincinnati, OH: NIOSH—Publications Dissemination; September 2004. **www.cdc.gov/niosh/docs/2004-165/**. Reviewed February 7, 2018. Accessed August 25, 2023

8. National Association of Boards of Pharmacy. *Model state pharmacy act and model rules of the national association of boards of pharmacy*. Published August 2022. **https://nabp.pharmacy/members/boardresources/model-pharmacy-act-rules/**. Accessed August 25, 2023.

9. USP <1197> Good distribution practices for bulk pharmaceutical excipients. In: *USP Compounding Compendium*. Rockville, MD: United States Pharmacopeial Convention; 2016.

10. USP <1072> Disinfectants and antiseptics. In: *USP 42–NF 37*. Rockville, MD: United States Pharmacopeial Convention; 2019.

11. USP <659> Packaging and storage requirements. In: *USP Compounding Compendium*. Rockville, MD: United States Pharmacopeial Convention; 2016.

12. USP <1066> Physical environments that promote safe medication use. In: *2015: USP Compounding Compendium*. Rockville, MD: The United States Pharmacopeial Convention. DOI: **https://doi.org/10.31003/USPNF_M3367_01_01**.

13. Health Level 7. Wikipedia, The Free Encyclopedia. **https://en.wikipedia.org/wiki/Health_Level_7**. Accessed August 29, 2023.

14. Barker KN, Allan EL, Kvancz DA. Facility planning and design. In: Brown TR, ed. *Handbook of Institutional Pharmacy Practice*. 4th ed. Bethesda, MD: American Society of Health-System Pharmacists; 2006:519–41.

15. The Drug Quality and Security Act (H.R. 3204) Section 503B of the Food, Drug and Cosmetic Act (November 18, 2013). **www.ashp.org/-/media/assets9/advocacy-issues/docs/drug-quality-and-securityact-section-503b-of-the-food-drug-cosmetic-act.ashx?la=en**. Accessed January 15, 2023.

16. USP <1151> Pharmaceutical dosage forms. In: 2022: *USP Compounding Compendium*. Rockville, MD: United States Pharmacopeial Convention; May 1, 2022. **https://doi.org/10.31003/USPNF_M99860_08_01**.

17. Columbia University Health Library. Repetitive motion injury. **https://www.cuimc.columbia.edu/rehab/staywell/repetitive-motion-injury**. Accessed August 29, 2023.

18. USP <1163> Quality assurance in pharmaceutical compounding. In: *2020: USP Compounding Compendium*. Rockville, MD: United States Pharmacopeial Convention; December 1, 2020. **https://doi.org/10.31003/USPNF_M1373_05_01**.

19. American Society of Health-System Pharmacists (ASHP), ASHP Section of Pharmacy Informatics and Technology. *Current state of IV workflow systems and IV robotics*. Bethesda, MD: American Society of Health-System Pharmacists; 2012.

Index

DOI 10.37573/9781585286492.BM

B

C

D

E

F

I

J

L

M

N

O

P

Q

R

U

V

W

Y